Empathy in Mental Illness

The lack of ability to empathize is central to many psychiatric conditions. Empathy (or social cognition) is probably affected by several factors, such as neurodevelopmental problems, brain damage and the onset of psychiatric illness. It is also amenable to manipulation and can be measured by neuropsychological assessment (both state and trait) and neuroimaging techniques. This book focuses specifically on the role of empathy in mental illness. It starts with the clinical psychiatric perspective and covers empathy in the context of mental illness, adult health, developmental course and explanatory models. Psychiatrists, psychotherapists and related mental health professionals will find this a very useful encapsulation of what is currently known about the role of empathy in mental health and illness.

Tom F. D. Farrow is a Lecturer in Psychiatric Neuroimaging at the University of Sheffield, and Honorary NHS Clinical Scientist for Sheffield Care Trust.

Peter W. R. Woodruff is Professor and Head of Academic Clinical Psychiatry and Director of the Sheffield Cognition and Neuroimaging Laboratory (SCANLab) at the University of Sheffield, and Honorary Consultant Psychiatrist for Sheffield Care Trust.

Empathy in Mental Illness

Tom F. D. Farrow
University of Sheffield

and

Peter W. R. Woodruff
University of Sheffield

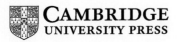
CAMBRIDGE
UNIVERSITY PRESS

CAMBRIDGE UNIVERSITY PRESS
Cambridge, New York, Melbourne, Madrid, Cape Town, Singapore, São Paulo

Cambridge University Press
The Edinburgh Building, Cambridge CB2 8RU, UK

Published in the United States of America by Cambridge University Press, New York

www.cambridge.org
Information on this title: www.cambridge.org/9780521847346

© Cambridge University Press 2007

First published 2007

Printed in the United Kingdom at the University Press, Cambridge

A catalogue record for this publication is available from the British Library

ISBN-13 978-0-521-84734-6 hardback

Contents

Foreword

Professor Peter W. R. Woodruff

Empathy literally means 'the power of understanding things outside ourselves' after the Greek *empatheia*, but has come to imply a reliance on 'inner feeling', from the German *ein* (in) *fuhlung* (feeling), and even an implied sense of 'cure' from 'em-pathy' the suffix-*pathy* meaning a 'method of cure'. It is after all through examination of our inner feelings that we gain a deeper understanding of ourselves. Our ability to relate to those feelings we see expressed by others depends on an ability to compare them with those we may have experienced ourselves, which allows us to infer 'what the other person must be going through'. The accuracy of our inference depends upon *empatheia*.

Much of psychotherapy depends on helping individuals to analyse and hence reach some emotional understanding of their inner world to enable them to relate more adaptively to people and events outside themselves. In this sense there is an assumption that individuals possess the 'capacity' to empathize. This capacity may be encouraged and developed through therapy. There is also an assumption that there may be individuals who lack such a capacity or, if they do possess it, may use it in a maladaptive way which can cause difficulties in their relationships. This raises the question of whether the 'psyche' or its substrate (the brain) lacks a necessary processing capacity or 'neural network' to empathize adequately. It would seem reasonable therefore to use current technology to uncover what brain mechanisms may underlie these deficits, and further investigate whether these mechanisms are sensitive to the effects of therapy. Hence we come back to the concept of 'therapy or cure' implied by the word itself.

Much of our understanding of 'normal' function relies upon the need to understand and treat mental conditions that result from 'abnormal' function, or 'dysfunction'. The clinical imperative is to understand the factors that lead to these conditions and hence treat them. With this in mind, we have started the book from the viewpoint of the clinical conditions that present to clinical psychiatrists: the 'dysempathy in psychiatric samples'. From the clinical position we move to a refined concept of empathy as applied to 'health' and, from that, proposed models for empathy and how to measure, monitor and regulate it in health and mental illness. Then more at a societal level the book explores how we detect concepts of empathy and their influence through literature.

This book attempts to bring together different ways of analysing the meaning of empathy from the point of view of 'normal' psychology, to how we can gain greater understanding of it by analysis of the behaviour of those in whom this facility is lacking (and impact of this on others). As with many aspects of normal psychology, we gain our understanding through examining examples where components are lacking. Much as studies of lesions in pathology can give us examples of what apparatus is necessary for the normal functioning of the body, studies of conditions where behaviour denotes a lack of empathy may give us insight into the necessary psychological, and possibly anatomical, substrate for its function.

Empathy is such a necessary means of every day communication between individuals and for social cohesion that we may take it for granted. However, as the contributors to the book make clear, because it is such a necessary component of healthy co-existence, its lack may lead to profound disturbance and dysfunction, both in causing mental illness itself and, through the resulting behavioural impact on others, may perpetuate the impact of the mental illness on the individual. Hence empathy is important to study. Its complexity requires the applied knowledge gained through the different approaches offered by the Arts, Medicine, Neuroscience and Psychology, and techniques that include neuroimaging and genetics.

Empathic dysfunction in psychiatric populations

Psychopathy

The clinical exploration of empathy begins with that in 'psychopathy'. Here, we have a disorder that encapsulates the essence of a *lack* of empathy, where we can gain an understanding of the nature of empathy through the behaviour of those who lack an appropriate 'empathic response'. James Blair sets the scene by distinguishing 'cognitive empathy' (Theory of Mind) from 'emotional empathy'. It appears that whereas some individuals with autism may show impaired performance on 'cognitive' Theory of Mind tasks, those with psychopathy (as well as other populations in whom antisocial conduct is prevalent) do not. On the other hand, he presents evidence that individuals with psychopathy have an impairment in processing facial emotional expression *selective* for fearful, sad and disgusted expressions (as distinct from angry, surprised or happy expressions) which he purports to be suggestive of amygdala dysfunction. He finally raises the prospect of improved long-term prognosis of psychopathy if treatment is aimed at increasing the empathic reaction of children with psychopathic tendencies. A greater understanding of the underlying basis for these psychological and neural mechanisms would take us further along this path.

Schizophrenia

The clinical picture is expanded into schizophrenia in the chapter by Kwang-Hyuk Lee. Here he draws a comparison between the autistic features and affective blunting in schizophrenia described by Bleuler and possible deficits in empathy observed in the disorder. Poor recognition of facial emotional expression and others' feelings, abnormal gaze patterns at faces, and emotional responsivity to the emotions of others may explain some of the associated 'negative' symptoms in schizophrenia. Likewise paranoid symptoms may be associated with an inappropriately exaggerated response to threat. He hints at some early work by the Sheffield Cognition and Neuroimaging Group that attempts to explore how neuroimaging can be used to map changes in prefrontal cortical response whilst performing tasks that invoke empathy processing in response to treatment. Here, for example, an enhanced response of prefrontal cortex correlated with improved social functioning.

Antisocial personality disorder

The clinical theme continues with Mairead Dolan and Rachael Fullam's exploration of the relationship between empathy, offending behaviour and antisocial personality disorder. They expose the complexities of empathy by disentangling its component processes (and by introducing the concept of sympathy as a possible further component responsible for 'feeling' concern for others). These definitions assume practical significance when studies report measures of empathy in clinical samples. For instance, how can we compare results from studies that report measures that differ in their relative weighting of cognitive and emotional aspects of empathy? Also, self-report measures may be unreliable in criminal populations. And some tasks, developed in young people with developmental disorders such as autism, may be insensitive at detecting subtle impairments in criminal samples. Despite these difficulties some meta-analyses support the suggestion that low levels of 'cognitive empathy' (as distinct from 'affective empathy') were particularly associated with offending. People with antisocial personality disorder (ASPD), however, appear not to have difficulties reading emotions from facial expressions. Empathy deficits seem to be generalized across sex offenders, and here may have a common association with those individuals with narcissistic personality disorder. Empathy is identified as an essential ingredient for effective parenting, and as a protective factor against the possibility of aggression by a mother directed at a distressed infant.

Depression

Following the theme of distress, Lynn O'Connor and colleagues explore how empathy may become turned on the self and lead to depression. Their starting point is that depression may be considered as a disorder of 'concern for others' where abnormally elevated levels of empathy could lead to excess self-blame and guilt for pain felt by others. Depression is increasingly prevalent worldwide, affecting 12% of women and 7% of men, with similar rates in children. Depression rates may be underestimated, however, in groups where the illness has an atypical presentation, e.g. in children (angry and defiant behaviour) and the elderly. To some extent, as recognition of these manifestations increases, reported rates of depression may also. One important facet of recognition is to identify vulnerability markers for depression. Here, empathy may play a part. For instance, O'Conner and colleagues cite work that reveals a correlation between empathy for distress in others and depression. They propose a model that links empathic concern to interpersonal guilt and both altruism and depression. Here, the concept of 'survivor guilt', following that felt by those who lost loved ones in the Nazi concentration camps and who became depressed, is extended to those with depression who feel guilt about their own fortune or happiness being at the expense of others, which may lead to submissive, self-destructive or altruistic behaviour. In turn, altruism may have some survival advantage in mate selection by giving the signal that the altruist has surplus resources in order to exercise this behaviour (and may therefore be a desirable mate). O'Conner and colleagues also attempt to disentangle the relationship between 'sub-scales' of empathy and survivor guilt and neuroticism. In doing so, they raise the possibility that empathic responses to others that aids social cohesion may also indirectly contribute to the current 'epidemic' of depression. On a positive note, empathy-induced guilt may act as an internal warning to let the person know that they need to help someone else, and hence may aid moral judgements.

Aggression

The idea that empathy may be protective against inter-personal aggression is further explored by Kaj Björkqvist, who makes the case for engaging empathic processes in children and adolescents as a means of reducing their aggression. He introduces the concept of indirect (non-physical) aggression, dependent upon social manipulation, which in turn is dependent on social intelligence. This form of aggression, considered more common in girls than boys, uses covert strategies and induces discomfort via psychological rather than direct physical means. On the other hand, direct verbal and physical aggression is more commonly employed by boys than girls. Social intelligence is considered to have perceptual, cognitive analytical and behavioural components, skills that may develop earlier in girls than boys. For instance, girls appear to develop the skills at decoding and encoding non-verbal signals faster than boys. Björkqvist presents compelling data that support the idea that, whereas social intelligence is required for conflict resolution, empathy is a necessary ingredient for peaceful (non-aggressive) conflict resolution. Hence empathy training may be useful for encouraging positive social behaviours.

Patients with brain lesions

The theme moves on in the chapter by Simone Shamay-Tsoory to the study of neuropsychological deficits in patients with localized brain lesions. Here she expands on the idea that the substrate for empathy resides in a network that depends on ventromedial (VM) prefrontal cortex. The story begins with the example of Phineas Gage and to more recent clinical examples that provide evidence for the central role of the VM prefrontal cortex in social cognition and empathy, through a discussion of cognitive models of VM cortex and social cognition towards an integrative view of the neuroanatomy of empathy. She reviews evidence from animal work and studies from patients with lesions that converge on the idea that empathic abilities of people with VM damage are most apparent when correct interpretation of social situations demands integration of cognitive and emotional processes. Shamay-Tsoory further suggests that right (posterior) hemisphere damage is particularly associated with difficulties with affective processing (voice intonation and facial expression identification), which is a prerequisite for feeling empathy. Right frontal damage may be responsible for difficulties in response expression. Hence, she concludes that the right VM plays a central role in mediating empathy through integrating inputs from dorsolateral cortex (affective processing, retrieval of past events, cognitive flexibility) as well as from the amygdala and autonomic nervous system.

Asperger's syndrome, attention deficit hyperactivity disorder and autism

Christopher Gillberg describes 'empathy disorder' in a wide range of (mainly developmental) non-autism clinical conditions such as Asperger's syndrome and attention deficit hyperactivity disorder (ADHD). He argues that empathy may be normally distributed in the population (like the intelligence quotient, IQ) and that those with certain disorders of empathy may lie at the extreme end of this spectrum. Despite sharing difficulties with empathy, autistic disorder, he argues, is associated with low verbal IQ, and Asperger's syndrome with higher verbal IQ. Apparent lack of empathy in children with ADHD may reflect their failing to attend to, rather than being impaired in their understanding of, other people's perspectives. The link he makes between extreme impulsivity in Tourette's syndrome patients and empathy problems in those with autism spectrum disorders being associated with severe cognitive dysfunction parallels the neuroanatomical discussion in the chapter by Shamay-Tsoory. It is clear from Gillberg's account that empathy deficits occur in a range of apparently disparate childhood disorders that share characteristics with autism spectrum disorders as well as in adult personality disorders that have their origins in early development.

Peter Hobson explores the nature of empathy through observations of behaviour in autism (where lack of empathy is a defining characteristic). He describes clinical examples which clearly illustrate how people with autism have profound difficulties relating to other people and engaging with them at a personal level. He emphasizes the point that our normal cognitive and social development depends upon understanding the world through other people. Here, Hobson asserts, a limit to the awareness of the emotional life of others restricts consciousness of themselves. He goes on to claim that identification with others' emotions, feeling the other's emotions and being 'moved to' the emotional stance of others are key facilities lacking in children with autism. He ends on the optimistic note that interventions may facilitate emotional engagement between children with autism and others.

From the clinical examples given, the book moves on to explore the concept of empathy in health. Throughout, we return to the clinical relevance of these concepts; for example, in understanding drug addictions, Asperger's syndrome and schizophrenia.

Empathy in health

Early development of empathy

Miguel Diego and Nancy Jones review the development of empathy from the neonatal period through infancy and childhood. They explore ideas that the imitation of emotions in newborns suggests the existence of the *capacity* for empathy upon which social experience can operate. Temperament indicates early predispositions in neonates, which allow them to evaluate the salience of different emotions. They present evidence that newborns of depressed mothers may already be biased in their (lack of) responses to the emotional expressions of others. Patterns of emotional responsiveness (and its physiological correlates) may be evident from the neonatal period, and hence the basis for social interactions and empathy may be established very early in brain development. Bonding between mother and child and the ability of the infant to discriminate features (voice, face, smell) of mother from those of others may be precursors for empathic responses later in life. 'Empathic competence' may depend on how well physiological and emotional processes between mother and infant are coordinated, or 'attuned'. The interaction of temperament and maternal characteristics are generally considered key factors in the development of empathy. Difficulties with these processes may be associated with autistic behaviour or depression later in life.

Evidence is presented for the existence of neural mechanisms underlying affect and empathy shortly after birth. For instance, newborn's distress is associated with hearing distress in another's cries as early as 18 months old. Maternal psychological state profoundly influences that of the infant, particularly during the early years when substantial re-modelling of synapses takes place. Maternal neglect and abuse both adversely affect empathy in later life. Emotionally neglected infants develop attachment problems, and are less able to differentiate between emotions in others and thus develop empathy. Abused infants may develop aberrant neural pathways that lead to aggressive rather than empathic means to achieve their ends. Help with parenting skills focused on mother–child interaction and heightened awareness that this intervention may help prevent the establishment of less desirable traits in later life may be worthwhile.

Evolution of empathy

James Harris approaches the concept of empathy from an evolutionary perspective. He refers to 'mutual aid' as a necessary prerequisite for social cooperation. Thus those groups that exhibit mutual aid are at an evolutionary advantage over those who do not. It may be for instance that the 'fittest' help others and hence altruism prevails in the population. It is possible that the evolution of social cooperation depended upon an advanced hearing mechanism and the sensitivity to higher frequencies of sounds akin to speech in mammals. Also, the evolution of the autonomic nervous system would allow awareness by individuals of their 'visceral tone', be it calmness induced in an infant rocked by their mother, or nausea associated with social distress. Mirror neurones are those that respond to performing an action and perceiving that same action performed (see Chapter 24). They thus provide a substrate for understanding the intentions of others. Applied to emotions this mechanism would allow for an understanding of other's emotions. Harris refers to work by Gallese and others that identifies the insula as a key brain region involved in both feeling and observing disgust and imitating facial expressions, hence his conclusion that 'empathic resonance takes place through communication between action representation networks and limbic areas via the insula'.

Empathy in healthy populations

John Nezlek and colleagues describe the variability of empathy in the general population. In particular they explore how empathy may depend on social environment. They refer to this variability as 'state empathy'. They present data from two major studies that measured empathic state, self-esteem depressogenic adjustment, mood and daily events over time. Intra-individual variability in empathy scores were as great as inter-individual variability, an observation they argue provides evidence for the existence of both trait *and* state empathy. Stronger daily (negative and positive) emotions were associated with greater empathy. The occurrence of social events was associated with increased empathy, including negative social events that were associated with negative emotions. Another study examined the interaction between the social setting of the event and the empathy of the interaction. Here, empathic ability was greatest when people were in pairs, and exchanged affection, and least in large gatherings and during focused work activity. In concluding, the authors question any assumption that empathy is always adaptive, and may in some circumstances actually lead to a negative effect on well-being, e.g. taking on the feelings of anxiety of those around. There may, therefore, be an 'optimal' level of state empathy which people need to regulate (see Chapter 21).

Sara Hodges and Robert Biswas-Diener shed light on the idea that we may need an optimal amount of empathy, i.e. it is not an unqualified 'good thing'. There may be a 'cost' if for instance a person experiences an excess of unpleasantness as a result of empathizing with another's misfortunes. We need strategies for regulating empathy if we are to succeed in human interactions. Possible mechanisms discussed include: suppression, reframing (to distance the empathiser from the empathisee) and controlling exposure to factors that cause us to feel empathy. Empathizing is hard work and relies on motivation. When these processes fail to regulate empathy optimally, individuals may suffer in various ways including by the development of mental distress or possibly illness.

In the chapter by Farrow he explains the approach common to many neuroimaging studies of trying to deconstruct the component cognitive processes thought to be responsible for the psychological response or behaviour. Functional neuroimaging depends on mapping the brain's response to a *difference* between two or more conditions. This approach is complicated when applying, to schizophrenia, as complex a facility as empathy. Farrow states that empathy depends on attention, a capacity for 'Theory of Mind', self-awareness, simulation of other's actions and appropriate emotional and autonomic responses. By reviewing neuroimaging literature on these key component processes, he concludes that there are likely to be 'core' brain regions such as the medial prefrontal cortex, posterior cingulate and temporal cortex involved in empathy, with other related regions such as the anterior cingulate, orbitofrontal cortices, amygdala, insula and precuneus brought into play as 'secondary' regions. In common with a number of authors, Farrow indicates that it is the connections between key regions that provide the substrate for the function. Connections such as those between superior temporal regions and inferior frontal cortexes to the limbic system via the insula may turn out to be crucial. Here, studies in patient groups who lack empathy or its components are important. Already some neuroimaging work in Asperger's syndrome, post-traumatic stress disorder and schizophrenia (as outlined in other chapters) has made a start in this direction.

Nancy Jones and Chantal Gagnon describe the neurophysiological basis of empathy. They outline evidence to suggest that empathy is linked to temperament (see Chapter 9). EEG changes during early brain development suggest that complex interaction between limbic and higher cortical regions becomes established in early childhood. They describe findings that link heart rate variability and emotional expressivity in newborns. Heart rate deceleration may be an index of other-orientated attention (empathy) whereas heart rate acceleration may be an index of self-orientated attention (anxiety and fear). Patterns of EEG responses may differ in groups defined by their empathic behaviours, particularly as observed in frontal cortex.

The cognitive neuropsychological approach attempts to simplify empathy into its component processes each underpinned by a purported neural system. Jean Decety and colleagues identify four basic components in their model: shared neural representations, self-awareness, mental flexibility and emotion regulation. Perception action coupling relies on mirror neurones (see Chapter 24). Facial expressions are accompanied by feeling the corresponding emotion. Empathy relies upon an intact executive system as well as a network involving inferior parietal, prefrontal and insula involved in the ability to discriminate between self and others. Medial paracingulate cortex is thought to reflect a 'de-coupling' mechanism that allows us to hold representations detached from their reality. Decety and colleagues propose that medial prefrontal cortex activation is related to the cognitive load associated with disengagement of the representation of others' feelings from explicit cues that are perceived. Drawing from neuroimaging and neuropsychological evidence, they argue that there are distinct neural underpinnings for cognitive and affective aspects of empathy.

Henrik Anckarsäter and Robert Cloninger review the genetics of empathy and its disorders. In doing so they acknowledge the difficulties of studying genetics of a characteristic that is dependent upon social context and subject to significant inter-individual variation. They approach the problem from the point of personality traits and the study of conditions associated with 'dysempathy' such as autism. Monozygotic twins are more concordant than dizygotic twins for traits relevant to empathy, such as: callousness, intimacy problems, restricted expression of affect and social avoidance. Twin studies show high levels of hereditability for altruistic traits. Genetic influences seem to be more important for temperamental, aggressive antisocial behaviour persistent into adulthood compared with non-aggressive behaviour limited to adolescence. It is likely that most genetic factors interact with environmental influences in modifying expression of the behaviour. For instance DRD4 polymorphisms are associated with high novelty-seeking behaviour; this behaviour is modified (reduced) by the level of cooperativeness in parenting. Hence their conclusion, that 'personality is comprised of multiple heritable dimensions of unique partially overlapping sets of epistatic genes, that modulate brain states by modifying the transitory connections between changing distributed networks of neurones', provides us with a model for further investigation.

Dan Velea and Michel Hautefeuille explore the relationship between drug-taking and the role drugs have in 'filling a gap' in the emotional life of people who take them. Here, alexithymia (inability to express emotions) and need for self-empathy (or self-acceptance) may be important predisposing factors to drug-taking, particularly those drugs with empathy-inducing properties such as ecstasy, MDMA, ketamine, phencyclidine and lysergic acid diethylamide (LSD). 'Raves' are an example of imitation where emotions and sensations are shared, and drug-taking may facilitate a 'quest for empathy' in addition to other sensations. They explore the hypothesis that those who are constitutionally deficient in serotonergic neurotransmitter activity (with associated anhedonia) may compensate by taking drugs that compensate (at least temporarily) for such deficiency.

Psychological processes

Marco Iacoboni brings to the theme of empathy the concept that to empathize successfully requires an appreciation of self versus other where we are able to internalize the feeling of what others feel rather than just imagine those feelings. We do this by imitating others, a process that commences at 18–30 months old. Here, the chameleon effect is discussed. This is a phenomenon that may result from non-conscious mimicry of postures, mannerisms and facial expressions of people while they interact with others in social situations. Also discussed is the idea that imitation of others leads to a liking of them. These ideas raise interesting testable hypotheses about which brain networks and regions are likely to underlie their function. For instance much evidence presented points to the insula as a key relay that connects and possibly coordinates sensory and association cortices with executive and limbic regions responsible for modulating a person's emotional response to situations that involve social interactions (see Chapter 24).

Nigel Goldenfeld and colleagues propose the idea that empathizing and systematizing balance one another. Systematizing is a process that occurs when a person analyses or constructs a system according to rules that govern that system. The authors maintain that empathizing and systematizing compete for common neural resources. Hence a balance between the two tendencies can be reached. Here, a combined score on both is taken as evidence of their competing with (or compensating for) each other. Generally they find that males tend to systematize at the expense of empathy, and females tend to empathize at the expense of systematizing. This pattern is also observed in patients with autism and Asperger's syndrome whereby systematizing predominates over empathy. They conclude that scores that represent the difference between systematizing and empathizing could be used to classify five different brain types between the extremes on the scale of systematizing tendency on one hand and empathizing tendency on the other.

India Morrison introduces the term 'vicarious responding' in place of empathy. She explains that vicarious responding is a requisite for emotional experience. For instance, vicarious responding to pain and disgust may depend upon learning and preparation of motivated, affectively valenced skeletomotor movements of aversion. She emphasizes the connection between somatosensory cortex, where bodily representations reside, and affectively laden material, related to others. She cites evidence for the concurrence of anterior cingulate and insula activations with the experience of pain and seeing pain inflicted on others. The sensory-discriminatory system, responsible for spatial localization of pain, is distinguished from the motivational-affective system (that determines affective unpleasantness).

Facial expressions coincident with the experience of disgust or pain also communicate a warning signal to others. Similarly such expressions may convey empathy with another's discomfort. Morrison emphasizes the importance of parietal cortex in integrating sensory input to the motor response in these aversive situations. Morrison postulates the existence of a motivational-affective (M-A) brain system that allows learning flexible responses to the properties of objects (will it bite?) together with a system concerned with kinaesthesis and discerning object proportions (where is it?). She asserts that it is 'too early to make the explanatory leap from vicarious responding to the rich scope of full-fledged affective experience evoked by the word "empathy"'.

Tony Atkinson also attempts to distinguish the perception of others' emotions from actually experiencing those emotions. He argues that emotions may be perceived either by computational (rule-based) systems that look for physical properties of the stimulus, or by processes specifically underpinning emotional experience. He then examines evidence for and against the idea that (1) we either perceive emotions through what he terms 'emotional contagion' whereby we engage primitive emotional systems within ourselves either directly or via facial mimicry, or (2) that we perceive emotion via body state (e.g. visceral sensations) or motor simulation (e.g. of facial movements).

The final section of the book concentrates on how we may model and measure empathy as well as educate students in empathy.

Modelling and measuring empathy

Marianne Schmid Mast and William Ickes describe methods for measuring empathic accuracy, for example by rating recorded interviews. They suggest ways of applying these techniques to help train therapists engaged in, for instance, couple therapy. Empathic accuracy is certainly central to social relationships, though they give examples of where knowing too much may destabilize a relationship, or trying too hard to know more (about the other) may lead to anxiety or suspiciousness and jealousy (that can in turn lead to aggression). They challenge some of what they refer to as 'clinical stereotypes', such as the assumption that autistic individuals are poor, and borderline personality disorder individuals good, at inferring other people's thoughts and feelings. On the other hand, they claim that the atypical nature of thoughts and feelings in people with borderline personality makes it difficult for others to make accurate inferences about them.

Stephanie Preston elaborates on the 'perception-action model' of empathy referred to in previous contributions. Here, she refers to a shared emotional experience occurring when a person feels a similar emotion to another as a result of perceiving the other's state. She uses behavioural and neuroimaging evidence to illustrate pertinent examples of how subjects use their own representations (such as shared past experiences, similarity and familiarity to the other's situation) to understand and feel the state of others. To succeed, subjects need to attend to the other, experience a similar emotional state as the other, and respond appropriately by inhibiting contagious distress and maintaining focus on the other. She ends by pointing out a number of interesting further aspects of empathy for us to investigate, such as differences between empathy for positive and negative states, imagining being (versus what it would be like to be another) and change in empathy over time.

Vittorio Gallese gives a definitive account of 'the shared manifold hypothesis'. He begins with the concept of 'embodied simulation' (a process that allows us a better understanding of events): first- and third-person experience of emotions and sensations and their neural underpinnings. He suggests ways in which these approaches may help us understand the 'whole brain' problem of schizophrenia and aspects of autism. He takes us through the 'mirror neurone' story with more recent examples of work in monkeys that elaborate the extent of mirror phenomena in everyday behaviour. For example, predictions about the goals of behaviour in others appear to be mediated by activity of motor neurones coding the goal of the same actions in the observer's brain. Hence it seems the mirror matching system maps the goals and purposes of others' actions. Embodied action simulation uses 'equivalence' of what is acted and perceived to predict the consequences of actions performed by others. Action observation automatically triggers action simulation. Studies on the appreciation of disgust converge on the insula being a key region involved in both the capacity to experience disgust, as well as the ability to recognize it in others. Hence this work supports the idea that first- and third-person experiences of a given emotion share a neural substrate. Another example given is that of a shared neural system involved in experiencing touch and observing others being touched. He extends the concept of empathy to that of a 'shared manifold' within which we establish meaningful links between ourselves and others. This he argues can occur at the levels of phenomena (e.g. sense of similarity): function (*as if* modes of interaction enable models of self/other) and subpersonal systems (mirror matching circuits for directly sharing the experiences we infer others are experiencing).

Once again, we return to the clinical problems associated with empathy which need unravelling. Patients with schizophrenia may have 'defective attunement'. Here, Gallese refers to an 'incapacity to engage oneself in meaningful relations with others and to establish non-inferential, intuitive interpersonal bonds'. In autism, he argues that some of what is observed is a compensatory mechanism for lack of the more elementary cognitive skills to enable an experience of the world of others. Thus, he concludes, embodied simulation, as a basic brain mechanism that gives us an experiential insight of others' minds, may provide the first unifying perspective of the neural basis of social cognition.

Finally, Johanna Shapiro concludes with a chapter that argues that medical education, rather than fostering empathy, may hinder it. Hence she makes a case for introducing the Arts to medical student teaching to facilitate their under-standing of others. This approach she argues is especially important in helping students understand mental illness, through, for example, subjective accounts written by those who have suffered mental illness in differing contexts. Involving readers in individual stories helps students see through the eyes of the patients, and, she states, has great potential to help learners understand how to be more empathic to their patients.

Hence, we move through from illness, to concepts and models and measure-ment of an elusive characteristic central to human understanding and interactions. Elusive it may be, but this book brings together experts in their fields in an attempt to elucidate the concept and to help us put the concept in the context of mental illness. Here we see in stark contrast to purely philosophical arguments about empathy, the ways in which loss of a core human faculty can cause such difficulty with social interactions and hence distress to patients and those close to them as well as the potential to perpetuate a vicious cycle of misunderstanding and stigma for those who suffer from mental illness. Much of the work refers to the neuroscience literature, and how our understanding of psychological processes relevant to empathy inform, and are informed by, recent developments in basic neuroscience. Understanding empathy relies on studying it from many sides, each complementing each other by shining light on the whole. The motivation for this search is continually driven by the clinical imperative of how we can help improve the lot of those who suffer from mental illness. Finally, we are presented with a perspective on medical education that some may find challenging. In this context, perhaps the challenge we face is in education more generally where a perceived need to 'teach' empathy may reflect the deficiencies of education in, and emphasis on, the Arts. After all, William Shakespeare described most of the human condition and psychopathology we encounter in clinical psychiatry, so why don't all psychiatrists (and medical students) have this as compulsory reading? Not as a substitute for William Shakespeare's *Complete Works*, but more as a complement to them, if this book helps us understand better the links between empathy and mental illness then it will have been worthwhile.

Contributors

Dr Henrik Anckarsäter
The Forensic Psychiatric Clinic, Malmö
University Hospital, University of Lund,
Sweden
Sege Park 8 A, S-205 02 Malmö, Sweden

Dr Chris Ashwin
Autism Research Centre, Department of
Psychiatry, University of Cambridge,
Douglas House, 18b Trumpington Road,
Cambridge CB2 2AH, UK

Dr Anthony P. Atkinson
Department of Psychology, University of
Durham, Science Site, South Road, Durham,
DH1 3LE, UK

Professor Simon Baron-Cohen
Autism Research Centre, Department of
Psychiatry, University of Cambridge,
Douglas House, 18b Trumpington Road,
Cambridge CB2 2AH, UK

Dr Jack W. Berry
Emotion, Personality and Altruism Research
Group, Samford University, 800 Lakeshore
Drive, Birmingham AL 35229, USA

Dr Robert Biswas-Diener
Department of Psychology, 1227 University
of Oregon, Eugene, Oregon 97403-1227,
USA

Dr Kaj Björkqvist
Department of Social Sciences,
Åbo Akademi University, PB 311,
FIN-65101, Vasa, Finland

Dr R. James R. Blair
Unit on Affective Cognitive Neuroscience,
Mood and Anxiety Disorders Program,
National Institute of Mental Health, 15 K
North Drive, Room 206, MSC 2670,
Bethesda, MD 20892-2670, USA

Dr Eric Brunet
Institute for Learning and Brain Sciences,
University of Washington, Box 357988,
Seattle, WA 98195-7988, USA

Dr Bhismadev Chakrabarti
Autism Research Centre, Department of
Psychiatry, University of Cambridge,
Douglas House, 18b Trumpington Road,
Cambridge CB2 2AH, UK

Professor C. Robert Cloninger
Washington University School of Medicine,
Department of Psychiatry 660
South Euclid Avenue, Campus Box 8134,
St Louis, MO 63110, USA

Dr Patrice S. Crisostomo
Emotion, Personality and Altruism Research Group, Wright Institute, 2728 Durant Avenue, Berkeley, CA 94794, USA

Professor Jean Decety
Department of Psychology, The University of Chicago, 5848 S. University Ave., Chicago, IL 60637, USA

Dr Miguel A. Diego
Department of Pediatrics, University of Miami, Room 7037A Mailman Center for Child Development, 1601 NW 12th Avenue, Miami, FL 33136, USA

Dr Mairead Dolan
University of Manchester, Department of Forensic Psychiatry, Edenfield Centre, Bolton Salford Trafford Mental Health Services NHS Trust, Bury New Road, Prestwich, Manchester, M25, 3BL, UK

Dr Tom F. D. Farrow
Academic Clinical Psychiatry, University of Sheffield, The Longley Centre, Northern General Hospital, Norwood Grange Drive, Sheffield, S5 7JT, UK

Dr Rachael Fullam
University of Manchester, Department of Forensic Psychiatry, Edenfield Centre, Bolton Salford Trafford Mental Health Services NHS Trust, Bury New Road, Prestwich, Manchester, M25 3BL, UK

Dr Chantal M. Gagnon
Department of Psychology, Florida Atlantic University, John D. Macarthur Campus, 777 Glades Road, Boca Raton, FL 33431-0991, USA

Dr Vittorio Gallese
Dipartimento dii Neuroscienze – Sezione di Fisiologia, Universita' di Parma, Via Volturno 39, I-43100 Parma, Italy

Professor Christopher Gillberg
Department of Child and Adolescent Psychiatry (University of Gothenburg, Sweden), Göteborgs Universitet, Avd för barn-ochungdomspsyk, Kungsgatan 12, 411 19, Göteborg, Sweden

Dr Nigel Goldenfeld
Department of Applied Mathematics and Theoretical Physics, Centre for Mathematical Sciences, University of Cambridge, Wilberforce Road, Cambridge CB3 0WA, UK
Department of Physics, University of Illinois at Urbana-Champaign, 1110 West Green Street, Urbana, IL 61801, USA

Professor James Harris
School of Medicine, CMSC 346, East Baltimore Campus, Johns Hopkins University, Baltimore, USA

Dr Michel Hautefeuille
Centre Médical Marmottan, Addictions Unit, 17–19 rue d'Armaillé, 75017, Paris, France

Professor Peter Hobson
Developmental Psychopathology Research Unit, Tavistock Clinic and Institute of Child Health, University College London, 120 Belsize Lane, London, NW3 5BA, UK

Dr Sara D. Hodges
Department of Psychology, 1227 University
of Oregon, Eugene, Oregon 97403-1227,
USA

Dr Marco Iacoboni
Ahmanson Lovelace Brain Mapping Center,
Brain Research Institute, David Geffen
School of Medicine at UCLA, 660 Charles E.
Young Drive South, Los Angeles, CA 90095,
USA

Dr William Ickes
Department of Psychology, University of
Texas at Arlington, Room 313, Life Science
Building, Box 19528, Arlington, Texas
76019-0528, USA

Dr Philip L. Jackson
Department of Psychology, The University
of Laval, Canada

Dr Nancy A. Jones
Department of Psychology, Florida Atlantic
University, John D. Macarthur Campus, 777
Glades Road, Boca Raton, FL 33431-0991,
USA

Dr Kwang-Hyuk Lee
Academic Clinical Psychiatry, University of
Sheffield, The Longley Centre, Northern
General Hospital, Norwood Grange Drive,
Sheffield, S5 7JT, UK

Dr Thomas Lewis
Emotion, Personality and Altruism Research
Group, University of California, San
Francisco, USA

Dr Paulo Lopes
Department of Psychology, University of
Surrey, Guildford, GU2 7XH, UK

Dr India Morrison
Centre for Cognitive Neuroscience, School
of Psychology, University of Wales, Adeilad
Brigantia, Penrallt Road, Gwynedd, LL57
2AS, UK

Dr Kathleen Mulherin
Emotion, Personality and Altruism Research
Group, Kaiser Permanente, South San
Francisco, California, USA

Professor John B. Nezlek
Department of Psychology, The College of
William and Mary, PO Box 8795,
Williamsburg, Virginia 23187, USA

Professor Lynn E. O'Connor
Emotion, Personality and Altruism Research
Group, Wright Institute, 2728 Durant
Avenue, Berkeley, CA 94794, USA

Dr Stephanie D. Preston
Department of Psychology, University of
Michigan, 3040 East Hall Ann Arbor,
MI 48109, USA

Dr Marianne Schmid Mast
University of Zurich, Social and Health
Psychology, Rämistrasse 66, CH-8001,
Zurich, Switzerland

Dr Astrid Schütz
Department of Psychology,
Chemnitz University of Technology,
Chemnitz, Germany

Dr Simone G. Shamay-Tsoory
Department of Psychology, University
of Haifa, Mount Carmel, Haifa, 31905,
Israel

Professor Johanna Shapiro
Department of Family Medicine, University of California at Irvine Medical Center, Building 200, Room 512, Route 81, 101 The City Drive South, Orange, CA 92868-3298, USA

Dr C. Veronica Smith
Department of Psychology, University of Delaware, 108 Wolf Hall, Newark, DE 19716, USA

Dr Dan Velea
Centre Médical Marmottan, Addictions Unit, 17–19 rue d'Armaillé, 75017, Paris, France

Dr Sally Wheelwright
Autism Research Centre, Department of Psychiatry, University of Cambridge, Douglas House, 18b Trumpington Road, Cambridge CB2 2AH, UK

Part I

'Dysempathy' in psychiatric samples

Empathic dysfunction in psychopathic individuals

R. James R. Blair

Mood and Anxiety Disorders Program, National Institute of Mental Health

1.1 Introduction

Psychopathy can be considered one of the prototypical disorders associated with empathic dysfunction. Reference to empathic dysfunction is part of the diagnostic criteria of psychopathy (Hare, 1991). The very ability to inflict serious harm to others repeatedly can be, and is (Hare, 1991), an indicator of a profound disturbance in an appropriate 'empathic' response to the suffering of another. The goal of this chapter will be to consider the nature of the empathic impairment in psychopathy.

First, I will consider the disorder of psychopathy and the definition of empathy. Second, I will consider whether individuals with psychopathy are impaired in 'cognitive empathy' or Theory of Mind. Third, I will consider the cognitive and neural architecture mediating 'emotional empathy'. Fourth, I will consider whether individuals with psychopathy are impaired in 'emotional empathy'.

1.1.1 The disorder of psychopathy

The origins of the concept of psychopathy probably originate in the writings of Pritchard (1837); see Pichot (1978). Pritchard developed the concept of 'moral insanity' to account for socially damaging or irresponsible behaviour that was not associated with known forms of mental disorder. He attributed morally objectionable behaviour to be a consequence of a diseased 'moral faculty'. While the notion of a 'moral faculty' has been dropped, modern psychiatric classifications such as the *American Psychiatric Association's Diagnostic and Statistical Manual* (currently, DSM-IV) make reference to syndromes associated with high levels of antisocial behaviour: conduct disorder (CD) in children and antisocial personality disorder (APD) in adults.

Empathy in Mental Illness, eds. Tom F. D. Farrow and Peter W. R. Woodruff. Published by Cambridge University Press. © Cambridge University Press 2007.

Unfortunately, the psychiatric diagnoses of CD and APD are flawed. Partly because they only focus on the presence of antisocial behaviour, these diagnoses tend to identify highly heterogeneous samples. This heterogeneity is even acknowledged in DSM-IV where two forms of CD are specified: childhood- and adolescent-onset types. Because of their lack of precision, the diagnostic rate of CD can reach 16% of boys in mainstream education (American Psychiatric Association, 1994) while the diagnostic rate of APD can reach over 80% in adult forensic institutions (Hare, 1991). Unsurprisingly, therefore, diagnoses of CD and APD are relatively uninformative regarding an individual's prognosis.

The classification of psychopathy, in contrast, is informative. This classification was introduced by Hare (1980; 1991) and has proved to be a useful predictor of future risk (Hare, 1991). The classification involves both affective-interpersonal (e.g. such as lack of empathy and guilt) and behavioural components (e.g. criminal activity and poor behavioural controls) (Frick & Hare, 2001; Hare, 1991). Psychopathy represents a developmental disorder. In childhood and adolescence, psychopathic tendencies are identified principally by either the use of the Antisocial Process Screening Device (Frick & Hare, 2001) or by the Psychopathy Checklist: Youth Version. In adulthood, psychopathy is identified through use of the Psychopathy Checklist – Revised (Hare, 1991).

As noted above, psychopathy can be considered one of the prototypical disorders associated with empathic dysfunction. In this chapter, I will consider the nature of the empathic impairment in psychopathy.

1.1.2 Defining empathy

Empathy has been defined as 'an affective response more appropriate to someone else's situation than to one's own' (Hoffman, 1987; p. 48); it is an emotional reaction in an observer to the affective state of another individual. This form of definition of empathy will underpin this paper. Unfortunately, however, the term empathy has been used in a variety of ways by a variety of authors (Hoffman, 1987). At least three different types of empathy can be considered. The differences between these types are important to identify as they must implicate notably different cognitive architectures. The three types of empathy are: (1) motor empathy where the individual mirrors the motor responses of the observed actor; (2) 'cognitive' empathy where the individual represents the internal mental state of the other (effectively Theory of Mind); (3) an emotional response to another individual that is congruent with the other's emotional reaction. In this chapter, I will briefly consider 'cognitive empathy', from here onwards referred to only as Theory of Mind, and emotional empathy with respect to psychopathy (a distinction will be made between the two forms outlined above later in the paper). I will not consider motor empathy in this chapter.

1.1.3 Theory of Mind and psychopathy

Theory of Mind refers to the ability to represent the mental states of others, i.e. their thoughts, desires, beliefs, intentions and knowledge (Frith, 1989). Theory of Mind allows the attribution of mental states to self and others in order to explain and predict behaviour.

The classic measure of Theory of Mind is the Sally-Anne task (Wimmer & Perner, 1983). In this task, the participant is shown two dolls, Sally and Anne, and a basket and a box. The participant watches as Sally places her marble in the basket and then leaves the room. While Sally is out, naughty Anne moves Sally's marble from the basket to the box. Then she, too, leaves the room. Now Sally comes back into the room. The participant is asked the test question: 'Where will Sally look for her marble?'. In order to pass this task, the participant must represent Sally's mental state, her belief that the marble is in the basket. Without this representation, the participant will answer on the basis of the marble's real location, i.e. the box. Most healthy developing individuals from the age of 4 years pass this task (Wimmer & Perner, 1983).

In addition to being considered a form of empathy in its own right, the ability to represent the mental states of others has been considered to be necessary for 'emotional empathy' to occur (Batson *et al.*, 1987; Feshbach, 1987). Within these positions, representations of the internal mental state of another are assumed to act as stimuli for the activation of the affective, empathic response (Batson *et al.*, 1987). Feshbach (1987), for example, viewed empathy to be a function of three processes: first, the cognitive ability to discriminate affective cues in others; second, the more mature cognitive skills entailed in assuming the perspective and role of another person; third, emotional responsiveness (i.e. the ability to experience emotions) (Feshbach, 1987). According to Feshbach (1987), 'empathy is conceived to be the outcome of cognitive and affective processes that operate conjointly' (p. 273).

There are no indications of Theory of Mind impairment in individuals with psychopathy. Three out of four studies assessing the ability of individuals with psychopathy on Theory of Mind measures have reported no impairment (Blair *et al.*, 1996; Richell *et al.*, 2003; Widom, 1978). Only one study has reported impairment and this used a rating scale that is not a typical measure of Theory of Mind (Widom, 1976).

Blair *et al.* (1996) assessed the ability of individuals with psychopathy to perform the Advanced Theory of Mind test (Happé, 1994). This is a story comprehension measure that assesses understanding of mental states. Individuals with autism, a population with known Theory of Mind impairment (Frith, 1989), are impaired on this measure (Happé, 1994). However, the individuals with psychopathy were not (Blair *et al.*, 1996).

Richell *et al.* (2003) examined the ability of individuals with psychopathy to perform the 'Reading the Mind in the Eyes' task. In this task, participants must judge the complex social emotion being displayed by an individual based on information only from the eye region (Baron-Cohen *et al.*, 1997). Individuals with autism are impaired on this task (Baron-Cohen *et al.*, 2001). However, again, the individuals with psychopathy were not (Richell *et al.*, 2003).

In addition to the above work with individuals with psychopathy, it is important to note that even in the broader spectrum of antisocial individuals, there are few data suggesting any link between Theory of Mind impairment and antisocial behaviour. Hughes and colleagues did find some indication of Theory of Mind impairment in their 'hard-to-manage' preschoolers relative to the comparison group (Hughes *et al.*, 1998). However, Happé and Frith found no impairment in their children with emotional and behavioural difficulties (Happé & Frith, 1996). Similarly a study of school bullies found no indications of Theory of Mind impairment (Sutton *et al.*, 1999). In addition, Sutton and colleagues also found no relationship between Theory of Mind performance on the advanced Eyes task and 'disruptive behaviour disorder' symptoms in children aged 11–13 years (Sutton *et al.*, 2000).

Summary

The profound empathic dysfunction reported in the clinical description of psychopathy (Hare, 1991) does not involve Theory of Mind impairment. Individuals with psychopathy are unimpaired on measures of Theory of Mind. Indeed, there are no indications that any populations who show heightened levels of antisocial behaviour are associated with Theory of Mind impairment.

1.2 Emotional empathy

Figure 1.1 represents a simple schematic of the cognitive processes that I consider to underpin empathy. Here empathy is being defined as the emotional response to another individual's visual or vocal expression of emotion. This schematic assumes that there may be at least two routes to the generation of an emotional empathic response: one which relies on the 'semantic processing' of the expression and one which does not. This follows suggestions that information on the emotional expressions of others can be conveyed either by a sub-cortical pathway (retinocollicular–pulvinar–amygdalar) or by a cortical pathway (retinogeniculostriate–extrastriate–fusiform) (Adolphs, 2002).

These two routes for expression processing mirror those previously suggested to be involved in aversive conditioning (LeDoux, 2000). The sub-cortical route is

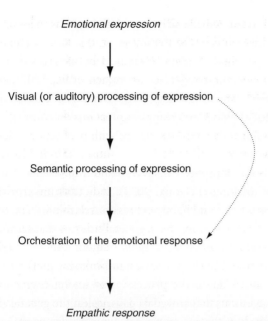

Figure 1.1. A schematic of the cognitive processes thought to underpin empathy. The dotted line refers to the suggested (sub-cortical) route that bypasses the semantic processing of the expression

thought to provide coarse stimulus processing while the cortical route is thought to allow more precise stimulus encoding and allow discrimination learning. The cortical route would underpin the 'semantic processing' of the expression; i.e. it would allow the expression to be named and would allow goal-directed behaviour to be initiated in response to the expression (e.g. initiate helping behaviour to a crying individual).

In Figure 1.1, there is reference to the systems involved in 'the orchestration of the emotional response'. I have stressed elsewhere that the facial expressions of emotion each have a communicatory function, that they impart specific infor-mation to the observer (Blair, 2003a). The systems involved in 'the orchestration of the emotional response' are those systems which respond automatically to the communicatory value of the expression. In short, an empathic response is a translation of a non-verbal communicatory signal. Because of the different implications of these communicatory signals, I have argued that they are translated in several separable systems (Blair, 2003a). I will consider this com-munication and the systems that orchestrate the response to this communication below.

I have suggested that fearfulness, sadness and happiness are reinforcers that modulate the probability that a particular behaviour will be performed in the future (Blair, 2003a). Indeed, fearful faces have been seen as aversive unconditioned stimuli that rapidly convey information to others that a novel stimulus is aversive and should be avoided (Mineka & Cook, 1993). Similarly, I have suggested that sad facial expressions also act as aversive unconditioned stimuli, discouraging actions that caused the display of sadness in another individual and motivating reparatory behaviours. Happy expressions, in contrast, are appetitive unconditioned stimuli which increase the probability of actions to which they appear causally related.

The amygdala has been implicated in aversive and appetitive conditioning including instrumental learning (LeDoux, 2000). It is thus unsurprising, given the suggested role of fearful, sad and happy expressions as reinforcers, that neuroimaging studies, with a few exceptions, have generally found that fearful, sad and happy expressions all modulate amygdala activity (see, for a review, Blair, 2003a). The neuropsychological literature supports the neuroimaging literature as regards the importance of the amygdala in the processing of fearful expressions. There have been occasional suggestions that amygdala damage leads to general expression-recognition impairment but these reports are typically from patients whose lesions extend considerably beyond the amygdala (Rapcsak *et al.*, 2000). Instead, amygdala lesions have been consistently associated with impairment in the recognition of fearful expressions (Adolphs, 2002; Blair, 2003a). Impairment in the processing of sad expressions is not uncommonly found in patients with amygdala lesions (Blair, 2003a). However, amygdala lesions rarely result in impairment in the recognition of happy expressions although this may reflect the ease with which happy expressions are recognized (Blair, 2003a).

Disgusted expressions are also reinforcers but are used most frequently to provide information about foods (Rozin *et al.*, 1993). In particular, they allow the rapid transmission of taste aversions; the observer is warned not to approach the food to which the emoter is displaying the disgust reaction. Thus, the suggestion is that the disgusted expressions of others activate in particular the insula allowing taste aversion [the disgust expression is the unconditioned stimulus (US) that is associated with the novel food conditioned stimulus (CS)] to occur (Blair, 2003a).

I have argued that displays of anger or embarrassment do not act as unconditioned stimuli for aversive conditioning or instrumental learning (Blair, 2003a). Angry expressions are known to curtail the behaviour of others in situations where social rules or expectations have been violated (Averill, 1982). Instead, they are important signals to modulate current behavioural responding, particularly in situations involving hierarchy interactions (Blair, 2003a). They appear to serve to inform the observer to stop the current behavioural action rather than to convey any information as to whether that action should be initiated in the future.

In other words, angry expressions can be seen as triggers for response reversal. Orbital and ventrolateral frontal cortex is crucially implicated in response reversal (Cools *et al.*, 2002). Interestingly, similar areas of lateral orbital frontal cortex are activated by angry expressions and response reversal as a function of contingency change (Blair, 2003b).

Summary

In short, emotional expressions are non-verbal communications. Empathy is a prime component of the translation of this communication within the observer. This translation is potentially reliant on both cortical and sub-cortical routes. These routes convey the communication to regions of the brain involved in emotional processing (the amygdala, insula and orbital and ventrolateral frontal cortex). These regions orchestrate a response to this communication; mediating emotional learning about objects or food or initiating response reversal.

1.3 Psychopathy and emotional empathy

As noted in the introduction, there can be no doubt that psychopathy is associated with empathic dysfunction. However, the question remains regarding the form of this dysfunction. I outlined above that the empathic dysfunction in psychopathy does not include impairment in Theory of Mind. What about emotional empathy? In Section 1.2, I outlined a schematic of the empathic process. Currently, no data exist regarding the two routes to the systems that allow the orchestration of the emotional response. We do not know whether psychopathy is associated with dysfunction in systems involved in face processing. However, one reason to believe that there is no obvious general dysfunction in the systems involved in facial processing is that while individuals with psychopathy are impaired in expression processing, their impairment appears to be selective. Given this selectivity (see below), it is unlikely that there is notable dysfunction in the systems involved in face processing.

Two main forms of paradigm have been used to index empathy in individuals with psychopathy: skin conductance responses (SCRs) to empathy-inducing stimuli and the ability to recognize facial expressions. Three studies have examined vicarious conditioning in individuals with psychopathy; i.e. the extent to which the participant will learn an autonomic response to a stimulus associated with another individual's distress (Aniskiewicz, 1979; House & Milligan, 1976; Sutker, 1970). Two of these three studies reported reduced vicarious conditioning in the individuals with psychopathy, the third did not.

Two studies have examined SCRs to sad faces in individuals with psychopathic tendencies: one examined adults with psychopathy, the other children with psychopathic tendencies (Blair, 1999; Blair *et al.*, 1997). In these studies, the participants were presented with images of sad faces, threatening stimuli (e.g. pointed guns but also including an angry face) or neutral stimuli (e.g. a book). Both the adults with psychopathy and the children with psychopathic tendencies showed reduced SCRs to the sad faces relative to their respective comparison populations. Interestingly, both adults with psychopathy and the children with psychopathic tendencies showed relatively appropriate SCRs to the angry face amidst the threatening stimuli. This was the first indication that the empathic impairment in individuals with psychopathy might be selective for particular expressions.

Studies have examined the ability of individuals with psychopathy to recognize the facial or vocal emotional expressions of others (Blair *et al.*, 2001, 2002, 2004, 2006a; Kosson *et al.*, 2002; Stevens *et al.*, 2001). In most of these studies, the children with psychopathic tendencies/adults with psychopathy have been impaired in the recognition of sad/fearful expressions. Typically, the children with psychopathic tendencies have shown impairment in the recognition of sad expressions (Blair *et al.*, 2001; Stevens *et al.*, 2001). However, this has not been found in the adults with psychopathy (with one exception; Dolan, personal communication). In all of the studies, except that of Kosson *et al.* (2002), the children with psychopathic tendencies and the adults with psychopathy have been impaired in the recognition of fearful expressions. Kosson *et al.* (2002) reported some difficulty with the recognition of disgusted expressions (but only when the participants were responding with the left hand). Blair *et al.* (2004) also found some impairment in the adults with psychopathy for the recognition of disgusted expressions, however this deficit was not present if the effect of intelligence quotient (IQ) was co-varied out.

The above data suggest a relative selectivity in the empathic dysfunction shown by individuals with psychopathy. Individuals with psychopathy are impaired when processing fearful, sad (in adulthood if responsiveness is indexed by SCRs, in childhood whether by SCR or recognition score) and possibly disgusted expressions. No study has yet reported that individuals with psychopathy show impairment in the processing of angry, happy or surprised expressions. The absence of impairment for angry expressions is particularly interesting. Neurological patients following lesions of orbital and ventral frontal cortex or psychiatric conditions which are thought to detrimentally affect orbital and ventrolateral regions, such as childhood bipolar disorder or intermittent explosive disorder, all show general difficulties with processing expressions but their difficulty is particularly marked for angry expressions (Best *et al.*, 2002; Blair & Cipolotti, 2000; Hornak *et al.*, 1996; McClure *et al.*, 2003).

In the Section 1.2, I suggested that there were at least three systems responsible for orchestrating responses to expressions; i.e. the core component of empathy

(Blair, 2003a). One system responsive to the aversive and appetitive unconditioned stimuli of fearful, sad and happy expressions and consequently modulating
the probability that any stimulus associated with these expressions will be avoided
or approached in the future. A second system responsive to the aversive unconditioned stimulus of a disgusted expression will reduce the probability that any
stimulus (particularly food) associated with this expression will be avoided in the
future. A third system is particularly responsive to displays of anger and embarrassment which modulates on-going social interactions (eliciting responses
according to the hierarchy level of the communicator amongst other factors).

I claim that individuals with psychopathy have dysfunction primarily in the
first system (that responsive to fearful, sad and happy expressions). They may
also have dysfunction in the second system (that responsive to disgusted expressions). However, in the absence of additional data that possibility will not be
considered here.

As noted above, the primary neural system responsible for orchestrating an
emotional response to fearful, sad and happy expressions is the amygdala (see
Blair, 2003a). This suggests amygdala dysfunction in psychopathy. There are
considerable data in line with this suggestion (Blair, 2003b). Thus, individuals
with psychopathy show reduced amygdaloid volume relative to comparison individuals and reduced amygdala activation during emotional memory and aversive
conditioning tasks. Human and animal neuropsychological work has informed
us that the effects of amygdala lesions include impairment in: (1) aversive conditioning; (2) the augmentation of the startle reflex to visual threat primes; and
(3) passive avoidance learning. If psychopathy is associated with amygdala dysfunction, the neuropsychological approach would predict that individuals with
psychopathy are impaired in the above tasks. Considerable data show that they are
(see, for a review, Blair, 2004).

While individuals with psychopathy are impaired in the processing of fearful
and sad expressions, they show no impairment for the processing of happy
expressions (Blair, 2003b; Blair *et al.*, 2001, 2002, 2006a; Kosson *et al.*, 2002;
Stevens *et al.*, 2001). While this is consistent with the neuropsychological literature
documenting the consequences of amygdala lesions, it is less consistent with the
neuroimaging literature (see above) which suggests a role for the amygdala in the
processing of happy expressions. Of course, the absence of impairment for happy
expressions in individuals with psychopathy might reflect the ease with which they
are recognized (i.e. an intact amygdala is not necessary for naming).

However, a more interesting possibility is that this absence of impairment
reflects the selectivity of their impairment. The amygdala is involved in the
formation of stimulus–reward and stimulus–punishment associations; animals
with amygdala lesions show impairment in both reward- and punishment-related

behaviour (Baxter & Murray, 2002). Yet, the impairment in individuals with psychopathy is far more marked for processing dependent on stimulus–punishment associations than for stimulus–reward associations (Levenston *et al.*, 2000). Thus, whereas individuals with psychopathy do not show augmentation of the startle reflex following a negative visual prime relative to comparison individuals, they do show a comparable reduction in startle reflex following a positive visual prime relative to comparison individuals (Levenston *et al.*, 2000). Moreover, in a decision-making study, individuals with psychopathy showed particular difficulty, relative to controls, when choosing between stimuli associated with different levels of punishment. Their impairment in choosing between stimuli associated with different levels of reward was far less marked (K. S. Peschardt, A. Leonard, J. Morton, & R. J. R. Blair, Differential stimulus–reward and stimulus–punishment learning in individuals with psychopathy. Submitted for publication). I argue that happy faces are appetitive unconditioned stimuli. In other words, the absence of impairment in individuals with psychopathy for happy expressions might also reflect the selectivity of their impairment for the processing of punishment information as opposed to reward information.

Summary

I assume that individuals with psychopathy have no impairment in the systems which convey facial expression information to those neural systems that are involved in orchestrating an emotional response to these expressions. This assumption is made because individuals with psychopathy show considerable selectivity in their facial-expression-processing impairment. They are not impaired for all expressions. They are not impaired when processing angry, surprised or happy expressions. They are, however, impaired when processing fearful, sad and, possibly, disgusted expressions. This impairment is likely related to the amygdala dysfunction seen in patients with this disorder.

1.4 Conclusion

Empathic dysfunction is one of the major features of psychopathy. The goal of this chapter was to consider the nature of this empathic dysfunction. Two main forms of empathy were considered: 'cognitive empathy' or Theory of Mind and 'emotional empathy'. Considerable work indicates that there is no Theory of Mind impairment in psychopathy. Moreover, it also appears clear that Theory of Mind impairment is not associated with more general populations of antisocial individuals.

Emotional empathy can be considered the results of the translation of the non-verbal communications that are the emotional expressions of others. It is potentially reliant on both cortical and sub-cortical face processing routes. These routes convey the communication to regions of the brain involved in emotional processing (the amygdala, insula and orbital and ventrolateral frontal cortex). These regions allow a dedicated response to the facial expressions of others. For example, fearful and sad expressions, processed by the amygdala, initiate emotional learning. In contrast, angry expressions, primarily processed by ventro-lateral prefrontal cortex, initiate the termination of on-going behaviour.

Individuals with psychopathy have a relatively selective empathy deficit. They are impaired in the processing of fearful, sad and possibly disgusted expressions. Impairment in the processing of particularly fearful expressions is a common consequence of amygdala lesions. Patients with psychopathy show many other impairments associated with amygdala dysfunction. In short, it appears likely that their reduced responsiveness to the fearful and sad expressions of others is related to their more general amygdala dysfunction.

I, and others, consider the empathy dysfunction seen in individuals with psychopathy to be at the heart of the disorder (Blair, 1995). Individuals who are indifferent to the fear and sadness of others are individuals who are difficult to socialize through effective socialization practices such as empathy induction. Empathy induction involves the socializer focusing the attention of the transgressor on the distress of the victim (and presumably heightens the salience of the aversive stimulus of the victim's distress). While the greater use of empathy induction and other positive forms of parenting reduce the probability of antisocial behaviour in healthy children, they have no significant effect on the probability of antisocial behaviour in children with psychopathic tendencies (Wootton *et al.*, 1997). In other words, if we could find means to increase the empathic reaction of children with psychopathic tendencies, we might be able to considerably improve the prognosis of this disorder. The investigation of such means is one of the main foci of our research at the moment.

REFERENCES

Adolphs, R. (2002). Neural systems for recognizing emotion. *Current Opinion in Neurobiology*, **12(2)**, 169–177.

American Psychiatric Association (APA). (1994). *Diagnostic and Statistical Manual of Mental Disorders* (4th edn.). Washington, DC: APA.

Aniskiewicz, A. S. (1979). Autonomic components of vicarious conditioning and psychopathy. *Journal of Clinical Psychology*, **35**, 60–67.

Averill, J. R. (1982). *Anger and Aggression: An Essay on Emotion*. New York: Springer-Verlag.

Baron-Cohen, S., Wheelwright, S., Hill, J., Raste, Y., & Plumb, I. (2001). The 'reading the mind in the eyes' test revised version: a study with normal adults, and adults with asperger syndrome or high-functioning autism. *Journal of Child Psychology and Psychiatry, and Applied Disciplines*, **42(2)**, 241–251.

Baron-Cohen, S., Wheelwright, S., & Joliffe, T. (1997). Is there a 'language of the eyes'? Evidence from normal adults, and adults with autism or asperger syndrome. *Visual Cognition*, **4(3)**, 311–331.

Batson, C. D., Fultz, J., & Schoenrade, P. A. (1987). Adults' emotional reactions to the distress of others. In N. Eisenberg & J. Strayer (eds.), *Empathy and its Development* (pp. 163–185). Cambridge: Cambridge University Press.

Baxter, M. G., & Murray, E. A. (2002). The amygdala and reward. *Nature Reviews Neuroscience*, **3(7)**, 563–573.

Best, M., Williams, J. M., & Coccaro, E. F. (2002). Evidence for a dysfunctional prefrontal circuit in patients with an impulsive aggressive disorder. *Proceedings of the National Academy of Sciences of the USA*, **99(12)**, 8448–8453.

Blair, R. J., Mitchell, D. G., Richell, R. A., *et al.* (2002). Turning a deaf ear to fear: impaired recognition of vocal affect in psychopathic individuals. *Journal of Abnormal Psychology*, **111(4)**, 682–686.

Blair, R. J. R. (1995). A cognitive developmental approach to morality: investigating the psychopath. *Cognition*, **57**, 1–29.

Blair, R. J. R. (1999). Responsiveness to distress cues in the child with psychopathic tendencies. *Personality and Individual Differences*, **27**, 135–145.

Blair, R. J. R. (2003a). Facial expressions, their communicatory functions and neuro-cognitive substrates. *Philosophical Transactions of the Royal Society of London. Series B, Biological Sciences*, **358(1431)**, 561–572.

Blair, R. J. R. (2003b). Neurobiological basis of psychopathy. *British Journal of Psychiatry*, **182**, 5–7.

Blair, R. J. R., Budhani, S., Colledge, E., & Scott, S. K. (2006a). Deafness to fear in boys with psychopathic tendencies. *Journal of Child Psychology and Psychiatry*, in press.

Blair, R. J. R., & Cipolotti, L. (2000). Impaired social response reversal: a case of 'acquired sociopathy'. *Brain*, **123**, 1122–1141.

Blair, R. J. R., Colledge, E., Murray, L., & Mitchell, D. G. (2001). A selective impairment in the processing of sad and fearful expressions in children with psychopathic tendencies. *Journal of Abnormal Child Psychology*, **29(6)**, 491–498.

Blair, R. J. R., Jones, L., Clark, F., & Smith, M. (1997). The psychopathic individual: a lack of responsiveness to distress cues? *Psychophysiology*, **34**, 192–198.

Blair, R. J. R., Mitchell, D. G. V., Colledge, E., *et al.* (2004). Reduced sensitivity to other's fearful expressions in psychopathic individuals. *Personality and Individual Differences*, **37**, 1111–1121.

Blair, R. J. R., Sellars, C., Strickland, I., *et al.* (1996). Theory of mind in the psychopath. *Journal of Forensic Psychiatry*, **7**, 15–25.

Cools, R., Clark, L., Owen, A. M., & Robbins, T. W. (2002). Defining the neural mechanisms of probabilistic reversal learning using event-related functional magnetic resonance imaging. *Journal of Neuroscience*, **22(11)**, 4563–4567.

Feshbach, N. D. (1987). Parental empathy and child adjustment/maladjustment. In N. Eisenberg & J. Strayer (eds.), *Empathy and its Development*. New York: Cambridge University Press.

Frick, P. J., & Hare, R. D. (2001). *The Antisocial Process Screening Device*. Toronto: Multi-Health Systems.

Frith, U. (1989). *Autism: Explaining the Enigma*. Oxford: Blackwell.

Happé, F. G. E. (1994). An advanced test of theory of mind: understanding of story characters' thoughts and feelings in able autistic, mentally handicapped, and normal children and adults. *Journal of Autism and Developmental Disorders*, **24**, 129–154.

Happé, F. G. E., & Frith, U. (1996). Theory of mind and social impairment in children with conduct disorder. *British Journal of Developmental Psychology*, **14(4)**, 385–398.

Hare, R. D. (1980). A research scale for the assessment of psychopathy in criminal populations. *Personality and Individual Differences*, **1**, 111–119.

Hare, R. D. (1991). *The Hare Psychopathy Checklist – Revised*. Toronto, Ontario: Multi-Health Systems.

Hoffman, M. L. (1987). The contribution of empathy to justice and moral judgment. In N. Eisenberg & J. Strayer (eds.), *Empathy and its Development* (pp. 47–80). Cambridge: Cambridge University Press.

Hornak, J., Rolls, E. T., & Wade, D. (1996). Face and voice expression identification in patients with emotional and behavioural changes following ventral frontal damage. *Neuropsychologia*, **34**, 247–261.

House, T. H., & Milligan, W. L. (1976). Autonomic responses to modeled distress in prison psychopaths. *Journal of Personality and Social Psychology*, **34**, 556–560.

Hughes, C., Dunn, J., & White, A. (1998). Trick or treat? Uneven understanding of mind and emotion and executive dysfunction in 'hard-to-manage' preschoolers. *Journal of Child Psychology and Psychiatry*, **39(7)**, 981–994.

Kosson, D. S., Suchy, Y., Mayer, A. R., & Libby, J. (2002). Facial affect recognition in criminal psychopaths. *Emotion*, **2(4)**, 398–411.

LeDoux, J. E. (2000). Emotion circuits in the brain. *Annual Review of Neuroscience*, **23**, 155–184.

Levenston, G. K., Patrick, C. J., Bradley, M. M., & Lang, P. J. (2000). The psychopath as observer: emotion and attention in picture processing. *Journal of Abnormal Psychology*, **109**, 373–386.

McClure, E. B., Pope, K., Hoberman, A. J., Pine, D. S., & Leibenluft, E. (2003). Facial expression recognition in adolescents with mood and anxiety disorders. *American Journal of Psychiatry*, **160(6)**, 1172–1174.

Mineka, S., & Cook, M. (1993). Mechanisms involved in the observational conditioning of fear. *Journal of Experimental Psychology: General*, **122**, 23–38.

Pichot, P. (1978). Psychopathic behavior: a historical review. In R. D. Hare & D. S. Schalling (eds.), *Psychopathic Behavior: Approaches to Research*. Chichester: Wiley.

Rapcsak, S. Z., Galper, S. R., Comer, J. F., *et al.* (2000). Fear recognition deficits after focal brain damage: a cautionary note. *Neurology*, **54**, 575–581.

Richell, R. A., Mitchell, D. G., Newman, C., *et al.* (2003). Theory of mind and psychopathy: can psychopathic individuals read the 'language of the eyes'? *Neuropsychologia*, **41(5)**, 523–526.

Rozin, P., Haidt, J., & McCauley, C. R. (1993). Disgust. In M. Lewis & J. M. Haviland (eds.), *Handbook of Emotions* (pp. 575–594). New York: The Guilford Press.

Stevens, D., Charman, T., & Blair, R. J. R. (2001). Recognition of emotion in facial expressions and vocal tones in children with psychopathic tendencies. *Journal of Genetic Psychology*, **162(2)**, 201–211.

Sutker, P. B. (1970). Vicarious conditioning and sociopathy. *Journal of Abnormal Psychology*, **76**, 380–386.

Sutton, J., Reeves, M., & Keogh, E. (2000). Disruptive behaviour, avoidance of responsibility and theory of mind. *British Journal of Developmental Psychology*, **18**(1), 1–11.

Sutton, J., Smith, P. K., & Swettenham, J. (1999). Social cognition and bullying: social inadequacy or skilled manipulation? *British Journal of Developmental Psychology*, **17**(3), 435–450.

Widom, C. S. (1976). Interpersonal and personal construct systems in psychopaths. *Journal of Consulting and Clinical Psychology*, **44**, 614–623.

Widom, C. S. (1978). An empirical classification of female offenders. *Criminal Justice and Behavior*, **5**, 35–52.

Wimmer, H., & Perner, J. (1983). Beliefs about beliefs: representation and the constraining function of wrong beliefs in young children's understanding of deception. *Cognition*, **13**, 103–128.

Wootton, J. M., Frick, P. J., Shelton, K. K., & Silverthorn, P. (1997). Ineffective parenting and childhood conduct problems: the moderating role of callous-unemotional traits. *Journal of Consulting and Clinical Psychology*, **65**, 292–300.

Empathy deficits in schizophrenia

Kwang-Hyuk Lee

Academic Clinical Psychiatry, University of Sheffield

2.1 Introduction

Schizophrenia affects about 1% of the population worldwide and its symptoms typically manifest in early adulthood (Jablensky *et al.*, 1992). Schizophrenia was first described by Kraepelin as dementia praecox and was re-designated as a disintegrative illness by Bleuler. Within this illness, the distinctiveness of paranoid, hebephrenic (disorganized) and catatonic subtypes has been continuously recognized from the time of Kraepelin, and is included in schizophrenia diagnosis in current diagnostic systems (American Psychiatric Association, 1994). Previous research on schizophrenia heterogeneity has emphasized the subtypes, focusing on paranoid symptoms (in a paranoid/non-paranoid distinction), thought disorder (in a thought-/non-thought-disorder distinction) and negative symptoms (in positive/negative and deficit/non-deficit distinctions), each of them being a cardinal feature of the classical subtypes. Nonetheless, patients often present with different combinations of symptoms with varying degrees of severity, stability and co-morbid features (Kraepelin, 1922). The aetiology(s) of this disorder has not yet been fully elucidated. It is possible that an additive effect of multiple genes confers susceptibility to schizophrenia, and that this vulnerability may interact with environmental factors (Tsuang, 2000).

Marked impairment in social functioning is a diagnostic feature of schizophrenia, and is one of the most disabling clinical features of the schizophrenic illness (American Psychiatric Association, 1994). An empathy deficit may underlie impaired social functioning in schizophrenia, as empathy mediates the understanding of others in social interactions, by representing or simulating other people's thoughts and feelings within the self. Indeed, some current models of schizophrenia postulate that the disorder can be understood as a disorder of representation of mental states (the inability to represent what others are thinking) (Frith, 1992) or, similarly, a disorder of intuitive attunement (the fundamental deficit in relationships with other people) (Stanghellini, 2000).

Empathy in Mental Illness, eds. Tom F. D. Farrow and Peter W. R. Woodruff. Published by Cambridge University Press. © Cambridge University Press 2007.

felt indirectly by imagining another person's experiences

In this chapter, the significance of affective cue perception, vicarious arousal and cognitive aspects of empathy are highlighted as a framework for the exploration of an empathy deficit in schizophrenia. Experimental psychopathological and neuroimaging studies relating the empathy deficit in schizophrenia are reviewed; each provides a different perspective on the empathy deficit in schizophrenia. Attention is also given to the relationship between an empathy deficit and symptom profiles. Finally, a theoretical consideration is presented.

2.2 Components of empathy

Empathy involves multiple affective and cognitive processes. Strayer (1987) used the term, 'components of empathy' to describe the multidimensional structure of empathy, and to emphasize the interaction between affective and cognitive factors. In this chapter, three processes, affective cue perception, vicarious arousal and cognitive aspects in empathy, are highlighted in the understanding of an empathy deficit in schizophrenia.

2.2.1 Affective cue perception

Attention to, and subsequently efficient perception of, affective cues may be an important factor for recognizing emotion of others and therefore fundamental to empathy. For example, a recent study demonstrated increased brain electrical activity in the visual cortex, prior to higher-order stimulus processing, in response to emotional compared to neutral images (Schupp *et al.*, 2003). This result suggests that emotionally salient stimulus perception requires a significant amount of attention and sensory processing resources. Individual differences in the ability to process social stimuli have been reported. People who were faster in discriminating facial expressions had higher scores on the Questionnaire Measure of Emotional Empathy (Martin *et al.*, 1996), a measure of responsiveness to another's emotional experience.

2.2.2 Vicarious arousal

The vicarious arousal of affect has been highlighted by Hoffman (1978) as the emotional basis for the development of empathy in children. In his model, conditioned affect arousal (mediated by direct caretaker handling) and motor mimicry (the activity of visceral and facial muscles) are involuntary, and these automatic processes form the basis of the emotional component of empathy. With the development of these processes, the observation of distress in others triggers inner bodily processes such as visceral and facial muscle activities to produce the same emotion within the self. Emotion and bodily processes become intimately linked together, to influence each other. For example, Levenson and colleagues showed that involuntarily produced facial muscle contractions, without eliciting events, produced a subjective experience of the associated emotion as well as changes in autonomic activity such as heart rate and skin conductance (Levenson *et al.*, 1990).

2.2.3 Cognitive empathy

Cognitive empathy (the cognitive understanding of mental states of others) has been referred to as 'Theory of Mind'. It has also been referred to as mind-reading or mentalizing. The term Theory of Mind implies that we employ a theory (analogous to a scientific theory) to make attributions of mental states of others. However, current neuroscience research supports the simulation theory positing that the ability to interpret the mental states of others depends on the ability to simulate another person's mind. For example, our brain may actually begin to function like the other's brain by generating similar processes in oneself.

Cognitive empathy requires a sense of others as having inner thoughts that are independent from self. The cognitive developmental model put forward by Perner (1991) distinguished three steps to achieving cognitive empathy, from primary representation (i.e. sensation), to secondary representation (holding and using primary representation) and finally to meta-representation (represen-tation of concept of representation). In children, meta-representation is consid-ered to be achieved when they understand another person's wrong belief. For example, in the classic 'Sally-Anne' false belief test (Baron-Cohen *et al.*, 1985), Sally has a basket and Anne has a box. Sally puts a marble into her basket, and then she leaves the scene. While she is outside, Anne takes the marble from the basket and puts it into her own box. Then Sally comes back and wants to play with her marble. Children are asked to predict where Sally will look for her marble. Four-year-old children tend to correctly predict that she will look for her marble in her basket. Cognitive empathy is also an active process, involving reconstruction of others' mental states from various social and emotional cues and comparison between the reconstructed other and similar experience from one's own past (episodic memory). Hence it is not surprising to know that the contributions of attention and memory resources (Bloom & German, 2000), and executive func-tion (Perner & Lang, 1999) are substantial in cognitive empathy. It is of interest as well that children's correct response to false-belief questions to 'other' and 'the self' showed the same developmental trajectory (Wellman *et al.*, 2001).

These three empathy processes, affective cue perception, vicarious arousal and cognitive empathy, should act in concert in 'normal' empathy. There is evidence that these processes can be dissociated differently in different clinical conditions. People with antisocial personality disorder are able to represent what other people think, but they are autonomically hyporesponsive to the distress of others

(Blair *et al.*, 1997). Sex offenders display a specific deficit in identifying the emotions experienced by victims of sexual abuse, while they are able to recognize the emotions of car accident victims (Marshall *et al.*, 1995). Finally, children with autistic disorders are capable of experiencing emotion, but they are impaired in making sense of feelings (cognitive empathy) (Gillberg, 1992). Section 2.3 considers some earlier understandings of empathy-related concepts in schizophrenia, followed by empirical studies on these three empathy components in this disorder.

2.3 Empathy in schizophrenia

2.3.1 Empathy-related concepts in earlier descriptive and phenomenological psychiatry

Difficulties with being engaged in relationships with another person in schizophrenia have been recognized since the earliest attempts to describe this disorder. Kraepelin (1919/1989) described the 'loss of sympathy' in patients with schizophrenia as being 'no share' of feelings with others. He speculated the loss of an emotional colouring mechanism in response to changes in social situation in the patients, so that their response became 'uniform'. Similarly, but in a wider context, Bleuler (1911/1950) described autism as a fundamental (but a complex symptom) in schizophrenia. Autistic thinking and affective disturbances were considered to be key features of autism. Affective disturbances included blunting of affect and inappropriate affective responses. In people with schizophrenia, feelings that regulate social interaction are blunted, and affective responses that would be expected from a social situation are often inappropriate. These cognitive (autistic thinking) and affective processes (affective blunting and inappropriate affect) manifested in social interactions may be closely related to the empathy deficit in schizophrenia.

Phenomenological psychiatry has contributed to the understanding of empathy or intersubjectivity phenomenon in schizophrenia. The phenomenological concept of intersubjectivity refers to the sharing of an object reference between separate conscious minds, and is established when the two minds undergo acts of empathy (Beyer, 2004). The lack of intersubjective or empathic experience in people with schizophrenia has been referred to as 'loss of vital contact with reality' (Minkowski), 'inconsistency of natural experience' (Binswanger), or 'a global crisis of common sense' (Blankenburg) (see Parnas & Bovet, 1991, for details). An observer, in turn, feels a lack of empathy towards a patient with schizophrenia. For example, the International Pilot Study of Schizophrenia (Carpenter *et al.*, 1973) reported that a psychiatrist's sense of poor rapport with patients, among several hundreds of variables, was the second most reliable discriminator of schizophrenia. This study supports the well-known idea in psychiatry that it is difficult to form or maintain rapport with patients with schizophrenia. The lack of rapport felt by the psychiatrist and similarly 'the praecox feeling' (the psychiatrist's inability to empathize with the patient) indicate patients' difficulty in establishing empathic relationships with other people (Parnas & Bovet, 1991; Schroder *et al.*, 1992).

2.3.2 Recent experimental studies of empathy components in schizophrenia

To date, empathic ability has not been experimentally examined in schizophrenia research, although a number of studies have indirectly supported an empathy deficit in this disorder. The paucity of direct schizophrenia research on empathy may primarily be due to the multidimensional nature of empathy and consequent lack of appropriate tests. However, empirical, experimental studies on the three components of empathy (affective cue perception, vicarious arousal and cognitive empathy) may provide clues to understanding empathy in schizophrenia.

A deficit in affect decoding from face stimuli has long been hypothesized to be a major contributing factor to empathy deficit in people with schizophrenia. People with schizophrenia often fail to identify facial affects. Facial affect recognition is also impaired in children and adolescent groups with schizophrenia (Walker *et al.*, 1980). Several studies have found that poor facial affect recognition is associated with impaired social functioning (Hooker & Park, 2002; Mueser *et al.*, 1996). Moreover, Penn and colleagues (Penn *et al.*, 1996) found that patients' performance on facial affect recognition and social stimuli sequencing tasks was related to a social functioning measure such as the evaluation of patients' ward behaviour. The severity of impairment in facial affect recognition has often been positively correlated with negative symptoms, especially 'blunting of affect' (Suslow *et al.*, 2003). Some other studies (Bozikas *et al.*, 2004) have found an association between a facial affect recognition deficit and disorganization syndrome (primarily characterized by thought disorder and 'inappropriate affect').

Facial emotion recognition dysfunction in schizophrenia can also be inferred from studies investigating scanning eye movements in schizophrenia. When patients with schizophrenia look at human faces, they show an abnormal viewing pattern. In a healthy sample, about half of face scanning time is focused on the eye region, with each of the remaining parts of the face (nose and mouth) being scanned less (Janik *et al.*, 1978). The concentration on the eyes becomes salient after 7 weeks of age (Haith *et al.*, 1977). While the importance of concentrating the eyes has not been formally analysed in face scanning studies in schizophrenia, there is a general agreement that people with schizophrenia, especially those with delusions or negative symptoms, show reduced attention to facial features during face scanning (Gordon *et al.*, 1992; Phillips & David, 1997; Streit *et al.*, 1997). When the face stimuli were not readily identifiable (degraded), schizophrenic patients scanned the facial features equally compared to normal controls (Williams *et al.*, 1999). Behavioural analysis has also shown that, similar to children with autism, schizophrenia patients showed partial gaze avoidance specific to human faces while they did not show gaze aversion when looking at non-human faces (Williams, 1974). It is possible that, especially in patients with delusions, hypersensitivity to another's gaze and subsequent misinterpretation would produce gaze aversion. For example, beliefs such as 'someone is spying on me' or 'people are staring at me' are very common in patients with delusions. If someone is perceived as staring, the person is interpreted as being hostile, and the most common strategy taken by the stared person is avoidance (see Kleinke, 1986, for a review of social psychology literature). However, the significance of gaze aversion in relation to the other cognitive and social functioning in schizophrenia has not been researched.

A number of studies suggest that people with schizophrenia have a deficit or dysregulation of vicarious arousal. As discussed in Section 2.2.2, autonomic processes (arousal and the activity of visceral and facial muscles) are significant factors in empathy, as these processes represent the generation of emotion in the self. In schizophrenia, behavioural and psychophysiological expression of emotion and subjective emotional experience are all impaired. First, children who later develop schizophrenia show abnormalities in facial expression of emotion (showing greater negative affect) as early as infancy (Walker *et al.*, 1993). Second, patients with schizophrenia also show abnormalities of skin conductance response (an autonomic system marker of emotional sweating) as early as 3 years of age (Venables, 1993). Finally, people with schizophrenia have abnormal subjective experience of emotion (Myin-Germeys *et al.*, 2000). Moreover, a disintegrative relationship among these emotional components has been observed. Kring and Neale (1996) observed that patients with schizophrenia showed diminished facial expression, but the patients reported the same degree of subjective emotional experience with an abnormally greater skin conductance response while they were viewing emotional film clips. Further, Blanchard and colleagues found that patients with schizophrenia showed more negative emotions and less intense expression of emotions compared with healthy controls, which was related to poor social functioning (Blanchard *et al.*, 1998).

A cognitive empathy impairment in schizophrenia has been documented in a number of studies (Lee *et al.*, 2004). The authors in most of these studies employed various false belief tasks (see the Sally-Anne task described in Section 2.2.3). When considered as a group, subjects with schizophrenia showed a deficit in this task, relative to non-psychiatric control subjects. Whether the cognitive empathy deficit in schizophrenia is a trait or influenced by mental state changes is not clear to date, but both children and chronically affected adults with schizophrenia exhibit the deficit (Pilowsky *et al.*, 2000). Some studies have revealed that symptom severity is, in fact, associated with the observed cognitive empathy deficit (Corcoran *et al.*, 1997; Doody *et al.*, 1998). These studies suggest the presence of an association between disturbed mental state and performance on cognitive empathy tasks. Symptoms posited to be related to cognitive empathy deficit include negative symptoms, thought disorder, or persecutory delusions (Frith & Corcoran, 1996).

To summarize, in people suffering from schizophrenia as a group, affective perceptual sensitivity, emotional arousal and cognitive empathy are all impaired. This would simply mean patients with schizophrenia have a generalized deficit manifesting across all domains of empathy-related processes. However, the pattern of impairment in empathy components appears to be dependent upon the configuration of symptoms and, moreover, the same deficit in a particular task may result from different sources. For example, patients with paranoid symptoms are hypersensitive to a potential threat (Fear *et al.*, 1996) and therefore they are likely to misinterpret another's facial expression and intention (such as jumping to conclusions). On the other hand, patients with negative symptoms of affective blunting may misidentify facial expressions because of their inability to feel what other people are feeling. Yet another source of variance would be 'dysfunction in emotional association' in patients with positive symptoms of inappropriate affect. In order to investigate a complex process such as empathy in this complex heterogeneous disorder, it is necessary to use a carefully designed battery of tasks assessing different aspects of empathy in a large sample of patients with schizophrenia or, alternatively, in patients with a specific symptom such as affective blunting or inappropriate affect. Section 2.4 considers the neural basis of empathy in healthy subjects and people with schizophrenia.

2.4 Neuroimaging empathy in schizophrenia

Empathy is a multidimensional construct involving the complex interaction between affective and cognitive factors. It is unlikely therefore that there is a single brain region dedicated to empathy. Brothers (1989) emphasized the role of the amygdala in empathy, as it projects to the sensory association cortex to process emotional and social information. A comprehensive review by Preston and de Waal (2002) suggests two empathy networks: (1) amygdala, cingulate and orbito-frontal cortices, involved in perception and emotion regulation, and (2) dorso-lateral and ventromedial prefrontal regions engaged in holding and manipulating this information. The medial prefrontal cortex may play a predominant role in cognitive empathy, as a number of neuroimaging studies have consistently reported medial prefrontal activation during a variety of tasks (Lee *et al.*, 2004). Interestingly, the medial prefrontal cortex is also activated when attention is directed to the self (self-awareness) (Johnson *et al.*, 2002). The common engagement of this area for representing the mental states of others as well as self-awareness may provide the neural basis for intersubjectivity (Frith, 2002). In addition, the fusiform gyrus, which is engaged in face processing, has also exhibited significant activation during the observation of human interactions (Castelli *et al.*, 2000; Schultz *et al.*, 2003).

Patients with schizophrenia show decreased activation in the amygdala and fusiform face area during facial affect recognition (Gur *et al.*, 2002; Quintana *et al.*, 2003). These findings might be closely related to volume reduction in the amygdala and fusiform gyrus in these patients (Joyal *et al.*, 2003; Onitsuka *et al.*, 2003). Consistent with these findings, patients with schizophrenia have an enduring difficulty with learning and recalling emotional facial pictures (Exner *et al.*, 2004). These functional and structural defects may have a significant impact during social interactions in schizophrenia.

Some recent studies have examined the neural mechanisms of cognitive empathy in people with schizophrenia. Russell and colleagues (Russell *et al.*, 2000) reported that people with schizophrenia made more errors in the mental state attribution of photographed eyes, and showed less activation in left prefrontal cortex, compared with controls. A positron emission tomography (PET) study by Brunet *et al.* (2003) used a sequencing task involving inferring the character's intention and choosing a card to complete sequences. In this task, in contrast to Russell *et al.*'s finding, people with schizophrenia showed decreased activation in right medial prefrontal cortex. It is possible that language material used by Russell *et al.* (2000) (matching words with photographs) might engage the left more than the right, whereas the non-verbal material used in Brunet *et al.* (2003) might have produced the opposite laterality.

We have recently investigated the neural basis of an empathy deficit in schizophrenia with an acute episode and its changes following recovery (Lee *et al.*, 2006). We were interested in whether deficient brain activation during empathy can 'recover' with clinical improvement. In a longitudinal design, 14 patients with schizophrenia experiencing an acute episode and 14 healthy controls were scanned twice within approximately two and half months. We employed empathy, forgiveness and baseline social reasoning scenarios in our social cognition functional magnetic resonance imaging (fMRI) paradigms (Farrow *et al.*, 2001). Schizophrenic symptoms, social functioning and illness insight scales, and the Wisconsin Card Sorting Test were used to examine whether improvement on these measures was predicted by recovery of brain activation in response to the social cognition paradigms. During an acute episode, compared with healthy volunteers, patients with schizophrenia had significantly reduced activation in left prefrontal cortex, thalamus and right posterior fusiform gyrus. Following recovery, patients showed increased activation in left medial prefrontal cortex which was, in turn, significantly correlated with improved insight and social functioning. These results suggest that medial prefrontal cortex underactivation in patients relative to healthy controls may reflect deficits in the representation of self and others, and that the recovery of medial prefrontal cortex activation may mediate improvement of insight and social functioning in patients with schizophrenia.

2.5 Empathy and symptomatology

Evidence suggests that impaired empathy might be more pronounced in certain types of schizophrenia. As highlighted by Bleuler (1911/1950), individual symptoms relevant to empathy deficit are those relating to affectivity: affective blunting and inappropriate affect. Both the positive/negative dichotomy and Liddle's three schizophrenia sub-syndrome model (disorganization, defined primarily by thought disorder and inappropriate affect; reality distortion, hallucinations and delusions; and psychomotor poverty, negative symptoms) (Liddle, 1987) have been widely used to address the issue of heterogeneity in schizophrenia. However, these models may not be suitable for empathy-related studies: affective blunting consists of negative symptoms or psychomotor poverty; on the other hand, inappropriate affect is included in negative symptoms or disorganization. It is not surprising therefore that studies have found associations of empathy-related variables with negative symptoms, psychomotor poverty, or disorganization. Other models that might be more relevant to account for the heterogeneity of schizophrenia with respect to empathy are the deficit syndrome or the disorder of relating.

'Deficit' negative symptoms refers to negative symptoms that are manifested as enduring traits, which are different from 'non-deficit' negative symptoms (reflecting transient 'pseudo negative' symptoms, which are secondary to a variety of factors such as medication side-effects, depression, or environmental understimulation) (Carpenter et al., 1988). Kirkpatrick and colleagues (Kirkpatrick & Buchanan, 1990; Kirkpatrick et al., 1989) have suggested that the impairment of empathy in people with schizophrenia with 'deficit' negative symptom may be associated with abnormalities in the circuit of social affiliation: the amygdala and the prefrontal cortex.

Similarly another subtype of schizophrenia suspected to be associated with an empathy deficit is Strauss et al.'s 'disorder of personal relationship' (Strauss et al., 1974). This subtype was distinct from positive and negative subtypes. It was characterized by poor social relationships and was associated with a poor recovery from the positive and negative symptoms of the disorder. Hoffmann and Kupper (1997) found an association between negative symptoms and deficits in social functioning, but this relationship was no longer present in a four-dimensional model (disorganization, psychomotor poverty, reality distortion, and disorder of relating). Instead, they found that both 'disorganization' and 'disorder of relating' (characterized by emotional and social withdrawal) predicted impaired social functioning. This study suggests the need for focusing upon the social domain of schizophrenic psychopathology as well as its positive and negative symptomatology.

2.6 Theoretical consideration

Two theories of schizophrenia briefly mentioned in the introduction of this chapter are now considered in detail to provide an attempt to integrate literature reviewed in this chapter. These are from a cognitive neuropsychological perspective by Frith (1992) and the phenomenological psychiatry tradition by Stanghellini (2000).

Frith (1992) postulates that schizophrenia can be understood as a disorder of representation of mental states (the inability to represent what others are thinking). He argued that a higher level prefrontal dysfunction (i.e. Shallice's supervisory attention system) might produce defects of awareness of one's own goals and intentions, and others' intentions, hence a disorder of conscious awareness. With neuroimaging evidence, he suggested that the medial prefrontal cortex (including anterior cingulate cortex) activity underlies awareness of our own intentions as well as intentions of others, to support our shared experience and consciousness (Frith, 2002). Stanghellini (2000), in line with the tradition of phenomenological psychiatry, proposed a disorder of intuitive attunement in the self and other relationships (the fundamental deficit to be involved in other people's mental lives) as a core disturbance in schizophrenia. Attunement is a precognitive, intuitive process to see another's mental life directly, and is a prerequisite for the familiarity feeling in everyday social situations. With the lack of intuitive attunement, patients with schizophrenia primarily have difficulties in relationships with other people. As their sense of reality is lost, they experience the sense of unfamiliarity or alienness.

The cognitive neuropsychological and the phenomenological approaches to understanding the empathy deficit in schizophrenia can be integrated as follows. In view of the converging evidence for the role of the medial prefrontal cortex in empathy, one might consider the implications for specific aspects of this impairment. The suggestion that dysfunction of the supervisory attention system may be a core feature of cognitive empathy deficit in schizophrenia is consistent with neuroimaging studies in healthy and schizophrenia subjects. However, the empathy deficit in schizophrenia includes not only cognitive empathy, but also affective cue perception and vicarious arousal that are more difficult to explain directly in terms of dysfunction of the supervisory attention system. An alternative possibility might be that different brain structures (e.g. the amygdala and fusiform face area), which should act together to produce empathy, may fail to interact with each other as a whole system in schizophrenia.

2.7 Future directions

One area in which future research is warranted is the development of new experimental tasks to assess different empathy components for people with schizophrenia. Examples of these tasks include the hinting task (Corcoran *et al.*, 1995) in which subjects are asked to infer the intention of a character in stories following a hint. The joke appreciation task (Corcoran *et al.*, 1997) requires subjects to explain jokes presented in cartoons. Each cartoon depicts a false-belief situation (the main character believes something that the subject knows to be false), and success in this task relies on using appropriate mental state language to interpret the jokes. Sarfati and colleagues (Sarfati *et al.*, 1997) developed a sequencing task involving inferring a character's intention and choosing the most likely card to complete comic strip sequences. A similar sequencing task has been developed by Brüne (2003) to assess a first-order false belief, a second-order false belief, and a tactical deception. The use of a sequencing paradigm has an advantage over tasks using stories, because verbal memory impairments in schizophrenia may be a potential confounding factor. The sequencing paradigm can potentially be used to assess a number of different empathy-related abilities such as forecasting a character's future emotional state.

2.8 Conclusion

In this chapter, perceptual, affective and cognitive processes are highlighted as components of empathy in the understanding of an empathy deficit in schizophrenia. Patients with schizophrenia have consistently showed abnormalities in these processes. The neural basis of empathy has recently been explored. The amygdala projection to the medial prefrontal cortex via anterior cingulate cortex may play a central role in empathy. Other modality-specific areas (notably fusiform face area) may contribute to empathy. Patients with schizophrenia have consistently shown decreased activation in the amygdala and fusiform gyrus during facial affect recognition, and the medial prefrontal cortex during cognitive empathy.

Elucidation of the nature of empathy in schizophrenia will require a substantial amount of further research, as empathy is an interaction of multiple processes of affect and cognition. In this regard, there is a pressing need for the development of empathy tasks in schizophrenia. Symptoms that are related to an empathy deficit (negative symptom of affective blunting and positive symptom of inappropriate affect) may require further attention.

REFERENCES

American Psychiatric Association. (1994). *Diagnostic and Statistical Manual of Mental Disorders* (4th edn.). Washington D.C.: American Psychiatric Association Press.

Baron-Cohen, S., Leslie, A. M., & Frith, U. (1985). Does the autistic child have a 'theory of mind'? *Cognition*, **21(1)**, 37–46.

Beyer, C. (2004). Edmund Husserl. In E. N. Zalta (ed.), *The Stanford Encyclopedia of Philosophy*. Stanford: Stanford University.

Blair, R. J., Jones, L., Clark, F., & Smith, M. (1997). The psychopathic individual: a lack of responsiveness to distress cues? *Psychophysiology*, **34(2)**, 192–198.

Blanchard, J. J., Mueser, K. T., & Bellack, A. S. (1998). Anhedonia, positive and negative affect, and social functioning in schizophrenia. *Schizophrenia Bulletin*, **24(3)**, 413–424.

Bleuler, E. (1911/1950). *Dementia Praecox or the Group of Schizophrenias* (translated by J. Zinkin). New York: International Universities Press.

Bloom, P., & German, T. P. (2000). Two reasons to abandon the false belief task as a test of theory of mind. *Cognition*, **77(1)**, B25–B31.

Bozikas, V. P., Kosmidis, M. H., Anezoulaki, D., Giannakou, M., & Karavatos, A. (2004). Relationship of affect recognition with psychopathology and cognitive performance in schizophrenia. *Journal of the International Neuropsychological Society*, **10(4)**, 549–558.

Brothers, L. (1989). A biological perspective on empathy. *American Journal of Psychiatry*, **146(1)**, 10–19.

Brüne, M. (2003). Theory of mind and the role of IQ in chronic disorganized schizophrenia. *Schizophrenia Research*, **60(1)**, 57–64.

Brunet, E., Sarfati, Y., Hardy-Bayle, M. C., & Decety, J. (2003). Abnormalities of brain function during a nonverbal theory of mind task in schizophrenia. *Neuropsychologia*, **41(12)**, 1574–1582.

Carpenter, W. T., Jr., Heinrichs, D. W., & Wagman, A. M. (1988). Deficit and nondeficit forms of schizophrenia: the concept. *American Journal of Psychiatry*, **145(5)**, 578–583.

Carpenter, W. T., Jr., Strauss, J. S., & Bartko, J. J. (1973). Flexible system for the diagnosis of schizophrenia: report from the WHO International Pilot Study of Schizophrenia. *Science*, **182(118)**, 1275–1278.

Castelli, F., Happe, F., Frith, U., & Frith, C. (2000). Movement and mind: a functional imaging study of perception and interpretation of complex intentional movement patterns. *Neuroimage*, **12(3)**, 314–325.

Corcoran, R., Cahill, C., & Frith, C. D. (1997). The appreciation of visual jokes in people with schizophrenia: a study of 'mentalizing' ability. *Schizophrenia Research*, **24(3)**, 319–327.

Corcoran, R., Mercer, G., & Frith, C. D. (1995). Schizophrenia, symptomatology and social inference: investigating 'theory of mind' in people with schizophrenia. *Schizophrenia Research*, **17(1)**, 5–13.

Doody, G. A., Gotz, M., Johnstone, E. C., Frith, C. D., & Owens, D. G. (1998). Theory of mind and psychoses. *Psychological Medicine*, **28(2)**, 397–405.

Exner, C., Boucsein, K., Degner, D., Irle, E., & Weniger, G. (2004). Impaired emotional learning and reduced amygdala size in schizophrenia: a 3-month follow-up. *Schizophrenia Research*, **71(2–3)**, 493–503.

Farrow, T. F., Zheng, Y., Wilkinson, I. D., *et al.* (2001). Investigating the functional anatomy of empathy and forgiveness. *Neuroreport*, **12(11)**, 2433–2438.

Fear, C. R., Sharp, H., & Healy, D. (1996). Cognitive processes in delusional disorders. *British Journal of Psychiatry*, **168**, 61–67.

Frith, C. (2002). Attention to action and awareness of other minds. *Consciousness and Cognition*, **11(4)**, 481–487.

Frith, C. D. (1992). *The Cognitive Neuropsychology of Schizophrenia*. Hove: Lawrence Erlbaum.

Frith, C. D., & Corcoran, R. (1996). Exploring 'theory of mind' in people with schizophrenia. *Psychological Medicine*, **26(3)**, 521–530.

Gillberg, C. L. (1992). The Emanuel Miller Memorial Lecture 1991. Autism and autistic-like conditions: subclasses among disorders of empathy. *Journal of Child Psychology and Psychiatry and Allied Disciplines*, **33(5)**, 813–842.

Gordon, E., Coyle, S., Anderson, J., *et al.* (1992). Eye movement response to a facial stimulus in schizophrenia. *Biological Psychiatry*, **31(6)**, 626–629.

Gur, R. E., McGrath, C., Chan, R. M., *et al.* (2002). An fMRI study of facial emotion processing in patients with schizophrenia. *American Journal of Psychiatry*, **159(12)**, 1992–1999.

Haith, M. M., Bergman, T., & Moore, M. J. (1977). Eye contact and face scanning in early infancy. *Science*, **198(4319)**, 853–855.

Hoffman, M. L. (1978). Toward a theory of empathic arousal and development. In M. R. Lewis, L. A. Rosenblum (ed.), *The Development of Affect* (pp. 227–256). New York: Plenum.

Hoffmann, H., & Kupper, Z. (1997). Relationships between social competence, psychopathology and work performance and their predictive value for vocational rehabilitation of schizophrenic outpatients. *Schizophrenia Research*, **23(1)**, 69–79.

Hooker, C., & Park, S. (2002). Emotion processing and its relationship to social functioning in schizophrenia patients. *Psychiatry Research*, **112(1)**, 41–50.

Jablensky, A., Sartorius, N., Ernberg, G., *et al.* (1992). Schizophrenia: manifestations, incidence and course in different cultures. A World Health Organization ten-country study. *Psychological Medicine. Monograph Supplement*, **20**, 1–97.

Janik, S. W., Wellens, A. R., Goldberg, M. I., & Dell'Osso, J. F. (1978). Eyes as the center of focus in the visual examination of human faces. *Perceptual and Motor Skills*, **47**, 857–858.

Johnson, S. C., Baxter, L. C., Wilder, L. S., *et al.* (2002). Neural correlates of self-reflection. *Brain*, **125(Pt 8)**, 1808–1814.

Joyal, C. C., Laakso, M. P., Tiihonen, J., *et al.* (2003). The amygdala and schizophrenia: a volumetric magnetic resonance imaging study in first-episode, neuroleptic-naive patients. *Biological Psychiatry*, **54(11)**, 1302–1304.

Kirkpatrick, B., & Buchanan, R. W. (1990). The neural basis of the deficit syndrome of schizophrenia. *Journal of Nervous and Mental Disease*, **178(9)**, 545–555.

Kirkpatrick, B., Carpenter, W. T., Jr., & Buchanan, R. W. (1989). Empathy and schizophrenia. *American Journal of Psychiatry*, **146(7)**, 945–946.

Kleinke, C. L. (1986). Gaze and eye contact: a research review. *Psychological Bulletin*, **100**(1), 78–100.

Kraepelin, E. (1919/1989). *Dementia Praecox and Paraphrenia Together with Manic-Depressive Insanity and Paranoia* (translated by R. Barclay). Birmingham: Classics of Medicine Library.

Kraepelin, E. (1922). Ends and means of psychiatric research. *Journal of Mental Science*, **68**, 115–143.

Kring, A. M., & Neale, J. M. (1996). Do schizophrenic patients show a disjunctive relationship among expressive, experiential, and psychophysiological components of emotion? *Journal of Abnormal Psychology*, **105**(2), 249–257.

Lee, K.-H., Brown, W. H., Egleston, P. N., *et al.* (2006). An fMRI study of social cognition in schizophrenia during an acute episode and following recovery. *American Journal of Psychiatry*, **163**(11), 1926–1933.

Lee, K.-H., Farrow, T. F. D., Spence, S. A., & Woodruff, P. W. R. (2004). Social cognition, brain networks and schizophrenia. *Psychological Medicine*, **34**, 391–400.

Levenson, R. W., Ekman, P., & Friesen, W. V. (1990). Voluntary facial action generates emotion-specific autonomic nervous system activity. *Psychophysiology*, **27**(4), 363–384.

Liddle, P. F. (1987). The symptoms of chronic schizophrenia. A re-examination of the positive-negative dichotomy. *British Journal of Psychiatry*, **151**, 145–151.

Marshall, W. L., Hudson, S. M., Jones, R., & Fernandez, Y. M. (1995). Empathy in sex offenders. *Clinical Psychology Review*, **15**, 99–113.

Martin, R. A., Berry, G. E., Dobranski, T., Horne, M., & Dodgson, P. G. (1996). Emotion perception threshold: individual differences in emotional sensitivity. *Journal of Research in Personality*, **30**, 290–305.

Mueser, K. T., Doonan, R., Penn, D. L., *et al.* (1996). Emotion recognition and social competence in chronic schizophrenia. *Journal of Abnormal Psychology*, **105**(2), 271–275.

Myin-Germeys, I., Delespaul, P. A., & deVries, M. W. (2000). Schizophrenia patients are more emotionally active than is assumed based on their behavior. *Schizophrenia Bulletin*, **26**(4), 847–854.

Onitsuka, T., Shenton, M. E., Kasai, K., *et al.* (2003). Fusiform gyrus volume reduction and facial recognition in chronic schizophrenia. *Archives of General Psychiatry*, **60**(4), 349–355.

Parnas, J., & Bovet, P. (1991). Autism in schizophrenia revisited. *Comprehensive Psychiatry*, **32**(1), 7–21.

Penn, D. L., Spaulding, W., Reed, D., & Sullivan, M. (1996). The relationship of social cognition toward behavior in chronic schizophrenia. *Schizophrenia Research*, **20**(3), 327–335.

Perner, J. (1991). *Understanding the Representational Mind*. Cambridge, Mass.: MIT Press.

Perner, J., & Lang, B. (1999). Development of theory of mind and executive control. *Trends in Cognitive Sciences*, **3**(9), 337–344.

Phillips, M. L., & David, A. S. (1997). Visual scan paths are abnormal in deluded schizophrenics. *Neuropsychologia*, **35**(1), 99–105.

Pilowsky, T., Yirmiya, N., Arbelle, S., & Mozes, T. (2000). Theory of mind abilities of children with schizophrenia, children with autism, and normally developing children. *Schizophrenia Research*, **42**(2), 145–155.

Preston, S. D., & de Waal, F. B. M. (2002). Empathy: its ultimate and proximate bases. *Behavioral and Brain Sciences*, **21**, 1–71.

Quintana, J., Wong, T., Ortiz-Portillo, E., Marder, S. R., & Mazziotta, J. C. (2003). Right lateral fusiform gyrus dysfunction during facial information processing in schizophrenia. *Biological Psychiatry*, **53**(12), 1099–1112.

Russell, T. A., Rubia, K., Bullmore, E. T., *et al.* (2000). Exploring the social brain in schizophrenia: left prefrontal underactivation during mental state attribution. *American Journal of Psychiatry*, **157**(12), 2040–2042.

Sarfati, Y., Hardy-Bayle, M. C., Besche, C., & Widlocher, D. (1997). Attribution of intentions to others in people with schizophrenia: a non-verbal exploration with comic strips. *Schizophrenia Research*, **25**(3), 199–209.

Schroder, J., Geider, F. J., Binkert, M., *et al.* (1992). Subsyndromes in chronic schizophrenia: do their psychopathological characteristics correspond to cerebral alterations? *Psychiatry Research*, **42**(3), 209–220.

Schultz, R. T., Grelotti, D. J., Klin, A., *et al.* (2003). The role of the fusiform face area in social cognition: implications for the pathobiology of autism. *Philosophical Transactions of the Royal Society of London. Series B: Biological Sciences*, **358**(1430), 415–427.

Schupp, H. T., Junghofer, M., Weike, A. I., & Hamm, A. O. (2003). Emotional facilitation of sensory processing in the visual cortex. *Psychological Science*, **14**(1), 7–13.

Stanghellini, G. (2000). Vulnerability to schizophrenia and lack of common sense. *Schizophrenia Bulletin*, **26**(4), 775–787.

Strauss, J. S., Carpenter, W. T., Jr., & Bartko, J. J. (1974). The diagnosis and understanding of schizophrenia. Part III. Speculations on the processes that underlie schizophrenic symptoms and signs. *Schizophrenia Bulletin*, (**11**), 61–69.

Strayer, J. (1987). Affective and cognitive perspectives on empathy. In N. Eisenberg & J. Strayer (eds.), *Empathy and its Development* (pp. 218–244). New York, N.Y.: Cambridge University Press.

Streit, M., Wolwer, W., & Gaebel, W. (1997). Facial-affect recognition and visual scanning behaviour in the course of schizophrenia. *Schizophrenia Research*, **24**(3), 311–317.

Suslow, T., Roestel, C., Ohrmann, P., & Arolt, V. (2003). Detection of facial expressions of emotions in schizophrenia. *Schizophrenia Research*, **64**(2–3), 137–145.

Tsuang, M. (2000). Schizophrenia: genes and environment. *Biological Psychiatry*, **47**(3), 210–220.

Venables, P. H. (1993). Electrodermal indices as markers for the development of schizophrenia. In J. C. Roy, W. Boucsein, D. C. Fowles & J. H. Gruzelier (eds.), *Progress in Electrodermal Research* (pp. 187–205). New York: Plenum.

Walker, E., Grimes, K. E., Davis, D. M., & Smith, A. J. (1993). Childhood precursors of schizophrenia: facial expressions of emotion. *American Journal of Psychiatry*, **150**(11), 1654–1660.

Walker, E., Marwit, S. J., & Emory, E. (1980). A cross-sectional study of emotion recognition in schizophrenics. *Journal of Abnormal Psychology*, **89(3)**, 428–436.

Wellman, H. M., Cross, D., & Watson, J. (2001). Meta-analysis of theory-of-mind development: the truth about false belief. *Child Development*, **72(3)**, 655–684.

Williams, E. (1974). An analysis of gaze in schizophrenics. *British Journal of Social and Clinical Psychology*, **13**, 1–8.

Williams, L. M., Loughland, C. M., Gordon, E., & Davidson, D. (1999). Visual scanpaths in schizophrenia: is there a deficit in face recognition? *Schizophrenia Research*, **40(3)**, 189–199.

Empathy, antisocial behaviour and personality pathology

Mairead Dolan and Rachael Fullam

Department of Forensic Psychiatry, University of Manchester

3.1 Introduction

This chapter will briefly explore the current definitions of empathy and report on studies looking at empathic deficits in antisocial and personality-disordered groups. To date, the literature on empathy, emotional-information-processing deficits and mentalizing ability is largely limited to studies in sex offenders or aggressive samples. There are few studies of empathy in DSM-IV personality-disordered samples although both antisocial and narcissistic personality disorders highlight empathy deficits in their criteria (see Tables 3.1 and 3.2).

3.1.1 Definitions of empathy

The experimental and theoretical literature on empathy has failed to agree on a single definition (Eisenberg & Miller, 1987); however, most theories about empathy have been based in trait psychology and empathy is seen as a fixed disposition evident over time and across situations and persons.

Empathy and sympathy have often been used interchangeably. Ohbuchi (1988) described the affective component of empathy as sympathy. Hogan (1969) used both terms when describing his empathy scale and Feshbach (1978) used the terms synonymously. By contrast, Miller and Eisenberg (1988) make a distinction between these concepts suggesting that empathy is the emotional response to another's distress while sympathy reflects feelings of concern.

Sympathy (e.g. Cooley, 1956) and empathy (e.g. Hogan, 1969) have both been defined as the ability to identify others' emotional states, i.e. to achieve a cognitive understanding of others' feelings. Others, however, have defined empathy (Feshbach, 1978; Mehrabian & Epstein, 1972) and sympathy (McDougall, 1950) primarily in affective terms.

Empathy in Mental Illness, eds. Tom F. D. Farrow and Peter W. R. Woodruff. Published by Cambridge University Press. © Cambridge University Press 2007.

Table 3.1: Diagnostic criteria for narcissistic personality disorder

A pervasive pattern of grandiosity (in fantasy or behaviour), need for admiration, and lack of empathy, beginning by early adulthood and present in a variety of contexts, as indicated by five (or more) of the following:
1. Has a grandiose sense of self-importance (e.g. exaggerates achievements and talents, expects to be recognized as superior without commensurate achievements)
2. Is preoccupied with fantasies of unlimited success, power, brilliance, beauty, or ideal love
3. Believes that he or she is 'special' and unique and can only be understood by, or should associate with, other special or high-status people (or institutions)
4. Requires excessive admiration
5. Has a sense of entitlement, i.e. unreasonable expectations of especially favourable treatment or automatic compliance with his or her expectations
6. Is interpersonally exploitative, i.e. takes advantage of others to achieve his or her own ends
7. *Lacks empathy: is unwilling to recognize or identify with the feelings and needs of others*
8. Is often envious of others or believes that others are envious of him or her
9. Shows arrogant, haughty behaviours or attitudes

Table 3.2: DSM-IV diagnostic criteria for antisocial personality disorder

Since the age of 15 years, the patient continues to display disregard for, and violation of, the rights of others, indicated by at least three of the following:
1. Failure to conform to social norms by repeatedly engaging in unlawful activity
2. Deceitfulness: repeated lying, use of aliases, or 'conning' others for personal profit
3. Impulsivity or failure to plan ahead
4. Irritability and aggressiveness, as indicated by repeated physical fights
5. Reckless disregard for the safety of self or others
6. Consistent irresponsibility: repeated failure to sustain consistent work behaviour
7. *Lack of remorse for any of the above behaviour and low empathy*
8. A history of some symptoms of conduct disorder before age 15 years as indicated by:
    A. Aggression to people and animals
    B. Destruction of property
    C. Deceitfulness or theft
    D. Serious violation of rules

Empathy is generally seen as having at least three qualities: (1) knowing what a person is feeling (Ickes, 1997); (2) feeling what another person is feeling (Eisenberg & Fabes, 1990); and (3) responding compassionately to another's distress (Batson *et al.*, 1983).

The ability to accurately perceive the feelings of another person is seen as a fundamental aspect of empathy (Levenson & Ruef, 1992). Williams (1990)

suggests that empathy is multidimensional and includes cognitive, emotional components as well as communicative and relational elements. Davis (1983) also suggested that empathy involves a multidimensional response, which involves:

1. Perspective taking – the ability to adopt the viewpoint of another (cognitive empathy).
2. Fantasy – which reflects the person's tendency to transpose themselves into the feelings of fictional characters (one aspect of affective empathy).
3. Empathic concern – which reflects feelings of concern for others (more sympathy than empathy).
4. Personal distress – which describes self-oriented feelings of distress.

Marshall *et al.* (1995) suggest that empathy is a staged process involving: (1) emotion recognition, (2) perspective taking, (3) emotion replication and (4) response decision.

1. The emotion recognition stage requires an ability to accurately discriminate the emotional state of another person. Feshbach (1987) and Miller and Eisenberg (1988) are the only two groups to have explored the issue of accuracy in the recognition of emotional responses in empathic and non-empathic individuals. They found empathic individuals were more skilled at discerning emotional states of others. Marshall *et al.* (1995) suggest that in order for someone to experience or feel the emotional state of another, they must first recognize the person's emotional state.
2. The second stage in the empathy process, according to Marshall *et al.* (1995), is perspective taking or the ability to put oneself in the observed person's place and view the world as they do. This is thought to be partly a function of how similar the observer and observed are and the issue of perceived similarity has been noted in the aggression literature.
3. The third stage – emotion replication – involves the replication of the emotional experience of the target person. Marshall *et al.* (1995) believe one cannot do stage 3 unless you are able to complete stages 1 and 2. It is also necessary to have the emotional repertoire to be able to replicate the observed state.
4. The final stage is response decision, which reflects the observer's decision to act on the basis of their feelings.

There are many definitions of empathy but the most current and inclusive one is that provided by Cohen and Strayer (1996, pp. 988), where they view empathy 'as the ability to understand and share in another's emotional state of context', as it encompasses both the cognitive and emotional aspects of this multidimensional construct.

Although there is a lack of consensus regarding its conceptualization there is some level of agreement about the following: there are individual differences in the level of this trait (Farrington & Jolliffe, 2001); it can be measured; and it influences antisocial behaviours (Miller & Eisenberg, 1988).

Empathy is an essential component of effective social communication and prosocial behaviour (Eisenberg & Strayer, 1987). It involves role or perspective taking (Perry et al., 2001) and the ability to attribute thoughts and feelings to self and others [i.e. 'Theory of Mind' (Premack & Woodruff, 1978) or 'mentalizing', (Frith et al., 1991)].

Hoffman (1982) speculated that empathic arousal follows a developmental pathway from infancy and is the central component of prosocial development in children and adolescents. Reviews of the child literature indicate a positive association between empathy and prosocial and socially competent behaviour (Eisenberg & Miller, 1987).

Research on empathy development in normal male and female adolescents has shown that, across age groups, females score higher on measures of empathy than males (e.g. Cohen & Strayer, 1996; Eisenberg & Fabes, 1990). Adolescent girls also have higher prosocial reasoning than boys when developmental stages are considered (Eisenberg et al., 1991). Feshbach (1982) reported that adolescent boys experiencing intense emotions such as sadness, anger and fear are more likely to engage in helping behaviours, be less aggressive and be more sensitive to the feelings of others compared with those experiencing less intense emotions.

3.1.2 Measures of empathy

There are currently a number of methods to assess empathy:

Picture/story assessments of empathy are primarily used to assess children's empathy. Examples include Feshbach and Roe's (1968) Affective Situations test for empathy in which children are presented with narratives and visual stimuli that are considered suitable to elicit empathic responses in the listener.

Self-report questionnaires

Questionnaire measures are generally used with adults and these are believed to be measures of a core personality trait.

The most commonly used measures include: Hogan's Empathy Scale (HES, Hogan, 1969), the Questionnaire Measure of Emotional Empathy (QMEE, Mehrabian & Epstein, 1972) and the Interpersonal Reactivity Index (IRI, Davis, 1983).

Hogan's Empathy Scale (HES, Hogan, 1969) is a 64-item scale measuring the cognitive aspect of empathy. Items are answered as true or false. The range of scores is 0–64, with higher scores reflecting greater empathy. According to Hogan (1969) the measure has good test-retest reliability ($r = 0.84$) with a mean score of 39.1 (sd 4.7) for college students and 30.4 for prison inmates.

The QMEE (Mehrabian & Epstein, 1972) is a 33-item scale assessing the emotional aspects of empathy. Each item is rated on a scale ranging from -4 to $+4$

giving a range of scores from -132 to $+132$. Higher positive scores indicate greater empathy.

The IRI (Davis, 1983) was designed to measure both cognitive and affective empathy. This 28-item measure consists of four 7-item subscales tapping at least one aspect of empathy (Davis, 1983, p. 113). Each item is scored on a 5-point Likert scale. The perspective taking (PT) scale is a cognitive measure of the ability to appreciate another's point of view. It is associated with high self-esteem but little emotion.

The Personal Distress (PD) scale measures the extent to which an individual can share negative emotions with others, anxiety, and the ability to cope with negative emotions.

The Fantasy Scale (FS) measures the ability to identify with imaginary characters in books and films and the ability to daydream or fantasize easily.

The Empathic Concern (EC) scale measures the ability to sympathize with less fortunate others and is related to prosocial behaviours.

Facial/gesture indexes of empathy

This method has been used to assess empathic responsiveness in children and it overcomes some of the problems in asking children to report their emotions verbally when they may not have the developmental capacity to do so.

3.2 Empathy and offending

A number of criminologists suggest that offenders have lower empathy than non-offenders (Burke, 2001; Bush *et al.*, 2000; Hogan, 1969). Farrington (1998, p. 275) suggests offenders have poor role-taking and perspective-taking ability and they may misinterpret others' intentions. Blackburn (1993, p. 34) suggests offenders have difficulty imagining the distress of others and therefore cannot inhibit harmful behaviour.

To date, there have been two meta-analytic studies looking at the relationship between empathy and antisocial/externalizing behaviours. The first by Miller and Eisenberg (1988) looked at 43 studies that used a variety of empathy measures including picture/story presentations; experimental induction procedures; facial/gesture responses and questionnaires. Aggressive and externalizing behaviours were defined broadly and included self-report and behavioural experimental measures. They reported moderate negative correlations and noted that the degree of association was influenced by age, mode of assessing empathy and method of assessing negative behaviour. They found empathy was negatively and significantly correlated with aggression when empathy was assessed using questionnaires but the effect was not as striking for facial affect, picture/story or experimental induction methods.

Jolliffe and Farrington (2004) conducted a more recent meta-analysis of studies using only questionnaire measures of empathy among criminal offenders and concentrating only on official or reported offences rather than non-adjudicated antisocial behaviours. They divided the empathy measures into cognitive and affective measures. Of the 21 studies using cognitive measures, 10 found that offenders had lower empathy than non-offenders but 11 found no differences. Of the 14 studies assessing affective empathy, 4 found that offenders had lower empathy but 9 did not. The results of the meta-analysis using the unbiased effect size indicated that there was a predictable link between low cognitive empathy and offending, but that between affective empathy and offending was unremarkable. For the 21 cognitive empathy studies there was a medium mean effect size of -0.48 (95% CI -0.56 to $+0.40$). The 14 affective empathy studies had a small but significant effect size of -0.11 (95% CI -0.19 to $+0.04$). The findings suggested that cognitive empathy had a stronger relationship with offending than affective empathy.

3.3 Empathy and aggression

Although there have been a number of studies looking at the relationship between picture/story assessments of empathy and aggression, the results indicate there is a reasonably low correlation particularly when adult and child samples are combined. One reason for the reported low correlation is the fact that few studies have separated positive from negative emotions on this task (Miller & Eisenberg, 1988). As it has been suggested that empathy with positive emotions is positively related to boys' aggression, whereas empathy with negative emotions is negatively related to aggression (Feshbach, 1982), the need to separate these emotions in the study of aggression is important.

The relationship between self-report measures of empathy and aggression has been examined in older children and adults. Overall, Miller and Eisenberg's (1988) meta-analyses suggested there was a significant negative relationship, which was consistent across the age range as well as level of aggression.

The relationship between facial/gesture indexes of empathy and aggression has generally been examined in younger cohorts where it has been found that negatively toned facial expression is associated with lower levels of aggression although the findings in meta-analytic studies indicate the association is generally non-significant.

3.4 Empathy, antisocial behaviour, and the antisocial personality disorders

Previous research has shown an inverse relationship between empathy and antisocial behaviour among young offenders (Ellis, 1982; Riley, 1986).

Studies looking at cognitive measures of empathy in delinquents, however, have produced inconsistent findings. Some (Ellis, 1982) report that delinquents had lower empathy scores on the HES than non-offenders. Others (Chandler & Moran, 1990; Hudak et al., 1980), however, found no significant differences on these measures in delinquent and non-delinquent samples.

Several studies of offender and non-offender youth suggest that male offenders with low empathy scores exhibit more aggression than those with higher empathy scores (Ellis, 1982). Kaplan and Arbuthnot (1985) utilized assessments of the cognitive aspects of empathy including emotion recognition in self and others and responses to stories of conflict, and found that delinquent adolescents produced lower scores than non-delinquent adolescents.

Bush et al. (2000) compared male and female offenders with male and female healthy controls on the IRI (Davis, 1983), a self-image scale, an index of social support index and a self-report altruism scale. They found that differences in empathy for offender and non-offender youth were minimal apart from the affective component of empathy, namely the emotional tone subscale of the self-image scale. There were no significant differences in the PT subscale of the IRI.

It has been proposed that the antisocial personality disorders (conduct disorder, antisocial personality disorder and psychopathy) may have deficits in empathy that are most striking in those with psychopathic traits (Blair, 1995). Dolan and Fullam (2004), however, found no striking differences between staff controls and psychopathic and non-psychopathic criminals with antisocial personality disorder (ASPD) on any of the IRI subscales including PT and EC. The latter finding may reflect the difficulty in assessing empathy-related constructs using a self-report measure in antisocial samples, as these measures are relatively transparent and potentially susceptible to response distortion. It is also possible, however, that the lack of an observed difference between the staff controls and criminal sample may reflect the impact on staff of working in penal settings on a long-term basis, as the controls had lower empathic concern scores than those reported for healthy male controls (Davis, 1983).

Role taking is a key component of mentalizing ability and has been defined as the 'imaginative transposing of oneself into the thinking and acting of another' (Feshbach, 1978). Gough (1948) suggested that a deficit in role-taking ability accounted for the under-socialization of psychopaths. However, several studies suggest that although role-taking impairments are observed in younger delinquents (Lee & Prentice, 1988) this effect is less apparent in older criminal samples (Widom, 1978) and it is possible that role-taking ability may be just as important in the ability to manipulate others. Previous studies specifically examining empathy based on self-report measures have produced inconsistent findings with some

(Ellis, 1982; Hogan, 1969) but not all (Kaplan & Arbuthnot, 1985; Lee & Prentice, 1988) reporting differences.

Overall, the literature suggests empathy is a multidimensional construct and reliance on self-report measures may be questionable in criminal populations (Eisenberg & Strayer, 1987).

3.5 Theory of Mind and the antisocial personality disorders

There have been a number of suggestions that a deficient or impaired Theory of Mind (ToM) might lead to the observed empathy deficits and ultimately aggressive or antisocial behaviour (e.g. Crick & Dodge, 1994; Feshbach, 1987). However, the results from studies across the age span have largely been inconsistent. Hughes *et al.* (1998) reported that 'hard to manage' preschoolers demonstrated impaired ToM compared to a healthy control comparison group. Povey (2005) found no significant differences between conduct-disordered offenders and healthy controls on first- and second-order (ToM) tasks devised by Stone *et al.* (1998) but the conduct-disordered group were impaired on higher-order ToM tasks such as the Faux Pas task (Baron-Cohen *et al.*, 1999).

The literature in adults is more variable, with some (Widom, 1978) but not all (Blair *et al.*, 1996) reporting ToM deficits. Work by Blair (1995, 1996) suggests subjects characterized as prototypical psychopaths using Hare's criteria have impairments in moral/conventional distinctions (Blair, 1995) but not on ToM stories compared with non-psychopathic criminals (Blair, 1996). Dolan and Fullam (2004) also examined ToM in those with ASPD and staff controls using stories devised by Stone *et al.* (1998) and the Faux Pas task. Similar to Blair *et al.* (1996), there were no differences between controls, psychopathic and non-psychopathic criminals on basic ToM tasks assessing first- and second-order false beliefs, confirming the notion that criminal ASPDs do not differ significantly from controls on basic mentalizing abilities. However, although the ASPD group were not impaired on the Faux Pas task, their responses to the empathy questions indicated an indifference to the impact of the Faux Pas on the speaker or the listener.

The inconsistent findings may be accounted for by differences in the complexity of the tasks. More recent work has questioned the validity of basic ToM tasks, which were developed for use in younger samples or patients with autistic spectrum disorders, suggesting that they may not be challenging enough to detect more subtle higher-order impairments in criminal samples.

The 'reading the mind in the eyes task' is a higher-order ToM task developed by Baron-Cohen *et al.* (2001) which requires subjects to view photographs of the eye-only region of the face and attribute a mental state to the person using a forced choice answer format taken from a group of mental state descriptors.

While Richell *et al.* (2003) found no significant differences between psycho-pathic and non-psychopathic criminals on this task Dolan and Fullam (2004) found non-psychopathic ASPDs were performing worse than controls and psychopathic ASPDs on some, but not all, basic emotions. The non-psychopathic ASPDs had particular difficulties in recognizing Distress versus Sadness and Arrogant versus Guilt in faces. Previous studies in criminal populations suggest that psychopathic offenders are more impaired in their emotional attributions relating to guilt as presented in story format (Blair *et al.*, 1995). Although Dolan and Fullam (2004) did not find this to be the case using the visual medium of facial expression the discrepant findings might be accounted for by differences in the modalities in which emotions were examined. Overall, the current literature suggests that ASPDs, including those with psychopathic traits, do not have marked difficulties in reading basic or complex emotions from facial expression.

3.6 Emotional information processing in the antisocial personality disorders

To date, there are relatively few data on emotional-information-processing deficits in the antisocial personality disorders. Povey (2005) used a multimorph face expression task to examine the recognition of positive and negative emotions in faces in healthy controls and conduct-disordered adolescents. Group comparisons indicated that the conduct-disordered sample were significantly worse at recognizing the negative emotions but not the positive emotions. When the specific emotions of sadness and fear were examined, the conduct-disordered group showed impairments in the recognition of these emotions but they were no more striking than the impairments shown in the recognition of other negative emotions such as anger and disgust. Previously studies specifically focusing on psychopathic traits have suggested that both adults (Blair *et al.*, 2004) and children with psychopathic tendencies (Blair, 2001; Blair & Coles, 2001) have deficits in the recognition of negatively valenced emotions such as sadness and fear. The latter findings add weight to the amygdala dysfunction theory of psychopathy (Blair, 2001), as neuroimaging studies indicate that the amygdala is a key component of the neural network involved in emotional information processing (Blair *et al.*, 1999), and reduced amygdala volume (Tiihonen *et al.*, 2000) and activation (Kiehl *et al.*, 2001) have been reported in psychopathic samples. See Chapter 1 on empathic dysfunction in psychopathic individuals for a fuller discussion of this area.

3.7 Empathy and emotion recognition in sex offenders

There is ample research suggesting that sex offenders are deficient in empathy assessed using psychometric measures (Marshall & Barbaree, 1990). Abel *et al.*

(1989) view these empathy deficits as part of the offenders' rationalization that permits them to engage in repetitive offending behaviour. There is some disagreement in the literature, however, on whether the observed empathy deficits are generalized or specific.

Studies looking at generalized empathy deficits have produced inconsistent findings, with some (Rice, 1994) but not all (Seto, 1992) reporting lower empathy scores in rapists compared with non-offender controls on questionnaire measures. Similar inconsistent findings have been reported in child molesters (Marshall & Maric, 1994). It is possible that the use of generalized measures of empathy obscures differences between sex offenders and non-offenders and between subtypes of sex offender.

Hudson *et al.* (1993) examined the emotion-recognition skills of sex offenders using Ekman and Freisen's (1975) photographic series in a mixed group of incarcerated sex and acquisitive offenders. The sexual and violent offenders had difficulty accurately discerning the emotional state of the target subjects, with the sex offenders showing greatest difficulty. The same report (Hudson *et al.*, 1993) found that child molesters had significantly less skill in recognizing emotional states in adults and children using the test of O'Sullivan and Guilford (1976), suggesting that they may have a more general deficit in emotional recognition. Later work by this group also indicated that child molesters did not experience the emotions that matched the distress felt by their victims, although they were able to replicate the distress of accident victims. The findings suggest that emotion-recognition skills may be generally deficient in sex offenders but there is some evidence that child molesters may have more person-specific problems. More recent studies (e.g. Marshall & Maric, 1994) confirm previous findings that child molesters are deficient in both the cognitive and emotional aspects of empathy compared to non-offenders and the findings highlight the need to develop therapeutic programmes that address both the cognitive and emotional aspects of empathy.

3.8 Empathy and child abuse

Research indicates that empathy is a significant variable in effective parenting. Studies have demonstrated a positive relationship between empathy and a variety of behaviours that successful parenting requires. These include the ability to comfort, being helpful and cooperative, being aware of need in others, being flexible and being sensitive to the needs of others (Ainsworth *et al.*, 1978). Studies suggest that there is an inverse relationship between parental empathy and child abuse in abusive mothers and that parents with limited empathic ability are more likely to respond aggressively or punitively in conflict situations

(LeTourneau, 1981). A number of studies have reported significantly lower scores on empathy scales in samples of abusive compared with non-abusive parents (Rosenstein, 1995). Indeed Frodi and Lamb (1980) concluded that an inability to empathize may be a key factor in abusive mothers' perceptions that infant attributes such as crying are aversive, and that this stimulates abusive mothers' aggression. It has also been demonstrated that abusive mothers have difficulties recognizing positive and negative emotions in slides of infants and this inability to perceive and identify emotions in infants may account for their observed empathy deficits (Kropp & Haynes, 1987). Although there are many factors that influence parenting style, empathy is recognized as a significant variable in effective parenting.

3.9 Empathy and narcissism

DSM-IV identifies a deficiency in empathy as one of the essential features of narcissistic personality disorder (American Psychiatric Association, 1994). These individuals 'generally have a lack of empathy and have difficulty recognising the desires, subjective experiences and feelings of others ... when recognised, the needs, desires and feelings of others are likely to be viewed disparagingly as signs of weakness or vulnerability'.

Watson *et al.* (1984) found empirical support for an inverse relationship between psychometric empathy measures and narcissism. They examined correlations between empathy questionnaires and the Narcissistic Personality Inventory (NPI) and found that the exploitativeness and entitlement subscales of the NPI were inversely correlated with all empathy scales.

Narcissism is often seen as a significant factor in perpetrators of child abuse and Gilgun (1988), in a review of the literature in this area, suggested sexual abuse perpetrators are characterized by self-centredness which she defines as 'a focus on the self so intense that it precludes consideration of the feelings and choices of others and which at times causes direct emotional and/or physical harm to others' (p. 223). There are now a number of studies indicating that perpetrators of child sexual abuse have elevated levels of narcissism and marked self-centredness (Hall *et al.*, 1991).

Wiehe (2003) examined narcissism and empathy in child abuse perpetrators and foster parents using the IRI, the NPI and the Hypersensitivity Narcissism Scale. Abusive parents had lower scores on three of the four IRI scales: PT, EC and PD. Although the abusive group had less self-confidence they had higher scores on authority, exhibitionism and entitlement, indicating that they were more narcissistic than non-abusive parents. Wiehe (2003) also noted that there were inverse correlations between scores on the PT component of the IRI and measures of entitlement and exhibitionism on the Narcissism measure, indicating the presence of an inverse relationship between empathy and the need for power, control and dominance.

3.10 Summary/Conclusions

Empathy is clearly a complex and multidimensional construct. It is a key factor in prosocial behaviour and in effective parenting, and empathy deficits have been reported in a number of areas and disorders associated with antisocial and aggressive behaviour. To date, there have been no longitudinal studies of empathy to establish a causal role for empathy deficits in personality pathology, offending and antisocial behaviour. There are currently a number of methods used to assess empathy, the most common of which are self-report measures. However, although many studies indicate that antisocial samples have lower scores on these measures a number of others have failed to detect differences between healthy controls and pathological populations. Many of the current questionnaire measures have been validated in university students and their utility in offender or criminal samples may be questionable given the transparency of the measures and the likelihood that these groups will respond in a socially desirable manner. There is a need to develop reliable and valid measures of empathy that detect the cognitive and emotional components of this construct. In recent years there has been a move towards using tasks that assess mentalizing ability and emotional information processing as proxy measures of empathy. The findings suggest that subjects with externalizing or antisocial behaviours do not have basic 'Theory of Mind' deficits but they may have subtle deficits in higher-order tasks that require empathic inference about how others feel. There is also some evidence that some antisocial groups, particularly those with psychopathic traits, have deficits in emotional information processing. As the amygdala and orbito-frontal cortex have been implicated in the neural network sub-serving empathic understanding and emotional recognition, functional imaging studies are likely to clarify the nature of any reported affective empathic deficits in antisocial populations.

REFERENCES

Abel, G. G., Gore, D. K., Holland, C. L., *et al.* (1989). The measurement of the cognitive distortions of child molesters. *Annals of Sex Research*, **2**, 135–152.

Ainsworth, M., Blehar, M., Waters, E., & Wall, S. (1978). *Patterns of Attachment: A Psychological Study of the Strange Situation*. Hillsdale, N.J.: Erlbaum.

American Psychiatric Association (APA). (1994). *Diagnostic and Statistical Manual of Mental Disorders* (4th edn.). Washington, DC: APA Press.

Baron-Cohen, S., O'Riordan, M., Stone, V., Jones, R., & Plaisted, K. (1999). Recognition of faux pas by normally developing children and children with Asperger syndrome or high-functioning autism. *Journal of Autism and Developmental Disorders*, **29**(5), 407–418.

Baron-Cohen, S., Wheelwrite, S., Hill, J., Raste, Y., & Plumb, I. (2001). The 'Reading the mind in eyes' test revised version: a study with normal adults, and adults with Asperger syndrome or high-functioning autism. *Journal of Child Psychology and Psychiatry and Allied Disciplines*, **42**, 241–251.

Batson, C. D., Oquin, K., Fultz, J., Vanderplas, M., & Isen, A. M. (1983). Influence of self-reported distress and empathy on egoistic versus altruistic motivation to help. *Journal of Psychology and Social Psychology*, **45**, 706–718.

Blackburn, R. (1993). *The Psychology of Criminal Conduct*. Chichester: Wiley, p. 34.

Blair, R. J. R. (1995). A cognitive developmental approach to morality: investigating the psychopath. *Cognition*, **57**, 1–29.

Blair, R. J. R. (1996). Brief report: morality in the autistic child. *Journal of Autism and Developmental Disorders*, **26**, 571–579.

Blair R. J. R. (2001). Neurocognitive models of aggression, the antisocial personality disorders and psychopathy. *Journal of Neurology, Neurosurgery and Psychiatry*, **71**, 727–731.

Blair R. J. R., & Coles, M (2001). Expression recognition and behavioural problems in early adolescence. *Cognitive Development*, **15**, 421–439.

Blair, R. J. R., Mitchell, D. G. V., Peschardt, K. S., *et al.* (2004). Reduced sensitivity to others' fearful expressions in psychopathic individuals. *Personality and Individual Differences*, **37(6)**, 1111–1122.

Blair R. J. R., Morris J. S., Frith, C. D., Perrett, D. I., & Dolan, R. (1999). Dissociable neural responses to facial expressions of sadness and anger. *Brain*, **122**, 883–893.

Blair, R. J. R., Sellars, C., Strickland, I., & Clark, F. (1995). Emotion attributions in the psychopath. *Personality and Individual Differences*, **19**, 431–437.

Blair, R. J. R., Sellars, C., Strickland, I., *et al.* (1996). Theory of mind in the psychopath. *The Journal of Forensic Psychiatry*, **7**, 15–25.

Burke, D. M. (2001). Empathy in sexually offending and nonoffending in adolescent males. *Journal of Interpersonal Violence*, **16**, 222–233.

Bush, C. A., Mullis, R. L., & Mullis, A. K. (2000). Differences between offender and non-offender youth. *Journal of Youth and Adolescence*, **29**, 467–478.

Chandler, M., & Moran, T. (1990). Psychopathy and moral development: a comparative study of delinquent and nondelinquent youth. *Development and Psychopathology*, **2**, 227–246.

Cohen, D., & Strayer, J. (1996). Empathy in conduct-disordered and comparison youth. *Developmental Psychology*, **32**, 988–998.

Cooley, C. H. (1956). *Two Major Works: Social Organization and Human Nature and the Social Order*. Glenco, IU.: Free Press. (Original work published 1902).

Crick, N. R., & Dodge, K. A. (1994). A review and reformulation of social information processing mechanisms in children's' social adjustment. *Psychological Bulletin*, **115**, 74–101.

Davis, M. H. (1983). Measuring individual differences in empathy: evidence for a multidimensional approach. *Journal of Personality and Social Psychology*, **44**, 113–126.

Dolan, M., & Fullam, R. (2004). Theory of Mind and mentalizing ability in antisocial personality disorder with and without psychopathy. *Psychological Medicine*, **34(6)**, 1093–1102.

Eisenberg, N., & Fabes, R. A. (1990). Empathy: conceptualization, measurement, and relation to prosocial behavior. *Motivation and Emotion*, **14**, 131–149.

Eisenberg, N., & Miller, P. A. (1987). The relation of empathy to prosocial and related behaviours. *Psychological Bulletin*, **101**, 91–119.

Eisenberg, N., Miller, P. A., Shell, R., McNally, S., & Shea, C. (1991). Prosocial development in adolescence: a longitudinal study. *Developmental Psychology*, **27**(5), 849–857.

Eisenberg, N., & Strayer, J. (eds.) (1987). *Empathy and its Development* (pp. 47–80). Cambridge: Cambridge University Press.

Ekman, P., & Freisen, W. V. (1975). *Unmasking the Face*. Enlgewood Cliffs, N.J.: Prentice Hall.

Ellis, P. L. (1982). Empathy: a factor in antisocial behaviour. *Journal of Abnormal Child Psychology*, **10**, 123–134.

Farrington, D. P. (1998). Individual differences and offending. In M. Tonry (ed.), *The Handbook of Crime and Punishment* (pp. 241–268). New York: Oxford University Press.

Farrington, D. P., & Jolliffe, D. (2001). Personality and crime. In N. J. Smelser, P. B. Baltes (eds.), *International Encyclopaedia of the Social and Behavioural Sciences* (pp. 11260–11264). Amsterdam: Elsevier.

Feshbach, N. D. (1978). Studies of empathic behaviour in children. In B. A. Maher (ed.), *Progress in Experimental Personality Research*. New York: Academic Press.

Feshbach, N. D. (1982). Sex differences in empathy and social behavior in children. In N. Eisenburg (ed.), *The Development of Prosocial Behaviour* (pp. 315–338). New York: Academic Press.

Feshbach, N. D. (1987). Parental empathy and child adjustment/maladjustment. In N. Eisenburg & J. Strayer (eds.), *Empathy and its Development* (pp. 271–291). New York: Cambridge University Press.

Feshbach, N. D. & Roe, K. (1968). Empathy in six- and seven-year-olds. *Child Development*, **39**, 133–145.

Frith, U., Morton, J., & Leslie, A. M. (1991). The cognitive basis of a biological disorder: autism. *Trends in Neuroscience*, **14**, 433–438.

Frodi, A., & Lamb, M. (1980). Child abusers' responses to infant smiles. *Child Development*, **51**, 238–241.

Gilgun, J. (1988). Self-centredness and the adult male perpetrator of child sexual abuse. *Contemporary Family Therapy*, **10**, 216–234.

Gough, H. G. (1948). A sociological theory of psychopathy. *American Journal of Sociology*, **53**, 359–366.

Hall, G. C., Shephard, J. B., & Mudrak, P. (1991). MMPI taxonomies of child sexual and non-sexual offenders: a cross-validation and extension. *Journal of Personality Assessment*, **58**, 127–137.

Hoffman, M. L. (1982). The measurement of empathy. In C. E. Izard (ed.), *Measuring Emotions in Infants and Children* (pp. 279–296). Cambridge, England: Cambridge University Press.

Hogan, R. (1969). Development of an empathy scale. *Journal of Consulting and Clinical Psychology*, **33**, 307–316.

Hudak, M. A., Andre, J., & Allen, R. O. (1980). Delinquency and social values: differences between delinquent and nondelinquent adolescents. *Youth and Society*, **11**, 353–368.

Hudson, S. M., Marshall, W. L., Wales, D., *et al.* (1993). Emotion recognition in sex offenders. *Annals of Sex Research*, **6**, 199–211.

Hughes, C., Dunn, J., & White, A. (1998). Trick or treat? Uneven understanding of mind and emotion and executive dysfunction in 'hard-to-manage' preschoolers. *Journal of Child Psychology and Psychiatry and Allied Disciplines*, **39**, 981–994.

Ickes, W. (1997). *Empathic Accuracy*. New York: The Guilford Press.

Jolliffe, D., & Farrington, D. P. (2004). Empathy and offending: a systematic review and meta-analysis. *Aggression and Violent Behavior*, **9**, 441–476.

Kaplan, P. J., & Arbuthnot, J. (1985). Affective empathy and cognitive role-taking in the delinquent and nondelinquent youth. *Adolescence*, **20**, 323–333.

Kiehl, K. A., Smith, A., Hare, R. D., *et al.* (2001). Limbic abnormalities in affective processing by criminal psychopaths as revealed by functional magnetic resonance imaging. *Biological Psychiatry*, **50**, 677–684.

Kropp, J., & Haynes, O. (1987). Abusive and nonabusive mothers' ability to identify general and specific emotion signals of infants. *Child Development*, **58**, 187–190.

LeTourneau, C. (1981). Empathy and stress: how they affect parental aggression. *Social Work*, **26**, 383–389.

Lee, M., & Prentice, N. M. (1988). Interrelations of empathy, cognition and moral reasoning with dimensions of juvenile delinquency. *Journal of Abnormal Child Psychology*, **16**, 127–139.

Levenson, R. W., & Ruef, A. M. (1992). Empathy: a physiological substrate. *Journal of Personality and Social Psychology*, **63**(2), 234–246.

Marshall, W. L., & Barbaree, H. E. (1990). An integrated theory of the etiology of sexual offending. In W. L. Marshall, D. R. Laws & H. E. Barbaree (eds.), *Handbook of Sexual Assault: Issues, Theories, and Treatment of the Offender* (pp. 257–275). New York: Plenum Press.

Marshall, W. L., Hudson, S. M., Jones, R., & Fernandez, Y. M. (1995). Empathy in sex offenders. *Clinical Psychology Review*, **15**, 99–113.

Marshall, W. L., & Maric, A. (1994). General empathy and self esteem in sex offenders. Unpublished manuscript, Queen's University, Kingston, Ontario.

McDougall, W. (1950). *An Introduction to Social Psychology* (30th edn.). London: Methuen. (Original work published 1908).

Mehrabian, A., & Epstein, N. A. (1972). A measure of emotional empathy. *Journal of Personality*, **40**, 523–543.

Miller, P. A., & Eisenberg, N. (1988). The relation of empathy to aggressive and externalising/antisocial behaviour. *Psychological Bulletin*, **103**, 324–344.

Ohbuchi, K. (1988). Arousal of empathy and aggression. *Psychologia: An International Journal of Psychology*, **31**, 177–186.

O'Sullivan, M., & Guilford, J. P. (1976). *Four Factor Tests of Social Intelligence (Behavioural Cognition): Manual of Instructions and Interpretations*. New York: Sheridan Psychological Services, Inc.

Perry, R. J., Rosen, H. R., Kramer, J. H., *et al.* (2001). Hemispheric dominance for emotions, empathy and social behaviour: evidence from right and left handers with frontotemporal dementia. *Neurocase*, **7**, 145–160.

Povey, A. (2005). Theory of mind deficits/mentalising ability in conduct disordered adolescents and healthy controls. Un-published master's thesis: University of Manchester, Manchester, UK.

Premack, D., & Woodruff, G. (1978). Does the Chimpanzee have a 'theory of mind'? *Behaviour and Brain Sciences*, **4**, 515–526.

Rice, M. E. (1994, March). Criminal and noncriminal history as an indicator of risk among sex offenders. Paper presented at Clarke Institution of Psychiatry's Conference on the Assessment and Management of Risk in Sex Offenders, Toronto.

Richell, R. A., Mitchell, D. G. V., Newman, C., *et al.* (2003). Theory of mind and psychopathology. Can psychopathic individuals read the 'language of the eyes'? *Neuropsychologia*, **4**, 523–526.

Riley, J. A. (1986). Empathy and criminal; behavior: a look at man's inhumanity to man. *Dissertation Abstracts International*, **47**, 1890–1891.

Rosenstein, P. (1995). Parental levels of empathy as related to risk assessment in child protective services. *Child Abuse and Neglect*, **19**, 1349–1360.

Seto, M. C. (1992). Victim, blame, empathy, and disinhibition of sexual arousal to rape in community males and incarcerated rapists. Unpublished master thesis, Queens University, Kingston, Ontario.

Stone, V. E., Baron-Cohen, S., & Knight, R. T. (1998). Frontal lobe contributions to theory of mind. *Journal of Cognitive Neuroscience*, **10**, 640–656.

Tiihonen, J., Hodgins, S., Vaurio, O., *et al.* (2000). Amygdaloid volume loss in psychopathy. *Society for Neuroscience, Abstracts*, 2017.

Watson, P, J., Grisham, S. O., Trotter, M, V., & Biderman, M. D. (1984). Narcissism and empathy: validity evidence for the narcissistic personality inventory. *Journal of Personality*, **48**, 301–305.

Widom, C. S. (1978). An empirical classification of female offenders. *Criminal Justice and Behaviour*, **5**, 35–52.

Wiehe, V. R. (2003). Empathy and narcissism in a sample of child abuse perpetrators and a comparison sample of foster parents. *Child Abuse and Neglect*, **27**, 541–555.

Williams, C. A. (1990). Biopsychology elements of empathy: a multidimensional model. *Issues in Mental Health Nursing*, **11**, 155–174.

4

Empathy and depression: the moral system on overdrive

Lynn E. O'Connor[1], Jack W. Berry[2], Thomas Lewis[3], Kathleen Mulherin[4] and Patrice S. Crisostomo[5]

[1] Emotion, Personality and Altruism Research Group, Wright Institute and University of California, Berkeley
[2] Emotion, Personality and Altruism Research Group, Samford University
[3] Emotion, Personality and Altruism Research Group, University of California, San Francisco
[4] Emotion, Personality and Altruism Research Group, Kaiser Permanente, San Francisco
[5] Emotion, Personality and Altruism Research Group, University of California, Berkeley

4.1 Introduction

This chapter describes the intimate connection between empathy and depression, the epidemic of our modern world. While depression has been described as a 'disorder of the self', it may be more accurately characterized as a disorder of 'concern for others'. People who are depressed most often have normal or elevated levels of empathy; however, their affect-directed, automatic causal interpretations of pain in others are often disturbed, leading to non-conscious assertions of blame, usually placed on themselves. Empathy, a socially organizing neural system, allows us to share others' feelings, to mimic without awareness, and forms the basis of our relationships and our social learning (Decety & Jackson, 2004).

A sophisticated Theory of Mind (ToM), or the ability to know what others are thinking, is sometimes considered a prerequisite for true empathy. The capacity for empathy, present in infants from the first days of life, may be independent of cognitive maturity and a developed ToM. Healthy empathy, however, requires an understanding of causality, undeveloped in very young children and affectively distorted in depression. The empathic reaction in depressives often leads to great distress because they tend to unrealistically blame themselves for pain felt by others. Thus, in mood disorders, the empathy system may be functional; however, an overly active and automatic moral system, connected to the empathic experience, tends to misinterpret attribution, and the guilt

Empathy in Mental Illness, eds. Tom F. D. Farrow and Peter W. R. Woodruff. Published by Cambridge University Press. © Cambridge University Press 2007.

felt at believing that you have caused pain in another leads to empathic distress, an exaggerated reaction.

Ubiquitous in mammalian species (Preston & de Waal, 2002), empathy is reflexive and non-conscious, occurring without awareness. The empathy system is active in all interpersonal encounters. Through a system of mirror neurones, people react to witnessing motor actions as well as to emotions, as if they themselves were having the same experiences and feelings. In empathic responses, people are literally feeling others' feelings, while maintaining a separate sense of self. While watching others, people mirror them as they engage in social conversations, experience emotions such as pain and distress, or participate in positive and pleasure-giving feelings and activities that bond people together, such as smiling, laughing, touching affectionately, reconciling after a break in connection, and forgiving after being harmed by another (Berry *et al.*, 2005; Farrow *et al.*, 2001; Keltner *et al.*, 2006). Blair (1997) observed that psychopaths have a deficit in the empathy system, leading to a lack of normal moral judgement. In contrast, people afflicted with depression are empathic, and yet they often fail to make normal moral assessments and this may be a fundamental dysfunction characterizing mood disorders.

The limbic and paralimbic system structures, found active in emotional empathy, automatic moral decision-making and guilt, are, broadly considered, those also found active or hyperactive in people suffering from depression. A deficit of empathy appears in a few mental disorders that have low prevalence rates, namely sociopathy, autism, Asperger's and some psychotic disorders, and in those with injury resulting from strokes, or other forms of damage. In contrast, people suffering from mood disorders are marked by functional and structural neural changes in the neural circuit associated with empathic responses; however, they exhibit a normal degree of empathy, or even a surplus in some cases. Depressives are rarely thinking exclusively about the self; instead, they are often dwelling on how they might endanger others, or on their beliefs – often false – that they have harmed others in the past. Depression is highlighted by excessive empathy-based guilt, and in our laboratory, we have repeatedly found empirical evidence of the connection (O'Connor *et al.*, 2002). Presently, multiple lines of evidence are converging to support the connection between depression, empathy and an overly active or misattributing moral system.

Advances in social, clinical and personality psychology, along with findings from neuroscience, psychiatry, molecular biology and psychopharmacology support a biological perspective of normal and abnormal sociability, with empathy at the centre of attachments. Empathy is perhaps the heart of mammalian development, limbic regulation and social organization (MacLean, 1985). The loss of attachments often initiates the onset of depression. Depressed individuals are eager to maintain relationships and to be of help when needed. However, they may fail in efforts to help and to remain socially connected, and often lose the affection needed for biological regulation. Their limited capacity to effectively help others is mirrored by their failure to help themselves or to routinely act in their own best interests, due to passivity, a symptom of depression. Failures in efforts to help and failures in relationships increase the severity of depression. Adding insult to injury, people suffering from depression interpret these failures as further evidence of their 'moral inferiority'.

Depressed patients often appear withdrawn and reclusive, their worries about others remaining silent and internal. Although it seems that no one understands the depth of their despair, their fear and sadness are reflected in the empathy system of their caretakers. However, instead of feeling more alert to the pain of those suffering from depression, caretakers may react like the depressive, by feeling overly responsible and guilty, resulting in their own withdrawal, and sometimes blaming depressives for their troubles. Like other pervasive, negative emotional states, depression is thus often contagious, first touching and then frustrating empathy in others. As multidisciplinary research continues to increase our knowledge of this isolating, chronic and relapsing illness, mental health providers, families and friends may be better able to maintain their natural empathy towards those afflicted with depression.

4.2 Depression: prevalence, costs and theories of aetiology

Depression is the most common mental disorder on our contemporary landscape, affecting millions of people worldwide. The World Health Organization has estimated that by 2020 depression will be the major source of disability in the developed world, and the second most important cause internationally (Ingleby, 2004). The prevalence of depression has been rising steadily since the middle of the last century; the rate in the United States has escalated from 2% of the population in the 1960s to 25% in the 1990s and 28.8% of Americans will experience a mood disorder sometime during their lifetime (Kessler *et al.*, 2005). It has been estimated that over 19 million people in the United States experience depression yearly, accounting for 4.7 million office visits and costing over $30 billion annually. Untreated depression costs billions annually. Suicide is the second leading cause of death for young people today, eclipsed only by motor vehicle accidents.

Rates of depression are consistently higher in women, with 12% affected by mood disorders each year compared to 7% of men. Mood disorders are afflicting our children and adolescents as well, with rates ranging from 2.5% to 8.3% in the United States. The criteria identifying depression in children have broadened, and now include the angry and defiant behaviours previously diagnosed as conduct and attention deficit hyperactivity disorders. Depression in the geriatric population is estimated to inflict 1% to 2% of people over the age of 65, and 13% to 24% of the elderly suffer from subclinical depression, placing them at risk for major depression and suicide (Kessler *et al.*, 2005).

The diagnosis of depression is complex, as clinicians are confronted with symptoms indicative of unipolar depression, bipolar I, bipolar II, or dysthymic disorder, with each diagnosis frequently associated with symptoms of anxiety disorders. Bipolar I and II are often misdiagnosed as unipolar depression and then under-treated, or treated with the wrong medications, resulting in rapid cycling or a worsening of depression (Strakowski, 2002). Patients suffering from bipolar disorders have also often been misdiagnosed as personality disordered and provided no psychopharmacological treatment, thus leading to a worsening of their condition.

The personal, social and economic costs of depression have resulted in international research efforts focused on aetiology, underlying biological and social mechanisms, effective treatments and prevention. Multiple biological factors have been associated with depression, including genetic heritability (Neumeister *et al.*, 2004) and distinct brain dysfunctions (Caetano *et al.*, 2004; Drevets, 2001; Goldapple *et al.*, 2004). Recent studies suggest that levels of brain-derived neurotrophic factor (BDNF), which functions to protect neurones, are lower in depressed people. Neuroticism, significantly associated with the BDNF gene, is a personality factor consisting of attributes such as high sensitivity to negative emotions, fear of rejection and proneness to worry. Heritable by 40% to 60%, neuroticism is also associated with depression, which is heritable by 35% to 50%. One of the two variants of the BDNF gene, the Val^{66} allele, is associated with higher scores on neuroticism and depression (Sen *et al.*, 2003). The Val allele is also implicated in bipolar disorder, impulse control syndromes, schizophrenia and addiction. BDNF protects hippocampal neurones in chronic stress conditions and in depression, which, if left untreated, results in neuronal death, with shrinkage of the hippocampus and prefrontal cortex. The other BDNF variant, Met, is associated with higher levels of BDNF, lower scores in Neuroticism and a significantly lower risk of depression. The BDNF gene appears to affect both serotonin and dopamine. While treatment with selective serotonin reuptake inhibitors (SSRIs) raises BDNF, lower levels are associated with the destruction of dopamine, central to the reward pathways. Using a scale consisting of attributes derived from psychiatrists' interviews of patients, we found high scores on the 'Low-Dopamine' subscale of the Neurotransmitter Attributes Questionnaire (NAQ; O' Connor *et al.*, 2005) to be associated with depression, along with high scores on neuroticism, and empathic guilt. This connection with high neuroticism supports the BDNF theory while the findings related to guilt provide the link to empathy (O'Connor *et al.*, 2005).

Various treatments, such as the SSRIs, monoamino oxidase (MAO) inhibitors, mood stabilizers including lithium and valproic acid, electroconvulsive therapy (ECT) and physical exercise, increase levels of BDNF (Russo-Neustadt *et al.*, 2001). Other genes related to the dopaminergic and serotonergic systems have been implicated in vulnerability to mood disorders, suggesting that they are polygenetic illnesses. Twin and sibling studies and research in molecular genetics, psychiatry and psychopharmacology are contributing to our understanding of the heritability of depression. Patients' genetic profiles in combination with symptoms will likely be the basis of diagnosis in the future. Stressors on pregnant women have been shown to have negative effects on the neural system in developing infants, including a lack of emotional support and traumatizing experiences during pregnancy such as terrorism and war. Neurotoxin exposure (Masters, 2001), and pre- and post-natal bacterial and viral infections are also associated with vulnerability to depression. Even a single neurotoxin may be implicated; for example, high blood mercury levels in dentists are associated with low BDNF, along with symptoms of mood disorders (Heyer *et al.*, 2004).

Negative childhood experiences are also related to the aetiology of depression (Westen, 1998). Family stressors, disturbed or embattled parents, and poor socio-economic conditions are found significant, and environmental factors are known to influence gene expression. Environmental conditions connecting high levels of empathy and depression were initially studied by developmental researchers (Eisenberg, 2000; Zahn-Waxler, 2000) and a few clinicians (Neiderland, 1961; Modell, 1971; Weiss, 1993). Some practitioners continue to consider childhood experiences primary in the aetiology of depression, while minimizing biological factors. Others explain depression as a function of an egocentric, antisocial and maladaptive unconscious mind, a fundamental construct in psychoanalytic theory. Biased by the belief in a maladaptive unconscious, it is easy to mistake the flat, anxious and passive responses of depressed patients as self-centred.

Depressed patients may also been seen as egocentric because they often fail to disclose their worry about others, and instead describe themselves as selfish. Clinicians from differing perspectives, including some who practise evidence-based therapy and biological psychiatrists dispensing medication, may refer to 'resistance to treatment', viewing depressed patients as hostile and lacking in empathy. However, as cognitive social neuroscience provides an empirically based replacement for the Freudian unconscious with the 'new unconscious', an adaptive and social mental framework will more likely guide the treatment of depression in the future (Hassin *et al.*, 2005; Kihlstrom, 1987).

4.3 Empathy and developmental pathways to depression

Over 30 years ago, developmental psychologists began to identify the links between high sensitivity to others' distress, proneness to worry, empathic guilt and vulnerability to depression. From observations of infants and their mothers in naturalistic and laboratory settings, associations between empathy, guilt and later proneness to depression, particularly in females, were noted (Nolen-Hoeksema *et al.*, 1999; Zahn-Waxler, 2000). Research designed to help parents teach their children empathic and prosocial responses to distress in others led to the discovery of significant links between guilt, empathy and moral development (Hoffman, 1975, 2000). Rosenfield *et al.* (2000) reported a correlation between empathy for distress in others and depression. Murray (2004) found that runaway adolescents in foster care had significantly more empathy-based guilt compared to non-troubled adolescents. Hay and Pawlby (2003) found that prosocial children worried about their families' well-being and suffered more than their less-worried peers from internalizing problems.

Zahn-Waxler (2000) described 'the presence of an early developmental pathway where surfeits of empathy, as well as guilt can place individuals at risk for later depression' (p. 226). The capacity to respond to others' distress appears early. Only one day after birth, infants react to the distress cry of other newborns with greater intensity than to the cry of a 5-month-old baby, a white noise, a synthetic cry, or a recording of their own distress cries (Martin & Clark, 1982; Sagi & Hoffman, 1976). From 4 months, infants attempt to engage depressed mothers (Cohn *et al.*, 1990); and between 12 and 18 months, they make overt efforts to help others in distress (Zahn-Waxler *et al.*, 1979). This sensitivity to people's emotions continues into adulthood. For example, Lane and DePaulo (1999) found that depressives exhibited heightened sensitivity to emotional dishonesty; the depressed subjects were better able to detect deception in dishonest feedback than the non-depressed sample.

Zahn-Waxler (2000) noted that early dysregulation of the moral system occurs when biologically vulnerable infants fail to engage depressed mothers, who appear to elicit a heightened sense of responsibility for others' emotions, along with chronic guilt. High empathy in children is a risk factor for later depression, if they are over-involved, self-blaming and distressed, with unregulated negative affect (Klimes-Dougan & Bolger, 1998). Recent findings suggest that the acquisition of a Theory of Mind in girls at an unusually early age is a predictor for high empathy-based guilt by adolescence, and may be associated with depression later (L. Rasco, personal communication, 2004).

The problems about which depressed patients feel like failures are ordinarily beyond their control; they can neither prevent nor resolve the distress they witness, but are feeling guilty for imaginary crimes. Despite intense concern for others, in depression empathic responses may fail to result in effective action even when it is possible. Symptoms such as passivity and withdrawal, common in depression, often inhibit altruistic behaviour and the ability to act in general. Nevertheless, in empirical studies we have found that empathy-based guilt, though associated with depression, is also associated with acts of altruism towards family members, friends and strangers (Crisostomo *et al.*, 2005). Figure 4.1 provides a structural model of these relationships.

Depression may render people unable to think clearly about helpful strategies or to carry out plans to come to the aid of others; thus, the connection between empathic concern and acts of altruism may sometimes be severed. Some suggest

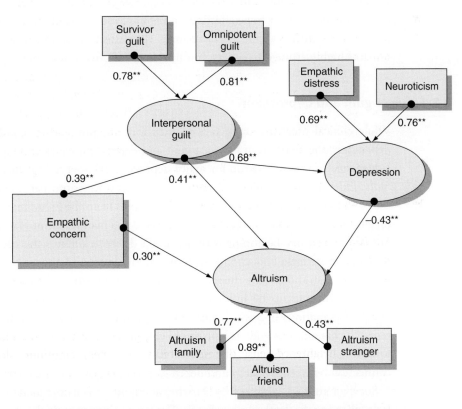

Figure 4.1.   Structural model: this presents a structural model illustrating that guilt (based on worry about others) appears to have a significant and positive influence on engaging in altruistic behaviours except when it leads to empathic distress and neuroticism. Neuroticism, a marker for brain-derived neurotrophic factor (BDNF) and a high risk factor for depression, appears to inhibit altruistic actions. The cumulative fit index = 0.96. All path coefficients were statistically significant at the 0.001 level

that excessive distress on witnessing distress in others results from overidentification and failure to distinguish self from others and, therefore, is not authentic empathy. However, it seems more likely that cognitive limitations accompanying depression have an impact on effective action at all levels: shrinkage of the hippocampus after a flood of excess cortisol and other stress hormones affects memory adversely. Furthermore, overactivity of the amygdala resulting from misunderstood input may lead to hyper-emotionality further disturbs cognitive processing. The dysfunctions of the prefrontal and orbitofrontal cortex found in depressives may impact other cognitive capacities, including planning and decision-making. Orbitofrontal and prefrontal cortex dysfunctions may increase inhibitions, in contrast to the uninhibited behaviour observed after brain-damaging accidents affecting the orbitofrontal cortex. Thus symptoms of withdrawal and passivity in part reflect the temporary decrease in cognitive competence in depression, and the associated inability to be effective contributes to the perception that depressed people are selfish. Despite these changes that affect cognition, the depressive remains highly attuned to others, but unable to effectively help them.

4.4 Survivor guilt and depression

While clinical literature often fails to mention empathy and its connection to depression, the association between guilt and depression has been long acknowledged, and guilt is a criterion for major depressive disorder in the *Diagnostic and Statistical Manual of Mental Disorders*, 4th edn., Text Revision. The failure to note the connection between guilt and empathy follows from the Freudian perspective on guilt. In psychoanalytic theory guilt is viewed as a manifestation of unconscious hostility and rivalry, beginning with the child's desire to kill his same-sex parent in the oedipal struggle and ending with an internalization of the avenging parent intent on castration. This theory, so pervasive in the middle to late twentieth century, continues to be influential throughout our culture, affecting psychological explanations of both normal and abnormal processes. However, current research characterizes guilt as a prosocial emotion tied to empathy and the desire to maintain social bonds (Baumeister & Leary, 1995; O'Connor, 2000). The connection between empathy and depression is highlighted in survivor guilt.

Survivor guilt was observed by Darwin and Freud as each described the guilt one feels following the death of a loved one. The term 'survivor guilt' came to life when Neiderland (1961) studied the severe depression and anxiety in survivors of Nazi concentration camps. He found them suffering from guilt, simply for being alive while their families had all been killed by the Nazis, as if their own survival had somehow caused the death of their families. Modell (1971) expanded the construct to include the guilt people feel when they believe they are harming others, by being successful, or happy. He noted that depressed patients often held the belief that if they had good fortune, success, or happiness, it was at the expense of other family members, who might then be less fortunate because there was a limit on how much 'good' could be had in a family. Weiss *et al.* (1986) followed with extensive clinical observations linking survivor guilt to depression and other psychological problems, forming the foundation for his theory of psychopathology and treatment, with altruism, the fundamental but often hidden human motivation, replacing the antisocial wishes and feelings held central by the Freudians. He proposed that people feel unconsciously compelled to help family and social group members, even when helping is at their own expense or personally costly. In line with these observations emphasizing human strengths rather than weaknesses, and in contrast to the psychoanalytic perspective, Weiss conveyed a positive view of human nature. He also observed that people think and plan non-consciously, much as they do consciously, which heralded discoveries in social cognitive neuroscience and positive psychology in the last decade.

Weiss *et al.* (1986) observed that patients enter psychotherapy with an unconscious plan to test grim and inhibiting pathogenic beliefs warning them not to pursue normal goals, for fear of surpassing someone in the family and thus making them feel inadequate by comparison. He proposed that patients' plans to test and change pathogenic beliefs were purposeful. Arguing that patients were not gratified by their problems, as proposed in analytic theory, Weiss held that patients were guided by the adaptive unconscious and determined to overcome their problems. In collaboration with Sampson, Weiss *et al.* (1986) supported his clinical observations upon which he built this more positive theory, with empirical single-case design psychotherapy research (Weiss *et al.*, 1986). Following Weiss, and in the context of the paradigm shift occurring in psychological science, we developed our programme of research to empirically test hypotheses derived from this new model of the mind and motivation (O'Connor *et al.*, 1997).

In our empirical research, we found significant associations between survivor guilt, empathy and depression. Survivor guilt is an empathic emotion often occurring without conscious awareness. We feel survivor guilt – albeit just slightly unconsciously – when we get a promotion or hear that a paper has been accepted for publication, while a friend just heard he was laid off or that he was going to be refused tenure. We feel survivor guilt when we are healthy and a friend calls one evening to tell us that she has been diagnosed with breast cancer. Survivor guilt is unusual in that we often fail to recognize it when we feel it most acutely; nor is it perceived by others watching our facial expressions or bodily movements. However, the presence of survivor guilt is often marked by submissive behaviour; we may put ourselves down and act as if we are lower in status than the person for whom we feel sorry. Survivor guilt may come to our attention only after we get self-destructive, in an effort to reduce its impact, by trying to 'level the playing field' and 'make things equal'.

The self-damaging behaviours resulting from survivor guilt may be self-defeating, but at the same time they are empathic acts of altruism aimed at preventing feelings of inadequacy in those perceived as less fortunate. The net result is a self-destructive but common cycle. The show of submissive behaviour often elicits negative reactions from others who then reevaluate the social ranking of the guilt-prone person. As witnesses look down on people who respond to survivor guilt with submission, they treat them as inferior. Though perhaps reducing guilt in the guilt-prone person, these social interactions are emotionally dysregulating and enhance feelings of depression if a mood disorder is already present or set off an episode in a vulnerable person. Thus, people who become submissive in an effort to help others often unwittingly become altruistic martyrs.

4.5 Programme of research: empathy, guilt and depression

Our programme of research on empathy, altruism, guilt and depression was initiated to test our biological, relational and affective theory of psychopathology and psychotherapy (Lewis *et al.*, 2000; O'Connor, 2000; Weiss, 1993). In line with our social and adaptive perspective on the mind, we hypothesized that people who suffer from depression and other common psychological problems score significantly higher in interpersonal guilt than those free of depression. In contrast to popular opinion, we also hypothesized that depressives are equal to or higher in empathy than non-depressed people.

We began our series of studies with the development of a measure designed to operationalize the constructs found useful in clinical work and central to our theory, placing altruism as a fundamental motivation, often manifested in survivor, separation, and overly responsible, omnipotent guilt. In prior single-case studies, it was found that survivor and separation guilt were the primary focus of each empirically developed case formulation and that interventions successful in reducing guilt were predictive of immediate and longer term positive outcome. The Interpersonal Guilt Questionnaire (IGQ-67: O'Connor *et al.*, 1997) was initiated by collecting statements typical of guilt-prone patients. These were categorized into four subscales: Survivor, Separation/Loyalty, Omnipotent Responsibility Guilt and Self-Hate. The first three subscales are other-focused, assessing guilt related to worry about others. The fourth subscale, Self-Hate, consists of negative self-focused statements, similar to items in cognitive measures of depression. The reliability and validity of the IGQ-67 was established in studies using several other validated measures of guilt, including scales of adaptive (Tangney *et al.*, 1992) and other measures of ruminative or maladaptive guilt.

As predicted, all measures of guilt were highly correlated with the first three IGQ-67 subscales (O'Connor *et al.*, 1997, 1999).

Other studies validated the underlying assumption that interpersonal guilt is based on human empathy, and indirectly, on altruism as a fundamental motivation. Results indicated that Survivor, Omnipotent and Separation Guilt are significantly correlated with Empathic Concern, Empathic Distress and Empathic Perspective-Taking, as measured by the Interpersonal Reactivity Index (IRI: Davis, 1980), demonstrating empirically that Survivor, Separation and Omnipotent Responsibility Guilt are empathy-associated emotions. We examined the correlations between various indexes of psychopathology, including depression, in order to test out the hypothesis that many clinical problems were associated with high levels of empathy-based guilt (O'Connor *et al.*, 1997, 2002). Empathy, Survivor Guilt and Neuroticism, described above as a high risk factor for depression, are modelled in Figure 4.2.

In another study, we compared patients hospitalized for depression with a non-clinical sample in order to determine if the two samples differed significantly in levels of guilt, if they differed significantly in self- versus other-focused concerns, and if the clinical sample was higher than or equal to the non-clinical sample in subscales of empathy (O'Connor *et al.*, 2002).

The results indicated that the depressed patients were equal to the non-clinical sample in Empathic Perspective-Taking and Concern and significantly higher than the non-clinical sample in Empathic Distress. These results demonstrate that

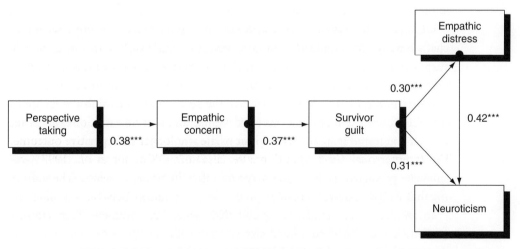

Figure 4.2.   Path analysis: the relationships of subscales of empathy, survivor guilt and neuroticism (as a marker of BDNF and high risk factor for depression). Several path models were tried, and Figure 4.2 was the best fitting model to our data. (Cumulative fit index = 0.95.) All path coefficients in the model are significant at 0.001

depressed patients do not differ from a normal sample in the ability to cognitively distinguish themselves from others. In order to compare self- and other-focused concerns in predicting depression in the depressed compared to non-depressed samples, we used instruments measuring worry about the self, including: Fear of Negative Evaluation (Brief-FNE; Leary, 1983); Fear of Envy Scale (FES; O'Connor *et al.*, 2002), a measure of worrying that others will feel jealous about one's success or happiness; the Social Comparison Scale (SCS; Allan & Gilbert, 1995), a measure of how people believe they rank in social status compared to others; and the Submissive Behaviour Scale (SBS; Allan & Gilbert, 1997), a measure of how submissive people believe themselves to be. Multiple regression analyses supported the hypothesis that, in depressed patients, other-focused concerns outweighed self-focused concerns in predicting depression, whereas in the non-clinical sample, both self- and other-focused concerns significantly predicted depression.

In other studies, interpersonal guilt significantly correlated with depression, assessed by a variety of measures: *Beck Depression Inventory*, Center for Epidemiological Studies Depression Scale (CES-D; Radloff, 1977), and subscales of the Brief Symptom Inventory, as well as indirect indicators of depression such as automatic thoughts, pessimistic explanatory style and Neuroticism. Still other studies conducted in our laboratory found significant associations between guilt and other psychological problems, for example jealousy (Webster *et al.*, 1997), addiction (Meehan *et al.*, 1996), obsessive compulsive disorder (OCD), perfectionism and pessimism.

In a recent experiment investigating survivor guilt in non-depressed college students, subjects read a story designed to induce survivor guilt in the story's hero, as the hero did better in a college class than did a second character in the story. The conditions varied only by the relationship between the main and the secondary characters; in one condition the hero surpassed his brother, in the second he surpassed a best friend, and in the third he surpassed a person with whom he had no personal relationship and who he never expected to see again. Subjects then wrote narratives about what they believed the hero would feel, think and do, under those conditions. Senior clinicians rated the narratives using a scale assessing levels of guilt and found it significantly lower in the stranger condition when compared to the family or friend conditions. We also found that scores on the IGQ-67 subscales predicted levels of guilt in the narratives written by each subject, indicating that IGQ-67 subscales reliably predict levels of guilt in behavioural indices.

In another recent study, we found that Generalized Anxious Temperament (GAT: Akiskal, 1998) correlated significantly with interpersonal guilt and with depression. According to Akiskal (1998), the GAT measures a personality type or style, typified by worries about self and others, that serves a protective function for the family and larger social group, and is therefore, from an evolutionary perspective, fitness enhancing at the level of the group.

The significant correlation between Survivor Guilt and depression has held up across cultures including Japan, Sweden and Germany, and across different cultural groups within the United States such as Filipino, Latin, African, Japanese, Middle Eastern and Chinese Americans. Figure 4.3 illustrates the correlations of the means of Survivor Guilt with the means of Depression across cultures.

In a study of 621 subjects, we examined the associations between guilt and self-reported acts of altruism. We found both Survivor and Omnipotent Guilt predictive of acts of altruism to family, friends and strangers. Comparing five cultures, significant differences were found in levels of altruism to family, with Asian, Middle Eastern and Hispanic subjects scoring significantly higher than European American subjects. In a study still underway with data collected from an internet sample, we are comparing Asian Americans to European Americans on guilt, empathy and altruism; with 348 subjects thus far, we have found no differences in major variables.

In another line of research related to depression, we conceptualize problematic temperament differences as reflecting low dopamine and/or low serotonin levels, instead of specific diagnoses, although we used diagnoses to validate a new measure, the Neurotransmitter Attributes Questionnaire (NAQ; O'Connor *et al.*,

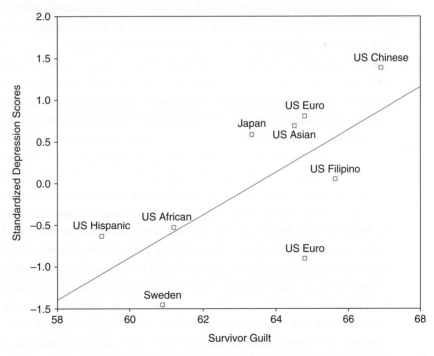

Figure 4.3. The correlations of the means of survivor guilt with the means of depression across cultures. (O'Connor, L. E. *Survivor Guilt Across Cultures*. University of Michigan, 2004)

2005). The NAQ consists of 51 items derived from questions used by psychiatrists in evaluating new patients for psychopharmacological treatment. Two clinicians knowledgeable about the effects of medications on particular symptoms placed each item in the Low-Dopamine and/or Low-Serotonin subscale. An internet study of 700 subjects from the general population resulted in several significant findings, related to guilt and depression, as well as to Neuroticism and Generalized Anxious Temperament, or 'Altruistic Anxiety'. We found both dopamine and serotonin significantly correlated with depression in both men and women, and each remained significant in a multiple regression predicting depression. We also found that Neuroticism significantly associated with guilt as well as both neurotransmitters when looked at alone; however, in a multiple regression, low serotonin remained significant while dopamine lost significance. Guilt-proneness was found to be associated significantly with both neurotransmitters.

4.6 Other empirical studies: empathy and depression

Findings in social and clinical psychology have supported the link between empathy and depression, connected to gender differences in empathy as well as depression. It is well established that females are at greater risk for depression, with rates at least three times that of males at all ages beyond puberty (Rosenfield *et al.*, 2000). In some studies females were also found higher than males in empathic concern and empathic distress (Bush *et al.*, 2000; Eisenberg, 2000).

Other studies found links between empathy, depression and stressful life conditions in various populations such as disabled children, adults with medical problems, people in helping professions, medical interns and others. Multiple studies demonstrate that individuals who are sensitive to distress in others are at risk for depression, anxiety and other symptoms of psychological distress (Griens *et al.*, 2002; Shieman & Turner, 2001), especially if they are female (Bandura *et al.*, 2003). Few studies failed to find an association between empathy and depression. For example, a cross cultural study of Iranian and American students found positive correlations between depression and empathic distress, but a negative relationship between depression and empathic concern (Ghorbani *et al.*, 2003).

Studies of adult samples have routinely found chronic guilt correlated with depressive symptoms (Jones & Kugler, 1993; O'Connor *et al.*, 2002; Quiles & Bybee, 1997). Situation-specific guilt in response to specific transgressions has been linked to empathic concern and other prosocial affects (Joireman, 2004; Quiles & Bybee, 1997; Tangney *et al.*, 1992). Situational guilt, assessed by measures designed to capture realistic, adaptive guilt, fails to significantly correlate with depressive symptoms as these measures do not include the dispositional, maladaptive and ruminative guilt common to both depression and anxiety disorders.

There remains a paradox in the findings on depression, empathy and guilt. On the one hand, empathy has been empirically linked to prosocial behaviour, moral maturity and emotional regulation, even among very young children. On the other hand, children who are high in empathy and other characteristics of maturity have higher rates of depressive symptoms in later years. In a longitudinal study of families conducted by Cowan and Cowan, it was found that survivor guilt, assessed in parents and adolescents followed since the children were about 4 years old, was significantly predicted for the adolescent girls by a behavioural test of ToM, administered at age 4 (L. Rasco, personal communication, 2004). It was considered unusually mature when these girls scored high on the test of ToM, and yet these findings suggest high ToM at a young age leads to problematic guilt-proneness. This adds another paradox to the already paradoxical findings that the empathic responses to others that hold our social groups together and enable cooperative group living are indirectly linked to the current epidemic of depression.

4.7 Evolutionary theories: empathy and depression

Over the past four decades sociobiologists, evolutionary psychologists and psychiatrists have attempted to fit depression into the adaptationist programme, explaining depression as a functional adaptation (Nesse, 2000). Price (1967) observed that symptoms found in psychiatric patients were similar to those seen in people who had lost status, making a connection between mental disorders and a dominance hierarchy. Price's dominance hierarchy theory of depression evolved into what is known as the ranking of depression, or 'an involuntary submission' in a losing situation, in order to avoid further futile conflicts, and to preserve one's self-interests by withdrawal from battle. Gilbert (1992) discussed depression as a method of signalling social group members that the depressed person is defeated, withdrawn and therefore no longer willing or able to fight. Gilbert and Allan (1994) gathered empirical evidence supporting this theory, examining social comparison and other self-focused variables related to social ranking, submission and depression. Our findings support both the concern for others theory of depression, and the social-ranking theory in a normal sample with minor symptoms. Hagen (2003) proposed that depressives use their illness as a means of social bargaining, with the intention of gaining resources.

Mismatch theory provides another evolutionary model of depression. While not suggesting that depression is adaptive, it explains it as the result of adaptations that were functional in the Era of Evolutionary Adaptation (EEA); that is, in the conditions in which our species evolved, but which have become maladaptive in present-day conditions. Some suggest that gender-specific attributes, adaptive for childrearing in a hunter-gatherer society, have become dysfunctional in the context of birth control and high technology, in which women commonly work outside of the home. Another example is seen in our current problem with obesity. The archaeological record suggests food supplies in the EEA were often variable, sometimes plentiful and sometimes scarce. Our species developed biological adaptations to ensure survival and reproduction when food was scarce, as in famines. To meet this condition we developed an energy-conserving metabolism with a capacity to store energy in fat cells, along with dietary tastes creating cravings for fat, sugar and salt, often scarce in the EEA. These adaptations, under modern conditions, have resulted in obesity, heart disease and other chronic modern illnesses. The link between rates of depression and the rise in obesity and dieting may have a functional connection. Deliberate food restriction is now found among young children; some begin dieting by age 6, establishing a life-long eating disorder, associated in numerous studies with depression.

The lifestyle of hunter-gatherers required large amounts of physical activity, along with living in close and stable social groups (Cosmides & Tooby, 1992). Exercise increases levels of BDNF, while lower levels are implicated in depression, and exercise has been found to be an effective antidepressant (Russo-Neustadt *et al.*, 2001). Lacking in natural opportunities for exercise, the contemporary lifestyle may be inherently harmful to genetically vulnerable people who respond with low BDNF and fall victim to depression. Studies of the hunter-gatherer groups remaining suggest that, in the distant past, people were social and cooperative by necessity. As small, slow moving mammals, we were 'Man the hunted' instead of 'Man the hunter'. Prey to numerous predators who viewed us as a source of protein, our developing brain and predilection for cooperative social living were our only defence. Privacy and ownership had not yet appeared. Singing, dancing, gossiping, hunting, gathering and child care were conducted in protective cooperative groups, conducive to intimate social interactions, and provided the level of physical and social activity required to maintain adequate BDNF and the limbic system regulation that prevent depression (Lewis *et al.*, 2000; McGuire & Troisi, 1987; Raleigh & McGuire, 1986).

4.8 The evolution of altruism and evolved mechanisms at work in depression

While theories of the adaptive function of depression abound, they have been limited to adaptation at the level of the individual or the 'selfish gene', and have neglected to consider fitness at the level of the group. Two explanations of altruism, kin selection (inclusive fitness theory) (Hamilton, 1964) and reciprocal altruism (Trivers, 1971), have dominated, despite their inability to account for altruism extended toward strangers. Both theories focus on within-group competition. Costly display, another theory explaining the evolution of altruism with individual fitness as the goal, proposes that altruistic acts serve to signal social group members that the altruist holds a surplus of resources and is a desirable mate in competition for reproductive partners.

Tooby and Cosmides (1996) described the 'the Banker's Paradox' theory, to explain altruism extended to friends, as well as to make sense of the evolution of our drive for recognition, or 'individual uniqueness'. Altruism extended to friends is analogous to a banker loaning money to a person in need at the moment, who is expected to pay it back later when resources may be scarce for others. They theorized that having unique skills makes the pay back more likely, and this contributed to the evolution of individuality, as well as to altruism between friends. Here too, kindness to strangers is neglected.

The insistence on viewing altruism as a deception, covering hidden selfishness and individual fitness while denying the existence of primary altruism, has been part of a four-decade-long bias against group selection and multilevel selection theory, which only now is finally lifting (Borrello, 2005). Although Darwin accepted group selection as a factor in the evolution of altruism and cooperation in humans and other species, the theory was rejected, beginning in the 1960s. Ignoring the 'science war' going on in evolutionary theory, group selection was kept alive by a small group of evolutionary scientists and theorists (Sober & Wilson, 1998; Wilson, 1975) through the gene-centric era, sometimes referred to 'ultra-Darwinism'. The recent reemergence of multilevel selection theory is joined and supported by the theory of gene-culture coevolution (Richerson & Boyd, 2004), in which cultural evolution, occurring more rapidly than genetically based evolution, provides the context for the evolution of group-focused cultural traditions that, in time, affect genetics, as genetics affect culture. As a mark of the end of the selfish gene era and the resurrection of group selection, at the 2005 meeting of the Human Behavior and Evolution Society, E. O. Wilson, the father of sociobiology, stated that group selection is the most important factor in the evolution of cooperation and altruism, including in our species. The results of our research on empathy, guilt and depression, and the presence of survivor guilt across cultures have also been best explained in terms of mechanisms operating at the level of the group and, ultimately, a function of group selection (O'Connor *et al.*, 2000).

Early human groups were relatively small, surviving by their 'wits' while prey to multiple predators, and engaged in intense warfare between groups, while developing the variations in customs known as culture, including traditions allowing groups to distinguish themselves from others. Cultural evolution is thus also a factor in competition between groups and was important in the evolution of altruism and cooperation. Prosocial emotions such as guilt, along with other emotional capacities that are in varied ways and degrees influenced by culture, serve as proximate motivators for altruism. Transmission of social norms limits within-group competition and promotes within-group levelling, leading to forms of social organization and ideologies such as monogamy and social sanctions against large income differentials (Gintis *et al.*, 2003).

Empirical studies of behaviour in economic games such as the 'Public Good', 'Ultimatum' and 'Prisoners' Dilemna', in vivo as well as in simulated computer experiments, demonstrate that groups with more altruists/cooperators do better in competition with groups who have fewer cooperators. Players are motivated to cooperate and will punish 'defectors', despite the personal cost. Several studies have demonstrated that guilt functions to increase cooperation in games. Guilt may function in two ways: first, it may serve as an internal warning signal, letting the person know that he or she is violating a social norm and is at risk of being punished. Second, guilt also serves as an internal signal letting the person know that he or she must take action to help someone else. This second function of guilt is based on the empathic response that begins with witnessing another's distress and, through the mirror neurone system, feeling it as one's own. This transforms into empathic concern, at which point the person feels compelled to help and, if failing, this becomes empathic distress, with guilt unresolved and often chronic. Therefore, guilt is the connector between empathy and the moral system; like a bell that goes off when action is needed, it is our form of alarm cry, telling us we must help a conspecific, and this becomes both an affective and a moral directive. Guilt may not always be reliable, as when it is exaggerated and unrealistic in depression. However imperfect our signal to act, it motivates the non-conscious moral judgements that help hold us together.

In a recent study we conducted in collaboration with Wilson (unpublished data, 2004) the Survivor Guilt subscale on the IGQ-67 significantly predicted cooperative behaviour in the Public Goods game. Across cultures, cooperation and fair play are expected, even when groups are temporary (Fehr & Fischbacher, 2003); thus both fear of being punished and empathic guilt are emotional capacities providing proximate motivation for automatic moral judgements, and then for cooperative and altruistic behaviour, while the ultimate cause is group level fitness.

While altruistic punishment infers a cost to the punisher as well as to the punished, a recent study demonstrated the punisher also receives a reward for punishing; as when cocaine or nicotine are administered, the punisher is rewarded by the activation of the caudate nucleus. Subjects who wished to punish maximally received an additional reward by activation of the thalamus and the dorsal striatum, associated with rewards gained from goal-directed activities (de Quervain *et al.*, 2004). Gintis *et al.* (2003) suggest that successful groups tend to have strong altruistic reciprocators who have received either altruistic rewards or altruistic punishments.

In order to distinguish the cooperator from the defector in a social group, people need to have a quick and implicit method of detecting cheaters (Cosmides & Tooby, 1992). 'Cheater detection', an evolved capacity forming what is referred to as a 'module' in our cognitive apparatus, enables people to detect and limit the invasion of cheaters in a community. Cheater detection and punishment of 'cheaters' (or altruistic punishment) are evolved capacities that blend into the area of empathy and moral judgement connected by guilt, that specifically become dysfunctional in mood disorders. People suffering from depression often exhibit hyper-moralistic standards and hyper-scrupulosity applied to others, but even more fiercely to themselves. In depression, cheater detection turns inward, unrealistic guilt signals the person of their so-called immoral intentions or actions, and altruistic punishment turns upon the self, providing one explanation for the self-destructive behaviours often seen in the clinic. Though arising with the evolution of cooperation, in depression these mechanisms, through the connecting emotion of guilt, have become dysfunctional and may sometimes render depressives victims of self-inflicted bodily injury.

The capacity to detect cheaters underlies survivor guilt. Cheater detection requires the ability to quantify and put value on something that a person gains, and then to determine if the value is deserved. Survivor guilt requires the capacity to detect cheaters, but instead of looking for cheating in others, the cheater to be detected is the self. People suffering from depression are looking at both others and themselves with suspicion, often believing whatever they have was obtained by cheating, and that it is more than they deserve. Depressives, burdened by moralistic standards, are harsh evaluators of both themselves and others. The self-punishment meted out by depressives is a common if disturbing symptom; while thinking 'I deserve this', they may engage in altruistic punishment turned upon the self. Just as altruistic punishers experience a neuronally based reward from punishing defectors, despite material costs, depressed patients report a sense of relief upon inflicting self-punishment. Patients who are 'cutters', describe relief from tension after cutting and depressives with suicidal ideation may describe the relief they felt when on the verge of attempting a suicidal action.

It is difficult to rationalize depression as adaptive from the point of view of the individual or even the group. However, from the perspective of an even higher level of organization, for example the species or whole eco-systems, depression may function to limit the growth of local populations, and to restrain depletion of worldwide resources, benefiting many species. In the most developed nations, increasing populations have settled in urban centres, resulting in local overcrowding. At the same time, rates of depression and rates of consumption of energy and other resources have been rising, while birth rates have been dropping for the past century. This situation resembles that of non-human animals living in overcrowded conditions, where they have been known to display socially aberrant behaviours, dropping rates of reproduction, rising rates of viral epidemics, destruction of their environments and, in some extreme cases, species extinction. In the ordinary time frame, the cost of depression is vast. However, at a higher level, evolution may be in action, with the rise in depression and dropping birth rates serving to limit the consumption of nations who are over-utilizing natural resources. The hidden benefit to rising rates of depression may go to multiple groups of people worldwide, as well as to numerous other species when looking from a long, evolutionary time frame.

4.9 Empathy, depression, and current neuroscience

As advances in neuroscience, including brain imaging, are applied to the study of depression and empathy, we are likely to also further study guilt. Serving as the mediator between depression and empathy, guilt is the moral emotion, based on empathic responses and our need for closely connected and stable social groups, manifested in our pain at witnessing pain in others, and our need to help those in distress. We are now able to compare normal people feeling empathic concern, or making morality-based decisions in experimental conditions, to brain activity in the sociopath, or autistic individuals with deficits in the capacity to feel empathy for others. Specific functional differences between depressed and non-depressed samples are compared through functional magnetic resonance imaging (fMRI), positron emission tomography (PET), single photon emission computed tomography (SPECT), magnetoencephalography (MEG) and other forms of imaging. In molecular biology genetic variables are also now being identified, including variations that appear correlated with vulnerabilities to depression, or expressed only when the vulnerable person is in adverse conditions. Moral reasoning is recognized as a function of non-conscious social emotions, and particularly guilt, driving decisions before there is awareness. The affective neural basis for social judgements, moral decisions and the detection of cheaters, all of which are connected by guilt, and mechanisms underlying empathy, compassion and altruism as well as depression are now under the gaze of brain imaging (Greene *et al.*, 2001; Greene & Haidt, 2002; Moll *et al.*, 2002a, 2002b).

Moll *et al.* (2002b) reported on an fMRI study in which subjects were presented with pictures representing six conditions: moral pictures portraying charged unpleasant scenes; pleasant scenes without a moral meaning; unpleasant scenes including an implicit moral connotation; neutral pictures with people and with landscapes; and scrambled images. When subjects viewed the moral in comparison to the non-morally tinged unpleasant pictures, findings demonstrated significantly increased activation in paralimbic structures also noted in fMRI studies of guilt.

In functional brain studies of depressed patients compared to normal samples, Lange and Irle (2004) found abnormal activation in limbic structures, including enlarged amygdalae in patients with recent major depression. Other studies of depressed patients find unusual activation of the amygdala, abnormally under-active in psychopathy, characterized by the absence of normal moral decision-making and guilt. Pagani *et al.* (2004) observed increased cerebral blood flow in the anterior temporal lobe of depressed patients, also a focus of activity in guilt. Abnormal limbic and paralimbic system activity has been observed with major depression, which returns to normal with successful antidepressant treatment, indicating that some portion of the pathophysiology of depression is connected to overactivity in limbic and paralimbic structures, affecting moral decision-making and guilt (Shin *et al.*, 2000).

Neumeister *et al.* (2004) reported that patients with a history of depression demonstrated chronic overactivity in the brain circuit central to emotion regulation. Hyperactivity was observed even when the patients were in remission, suggesting that dysfunctions in emotion regulation highlighted in this study may be genetic. Between depressive episodes, hyperactivity in the emotion regulation circuit included these same limbic and paralimbic structures associated with morality and empathy. The associations between empathy, guilt and depression were established using older research methods; however, brain imaging technology provides a detailed picture of both normal and abnormal activity in limbic and paralimbic structures and connected cortices that form the neural network of the social brain, the home of empathy and guilt. Imaging research allows us to begin to understand the mechanism by which the results of empathy become dysfunctional, when interpreted through the lens of chronic and unrealistic guilt found in depressive illness.

4.10 Conclusions

The review of research in this chapter brings together evidence from multiple areas in psychology and neuroscience demonstrating the connection between empathy, morality, guilt and depression. The neuroscience of empathy describes a complex network, beginning in limbic structures and leading to automatic moral decision-making, that appears also focused in the paralimbic system, associated with executive control and planning. Brain regions associated with the empathy system are also involved in other mental disorders characterized by a high proneness to empathy in combination with an overly active and even harsh moral system, such as obsessive compulsive disorder and addiction. Against the background of this network of inter-connected structures, we are able to place our empirical findings, connecting guilt and depression across cultures. Empirical studies of the social brain, in its normal and abnormal states, are paving the way for a more patient-friendly and positive perspective on human motivation, and therefore also on depressives. In most studies, depressives are found to have similar empathic responses to non-clinical samples, with depressives differing only in that they are prone to feeling greater guilt leading to greater distress upon witnessing distress felt by others.

The early work of developmental scientists has been confirmed by numerous studies demonstrating the connection between empathy and depression, connected by guilt which, in those vulnerable, tends to transform empathic concern into empathic distress. Paradoxically, guilt serves as a proximate motivation for altruistic actions. While playing economic games in experimental conditions, it is found that people usually expect cooperative behaviour from others, and behave cooperatively themselves. Those who express feeling guilty after failing to follow the social norm of cooperative behaviour in the first round of a game tend to behave more altruistically in the next round, compared to those who express no feelings of guilt at their failure to follow the norm of cooperation.

A shift in focus from a self- to other-centred view of depression is likely to encourage more positive attitudes in treatment providers, and thus to improve treatments as well as modes of prevention. The connection between depression and empathy is found in guilt – the moral emotion, the signal that makes us so uneasy when witnessing unfairness and inequity. The rapid rise in depression suggests that our current lifestyle may be less than ideal for the social brain; assuming the human brain evolved for life in cooperative and empathic social units, overcoming depression may require the development of social environments better suited to the nature of our species.

AUTHORS' NOTE

The authors wish to thank the Terrence and Emily Meehan Foundation and the Miriam F. Meehan Charitable Trusts, for supporting our research at the Emotion, Personality and Altruism Research Group at the Wright Institute, Berkeley, and the writing of this paper. In addition, thanks to Kelly McCoy, Laura Cayan, Anders Greenwood and Steven O'Connor for their careful reading of the manuscript and great recommendations. We also thank Stephen Hinshaw for reading the manuscript in a very early phase and David Stiver, for translating our models into readable graphics. Finally, we thank Tom Farrow for the invitation to tackle the job of integrating the many disciplines required to understand the link between depression, empathy and guilt, and then for his patience while everything took much longer than expected.

REFERENCES

Akiskal, H. S. (1998). Toward a definition of generalized anxiety disorder as an anxious temperament type. *Acta Psychiatrica Scandinavica*, **98(393)**, 66–73.

Allan, S., & Gilbert, P. (1997). Submissive behaviour and psychopathology. *British Journal of Clinical Psychology*, **36**, 467–488.

Bandura, A., Caprara, G. V., Barbaranelli, C., Gerbino, M., & Pastorelli, C. (2003). Role of affective self-regulatory efficacy in diverse spheres of psychosocial functioning. *Child Development*, **74(3)**, 769–782.

Baumeister, R. F., & Leary, M. R. (1995). The need to belong: desire for interpersonal attachments as a fundamental human motivation. *Psychological Bulletin*, **117(3)**, 497–529.

Berry, J. W., Worthington, E. L., O'Connor, L. E., Parrott, L., & Wade, N. G. (2005). Forgivingness, vengeful rumination, and affective traits. *Journal of Personality*, **73**, 183–226.

Blair, R. J. R. (1997). Moral reasoning and the child with psychopathic tendencies. *Personality and Indifferences*, **22**, 731–739.

Borrello, M. E. (2005). The rise, fall and resurrection of group selection. *Endeavor*, **2(1)**, 43–47.

Bush, C. A., Mullis, R. L., & Mullis, A. K. (2000). Differences in empathy between offender and non-offender youth. *Journal of Youth and Adolescence*, **29**, 467–478.

Caetano, S. C., Hatch, J. P., Brambilla, P., *et al.* (2004). Anatomical MRI study of hippocampus and amygdala in patients with current and remitted major depression. *Psychiatry Research: Neuroimaging*, **132(2)**, 141–147.

Cohn, J. F., Campbell, S. B., Matias, R., & Hopkins, J. (1990). Face-to-face interactions of postpartum depressed and nondepressed mother-infant pairs at 1 months. *Developmental Psychology*, **26**, 15–23.

Cosmides, L., & Tooby, J. (1992). Cognitive adaptations for social exchange. In J. H. Barkow, L. Cosmides & J. Tooby (eds.), *The Adapted Mind: Evolutionary Psychology and the Generation of Culture* (pp. 163–228). Oxford: Oxford University Press.

Crisostomo, P. S., Yi, E., O'Connor, L. E., & Tsai, M. (2005). Cross-cultural studies of empathy based guilt and altruism: differences among European – and Asian American females. *Poster Session at the Annual Meeting of the American Psychological Society*. Los Angeles, Calif.

Davis, M. H. (1980). A multidimensional approach to individual differences in empathy. *Catalog of Selected Documents in Psychology*, **10**, MS. 2124, p. 85.

de Quervain, D. J. F., Fischbacher, U., Treyer, V., *et al.* (2004). The neural basis of altruistic punishment. *Science*, **305(5688)**, 1254–1258.

Decety, J., & Jackson, P. L. (2004). The functional architecture of human empathy. *Behavioral and Cognitive Neuroscience Reviews*, **3(2)**, 71–100.

Drevets, W. C. (2001). Neuroimaging and neuropathological studies of depression: implications for the cognitive-emotional features of mood disorders. *Current Opinion in Neurobiology*, **11**, 240–249.

Eisenberg, N. (2000). Emotion, regulation, and moral development. *Annual Review of Psychology*, **51**, 665–697.

Farrow, T. F. D., Zheng, Y., Wilkinson, I. D., *et al.* (2001). Investigating the functional anatomy of empathy and forgiveness. *NeuroReport*, **12(11)**, 2433–2438.

Fehr, E., & Fischbacher, U. (2003). The nature of human altruism. *Nature*, **425**, 785–791.

Ghorbani, N., Bing, M. N., Watson, P. J., Davison, H. K., & LeBreton, D. L. (2003). Individualist and collectivist values: evidence of compatibility in Iran and the United States. *Personality and Individual Differences*, **35**, 431–447.

Gilbert, P. (1992). *Depression: The Evolution of Powerlessness*. New York: The Guilford Press.

Gilbert, P., & Allan, S. (1994). Assertiveness, submissive behavior, and social comparison. *British Journal of Clinical Psychology*, **33**, 295–306.

Gintis, H., Bowles, S., Boyd, R., & Fehr, E. (2003). Explaining altruistic behavior in humans. *Evolution and Human Behavior*, **24**, 153–172.

Goldapple, K., Segal, Z., Carson, C., *et al.* (2004). Modulation of cortical-limbic pathways in major depression. *Archives of General Psychiatry*, **61**, 34–41.

Greene, J. D., & Haidt, J. (2002). How (and where) does moral judgment work? *Trends in Cognitive Sciences*, **6(12)**, 517–523.

Greene, J. D., Sommerville, R. B., Nystrom, L. E., Darley, J. M., & Cohen, J. D. (2001). An fMRI investigation of emotional engagement in moral judgment. *Science*, **293**, 2105–2108.

Griens, A. M. G. F., Jonker, K., Spinhoven, P., & Blom, M. B. J. (2002). The influence of depressive state features on trait measurement. *Journal of Affective Disorders*, **70**.

Hagen, E. H. (2003). The bargaining model of depression. In P. Hammerstein (ed.), *Genetic and Cultural Evolution of Cooperation. Dahlem Workshop Reports* (pp. 95–124). Cambridge, Mass.: MIT Press.

Hamilton, W. D. (1964). The evolution of social behavior. *Journal of Theoretical Biology*, **7**, 1–52.

Hassin, R. R., Uleman, J. S., & Bargh, J. A. (eds.). (2005). *The New Unconscious*. New York: Oxford University Press.

Hay, D. F., & Pawlby, S. (2003). Prosocial development in relation to children's and mothers' psychological problems. *Child Development*, **74(5)**, 1314–1327.

Heyer, N. J., Echeverria, D., Bittner, A. C., *et al.* (2004). Chronic low-level mercury exposure, BDNF polymorphism, and associations with self-reported symptoms and mood. *Toxicological Sciences*, **81(2)**, 354–363.

Hoffman, M. L. (1975). Developmental synthesis of affect and cognition and its implications for altruistic motivation. *Developmental Psychology*, **11**, 607–622.

Hoffman, M. L. (2000). *Empathy and Moral Development: Implications for Caring and Justice*. Cambridge, UK: Cambridge University Press.

Ingleby, D. (ed.). (2004). *Critical Psychiatry: The Politics of Mental Health*. London: Free Association.

Joireman, J. (2004). Empathy and the self-absorption paradox. II: Self-rumination and self-reflection as mediators between shame, guilt, and empathy. *Self and Identity*, **3**, 225–238.

Jones, W. H., & Kugler, K. E. (1993). Interpersonal correlates of the Guilt Inventory. *Journal of Personality Assessment*, **61(2)**.

Keltner, D., Haidt, J., & Shiota, M. N. (2006). Social functionalism and the evolution of emotions. In M. Schaller, J. A. Simpson, & D. T. Kenrick (eds.), *Evolution and Social Psychology*. Hore: Psychology Press.

Kessler, R. C., Berglund, P., Demler, O., *et al.* (2005). Lifetime prevalence and age-of-onset distributions of DSM-IV disorders in the National Cormorbidity Survey Replication. *Archives of General Psychiatry*, **62(6)**, 593–602.

Kihlstrom, J. F. (1987). The cognitive unconscious. *Science*, **237**, 1445–1452.

Klimes-Dougan, B., & Bolger, A. K. (1998). Coping with maternal depressed affect and depression: adolescent children of depressed and well mothers. *Journal of Youth and Adolescence*, **27(1)**, 1–15.

Lane, J. D., & DePaulo, B. M. (1999). Completing Coyne's cycle: dysphorics' ability to detect deception. *Journal of Research in Personality*, **33**, 311–329.

Lange, C., & Irle, E. (2004). Enlarged amygdala volume and reduced hippocampal volume in young women with major depression. *Psychological Medicine*, **34(6)**.

Leary, M. R. (1983). A brief version of the Fear of Negative Evaluation Scale. *Personality and Social Psychology Bulletin*, **9**, 371–376.

Lewis, T., Amini, F., & Lannon, R. (2000). *A General Theory of Love*. New York: Random House.

MacLean, P. D. (1985). Brain evolution relating to family, play, and the separation call. *Archives of General Psychiatry*, **42**, 405–417.

Martin, G. B., & Clark, III, R. D. (1982). Distress crying in neonates: species and peer specificity. *Developmental Psychology*, **18**, 3–9.

Masters, R. (2001). Biology and politics: linking nature and nurture. *Annual Review of Political Science*, **4**, 345–369.

McGuire, M. T., & Troisi, A. (1987). Physiological regulation-deregulation and psychiatric disorders. *Ethology and Sociobiology*, **8**, 9S–25S.

Meehan, W., O'Connor, L. E., Berry, J. W., *et al.* (1996). Guilt, shame, and depression in clients in recovery from addiction. *Journal of Psychoactive Drugs*, **28**, 125–134.

Modell, A. H. (1971). The origin of certain forms of pre-oedipal guilt and the implications for a psychoanalytic theory of affects. *International Journal of Psychoanalysis*, **52**, 337–346.

Moll, J., de Oliveira-Souza, R., Bramati, I. E., & Grafman, J. (2002a). Functional networks in emotional moral and nonmoral social judgments. *NeuroImage*, **16**, 696–703.

Moll, J., de Oliveira-Souza, R., Eslinger, P. J., *et al.* (2002b). The neural correlates of moral sensitivity: a functional magnetic resonance imaging investigation of basic and moral emotions. *The Journal of Neuroscience*, **22(7)**, 2730–2736.

Murray, R. (2004). Interpersonal guilt and self-defeating behavior of foster youth. Unpublished doctoral dissertation, Wright Institute, Berkeley, Calif.

Neiderland, W. G. (1961). The problem of the survivor. *Journal of Hillside Hospital*, **10**, 233–247.

Nesse, R. M. (2000). Is depression an adaptation? *Archives of General Psychiatry*, **57**, 14–20.

Neumeister, M. D., Charney, D., & Drevets, W. C. (2004). NIMH Mood and Anxiety Disorders Program, and colleagues, report on their positron emission tomography (PET) scan study. From http://www.nih.gov/news/pr/aug2004/nimh-03.htm.

Nolen-Hoeksema, S., Larson, J., & Grayson, C. (1999). Explaining the gender difference in depression. *Journal of Personality and Social Psychology*, **77**, 1061–1072.

O'Connor, L. E. (2000). Pathogenic beliefs and guilt in human evolution: implications for psychotherapy. In P. Gilbert & K. G. Bailey (eds.), *Genes on the Couch: Explorations in Evolutionary Psychology* (pp. 276–303). London: Brunner-Routledge.

O'Connor, L. E., Berry, J. W., Lewis, T., Wilson, & Yi, E. (2005). Neurotransmitter Attributes Questionnaire (NAQ): Personality on the Internet and in the Classroom. Poster presentation, American Psychological Society, May, Los Angeles, Calif.

O'Connor, L. E., Berry, J. W., & Weiss, J. (1999). Interpersonal guilt, shame, and psychological problems. *Journal of Social and Clinical Psychology*, **18**, 181–203.

O'Connor, L. E., Berry, J. W., Weiss, J., Bush, M., & Sampson, H. (1997). Survivor guilt. The development of a new measure. *Journal of Clinical Psychology*, **53(1)**, 73–89.

O'Connor, L. E., Berry, J. W., Weiss, J., & Gilbert, P. (2002). Guilt, fear submission, and empathy in depression. *Journal of Affective Disorders*, **71**, 19–27.

O'Connor, L. E., Berry, J. W., Weiss, J., Schweitzer, D., & Sevier, M. (2000). Survivor guilt, submissive behaviour, and evolutionary theory: the down-side of winning in social comparison. *British Journal of Medical Psychology*, **73**, 519–530.

Pagani, M., Gardner, A., Salmaso, D., *et al.* (2004). Principal component and volume of interest analyses in depressed patients imaged by 99mTc-HMPAO SPET: a methodological comparison. *European Journal of Nuclear Medicine and Molecular Imaging*, **31(7)**, 995–1004.

Preston, S. D., & de Waal, F. B. M. (2002). Empathy: its ultimate and proximate bases. *Behavioral and Brain Sciences*, **25(1)**, 1–72.

Price, J. S. (1967). The dominance hierarchy and the evolution of mental illness. *Lancet* (27 July), 243–246.

Quiles, Z. N., & Bybee, J. (1997). Chronic and predispositional guilt: relations to mental health, prosocial behavior, and religiosity. *Journal of Personality Assessment*, **69**, 104–126.

Radloff, L. S. (1977). The CES-D scale: a self-report depression scale for research in the general population. *Applied Psychology Measures*, **1**, 385–401.

Raleigh, M. J., & McGuire, M. T. (1986). Animal analogues of ostracism: biological mechanisms and social consequences. *Ethology and Sociobiology*, **7**, 201–214.

Richerson, P. J., & Boyd, R. (2004). *Not by Genes Alone: How Culture Transformed Human Evolution*. Chicago: Chicago University Press.

Rosenfield, S., Vertefuille, J., & McAlpine, D. D. (2000). Gender stratification and mental health: an exploration of dimensions of the self. *Social Psychology Quarterly*, **63**, 208–223.

Russo-Neustadt, A., Ha, T., Ramirez, R., & Kesslak, J. P. (2001). Physical activity-antidepressant treatment combination: impact on brain-deprived neurotropic factor and behavior in an animal model. *Behavioural Brain Research*, **120**, 87–95.

Sagi, A., & Hoffman, M. L. (1976). Empathic distress in the newborn. *Developmental Psychology*, **12**, 175–226.

Sen, S., Nesse, R. M., Stoltenberg, S. F., *et al.* (2003). A BDNF coding variant is associated with the NEO Personality Inventory Domain Neuroticism, a risk factor for depression. *Neuropsychopharmacology*, **28**, 397–401.

Shieman, S., & Turner, H. A. (2001). When feeling other people's pain hurts: the influence of psychosocial resources on the association between self-reported empathy and depressive symptoms. *Social Psychology Quarterly*, **64**, 376–389.

Shin, L. M., Dougherty, D. D., Orr, S. P., *et al.* (2000). Activation of the anterior paralimbic structures during guilt-related script-driven imagery. *Society of Biological Psychiatry*, **48**, 43–50.

Sober, E., & Wilson, D. S. (1998). *Unto Others: The Evolution and Psychology of Unselfish Behavior*. Cambridge, Mass.: Harvard University Press.

Strakowski, S. M. (2002). Narrowing and broadening diagnostic criteria for bipolar disorder: competing demands of research and clinical practice. In M. Maj, H. S. Akiskal, J. J. Lopez-Ibor & N. Sartorius (eds.), *Bipolar Disorder* (pp. 57–59). New York: John Wiley & Sons, Ltd.

Tangney, J. P., Wagner, P., & Gramzow, R. (1992). Proneness to shame, proneness to guilt, and psychopathology. *Journal of Abnormal Psychology*, **101(3)**, 469–478.

Tooby, J., & Cosmides, L. (1996). Friendship and the banker's paradox: other pathways to the evolution of adaptations for altruism. *Proceedings of the British Academy*, **88**, 119–143.

Trivers, R. L. (1971). The evolution of reciprocal altruism. *Quarterly Review of Biology*, **46**, 35–57.

Webster, R. G., Berry, J. W., O'Connor, L. E., Mulherin, K., & Weiss, J. (1997). Interpersonal guilt, envy, and jealousy in sibling childhood relationships. Unpublished manuscript.

Weiss, J. (1993). *How Psychotherapy Works: Process and Technique*. New York: Guilford Press.

Weiss, J., Sampson, H., & Mount Zion Psychotherapy Research Group (1986). *The psychoanalytic Process: Theory, Clinical Observation and Empirical Research*. New York: Guilford Press.

Westen, D. (1998). The scientific legacy of Sigmund Freud: toward a psychodynamically informed psychological science. *Psychological Bulletin*, **124(3)**, 333–371.

Wilson, D. S. (1975). A theory of group selection. *Proceedings of the National Academy of Sciences*, **72**, 143–146.

Zahn-Waxler, C. (2000). The development of empathy, guilt, and internalization of distress: implications for gender differences in internalizing and externalizing problems. In R. J. Davidson (ed.), *Anxiety, Depression, and Emotion*. New York: Oxford University Press.

Zahn-Waxler, C., Radke-Yarrow, M., & King, R. A. (1979). Child rearing and children's prosocial initiations towards victims of distress. *Child Development*, **50**, 319–330.

Empathy, social intelligence and aggression in adolescent boys and girls

Kaj Björkqvist

Department of Social Sciences, Åbo Akademi University

5.1 Introduction

My first insight into the possibility of a negative relationship between empathy and aggressiveness dates back to the early 1980s, when I was conducting research on the effects of violent film viewing on subsequent aggressive behaviour in children. There is good evidence that violent films indeed increase aggressive behaviour, at least among some viewers, and especially so if the viewer identifies with an aggressive hero (cf. Huesmann & Eron, 1986). However, in my readings of the research literature, I came across a few reports (e.g. Baron, 1971; Hartman, 1969; see also Bramel *et al.*, 1968) in which violent films actually *reduced* the aggressiveness of viewers. In these cases, empathy towards the victim appears to have been the crucial intervening variable. In these films, pain cues of victims of violence were presented in a way that awakened feelings of empathy, and the viewer identified with the victim rather than with the perpetrator of aggression. Such films are regrettably few, however, within the violent film entertainment business. In my own research (Björkqvist, 1985), I found that film violence presented in a humorous way, making the viewer laugh at the victim, increased the aggressiveness of viewers more than realistic presentation of violence did. In films with a humorous aggressive content, the victim is objectified and dehumanized, and empathy is reduced. Also Feshbach (1988) suggests that regular television is not likely to increase empathy, rather the opposite. Violent films typically portray the villain of the plot in very negative terms, in order to make the viewers dislike him; thus, the violence directed by the hero towards the villain appears justified.

However, I did not pursue the investigation of the negative relationship between empathy and aggression further at that point. Instead, my focus of interest turned to aggressive behaviour among children in school settings and, in particular, the

Empathy in Mental Illness, eds. Tom F. D. Farrow and Peter W. R. Woodruff. Published by Cambridge University Press. © Cambridge University Press 2007.

phenomenon of indirect aggression and sex differences with respect to this type of aggression. These studies suggested that social intelligence was a necessary pre-requisite for indirect aggression and, in order to understand and study the role of social intelligence in this respect, it became important to separate out empathy from social intelligence, since empathy seemed to inhibit aggression. The circle was closed, and it became necessary to study the role and impact of empathy in aggression as well as in peaceful means of problem solving.

5.2 Sex differences in indirect aggression

In the latter part of the 1980s, our research group in Finland, consisting mainly of Kirsti Lagerspetz, Karin Österman, Ari Kaukiainen and myself, had become increasingly dissatisfied with the general conception of that time that girls and females were non-aggressive – to a point that even a leading researcher on school bullying, Dan Olweus, suggested that bullying among girls was so rare that it was not worth studying (Olweus, 1978). We collected interview data, suggesting that girls indeed bullied and were quite aggressive towards each other, but they were so in different ways than boys: they tended to use non-physical, indirect means of aggression, such as malicious gossiping, 'bitching', etc. We labelled this type indirect aggression, and defined it as social manipulation, attacking the target circuitously. We decided to examine the phenomenon by quantitative means, using the peer estimation paradigm, since many forms of interpersonal aggression will simply go unnoticed if only self reports or beha-vioural observations are used (for a review of the development of peer estimations in aggression research, see Björkqvist et al., 1992c). Through a series of studies, an instrument based on peer estimations was developed, by which it was possible to distinguish between three types of aggression: physical, verbal and indirect aggression. It was called the Direct & Indirect Aggression Scales (DIAS) (Björkqvist et al., 1992b). We found as predicted that girls in Finland indeed exceeded boys in indirect aggression (e.g. Björkqvist, 1992; Björkqvist et al., 1992a, 1992c; Lagerspetz et al., 1988). Österman et al. (1994) replicated the findings in Israel, Italy and Poland with the same methodology. Owen (1996), in turn, replicated the study in Australia, applying DIAS in a version based on self-estimations; the findings were similar. Rivers and Smith (1994) found that British girls exceed British boys in indirect bullying in schools. Crick (1995), using corresponding items as those of DIAS, made similar findings with a North American sample, although she referred to the phenomenon as relational aggres-sion. A female preference for indirect aggression has been found not only among adolescents, but also among adults. Fry and Hines (1993) found adult women in Argentina to use indirect aggression more than males, and Björkqvist et al.

(1994) found adult women in Finland to apply more covert strategies than males in workplace conflicts.

Accordingly, there is now a substantial body of research indicating that females of different ages indeed use indirect means of aggression to a significantly greater extent than males. Females also prefer to induce psychological rather than physical harm to their opponents (Hyde, 1984).

There may be multiple reasons for this sex difference in human aggressive behaviour. It has been suggested (Lagerspetz et al., 1988) that differences in the structure of friendship groups formed by adolescent boys and girls, respectively, facilitate the growth of the observed sex difference. While boys socialize in large groups with loose boundaries, girls prefer small, tight friendship groups, typically dyads, i.e. having a close best friend. They discuss emotions and relations more than adolescent boys do and they use 'she said . . . and then he said . . .' expressions frequently. This specific friendship pattern is likely to be fertile soil for the development of indirect, socially manipulative aggressive strategies.

In accordance with another line of thinking, individual differences in power and skills – not only physical strength, but also mental faculties – influence the choice of aggressive strategy. Björkqvist et al. (1994) suggested that a principle which we referred to as the effect/danger ratio may be in operation, and that each individual (when controlled enough to behave rationally) learns to apply conflict strategies having the most advantageous ratio in his/her particular case. Since males are physically stronger than females, they are more likely to apply physical means, which are more effective and less dangerous for them than for females. Reviews also agree on the fact that males in general are physically more aggressive than females (e.g. Björkqvist & Niemelä, 1992; Frodi et al., 1977; Hyde, 1984). In regard to direct verbal aggression, some authors report greater frequency among boys than among girls (e.g. Whiting & Edwards, 1973), while others find no sex differ-ence (e.g. Björkqvist et al., 1992a) or slight variation due to culture or age (Österman et al., 1994). Frodi et al. (1977), reviewing 26 studies, came to the conclusion that no sex difference could be discerned in 16 of them, while males were more aggressive in a direct verbal way in 9 studies, and females in 1. The review by Hyde (1984) is inconclusive. That is, the majority of studies do not report a sex difference with respect to verbal aggression, and when a sex difference is found, it usually indicates higher scores of direct verbal aggression among males. This relatively minor sex difference is understandable in the light that males and females, according to recent reviews (e.g. Hyde 1990), are equals with respect to verbal intelligence. If males have a slight edge in direct verbal aggression, this circumstance may be explained by the fact that, due to their greater physical strength, verbal threats from their part may appear more credible and frightening than similar threats by females.

5.3 Indirect aggression and social intelligence

Björkqvíst *et al.* (1992a, 1992c) suggested a developmental theory in regard to styles of aggressive behaviour: physical, direct verbal and indirect aggression are not only three different strategies, but they also constitute three developmental phases, partly following, partly overlapping each other during childhood and adolescence. Small children, who have not yet developed verbal and social skills to any considerable degree, will have to resort to physical aggression. In this respect, they are like members of subhuman species, who do not possess a language. When verbal and social skills develop, these facilitate the expression of aggression without having to resort to physical force. When social intelligence develops sufficiently, the individual is fully capable of indirect aggressive behaviour: s/he is able to induce psychological, sometimes even physical, harm to a target person by mere social manipulation, without putting him/herself at direct risk of retaliation. A consequence of the theory is that social intelligence should be expected to correlate more with indirect than with direct forms of aggression, since indirect aggression by definition requires skills at social manipulation.

The concept of social intelligence was coined as early as 1920 (Thorndike 1920, p. 228). However, Thorndike was not able to verify the existence of such a domain of intelligence through psychometric studies (Thorndike & Stein, 1937), and the concept fell into oblivion. Half a century later, a renewed interest in social intelligence emerged, with most authors claiming that there is, indeed, evidence for the existence of this domain (e.g. Cantor & Kihlstrom, 1989; Ford & Tisak, 1983), with others being critical (e.g. Keating, 1978). Social intelligence has a connotation closely related to concepts such as social skills and competence. Emotional intelligence (Goleman, 1995) clearly is a partly overlapping concept, and interpersonal intelligence (Hatch & Gardner, 1993) another. Social intelligence has a perceptual, a cognitive-analytical and a behavioural (skills) component. Cleverness in analysing the social behaviour of others is central and, reciprocally, so is the ability to recognize motives and cognitive traps of one's own. Furthermore, the socially intelligent individual is capable of perpetrating adequate behaviour for the purpose of achieving desired social goals. As far as goals with respect to conflicts are concerned, these may be hostile, but also aiming at peaceful resolution of conflicts. Social intelligence should be an asset in conflict situations, whether the individual chooses to be aggressive or peaceful. The choice between these two types of conflict behaviour is, for the socially intelligent individual, optional.

Levels of peer-estimated conflict are, among adolescents, optimal at ages 11–12 (Björkqvist *et al.*, 1992a; Österman *et al.*, 1997). Österman *et al.* (1997) suggest this fact to be related to the circumstance that adolescents of this age are transiting from level 3 to level 4, according to Selman's (1980) stage theory of socio-cognitive development: not only are adolescents of this age able to take a third-person, mutual perspective in dyadic social interaction, but they are also reaching a level at which they are mentally able to step outside of the situation altogether, looking at it with a societal-symbolic perspective. According to Flavell's (1979) somewhat similar stage theory, adolescents of this age reach level C of meta-cognition: 'I know that you know that I know'. This particular age period (11–12 years) appears to be one of intensive small group interaction; the individual learns about both immediate and symbolic implications of different behaviours in conflict situations, and girls appear to develop socially somewhat faster than boys, at this age (Cohn, 1991).

Not only do girls exceed boys in indirect aggression, but they are also better at peaceful interpersonal conflict resolution (Österman *et al.*, 1997). Both types of conflict behaviour require a relatively high degree of social intelligence. Females have been shown to be better than males at both decoding and encoding of non-verbal signals (Hall, 1978, 1990; Hyde, 1990). According to Cohn (1991), girls mature socially faster than boys, but the difference declines by age. If adolescent girls are socially more competent than boys, these skills may be utilized for both aggressive and peaceful purposes. This finding may contribute to the explanation of why adolescent girls exceed boys in both indirect aggression and peaceful conflict resolution (Österman *et al.*, 1997).

Social intelligence has mostly been measured by self-reports, such as the Six Factors Test of Social Intelligence (O'Sullivan & Guilford, 1966). The validity of self-reports is always somewhat questionable if the measured ability or trait is clearly socially either desirable (such as social intelligence) or undesirable (such as aggression) and, accordingly, peer-estimated measures are recommended in such cases. There are few peer-estimated measures of social intelligence; Ford and Tisak (1983) included a peer *nomination* measure (which is not the same as peer estimations, in a strict sense) in their test battery. In order to cover this lack, our research team (Kaukiainen *et al.*, 1995b) developed an instrument labelled *Peer-Estimated Social Intelligence* (PESI).

5.4 Social intelligence and empathy

In the literature published to date, it has been taken more or less for granted that empathy constitutes an integral part of social intelligence, and that the two are overlapping concepts, difficult to separate from each other. For instance, Ford and Tisak (1983) chose Hogan's (1969) Empathy Scale as one of six measures of social intelligence in their test battery. However, the ability to feel empathy is at least logically distinct from social intelligence, although the two are likely to correlate significantly.

Levels of empathy have usually been assessed by self-reports, projective methods, experimental procedures, or the recording and interpretation of non-verbal signals (Miller & Eisenberg, 1988). Our research group (Kaukiainen *et al.*, 1995a) developed the first instrument intended to measure empathy by use of peer estimations, *Peer-Estimated Empathy* (PEE).

For the sake of investigating their relationship to aggression, it is meaningful to make a distinction between empathy and social intelligence, not only conceptually but also at the level of operationalization. When we factor-analysed the items of PEE and PESI, i.e. peer-estimated measures of empathy and social intelligence, we found that the concepts clustered into two separate factors as predicted.

The concept of empathy was introduced into North American psychology by Titchener (1909), who received part of his training in Germany. The German notion of *Eingefühlung* was translated into empathy, and *Mitgefühlung* into sympathy (for a discussion of the history of the concept, see Wispe, 1987). Empathy and sympathy are not identical, although sympathy is the common consequence of empathy. While empathy is the sharing of the perceived emotion of another, sympathy mirrors the willingness to alleviate the sufferings of another (Eisenberg & Miller, 1987). However, in the literature, these two terms have been used as almost interchangeable concepts.

There are both affective and cognitive aspects to empathy. According to Feshbach and Feshbach (1982), empathy comprises three essential components: (1) perception and discrimination, i.e. the ability to use relevant information in order to recognize, identify and label emotions; (2) perspective and role taking, i.e. the ability to assume and experience another's viewpoint; and (3) emotional responsiveness, i.e. the ability to share another's feelings. Empathy increases with age, with the exception of puberty, and girls are, in general, more empathic than boys (Lennon & Eisenberg, 1987).

5.5 Relationships between social intelligence, empathy and conflict behaviour

Kaukainen *et al.* (1994, 1996) investigated whether social intelligence was related to the use of indirect aggression, while empathy was predicted to mitigate such behaviour. Social intelligence was measured by peer estimations (PESI); empathy, on the other hand, was measured by self estimations – PEE had not been constructed at the time of data collection. The findings suggested evidence in support of the hypothesis. The results encouraged a study in which all variables would be measured by peer estimations, and PEE was developed for this very purpose. The findings of the new study (Kaukiainen *et al.*, 1999) corroborated the hypothesis.

One may ask how social intelligence and empathy relate not only to indirect aggression, but to a variety of forms of conflict behaviour, prosocial as well as antisocial. This issue was investigated by Björkqvist, Österman, & Kaukiainen (1992c). PESI, PEE and DIAS were used as measures, and 203 adolescents (mean age = 12 years, SD = 0.8) participated in the study. The Cronbach's α-scores of the different measures were as follows: *social intelligence*, 0.95; *empathy*, 0.96; *physical aggression*, 0.96; *verbal aggression*, 0.94; *indirect aggression*, 0.97; *peaceful conflict resolution*, 0.86; and *withdrawal from conflicts*, 0.73. The relationships between the measures are summarized in Tables 5.1 and 5.2.

As shown in Table 5.1, social intelligence correlates significantly with all forms of conflict behaviour, aggressive as well as peaceful. Starting with the bivariate correlations, it is noteworthy that the correlation between social intelligence and the various types of aggressive behaviour is strongest in the case of indirect

Table 5.1: Bivariate and partial correlations (empathy partialed out) between Peer-Estimated Social Intelligence and different types of conflict behaviour (n = 203; ♀ = 110, ♂ = 93)

	Social intelligence	
	Bivariate correlations	Partial correlations (empathy controlled)
Indirect aggression	0.55***	0.65***
Verbal aggression	0.39***	0.54***
Physical aggression	0.22**	0.38***
Peaceful conflict resolution	0.80***	0.51***
Withdrawal	0.48***	0.23***

$p < 0.05$, **$p < 0.01$, ***$p < 0.001$

Table 5.2: Bivariate and partial correlations (social intelligence partialed out) between Peer-Estimated Empathy and different types of conflict behaviour (n = 203; ♀ = 110, ♂ = 93)

	Empathy	
	Bivariate correlations	Partial correlations (social intelligence controlled)
Indirect aggression	0.15*	−0.45***
Verbal aggression	0.05	−0.40***
Physical aggression	−0.04	−0.32***
Peaceful conflict resolution	0.80***	0.51***
Withdrawal	0.47***	0.18**

*$p < 0.05$, **$p < 0.01$, ***$p < 0.001$

aggression, weaker in the case of verbal aggression and weakest in the case of physical aggression. The correlation coefficient with peaceful conflict resolution is larger than any other.

When empathy is partialed out, correlations pertaining to indirect, verbal and physical aggression increase, while correlations with peaceful conflict resolution and withdrawal decrease (see Table 5.1).

Empathy, on the other hand, correlates strongly with peaceful conflict resolution and withdrawal, but not significantly with verbal or physical aggression, and only weakly with indirect aggression. When social intelligence is partialed out, correlations with the various types of aggression turn significantly negative, while correlations with peaceful conflict resolution and withdrawal decrease (see Table 5.2).

Social intelligence, thus, is required for aggressive as well as for peaceful conflict behaviour, but empathy clearly reduces aggression. Social intelligence (without controlling for empathy) correlates with the various types of conflict behaviour in the following order: (1) peaceful means of conflict resolution, (2) indirect aggression, (3) withdrawal, (4) verbal aggression and (5) physical aggression. The order is most likely no coincidence – the various types of conflict behaviour are ordered in accordance with how 'safe' they are. This circumstance suggests that socially intelligent individuals choose methods which expose them to as little direct danger as possible. Solving conflict peacefully is the least dangerous, and also the most advantageous method; it has the best effect/danger ratio. Peaceful conflict resolution de-escalates aggression and, thereby, reduces risks of future harm. Indirect aggression may have advantages, but it also encompasses risks and may escalate conflict. Withdrawal is a strategy including little effect, but also little danger. And, direct verbal and, especially, physical aggression involve risks.

With respect to the three types of aggression, social intelligence correlates most strongly with indirect aggression, somewhat weaker with verbal aggression and weakest with physical aggression. This fact is in line with the developmental theory suggested by Björkqvist *et al.* (1992a, 1992c), according to which indirect aggression requires more social intelligence than direct verbal aggression, which, in turn, requires more intelligence than physical aggression.

5.6 Empathy training as an inhibitor of aggression

Our studies of the negative relationship between empathy and aggression have been correlational ones. Richardson *et al.* (1994) reported three other studies in which empathy was negatively related to aggression. However, there are also studies which more directly show empathy to be an inhibitor of aggression; such as the meta-analysis by Miller and Eisenberg (1988), suggesting empathy to inhibit and mitigate aggressive behaviour. Accordingly, it is logical to suggest that empathy training may be a valuable tool to reduce aggression in school settings. The first one to develop empathy training techniques aimed at school children was Norma Feshbach of UCLA (e.g. Feshbach & Feshbach, 1982; Feshbach, 1989), who developed the so-called Empathy Slide Series. Empathy training may encompass the presentation of slides or films in which violence is not glorified, but the viewer identifies with the victim rather than with the aggressor, and negative consequences of aggression are presented clearly. A variant of this theme, reported by Björkqvist and Österman (1999), was the victim slide show by Timo Nuutinen, a male nurse at a Finnish polyclinic, who was shocked to find how frequently young victims of other adolescents' violent behaviour were admitted, and how easily severe injuries were inflicted: tripping a victim in the school yard, a snowball aimed at the eyes, or a single blow to the nose. Seemingly harmless bullying often caused broken teeth, damaged eyes, broken noses, concussion of the brain or even irreversible brain damage. He compiled a slide show, presenting photographs and radiographs of real-life cases of injured young victims. The slides were quite shocking. He presented this slide show to pupils in schools, accompanied by descriptions of how the injuries were produced. The slide show became very popular all over the nation, and we evaluated it (Björkqvist & Österman, 1999), finding it to have both short- and long-term (according to a 5-month follow-up assessment) effects. Another successful empathy training project conducted in Finland, among preschoolers, was reported by Kalliopuska and Tiitinen (1991). Their training included role-playing, acting and storytelling. Role play is perhaps the most common technique of empathy training today.

Feshbach and Feshbach (1982) conducted a field experiment with 98 aggressive and non-aggressive third to fourth graders who participated in empathy training, a problem-solving control activity, or a no-intervention control condition. The results indicated that the empathy training helped bring about more positive social behaviours and a more positive self-evaluation in both aggressive and non-aggressive children.

Two Chinese studies also report the usefulness of empathy training. Li (1990) found empathy training to increase prosocial behaviour in 12- to 16-year-old adolescents, and Wei and Li (2001) found that empathy training increased sharing behaviour among 5- to 9-year-old children. Pecukonis (1990) has reported the usefulness of empathy training among 14- to 17-year-old aggressive females in a residential treatment centre. He combined the empathy training with cognitive training, a combination which is quite common in treatment programmes. For instance the Aggression Replacement Training (ART) developed by Arnold Goldstein combines cognitive techniques with the teaching of impulse control and moral reasoning. The latter aims not only at moral understanding, but also at increasing empathy towards one's enemies. ART has been shown to be quite effective in reducing aggression (Goldstein, 1999).

Conclusively, empathy appears to be a mitigator and in the best cases an inhibitor of aggression. It would probably be going too far to claim empathy to be the opposite of aggressiveness; they are after all two different traits, and an empathic individual may of course be aggressive in certain situations. But the capacity to understand and feel how a potential victim of one's own aggression may suffer is in most cases likely to create enough sympathy for the victim to stop the aggressive encounter before it has even started. Since empathy mitigates interpersonal aggression, empathy training is likely to be a useful contribution to programmes aiming at reducing aggression in children and adolescents.

REFERENCES

Baron, R. A. (1971). Aggression as a function of magnitude of victim's pain cues, level of prior anger arousal, and aggressor-victim similarity. *Journal of Personality and Social Psychology*, **18**, 48–54.

Björkqvist, K. (1985). *Violent Films, Anxiety, and Aggression*. Helsinki, Finland: Commentationes Scientiarium Socialum.

Björkqvist, K. (1992). Sex differences in physical, verbal, and indirect aggression: a review of recent research. *Sex Roles*, **30**, 177–188.

Björkqvist, K., Lagerspetz, K. M. J., & Kaukiainen, A. (1992a). Do girls manipulate and boys fight? Developmental trends regarding direct and indirect aggression. *Aggressive Behaviour*, **18**, 117–127.

Björkqvist, K., Lagerspetz, K. M. J., & Österman, K. (1992b). *The Direct & Indirect Aggression Scales*. Vasa, Finland: Department of Social Sciences, Åbo Akademi University.

Björkqvist, K., & Niemelä, P. (1992). New trends in the study of female aggression. In K. Björkqvist & P. Niemelä (eds.), *Of Mice and Women: Aspects of Female Aggression* (pp. 3–16). San Diego, Calif.: Academic Press.

Björkqvist, K., & Österman, K. (1999). Finland. In P. K. Smith, Y. Morita, J. Junger-Tas, D. Olweus, R. Catalano & P. Slee (eds.), *The Nature of School Bullying: A Cross-National Perspective* (pp. 56–67). London: Routledge.

Björkqvist, K., Österman, K., & Kaukiainen, A. (1992c). The development of direct and indirect aggressive strategies in males and females. In K. Björkqvist & P. Niemelä (eds.), *Of Mice and Women: Aspects of Female Aggression* (pp. 51–64). San Diego, Calif.: Academic Press.

Björkqvist, K., Österman, K., & Lagerspetz, K. M. J. (1994). Sex differences in covert aggression among adults. *Aggressive Behavior*, **20**, 27–33.

Bramel, D., Taub, B., & Blum, B. (1968). An observer's reaction to the suffering of his enemy. *Journal of Personality and Social Psychology*, **8**, 384–392.

Cantor, N., & Kihlstrom, J. F. (1989). Social intelligence and cognitive assessments of personality. In R. S. Wyer, Jr., & T. K. Srull (eds.), *Social Intelligence and Cognitive Assessments of Personality. Advances in Social Cognition* (Vol. 2) (pp. 1–59). Hillsdale, N.J.: Lawrence Erlbaum.

Cohn, L. D. (1991). Sex differences in the course of personality development: A meta-analysis. *Psychological Bulletin*, **109**, 252–266.

Crick, N. R. (1995). Relational aggression: the role of intent attributions, feelings of distress, and provocation type. *Development and Psychopathology*, **7**, 313–322.

Eisenberg, N., & Miller, P. A. (1987). Empathy, sympathy, and altruism: empirical and conceptual links. In N. Eisenberg, & J. Strayer (eds.), *Empathy and its Development. Cambridge Studies in Social and Emotional Development* (pp. 292–316). New York: Cambridge University Press.

Feshbach, N. D. (1988). Television and the development of empathy. In S. Oskamp (ed.), *Television as a Social Issue. Applied Social Psychology Annual* (Vol. 8) (pp. 261–269). Beverly Hills, Calif.: Sage.

Feshbach, N. D. (1989). Empathy training and prosocial behaviour. In J. Groebel, & R. A. Hinde (eds.), *Aggression and War: Their Biological and Social Bases* (pp. 101–111). Cambridge, UK: Cambridge University Press.

Feshbach, N. D., & Feshbach, S. (1982). *Learning to Care*. San Francisco, Calif.: Scott, Foresman & Co.

Flavell, J. H. (1979). Metacognitive development and cognitive monitoring: a new area of cognitive development inquiry. *American Psychologist*, **34**, 906–911.

Ford, M. E., & Tisak, M. S. (1983). A further search for social intelligence. *Journal of Educational Psychology*, **75**, 196–206.

Frodi, A., Macaulay, J., & Thome, P. R. (1977). Are women always less aggressive than men? *Psychological Bulletin*, **84**, 634–660.

Fry, D. P., & Hines, N. (1993, July). Sex differences in indirect and direct aggression in Argentina. Paper presented at the 3rd European Congress of Psychology, Tampere, Finland.

Goldstein, A. (1999). Aggression reduction strategies: effective and ineffective. *School Psychology Quarterly*, **14**, 40–58.

Goleman, D. (1995). *Emotional Intelligence*. New York: Bantam Books.

Hall, J. A. (1978). Gender effects in decoding nonverbal cues. *Psychological Bulletin*, **85**, 845–857.

Hall, J. A. (1990). *Nonverbal Sex Differences: Accuracy of Communication and Expressive Style*. Baltimore, Md.: Johns Hopkins University Press.

Hartman, D. P. (1969). Influence of symbolically modelled instrumental aggression and pain cues on aggressive behaviour. *Journal of Personality and Social Psychology*, **11**, 280–288.

Hatch, T., & Gardner, H. (1993). Finding cognition in the classroom: an expanded view of human intelligence. In G. Salomon (ed.), *Distributed Cognitions: Psychological and Educational Considerations. Learning in Doing: Social, Cognitive, and Computational Perspectives* (pp. 164–187). New York: Cambridge University Press.

Hogan, R. (1969). Development of an empathy scale. *Journal of Consulting and Clinical Psychology*, **33**, 307–316.

Huesmann, L. R., & Eron, L. D. (eds.) (1986). *Television and the Aggressive Child: A Cross-National Comparison*. Hillsdale, N.J.: Lawrence Erlbaum.

Hyde, J. S. (1984). How large are gender differences in aggression? A developmental meta-analysis. *Developmental Psychology*, **20**, 722–736.

Hyde, J. S. (1990). Meta-analysis and the psychology of sex differences. *Signs*, **16**, 55–73.

Kalliopuska, M., & Tiitinen, U. (1991). Influence of two developmental programmes on the empathy and prosociability of preschool children. *Perceptual and Motor Skills*, **72**, 323–328.

Kaukiainen, A., Björkqvist, K., Lagerspetz, K. M. J., *et al.* (1999). The relationships between social intelligence, empathy, and three types of aggression. *Aggressive Behavior*, **25**, 81–89.

Kaukiainen, A., Björkqvist, K., Österman, K., & Lagerspetz, K. M. J. (1996). Social intelligence and empathy as antecedents of different types of aggression. In C. F. Ferris & T. Grisson (eds.), *Understanding Aggressive Behaviour in Children. Annals of the New York Academy of Sciences*, **794**, 364–366.

Kaukiainen, A., Björkqvist, K., Österman, K., Lagerspetz, K. M. J., & Forsblom, S. (1995a). *Peer-Estimated Empathy (PEE)*. Turku, Finland: Department of Psychology, University of Turku.

Kaukiainen, A., Björkqvist, K., Österman, K., Lagerspetz, K. M. J., & Forsblom, S. (1995b). *Peer-Estimated Social Intelligence (PESI)*. Turku, Finland: Department of Psychology, University of Turku.

Kaukiainen, A., Björkqvist, K., Österman, K., Lagerspetz, K. M. J., & Niskanen, L. (1994). Social intelligence and the use of indirect aggression. Presented at the XIII Biennal Meetings of the International Society for the Study of Behavioural Development, June 28 to July 2, Amsterdam, The Netherlands.

Keating, D. P. (1978). A search for social intelligence. *Journal of Educational Psychology*, **70**, 218–233.

Lagerspetz, K. M. J., Björkqvist, K., & Peltonen, T. (1988). Is indirect aggression typical of females? Gender differences in 11- to 12-year old children. *Aggressive Behaviour*, **14**, 403–414.

Lennon, R., & Eisenberg, N. (1987). Gender and age differences in empathy and sympathy. In N. Eisenberg, & J. Strayer (eds.), *Empathy and its Development. Cambridge Studies in Social and Developmental Development* (pp. 195–217). New York: Cambridge University Press.

Li, L. (1990). The relationship between empathy and prosocial behavior in adolescents. *Acta Psychologica Sinica*, **22**, 72–79.

Miller, P. A., & Eisenberg, N. (1988). The relationship of empathy to aggressive and externalising/antisocial behaviour. *Psychological Bulletin*, **103**, 324–344.

Olweus, D. (1978). *Aggression in the Schools: Bullies and Whipping Boys*. New York: John Wiley.

Österman, K., Björkqvist, K., Lagerspetz, K. M. J., *et al.* (1994). Peer and self estimated aggression in 8-year old children from five ethnic groups. *Aggressive Behavior*, **20**, 411–428.

Österman, K., Björkqvist, K., & Lagerspetz, K. M. J., with Kaukianen, A., Landau, S. F., Fraczek, A., & Pastorelli, C. (1997). Sex differences in styles of conflict resolution: a developmental and cross-cultural study with data from Finland, Israel, Italy, and Poland. In D. P. Fry, & K. Björkqvist (eds.), *Cultural Variation in Conflict Resolution: Alternatives to Violence* (pp. 185–197). Mahwah, N.J.: Lawrence Erlbaum.

O'Sullivan, M., & Guilford, J. P. (1966). *Six Factors Test of Social Intelligence: Manual of Instructions and Interpretations*. Beverly Hills, Calif.: Sheridan Psychological Services.

Owen, L. D. (1996). Sticks and stones and sugar and spice: girls' and boys' aggression in schools. *Australian Journal of Guidance and Counselling*, **6**, 45–55.

Pecukonis, E. D. (1990). A cognitive/affective empathy training program as a function of ego-development in aggressive adolescent females. *Adolescence*, **25**, 59–76.

Richardson, R., Hammock, G. S., Smith, S. M., Gardner, W., & Signo, M. (1994). Empathy as a cognitive inhibitor of interpersonal aggression. *Aggressive Behavior*, **20**, 275–289.

Rivers, I., & Smith, P. K. (1994). Types of bullying behaviour and their correlates. *Aggressive Behaviour*, **20**, 359–368.

Selman, R. (1980). *The Growth of Interpersonal Understanding*. Orlando, Fla.: Academic Press.

Titchener, E. (1909). *Experimental Psychology of Thought Processes*. New York: MacMillan.

Thorndike, E. L. (1920). Intelligence and its use. *Harper's Magazine*, **140**, 227–235.

Thorndike, E. L., & Stein, S. (1937). An evaluation of the attempts to measure social intelligence. *Psychological Bulletin*, **34**, 275–285.

Wei, Y., & Li, Y. (2001). The experimental research on the influence of different empathy training methods on children's sharing behavior. *Psychological Science (China)*, **24**, 557–562.

Whiting, B., & Edwards, C. P. (1973). Cross-cultural analysis of sex differences in the behaviour of children aged three to eleven. *Journal of Social Psychology*, **91**, 171–188.

Wispe. L. (1987). History of the concept of empathy. In N. Eisenberg, & J. Strayer (eds.), *Empathy and its Development. Cambridge Studies in Social and Developmental Development* (pp. 17–37). New York: Cambridge University Press.

Impaired empathy following ventromedial prefrontal brain damage

Simone G. Shamay-Tsoory

Department of Psychology, University of Haifa

6.1 Introduction

The study of the neurobiological bases of social cognition is currently one of the most prominent areas of research in behavioural neurology and in neuropsychology. Similar to many other areas of contemporary neuropsychological research, it was first characterized by single case reports of patients suffering from brain damage. One of the first descriptions of impaired social cognition following brain damage was provided by Harlow (1868). In his famous case report, Harlow portrays the case of Phineas Gage, a railroad employee, who suffered severe frontal lobe injury due to an iron bar that penetrated his frontal lobes. Although he survived, recovered physically and had many preserved cognitive abilities, his social behaviour was so impaired that his acquaintances said he was 'no longer Gage'. Harlow does not refer directly to Gage's empathic ability yet he describes him as '. . . fitful, irreverent, indulging at times in the grossest profanity, manifesting but little deference for his fellow . . .' (Harlow, 1868). In the following years, similar clinical reports have offered accumulating evidence regarding the role of the frontal lobes in emotions and behaviour regulation, and the past 10 years have seen tremendous resurgence of interest in this area. Studies have consistently suggested that acquired damage to the prefrontal cortex may result in severe impairment in interpersonal behaviour (Damasio et al., 1991; Mesulam, 1985; Stuss and Benson, 1986; Stuss et al., 2001). In particular, damage to the ventral prefrontal cortex (PFC) has been associated with misinterpretation of social situations and socially inappropriate behaviour (Rolls, 1996). This chapter provides an overview of the research on empathy and the ventromedial (VM) PFC as well as an orientation to the major theoretical frameworks aimed at accounting for impaired social cognition following frontal brain lesions. The first section of the chapter will briefly discuss the neuroanatomy of the VM PFC. The second

Empathy in Mental Illness, eds. Tom F. D. Farrow and Peter W. R. Woodruff. Published by Cambridge University Press. © Cambridge University Press 2007.

section will then present several lesion studies that examined directly the relationship between VM damage and impaired empathy. In addition, related studies of impaired Theory of Mind following PFC damage will be outlined. The third section will provide an overview of some of the leading theories concerning the role of the VM cortex in social cognition. The final section will attempt to bridge the gaps between the various accounts of the social-behavioural disturbances observed following PFC damage, and will lay the groundwork for an integrative view of the neuroanatomy of empathy.

6.2 The anatomy of the ventromedial prefrontal cortex

The frontal lobes are the anterior portion of the cerebral cortex in front of the central sulcus. The posterior of the frontal lobe consists of the premotor and motor areas. The area between the central and the precentral sulci is primary motor cortex (Brodmann area 4). Anterior to the motor area is the premotor cortex and the supplementary motor area (SMA), both subregions of Brodmann area 6 that have a major part in the modification of movement. The PFC is the area located anterior to the SMA and the premotor areas.

Alexander *et al.* (1986) described a parallel organization of functionally segregated circuits linking basal ganglia and cortex in five frontal-subcortical circuits. Two of the circuits are associated with motor activity and three subserve cognitive and emotional functions. Each of the circuits involves the same member structures including the frontal lobe, striatum, globus pallidus, substantia nigra and thalamus.

According to Alexander *et al.* (1986), the circuits associated with cognitive and emotional functions are the dorsolateral (DLC), the orbitofrontal (OFC) and the medial circuits (Figure 6.1).

The OFC lies superior to the orbit of the eyes. This area plays an important role in emotional behaviour. The OFC receives direct inputs from the dorsomedial thalamus, temporal cortex, ventral tegmental area, olfactory system and the amygdala. Its outputs go to several brain regions, including the cingulate cortex, hippocampal formation, temporal cortex, lateral hypothalamus and amygdala. Behaviourally, the OFC is involved in emotion regulation, inhibition of behaviour, decision-making and rewards learning. Its communication with other regions of the frontal cortex provides it with information about what is happening in the environment and what plans are being made by the rest of the frontal lobes. Its output permits it to affect a variety of behaviours and physiological responses, including emotional responses organized by the amygdala. Lesions in OFC have been reported to lead to impulsive and inappropriate behaviour (Berlin *et al.*, 2004), impaired reversal learning (Rolls, 1996), personality changes (Stuss &

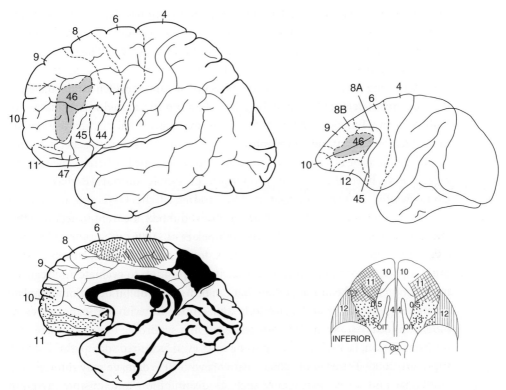

Figure 6.1.   Cytoarchitectonic areas of human brain (Brodmann, 1909) and the frontal lobes of a Rhesus monkey (From Goldman-Rakic, 1987)

Benson, 1986), 'myopia for the future' (Bechara *et al.*, 2000) and difficulties in emotional processing (Adolphs, 2001).

The medial parts of the PFC include the anterior cingulate gyrus (Brodmann area 24 and posterior Brodmann areas 23, 31), the supplementary motor area 6, the prefrontal regions 8, 9, 10 and the Rolandic regions 4, 3, 1,2 (Damasio & Damasio, 1989). The cingulate gyrus is located in the medial part of the cortex. It partially wraps around corpus callosum and is limited by the cingulate sulcus. Recent evidence by Bush *et al.* (2000) suggests that the anterior cingulate plays a major role as an interface for the regulation between emotional and cortical messages. This circuit is involved in motivation, initiation of activity and emotional processes. Lesions in this region often result in a syndrome that is characterized by apathy.

Finally, the DLC circuit includes the frontal operculum (44, 45), the prefrontal region (8, 9, 46) the dorsal premotor region (6), the dorsal Rolandic region (4, 3, 1,2), the paraventricular and the supraventricular area (Damasio & Damasio, 1989). The DLC receives input from the motor cortex as well as from the multimodal sensory areas of the parietal and temporal lobes. This circuit is mainly involved in executive functions, attention and working memory. Damage to the DLC may produce deficits in cognitive flexibility, set shifting (Dias *et al.*, 1996) and working memory (Goldman-Rakic, 1987).

When taking into consideration the spectrum of clinical evidence it is suggested that the dorsolateral circuit may be relatively more specialized for regulation of high cognitive functions, whereas the OFC and the medial circuits are mainly involved in emotional and motivational aspects of behaviour. A general rostro-caudal gradient of limbic innervations has been described, whereby medial and orbital PFC have the highest proportion of limbic output (Barbas, 1992). Consequently, several investigators have addressed the OFC and the medial circuits as one functional unit that has been dubbed the ventromedial (VM) prefrontal cortex (Bechara *et al.*, 2000; Hornak *et al.*, 1996).

The intimate connections of the VM PFC to the anterior insula, temporal pole, inferior parietal lobe and amygdala place it in a position to evaluate and regulate information from the limbic system that can be used to inhibit behaviour, regulate emotions, personality and behaviour and empathize with the experiences of others. Indeed, lesions in VM cortexes result in a syndrome that is characterized by disinhibition, lack of tact and in some cases even 'acquired sociopathy' (Blair & Cipolotti, 2000; Tranel *et al.*, 2002). Patients with PFC damage may show altered emotional and social behaviour, such as disinhibition and misinterpretation of social situations, especially when the damage involves the VM (Rolls, 1996; Stuss & Benson, 1986). Clinical observations and experimental evidence indicate that these patients develop a severe impairment in personal and social decision-making, despite relatively intact intellectual abilities (Damasio *et al.*, 1991; Eslinger & Damasio, 1985). Such behavioural deficits are most evident in social situations. However, there is a scarcity of laboratory probes to measure this deficit, and few satisfactory accounts of the neural and cognitive mechanisms underlying it. Recently, attempts to explain the behavioural disturbances following VM damage have emphasized the breakdown in these patients' ability to empathize with the experiences of other individuals.

6.3 The neuroanatomical basis of empathy: the role of the frontal lobes

Impaired social behaviour has been consistently observed in patients with pre-frontal lobe dysfunction, and was found to dissociate from other cognitive functions and in some instances from moral knowledge. Eslinger and Damasio (1985) have described a patient (E.V.R.) who underwent bilateral ablation of orbital and lower mesial frontal cortexes and similarly to Phineas Gage, and suffered from extensive behavioural changes. It is reported that E.V.R. was previously successful in his professional occupation, happily married and the father of two children. After a VM ablation he had many difficulties in meeting personal and professional responsibilities. He was fired from several jobs and his wife left home with the children and filed for divorce after 17 years of marriage. Despite these behavioural problems he was described as having superior intelligence. It is reported that although he remembered social norms and had intact moral judgement, his behaviour was profoundly inappropriate. In concordance with this, Price *et al.* (1990) have described two patients who suffered bilateral prefrontal damage early in life. These patients were under psychiatric attention following several incidences of aberrant behaviour. A neuropsychological examination has revealed deficits in moral judgement, lack of insight, foresight, impaired social judgement, impaired empathy and difficulties in complex reasoning.

Similar evidence of impaired social cognition after early damage to the VM was provided by Anderson *et al.* (1999), who characterized the long-term consequences of early PFC lesions in two adults, who had suffered prefrontal damage before they had reached the age of 16 months. In accordance with Price *et al.* (1990) these patients showed impaired social behaviour despite normal basic cognitive abilities. They showed insensitivity to future consequences of decisions, defective auto-nomic responses to punishment contingencies and a failure to respond to beha-vioural interventions. However, as opposed to adult-onset patients (such as E.V.R.), these patients had profound deficits in moral reasoning, suggesting that early VM damage impairs social behaviour as well as social perception and moral judgement.

The aforementioned studies clearly indicate that the VM mediates behaviours that involve social interactions. One concept that appears to have great utility in understanding personality alterations in the neurological population is that of empathy.

6.3.1 What is the empathic ability comprised of?

In the broadest sense empathy refers to the reactions of one individual to the observed experiences of another (Davis, 1994). Some investigators have consid-ered empathy to be a cognitive phenomenon, emphasizing the ability to engage in the cognitive process of adopting another's psychological point of view, with a resulting research focus on intellectual processes such as accurate perception of others (DeKosky *et al.*, 1980). This process, which may be termed 'cognitive empathy', involves perspective taking (Eslinger, 1998), and has been reported to be dependent upon several cognitive capacities (Davis, 1994; Eslinger, 1998; Grattan *et al.*, 1994).

Other investigators have used a definition of empathy stressing its affective facets. These investigators studied aspects such as helping behaviour, referring to the capacity to experience affective reactions to the observed experiences of others as 'affective empathy' (Davis, 1994).

The critical difference between cognitive empathy and emotional empathy is that the former involves cognitive understanding of the other person's point of view whereas the latter also includes sharing of those feelings, at least at the gross affect (pleasant-unpleasant) level (Mehrabian & Epstein, 1972). Since it has been previously suggested that the different aspects of empathy are related and interact throughout development (Hoffman, 1978), recent theories of empathy have introduced multidimensional (Davis, 1994) and integrative (Preston & de Waal, 2002) models that combine several aspects of empathy and empathic-related behaviours. However, it appears that while historical definitions of empathy have emphasized the emotional aspects of sharing an experience with the other (Mehrabian & Epstein, 1972), more recent accounts of empathy have underscored its cognitive aspects, emphasizing the importance of cognitive perspective taking (Davis, 1994) in the understanding of the other. Thus, alterations in the empathic response may reflect impairment in a number of cognitive and affective processes that may depend upon the integrity of the frontal lobes.

In concordance with the conflicting definitions of empathy, competing views have been proposed as to how we basically understand the behaviour of others. Two different approaches attempt to account for the cognitive mechanisms that subserve the ability by which we represent and predict another person's behaviour. The 'Theory of Mind' theorists (ToM theorists) maintain that mental states attributed to other people are conceived as unobservable, theoretical posits, invoked to explain and predict behaviour, something akin of a scientific theory (Gopnik & Meltzoff, 1998). According to Wellman (1990) and other proponents of the ToM position, this kind of process is actually a 'theory' of mind because beliefs and desires form the basic theoretical constructs that we combine through a system of rules to predict and explain behaviours and thoughts of other people.

On the other hand, the 'simulation' perspective (Gallese & Goldman, 1999) emphasizes the first-person perspective consciousness and suggests that the others' mental states are represented by tracking or matching their states with resonant states of one's own. Thus, the attributor tries to covertly mimic the mental activity of the target. The simulation perspective is based on findings regarding 'mirror' neurones in the monkey's ventral precentral motor cortex that respond both when a particular action is performed by the recorded monkey and when the same action, performed by another monkey, is observed (Gallese & Goldman, 1999).

It appears that the core difference between ToM and simulation approaches to empathy is that while ToM may view empathy as a thoroughly 'detached' theoretical analysis that will involve cortexes that are usually activated during mental state attribution, simulation may depict empathy as incorporating an attempt to replicate the other affective mental state via emotion-processing-related neural networks. It might be interesting to speculate that whereas cognitive empathy involves ToM processes, affective empathy involves a process of simulation.

6.3.2 Impaired empathic ability following prefrontal lesions

In concordance with these various definitions of empathy, several lesion studies, commencing with the work of Grattan and Eslinger (1989), have studied the empathic abilities of patients with brain damage. Grattan and Enlinger (1989) found that cognitive empathic ability was correlated with cognitive flexibility, an aspect of executive functions which is considered to be mediated by the PFC. These results led the authors to consider the hypothesis that impaired empathic behaviour is associated with frontal lobe damage (Grattan *et al.*, 1994). Interestingly, they did not find significant differences in the overall empathy scores between patients with lesions restricted to the PFC and patients with other cortical lesions (Grattan *et al.*, 1994). However, when the authors divided the PFC into subgroups according to PFC damage in the OFC, medial and dorsolateral sections a dissociable pattern of impairment in empathy and cognitive flexibility emerged. Apparently, impaired empathy was significantly related to cognitive flexibility in patients with dorsolateral PFC damage but not in the OFC and the medial subgroups. In the medial subgroup empathic ability was preserved while cognitive flexibility was impaired, whereas in the OFC subgroup empathic ability was impaired while cognitive flexibility was preserved. The authors concluded that impaired empathy in this group was independent of cognitive flexibility and reflected an inability to activate the appropriate somatic or autonomic states required for empathic processing.

Extending these initial efforts, Shamay-Tsoory *et al.* (2003) have compared the empathic response of patients with localized lesions in the PFC to responses of patients with posterior lesions and healthy control subjects. To examine the cognitive processes that underlie the empathic ability, the relationships between empathy scores and the performance on tasks that assess processes of cognitive flexibility, affect recognition and ToM were also examined.

The findings of Shamay-Tsoory *et al.* (2003) indicated that patients with lesions restricted to the PFC and patients with damage to the right hemisphere were significantly impaired in empathic ability, as assessed using a cognitive empathy scale. Furthermore, lesions in the VM region appeared to be associated with a greater deficit in empathy (Figure 6.2).

These findings also suggested that the localization of the lesion along the anterior–posterior axis is not the only factor. When the lesion is confined to the posterior cortex, involvement of the *right*, but not left, hemisphere is associated with impaired empathic responses (Figure 6.3).

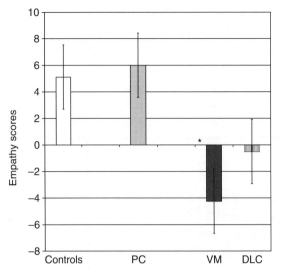

Figure 6.2. Empathy scores in patients with lesions limited to subregions of the prefrontal cortex (PFC), compared to posterior (PC) lesions and healthy controls. * Significantly different from PC and controls, $p < 0.05$

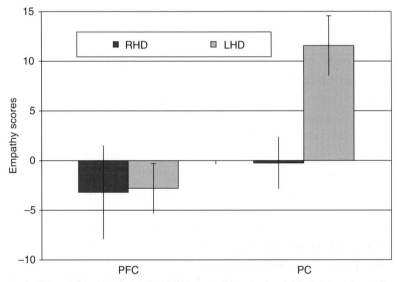

Figure 6.3. Empathy scores in patients with unilateral lesions RHD, right hemisphere damage; LHD, left hemisphere damage. * Significantly different from all other groups, $p < 0.05$

However, *both* left and right prefrontal lesions resulted in equally severe deficits in empathy. Despite this apparent lack of asymmetry within the PFC, the most severe deficit in empathy in this group was noted among patients whose lesion involved the right VM region, again suggesting that both the asymmetry of the

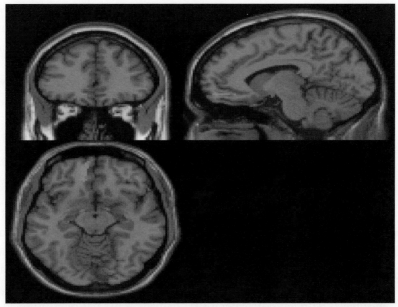

Figure 6.4.   Lesions associated with impaired empathy: overlap of lesions in 7 of the 8 patients with the most impaired empathy scores shown; all 7 lesions included the right ventromedial region

lesion and the localization within the hemisphere are important in determining the degree of deficit in empathy (Figure 6.4).

When compared to the healthy control group, the PFC patients were impaired on the various measures of cognitive flexibility employed in this study. Of greater interest, however, is the finding that the relationships between empathy scores and performance on measures of cognitive flexibility, affect recognition and ToM (assessed with the faux pas task) revealed a differential pattern in the two subgroups of PFC lesions. Thus, in the DLC group, empathic ability was related to cognitive flexibility but not to ToM, whereas in the VM group empathy was related to ToM but not to cognitive flexibility. In fact, the VM group had both the lowest empathy scores and the greatest number of errors in the ToM task. These results suggest that deficits in the ability to make an inference regarding another person's mental state may account for the profound deficit in empathic ability observed in the VM group.

6.3.3 Impaired 'mindreading': the case of ToM

The above-mentioned studies highlight the role of involvement of the VM in empathic abilities. In line with the ToM perspective Baron-Cohen suggested that the impairment of PFC patients with 'acquired sociopathy' can be accounted for in terms of damage to neural circuits that mediate ToM (Baron-Cohen, 1995). Failure to represent the other person's beliefs, knowledge and intentions may result in failure to see things from another person's perspective and thus interfere with the empathic response. By demonstrating a selective ToM impairment in autistic children, Baron-Cohen *et al.* (1985) have put forward the possibility of a specific brain basis for 'mindreading'. Operationally, subjects are credited with ToM if they succeed in tasks designed to test their understanding that an individual may hold a false belief. Tests of first-order false belief measure the ability of an individual to understand that another person can hold a belief that is mistaken, whereas tests of second-order false belief test 'belief about belief' (Perner & Wimmer, 1985).

Rowe *et al.* (2001) have reported that subjects with either right or left prefrontal lesions were impaired in ToM ability, as assessed by first- and second-order false-belief tests. Stone *et al.* (1998), however, have reported good performance on first-order and second-order ToM tests and impairment only on a more advanced ToM test (identifying a social 'faux pas'), in subjects with bilateral OFC lesions but not in subjects with left dorsolateral PFC damage. Faux pas refers to incidents where someone said something they should not have said, not knowing or not realizing that they should not have said it. As mentioned before in Shamay-Tsoory *et al.* (2003) performance in the faux pas task significantly predicted the levels of empathic ability of patients with VM lesions.

In a later study Shamay-Tsoory *et al.* (2005) has examined the hypothesis that patients with VM frontal lesions are impaired in the *affective* rather than *cognitive* facets of ToM. In this study three ToM tasks differing in the level of emotional processing involved were used on patients and controls: second-order false-belief task, understanding ironic utterances and identifying social faux pas. The results indicated that patients with VM prefrontal lesions were significantly impaired in irony and faux pas but not in second-order false belief, as compared to patients with posterior lesions and healthy controls. Furthermore, among the patients with the most impaired ToM, lesions in the right VM area were significantly larger than the lesions in the left VM, right and left dorsolateral regions.

One explanation for the difference in performance of patients in the false-belief task, the irony detection task and the faux pas task is that the tasks used in the study differed qualitatively. In order to understand irony and even more so in order to detect faux pas, one is required not only to understand the knowledge of the others, but also to have empathic understanding of their feelings. Thus, good performance of these tasks requires integration between the cognitive and affective facets of a given situation, whereas in the false-belief task no affective processing is needed. In this study, the VM patients performed without difficulty a task that requires understanding belief about belief but were impaired in tasks that involved understanding belief about emotions. This was not due to difficulty in identifying emotions (either through facial expression or through prosody). It might be suggested that the performance of patients with damage to the VM reflects impaired 'affective' ToM rather than 'cognitive' ToM.

Moreover, in this study the relationship between ToM and cognitive and affective empathy was examined. The correlation between the poor performance of the 'affective' ToM tasks and impaired empathy was significant, suggesting that affective 'mindreading' may, in fact, be an empathic response. However, the significant correlation between 'affective ToM' and 'cognitive empathy' (and insignificant correlation with 'affective empathy') implies that although inferences of feelings and emotional experiences in other people involve affective processes, they are nonetheless still cognitive. It has been previously suggested that whereas affectively based empathy involves vicarious arousal and experience of another's feeling state, cognitively based empathy involves the ability to take another's viewpoint and infer that person's feelings (Eslinger, 1998). On the basis of this, it may be assumed that 'affective ToM' has to do with processes of cognitive empathy, which are involved in the inference of other people's emotions.

Another ability that relies on ToM is the ability to understand deception. Deception is relevant to ToM because it involves trying to make someone else believe that something is true when in fact it is false (Baron-Cohen, 2000). Stuss *et al.* (2001) examined the performance of patients with focal frontal lesions in a task designed to assess an individual's ability to infer that someone was trying to deceive them. In this task the subjects were required to point to the cup where he or she thought a coin was hidden. However, an assistant, who was supposed to deceive the subject, always pointed to the wrong cup, the one without the hidden coin. The authors report that patients with right PFC damage made more errors in this task, suggesting that it is the right, rather than left, frontal lobe that plays an important role in assessing an individual's ability to infer that someone was trying to deceive them.

6.3.4 Further evidence for the role of the PFC in empathy: frontotemporal dementia studies

In keeping with the above-mentioned lesion studies, recent evidence from studies of patients suffering frontal lobe degeneration have supported the role of the PFC in empathy and ToM. Lough *et al.* (2001) presented the case of J.M., a 47-year-old man diagnosed with frontal variant of frontotemporal dementia. J.M. was described as exhibiting severe antisocial behaviour. His neuropsychological assessment indicated relatively intact general neuropsychological and executive function, but extremely poor performance on tasks of ToM.

In a later study, Gregory *et al.* (2002) examined ToM abilities (first-order false belief; second-order false belief; faux pas detection; and reading the mind in the eyes) in a group of patients with frontal variant of frontotemporal dementia and in patients with Alzheimer's disease. The authors report that the frontotemporal patients were impaired on all tests of ToM, but had no difficulty with control questions designed to test general comprehension and memory. However, the Alzheimer's disease group showed impaired performance on only one ToM task (second-order false belief), a task that involves more working memory than the other ToM tasks. In addition, the authors report a double dissociation in performance of the faux pas task: the frontotemporal group was impaired on ToM-based questions, whereas the Alzheimer's disease group was impaired on questions that assessed memory of the stories. Furthermore, it is reported that in the frontotemporal group, evident correlation between the magnitude of impairment on tests of ToM and their degree of ventromedial frontal damage was observed.

Another example linking the impaired social cognition with neurodegenerative diseases comes from the work of Snowden *et al.* (2003) with patients suffering from frontotemporal dementia and patients with Huntington's disease. The authors selected these physical conditions because frontotemporal dementia involves predominantly frontal degeneration, while Huntington's disease involves mainly degeneration of the striatum. In this study several tests of ToM were used: interpretation of cartoons and stories and judgement of preference based on eye gaze. The authors indicate that both groups showed impaired performance in the ToM task, however each group's performance was characterized by different errors. While the frontotemporal group was severely impaired on all tasks, mainly due to concrete interpretations, the Huntington disease group showed a milder impairment in cartoon and story interpretation, mainly due to misinterpretation of social situations.

To summarize, the aforementioned case reports, lesions experiments and neurodegenerative studies clearly indicate that the deficit in empathy is associated with VM lesions (especially in the right hemisphere) rather than damage to other brain areas. However, it is not claimed that empathy is localized to the right VM. Rather, it implies that the right VM region plays a major part in a network mediating empathy. Indeed, Brothers (1995) has described a neural circuit including the orbitofrontal cortex, the amygdala, the anterior cingulate gyrus and the temporal pole, suggesting that this circuit functions as a unitary social 'editor' specialized in the processing of others in a social interaction.

Given the considerable evidence then that VM damage may impair empathy and the affective aspects of ToM, attempts are being made to replicate the results of lesion studies using imaging techniques and normal subjects. To date, there has been only one published report examining directly the functional brain imaging of empathic judgement (Farrow *et al.*, 2001). In congruence with reports regarding sympathy (Decety & Chaminade, 2003b) these authors report mainly inferior frontal activation as well as middle, temporal, premotor and VM prefrontal involvement. These imaging results confirm yet again that the role of the VM is empathic response processing and highlight the concept of a neural network that mediates empathic ability.

6.4 The role of the VM PFC in social cognition

It is well established that the VM cortex plays an important role in a network that mediates empathic abilities. But how can we explain the particular role of the VM in empathic behaviour?

Several attempts have been made to delineate the role of the VM PFC in social behaviour. One of the leading theories that attempted to examine the learning deficits that may underpin behavioural disturbance in VM patients has been formulated by Rolls (2000). Rolls hypothesized that the OFC cortex is particularly involved in correcting behavioural responses made to stimuli previously associated with reinforcement. By looking at recordings from single neurones in the OFC cortex, Rolls has shown that some neurones respond to primary reinforcers such as taste and touch; that others respond to learned secondary reinforcers, such as the sight of a rewarded visual stimulus; and that the rapid learning of associations between previously neutral visual stimuli and primary reinforcers is reflected in the responses of the OFC neurones.

These findings led Rolls (1990) to consider that the OFC cortex is involved particularly in emotion-related learning. The learning deficits associated with damage to the OFC cortex in non-human primates include impaired extinction and impaired visual discrimination reversal. These impairments in human subjects may result in continued responding to a previously rewarded stimulus, leading to inappropriate emotional and social behaviour (Rolls, 1996).

Indeed, recent investigations in macaques have shown that neurones in the OFC cortex reverse their visual and olfactory responses during reversals (Rolls, 2004), and that lesions of this region impair reversal (Dias *et al.*, 1996; Iversen & Mishkin, 1970). In agreement with this concept, Hornak *et al.* (1996) have suggested that voice or face expression may serve as reinforcers to which VM patients fail to respond. The authors demonstrated impairments in the identification of facial and vocal emotional expression in patients with ventral PFC damage who had socially inappropriate behaviour. They concluded that impaired social behaviour in these patients is related to their inability to rapid learning of associations between previously neutral stimuli and primary reinforcers.

This view may explain deficits in empathic abilities in patients with VM lesions as resulting from their inability to adapt to other individual's changing emotional experiences. However, it is not obvious that a deficit in reversal learning necessarily affects empathic ability.

In the 'inhibition hypothesis', proposed by Sahakian and colleagues to account for the social cognition deficits observed in patients with frontal lobe dysfunction (Plaisted & Sahakian, 1997; Rahman *et al.* 1999), the reversal learning deficits are also considered. The Plaisted and Sahakian (1997) hypothesis is based on an established non-human finding that damage to the PFC results in loss of inhibitory control over inappropriate responses to any current situation. Recently, in the primate literature, Dias *et al.* (1996) have reported a double dissociation in the PFC of affective and attentional shifts following excitotoxic lesions to the lateral cortex and OFC. The authors report that whereas damage to the lateral PFC (Brodmann area 9) in monkeys caused a loss of inhibitory control in attentional selection, damage to the OFC in monkeys causes a loss of inhibitory control in 'affective' processing. Similar findings were found in human patients by Rahman *et al.* (1999). By examining patients with the frontal variant of frontotemporal dementia, the authors argued that these patients' aberrant social behaviour is related to the inability of their orbitofrontal inhibitory mechanisms to suppress inappropriate behaviours elicited by the immediate environment. The authors suggest that these patients' behaviour is predominantly controlled by immediate emotional evaluation of the stimuli and, therefore, such disinhibition disturbs the selection of alternative and more appropriate action plans which are dictated by long-term goals.

This view may regard the empathy deficit observed in these patients as stemming from a difficulty in inhibiting their own perspective and adopting alternative perspectives of others.

Blair and Cipolotti (2000) have also put forward the role played by the VM in generating behavioural alternatives in social situations. The authors reported a single case study of a patient suffering from PFC damage including the VM who specifically showed impairment in the recognition of, and autonomic responding to, angry and disgusted expressions. They concluded that this impairment was due to a reduced ability to generate expectations of others' negative emotional reactions, in particular anger, and proposed that the VM may be implicated specifically either in the generation of these expectations or the use of these expectations to suppress inappropriate behaviour.

According to this hypothesis impaired empathy is therefore based on these patients' deficits in anticipating the emotional reactions of other people, particularly negative reactions. This explanation focuses on understanding the negative emotions of others and says very little about these patients' lack of understanding of other mental states.

An alternative view of the role of the VM in social behaviour has been proposed by Damasio *et al.* (1991), who suggested a 'somatic marker hypothesis' for processes of decision-making. Damasio and colleagues argue that somatic feedback to the brain influences higher cognitive processes, in particular decision-making in humans. The 'somatic marker hypothesis' (Damasio *et al.*, 1991) proposes that the VM cortex participates in integrating information regarding body states evoked by experiences, and the outcome of these experiences. The VM, through its connections with the limbic system and the autonomic nervous system, 'marks' internal representations with somatic markers. These are the convergence zones for knowledge about the categorization of previous experiences, and different profiles of emotional or biological states. Damasio proposes that when choosing between options that differ in relative risk, a somatic marker (for example, a 'gut feeling') feeds back to the brain and influences cognitive appraisal, often without conscious awareness.

In line with the somatic marker hypothesis, Bechara and colleagues (1994) have developed a card task known as 'the gambling task'. The gambling task intends to simulate real-life situations in the way it engages in uncertainty, reward and punishment. The task involves selections of decks of cards that are rewarded and punished with monetary gains and losses. The schedules of rewards and punishments are planned in a manner such that in the short term two decks appear advantageous but in the long term these decks are disadvantageous, whereas the other decks first appear unfavourable but in the long term are more profitable (Bechara *et al.*, 1994). According to Bechara, normal subjects gradually make more selections of cards from the good decks and fewer selections from the bad decks. However, patients with bilateral lesions of the VM do not increase the number of selection of cards from the good decks and persist in selecting more cards from the bad decks. Furthermore, Bechara *et al.* (1998) have reported that the gambling task is independent of working memory. The authors found that while VM subjects with more anterior lesions performed defectively on the gambling but not the delay task, subjects with right dorsolateral cortex lesions were impaired on the delay task but not the gambling task. Moreover, in previous studies the authors have shown that in patients with VM damage, choosing disadvantageously correlates with failure to acquire anticipatory skin conductance response, compared to healthy controls.

The authors concluded that the VM patients' performance profile is comparable to their real-life inability to learn from their previous mistakes (Bechara *et al.*, 2000). Thus, according to the somatic marker hypothesis damage to the VM results in a failure to respond appropriately to a given situation, which – in social situations – may be expressed as lack of empathy.

Taken together the various hypotheses raised in this section share several components. It appears that the difficulties in empathic abilities of people with VM damage are most apparent when integration or association of cognition and emotions is required. Sahakian and colleagues' argument for lack of inhibitory control in 'affective' processing, as well as Blair and Cipolottis' explanations of deficits in the generation of expectation of other's feelings may actually refer to a cognitive deficit in affective processing. Damasio's somatic marker hypothesis of impaired associations between the situation and the appropriate emotional state clearly indicates a deficit in integration of emotion with cognition.

Perhaps these patients' difficulty is particularly evident when cognition and affect are interwoven and it is this key connection – the interplay between cognition and emotion – that is particularly problematic for these individuals.

6.5 A neural network for the organization of the empathic response: an integrative view

Considering the multifaceted nature of empathy, it is only to be expected that it should be mediated by a complex neural network. A decreased empathic response may be due to deficits in a variety of cognitive and emotional processes, mediated by different neural systems. The various findings mentioned in the second section suggest that the VM cortex is involved in empathic ability. In addition it is suggested that the right hemisphere plays an important role in the mediation of empathy. This is not surprising, considering that the right hemisphere contains essential components of systems specialized in the processing of emotion (DeKosky et al., 1980). In Shamay-Tsoory et al. (2003), affective processing (as measured by prosody and facial expression identification) was associated with right hemisphere damage. These results confirm yet again the role of the right hemisphere in social interactions (Adolphs, 2001) and are in concordance with imaging data indicating the role of the right inferior parietal cortex in feeling sympathy (Decety & Chaminade, 2003a) and in imitation (Meltzoff & Decety, 2003). Furthermore, it has been recently suggested that the ability to identify with other individuals, an ability that is considered a prerequisite for feeling empathy, involves the right parietal cortex (Decety & Chaminade, 2003b).

While empathy is reduced following right hemisphere damage, the empathic response is most severely impaired following lesions within the right frontal structures, and most notably the right VM region of the PFC, suggesting a greater role for right PFC structures in the mediation of empathy. Posterior right hemisphere regions are involved in emotional perception whereas the right frontal lobe is crucial for choosing the appropriate emotional response to situations, as well as the expression of mood and emotions (Edwards-Lee & Saul, 1999). It is suggested, therefore, that right posterior damage results in impaired empathy due to deficits in affect recognition whereas right frontal damage influences the expression of the response.

Another cognitive process which may be important for the empathic response involves reactivating one's past experiences, which may then be related to the other person's experience. The right frontal lobe has been associated with processes of episodic retrieval (Tulving *et al.*, 1994). It has been suggested that a right hemispheric network of temporal, together with posterior, cingulate and PFC, areas is engaged in the retrieval of autobiographical information (Fink *et al.*, 1996). Thus, it might be suggested that the PFC mediates the empathic response by integrating reactivated past scenarios (which are processed in the right hemisphere) with other affective and cognitive processes mediated by the PFC.

The right VM region plays a major part in a neural network mediating the empathic ability. The components of this network (see Figure 6.5) include the processing of affective information (posterior right hemisphere), the retrieval of past personal events (right prefrontal cortex) and aspects of executive functions (such as cognitive flexibility, among others) which are mediated by the DLC. Therefore, a lesion in any of these regions may result in impaired empathic response. The importance of the VM area reflects its major role in integrating these various processes (together with input from other brain regions, most importantly the amygdala and the autonomic nervous system), thus facilitating the formation of the empathic response.

This network may be divided into a core system and an extended system. The core system is comprised of the VM region of the PFC, where integration of several cognitive and affective processes takes place. The extended system includes the

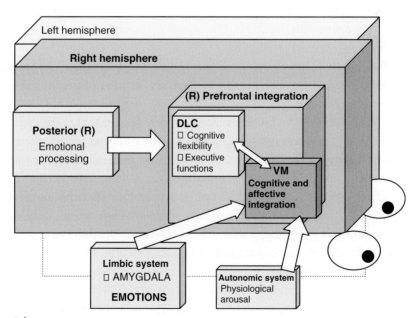

Figure 6.5   Scheme 1

DLC region of the PFC, and circuits within the right hemisphere, which are involved in the identification and processing of affective information. Each component in this system has some specialization, yet this specialization is not absolute because lesions to different parts of the network can have similar effects on the empathic ability. Each region plays a prominent, but not exclusive role in controlling a certain aspect of empathy.

Other regions of the brain may also be involved in this network. Specifically, the amygdala has been shown to play an important role in the mediation of social behaviour. Baron-Cohen (1995) has also suggested a neural circuit including the amygdala and the VM, which is involved in the mediation processes of ToM. In addition, the amygdala has been shown to respond to negative emotions such as fear and sadness (Blair *et al.*, 1999).

Interestingly, neuroantomical data suggest that the VM region of the PFC is one station in an extensive circuitry (including the ventral striatum and amygdala) which is implicated in the processes of reinforcement and incentive motivation and is strongly influenced by mesocorticolimbic dopamine input (Koob & Bloom, 1988). In addition, the OFC cortex is known to receive strong inputs from the amygdala and projects back to temporal lobe areas (Price *et al.*, 1996). Thus, empathy deficits after amygdala damage may be similar to those observed after VM damage. This suggestion is supported by several single cases and lesion studies regarding the role of the amygdala in social behaviour and emotion (Adolphs *et al.*, 2002).

6.6 Summary

The chapter reviewed the social-emotional consequences of VM prefrontal brain damage, particularly as revealed by the characteristics of empathy deficits following brain damage.

Examining the VM neuroanatomy, it is suggested that these cortexes are in a position to evaluate and regulate information from the limbic system that can be used to inhibit behaviour, regulate emotions, integrate emotion with cognition and thus may subserve empathizing with the experiences of others.

It is proposed that the VM is part of a neural network that mediates empathic abilities. The VM mediates empathy by integrating emotional processing and cognition. It is suggested that whereas the right hemisphere and the amygdala contribute to the processing of affective information, the prefrontal lobes contribute to the processing of ToM and executive functions. These distinct processes overlap and are integrated by a core system located at the right VM frontal cortex, allowing correct understanding of other people's affective and cognitive mental states.

REFERENCES

Adolphs, R. (2001). The neurobiology of social cognition. *Current Opinion in Neurobiology*, **11**(2), 231–239.

Adolphs, R., Baron-Cohen, S., & Tranel, D. (2002). Impaired recognition of social emotions following amygdala damage. *Journal of Cognitive Neuroscience*, **14**(8), 1264–1274.

Alexander, G. E., DeLong, M. R., & Strick, P. L. (1986). Parallel organization of functionally segregated circuits linking basal ganglia and cortex. *Annual Review of Neuroscience*, **9**, 357–381.

Anderson, S. W., Bechara, A., Damasio, H., Tranel, D., & Damasio, A. R. (1999). Impairment of social and moral behavior related to early damage in human prefrontal cortex. *Nature Neuroscience*, **2**(11), 1032–1037.

Barbas, H. (1992). Architecture and cortical connections of the prefrontal cortex in the rhesus monkey. *Advances in Neurology*, **57**, 91–115.

Baron-Cohen, S. (1995). *Mindblindedness: An Essay on Autism and Theory of Mind*. Cambridge, Mass.: MIT Press.

Baron-Cohen, S. (2000). Theory of mind and autism: a fifteen year review. In S. Baron-Cohen, H. Tager-Flusberg, D. Cohen (eds.), *Understanding Other Minds Perspectives From Developmental Cognitive Neuroscience*. Oxford: Oxford University Press.

Baron-Cohen, S., Leslie, A. M., & Frith, U. (1985). Does the autistic child have a 'Theory of Mind'. *Cognition*, **21**, 37–46.

Bechara, A., & Damasio, H. (2002). Decision-making and addiction (part I): impaired activation of somatic states in substance dependent individuals when pondering decisions with negative future consequences. *Neuropsychologia*, **40**(10), 1675–1689.

Bechara, A., Damasio, A. R., Damasio, H., & Anderson, S. W. (1994). Insensitivity to future consequences following damage to human prefrontal cortex. *Cognition*, **50**(1–3), 7–15.

Bechara, A., Damasio, H., Tranel, D., & Anderson, S. W. (1998). Dissociation of working memory from decision making within the human prefrontal cortex. *Journal of Neuroscience*, **18**(1), 428–437.

Bechara, A., Tranel, D., & Damasio, H. (2000). Characterization of the decision-making deficit of patients with ventromedial prefrontal cortex lesions. *Brain*, **123** (Pt 11), 2189–2202.

Berlin, H. A., Rolls, E. T., & Kischka, U. (2004). Impulsivity, time perception, emotion and reinforcement sensitivity in patients with orbitofrontal cortex lesions. *Brain*, **127**(Pt 5), 1108–1126.

Blair, R. J. R., & Cipolotti, L. (2000). Impaired social response reversal: a case of 'acquired sociopathy'. *Brain*, **123**, 1122–1141.

Blair, R. J., Morris, J. S., Frith, C. D., Perrett, D. I., & Dolan, R. J. (1999). Dissociable neural responses to facial expressions of sadness and anger. *Brain*, **122** (Pt 5), 883–893.

Brothers, L. (1995). Neurophysiology of the perception of intentions by primates. In M. S. Gazzaniga (eds.), *The Cognitive Neurosciences* (pp. 1107–1115). Cambridge, Mass.: MIT Press; pp. 1107–1115.

Bush, G., Luu, P., & Posner, M. I. (2000). Cognitive and emotional influences in anterior cingulate cortex. *Trends in Cognitive Science*, **4**(6), 215–222.

Damasio, H., & Damasio, A. (1989). *Lesion Analysis in Neuropsychology*. New York: Oxford University Press.

Damasio, A. R., Tranel, D., & Damasio, H. C. (1991). Somatic markers and guidance of behavior: theory and preliminary testing. In H. S. Levin, H. M. Eisenberg, A. L. Benton (eds.), *Frontal Lobe Function and Dysfunction* (pp. 217–229). New York: Oxford University Press.

Davis, M. H. (1994). *Empathy*. Madison, Wi.: Brown and Benchmark.

Decety, J., & Chaminade T. (2003a). When the self represents the other: a new cognitive neuroscience view on psychological identification. *Consciousness and Cognition*, **12(4)**, 577–596.

Decety, J., & Chaminade T. (2003b). Neural correlates of feeling sympathy. *Neuropsychologia*, **41(2)**, 127–138.

DeKosky, S. T., Heilman, K. M., Bowers, D., & Valenshtein, E. (1980). Recognition and discrimination of emotional faces and pictures. *Brain and Language*, **9(2)**, 206–214.

Dias, R., Robbins, T. W., & Roberts, A. C. (1996). Dissociation in prefrontal cortex of affective and attentional shifts. *Nature*, **38**, 69–72.

Edwards-Lee, T. A., & Saul, R. E. (1999). Neuropsychiatry of the right frontal lobe. In B. L. Miller, J. L. Cummings (eds.), *The Human Frontal Lobes: Functions and Disorders. The Science and Practice of Neuropsychology Series*. New York: Guilford Press.

Eslinger, P. J. (1998). Neurological and neuropsychological bases of empathy. *European Neurology*, **39**, 193–199.

Eslinger, P. J., & Damasio, A. R (1985). Severe disturbance of higher cognition after bilateral frontal lobe ablations: patient EVR. *Neurology*, **35**, 1731–1741.

Farrow, T. F., Zheng, Y., Wilkinson, I. D., *et al.* (2001). Investigating the functional anatomy of empathy and forgiveness. *Neuroreport*, **8;12(11)**, 2433–2438.

Fink, G. R., Markowitsch, H. J., Reinkemeier, M., Bruckbauer, T., Kessler, J., & Heiss, W. (1996). Cerebral representation of one's own past: neural networks involved in autobiographical memory. *Journal of Neuroscience*, **16(13)**, 4275–4282.

Gallese, V., & Goldman, A. (1999). Mirror neurons and the simulation theory of mind-reading. *Trends in Cognitive Sciences*, **2;12**, 493–501.

Goldman-Rakic, P. S. (1987). In F. Plum, V. Mountcastle (eds.), *Handbook of Physiology: The Nervous System* (Vol. 5) (pp. 373–417). Bethesda, Md.: American Physiological Society.

Gopnik, A., & Meltzoff, A. N. (1998). *Words, Thoughts, and Theories*. Cambridge, Mass.: MIT Press.

Grattan, L. M., Bloomer, R. H., Archambault, F. X., & Eslinger, P. J. (1994). Cognitive flexibility and empathy after frontal lobe lesion. *Neuropsychiatry, Neuropsychology and Behavioral Neurology*, **7**, 251–257.

Grattan, L. M., & Eslinger, P. J. (1989). Higher cognition and social behavior: changes in cognitive flexibility and empathy after cerebral lesions. *Neuropsychology*, **3**, 175–185.

Gregory, C., Lough, S., Stone, V., *et al.* (2002). Theory of mind in patients with frontal variant frontotemporal dementia and Alzheimer's disease: theoretical and practical implications. *Brain*, **125**(Pt 4), 752–764.

Harlow, J. M. (1868). Recovery from the passage of an iron bar through the head. *Publications of the Massachusetts Medical Society*, **2**, 327–347.

Hoffman, M. L. (1978). Toward a theory of empathic arousal and development. In M. Lewis, & L. Rosenblum (eds.) *The Development of Affect*. New York: Plenum.

Hornak, J., Rolls, E. T., & Wade, D. (1996). Face and voice expression identification in patients with emotional and behavioural changes following ventral frontal lobe damage. *Neuropsychologia*, **34(4)**, 247–261.

Iversen, S. D., & Mishkin, M. (1970). Perseverative interference in monkeys following selective lesions of the inferior prefrontal convexity. *Experimental Brain Research*, **11(4)**, 376–386.

Koob, G. F., & Bloom, F. E. (1988). Cellular and molecular mechanisms of drug dependence. *Science*, **242(4879)**, 715–723.

Lough, S., Gregory, C., & Hodges, J. R. (2001). Dissociation of social cognition and executive function in frontal variant frontotemporal dementia. *Neurocase*, **7(2)**, 123–130.

Mehrabian, A., & Epstein, N. (1972). A measure of emotional empathy. *Journal of Personality*, **40**, 523–543.

Meltzoff, A. N., & Decety, J. (2003). What imitation tells us about social cognition: a rapprochement between developmental psychology and cognitive neuroscience. *Philosophical Transactions of the Royal Society of London Series B Biological Sciences*, **29;358(1431)**, 491–500.

Mesulam, M. M. (1985). *Principles of Behavioral Neurology*. Philadelphia: F. A. Davis.

Perner, J., & Wimmer, H. (1985). 'John thinks that Mary thinks that . . .': attribution of second-order false beliefs by 5- to 10-year-old children. *Journal of Experimental Child Psychology*, **39**, 437–471.

Plaisted, K. C., & Sahakian, B. J. (1997). Dementia of frontal type – living in the here and now. *Aging and Mental Health*, **1**, 293–295.

Premack, D., & Woodruff, G. (1978). Chimpanzee problem-solving: a test for comprehension. *Science*, **3;202(4367)**, 532–535.

Preston, S. D., & de Waal, F. B. (2002). Empathy: its ultimate and proximate bases. *Behaviour and Brain Science*, **25(1)**, 1–20; discussion 20–71.

Price, B. H., Daffner, K. R., Stowe, R. M., & Mesulam, M. M. (1990). The comportmental learning disabilities of early frontal lobe damage. *Brain*, **113** (Pt 5), 1383–1393.

Price, J. L., Carmichael, S. T., & Drevets, W. C. (1996). Networks related to the orbital and medial prefrontal cortex; a substrate for emotional behavior? *Progress in Brain Research*, **107**, 523–536.

Rahman, S., Sahakian, B. J., Hodges, J. R., Rogers, R. D., & Robbins, T. W. (1999). Specific cognitive deficits in mild frontal variant frontotemporal dementia. *Brain*, **122** (Pt 8), 1469–1493.

Rolls, E. T. (1990). A theory of emotion, and its application to understanding the neural basis of emotion. *Cognition and Emotion*, **4**, 161–190.

Rolls, E. T. (1996). The orbitofrontal cortex. *Philosophical Transactions of the Royal Society of London*, **29;351(1346)**, 1433–1443.

Rolls, E. T. (2000). The orbitofrontal cortex and reward. *Cerebral Cortex*, **10(3)**, 284–294.

Rolls, E. T. (2004). Convergence of sensory systems in the orbitofrontal cortex in primates and brain design for emotion. *The Anatomical Record. Part A: Discoveries in Molecular, Cellular, and Evolutionary Biology*, **1**, 1212–1225.

Rowe, A. D., Bullock, P. R., Polkey, C. E., & Morris, R. G. (2001) 'Theory of mind' impairments and their relationship to executive functioning following frontal lobe excisions. *Brain*, **124**, (Pt 3), 600–616.

Shamay, S. G., Tomer, R., Berger, B. D., & Aharon-Peretz, J. (2005). Impaired affective 'theory of mind' is associated with right ventromedial prefrontal damage. *Cognitive and Behavioral Neurology*, **18(1)**, 55–67.

Shamay-Tsoory, S. G., Tomer, R., Berger, B. D., & Aharon-Peretz, J. (2003). Characterization of empathy deficits following prefrontal brain damage: the role of the right ventromedial prefrontal cortex. *Journal of Cognitive Neuroscience*, **15(3)**, 324–337.

Snowden, J. S., Gibbons, Z. C., Blackshaw, A., *et al.* (2003). Social cognition in frontotemporal dementia and Huntington's disease. *Neuropsychologia*, **41(6)**, 688–701.

Stone, V. E., Baron-Cohen, S., & Knight, R. T. (1998). Frontal lobe contributions to theory of mind. *Journal of Cognitive Neuroscience*, **10(5)**, 640–656.

Stuss, D. T., & Benson, D. F. (1986). *The Frontal Lobes*. New York: Raven Press.

Stuss, D. T., Gallup, G. G., & Alexander, M. P. (2001). The frontal lobes are necessary for 'theory of mind'. *Brain*, **124**(Pt 2), 279–286.

Tranel, D., Bechara, A., & Denburg, N. L. (2002). Asymmetric functional roles of right and left ventromedial prefrontal cortices in social conduct, decision-making, and emotional processing. *Cortex*, **38(4)**, 589–612.

Tulving, E., Kapur, S., Craik, F. L., Moscovitch, M., & Houle S. (1994). Hemispheric encoding/ retrieval asymmetry in episodic memory: positron emission tomography findings. *Proceedings of the National Academy of Science of the USA*, **91**, 2016–2020.

Wellman, H. M. (1990). *The Child's Theory of Mind*. Cambridge, Mass.: MIT Press.

Non-autism childhood empathy disorders

Christopher Gillberg

Department of Child and Adolescent Psychiatry, University of Gothenburg, Sweden

7.1 Introduction

Autism – first described by Itard in 1828 as 'intellectual mutism' (Carrey, 1995) – is considered the most typical example of a disorder of empathy (Gillberg, 1992). 'Classic' autism, i.e. autistic disorder (American Psychiatric Association, 1994) also known as childhood autism (World Health Organization, 1993), is the subject of a separate chapter in this book. This chapter, instead, focuses on other disorders of empathy, ranging from so-called Asperger's syndrome and 'pervasive developmental disorder not otherwise specified' (PDDNOS) through a number of syndromes and disorders that have a substantial subgroup affected by clinically important empathy problems. First, however, follows a brief section on how I envisage 'empathy' and 'disorders of empathy' based on my own writings in the field since I first coined the term 'disorders of empathy' in my Emanuel Miller memorial lecture held in 1991 (Gillberg, 1992).

7.2 Empathy and 'disorders of empathy'

The word empathy (constructed on the Greek roots of 'em' and 'pathos') probably goes back to the early 1900s, when a group of German doctors used it to describe 'Einfühlung' or the ability to put oneself in the mind of another person (Gillberg, 1993). It is in this way that Sigmund Freud later used it when he referred to the ability – that he believed existed in all people – to intuitively take the perspective of other people. In this sense, empathy is not the same as sympathy, but rather a prerequisite for both sympathy and antipathy. Sympathy and antipathy are cognitive states coloured by emotions, whereas empathy is an emotionally more neutral construct that refers only to the actual ability to take the mental perspective of other people.

Defined as in the foregoing, empathic ability is obviously very similar – perhaps identical – to the construct of mentalizing and Theory of Mind (ToM) skills. I have

Empathy in Mental Illness, eds. Tom F. D. Farrow and Peter W. R. Woodruff. Published by Cambridge University Press. © Cambridge University Press 2007.

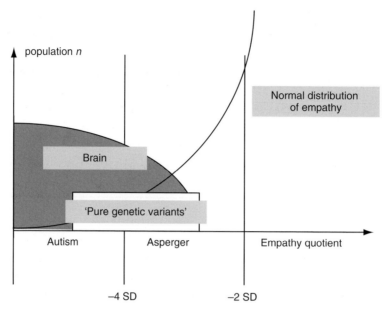

Figure 7.1.   Normal distribution of empathy, 'pure genetic variants' and brain dysfunction in autism and Asperger's syndrome

argued elsewhere that empathy/ToM skills are probably, at least partly for genetic/constitutional reasons, a normally distributed function, in much the same way as 'intelligence' (Gillberg, 1992). Empathy quotients (EQs) could be constructed on the basis of empathy/ToM tests in accordance with intelligence quotients (IQs) based on intelligence tests. As with IQ, EQ would probably show a similar 'hump' as IQ in the very 'subnormal' range of functioning (Figure 7.1). This extra prevalence would not be accounted for by simple normal distribution, but by pathological factors (including brain damage and genetic syndromes/variation/abnormality) affecting the central nervous system in neural circuitries subserving functions crucial for the development of empathy/ToM skills.

Theoretically, under a model of this kind, autistic disorder would be associated with very low EQ (perhaps under about 50) whereas milder disorders in the so-called autism spectrum might be associated with EQs in the 50–70 range.

Alternatively, all disorders in the autism spectrum (including Asperger's syndrome) could be conceptualized as falling in the EQ 50 or under range, with only IQ determining whether an individual is classified as having autism (IQ < 70) or Asperger's syndrome/atypical autism (IQ > 70). Using this latter theoretical model for the purpose of the present chapter, empathy disorders that do not even fall into the autism spectrum would probably best be seen as those disorders with an EQ in the range 50–70 (or even 85), quite regardless of overall IQ. There is some evidence to uphold this model when it comes to autism spectrum disorders (see Gillberg, 1999; Gillberg & Coleman, 2000), and the subdivision of autism and Asperger's syndrome, in clinical practice, is usually made more on the basis of IQ than on 'EQ' (which may indeed be very low in Asperger's syndrome). When it comes to other disorders of empathy (such as encountered in attention-deficit/hyperactivity disorder and Tourette syndrome), there is – to my knowledge – no systematic underpinnings to suggest that the model is relevant, and, so, what follows is my own tentative subdivision of disorders of empathy based on 30 years of very considerable clinical experience with all sorts of people at all ages, particularly from the field of so-called neuropsychiatry (see Gillberg, 1995 for a definition).

Empathy disorder was recently defined by our group as 'a history since early childhood as well as persistent difficulties (at the time of diagnosis) in (i) reciprocal interaction with same aged peers, (ii) taking the social perspective of other people, (iii) empathizing with other people, and (iv) difficulty in relating in an empathic way – including poor eye contact, mime and gesturing – with the psychiatrist (or other diagnostician) at the time of the interview' (Råstam et al., 1997).

7.3 Diagnostic conditions that contain an important subgroup with empathy disorder

A very considerable number of psychiatric/mental health problems are linked to (though not necessarily caused by) empathy problems. Table 7.1 lists some of the most obvious examples of diagnosable conditions that contain a large subgroup with empathy disorder. In the following, all of these conditions will be briefly reviewed.

7.4 Asperger's syndrome and the inappropriate label of high-functioning autism

Even though most authorities in the field believe that many (indeed probably most) individuals diagnosed with Asperger's syndrome have a disorder which is clearly strongly related (genetically, familially and clinically) to autistic disorder, some (such as myself) also have a clinical conviction that there are subgroups within the Asperger's group that might not be as closely related to the core autism phenotype as currently taken for granted. For instance, I have come across at least three different 'familial' subtypes of families with so-called autism spectrum disorders. The first is a family in which there are occasional members affected by classic autism, but no individuals with Asperger's syndrome. The second is a more

Table 7.1: Diagnoses (other than autistic disorder) that confer a high risk of an associated empathy disorder

Diagnosis in the DSM-IV	Important reference
Asperger's disorder	Frith (1991)
Attention deficit/hyperactivity disorder (ADHD)	Gillberg et al. (2006)
Developmental coordination disorder (DCD)	Kadesjö & Gillberg (1999)
Pervasive developmental disorder NOS	Gadow (2005)
Tourette's disorder	Kadesjö & Gillberg (2000)
Obsessive-compulsive personality disorder (OCPD)	Wentz Nilsson et al. (1999)
Other personality disorders	Söderström et al. (2005)
Eating disorders	Wentz et al. (2005)
Selective mutism	Kopp & Gillberg (1997)
Childhood schizophrenia	Asarnow & Ben-Meir (1988)
Bipolar disorder	deLong et al. (2002)
Conduct disorder/oppositional defiant disorder	Green et al. (2000)

common subtype, in which occasional members of the extended family have classic autism and a larger number of members have Asperger's syndrome and an even larger group have autistic features not meeting full criteria for a diagnosis of autism or Asperger's syndrome. The third type of family is one in which a very large number of individuals have Asperger's syndrome, but there is no member even of the very extended family tree who have ever met full criteria for autism. It is this latter group that I sometimes wonder is maybe (even, to some extent clinically) neurobiologically very different from the first two.

Asperger's syndrome of the latter type is only associated with some impairment in the social domain, and very often the 'total' picture does not amount to clear-cut clinical impairment. The first two variants are usually associated with more impairment, usually even severe functional disability. However, all three variants do meet the symptom criteria suggested by my own group (Gillberg, 1991; Gillberg & Gillberg, 1989) (Table 7.1). Incidentally, the variant of Asperger's syndrome described by Hans Asperger (1944) does not meet the DSM-IV or ICD-10 criteria for Asperger's disorder or Asperger syndrome (Miller & Ozonoff, 1997). There is, in fact, good evidence that, if the diagnostic criteria of the ICD-10 or DSM-IV are strictly adhered to, Asperger's syndrome does not exist or is so extremely rare as to be clinically almost meaningless (Leekam et al., 2000, one further reference to the non-usefulness of these criteria).

Whether Asperger's syndrome is the same as or different to 'high-functioning autism' is a topical issue, currently much debated. Personally I do not believe that the concept 'high-functioning autism' is appropriate. It is not the autism that is high functioning in individuals given this diagnosis. The autism symptoms are very often as severe as in so-called low-functioning autism. If this concept is to be used at all, it is better applied to the individual (who may have an IQ in the normal range compared to a more 'low-functioning' individual with an IQ in the mentally retarded range) than to the autism per se. If used in this way, it is my contention that 'high-functioning autism' and Asperger's syndrome are very often one and the same and it is not clinically meaningful to make a distinction between the two.

Of course, on the basis of what has been said in the foregoing, it would probably make most sense to refer to both autistic disorder and Asperger's syndrome as 'autism' (or 'autism spectrum disorder'), the former variant being associated with low IQ (particularly low verbal IQ), and the latter being linked to higher IQ (especially much higher verbal IQ). Put another way, autistic disorder would be autism with a verbal learning disability, and Asperger's syndrome would be the same condition in individuals with a non-verbal learning disability (Cederlund & Gillberg, 2004) or – at least – no verbal learning disability.

7.5 Attention-deficit/hyperactivity disorder (ADHD) with and without developmental coordination disorder (DCD)

Children with ADHD often have empathy problems (Kadesjö & Gillberg, 1998), and a subgroup meet symptomatic diagnostic criteria either for autistic disorder or Asperger's syndrome (Kadesjö & Gillberg, 2001). Children with ADHD (with and without DCD), on average, have very few friends (Barkley, 1990; Gillberg, 1983; Taylor *et al.*, 2004) compared to age peers without ADHD. A number of Swedish studies (e.g. Gillberg, 1983, Kadesjö & Gillberg, 2001; Sturm *et al.*, 2004) have shown that the overlap of ADHD, DCD and autism spectrum disorders is very considerable, and at least one study (Kadesjö & Gillberg, 1999) has suggested that it is the interaction of ADHD with DCD that is strongly associated with autistic symptomatology, ADHD without DCD only very rarely showing 'comorbidity' with autism spectrum disorders.

In an early study of the general population of 7 year olds, Gillberg (1983) reported that a substantial proportion (57%) of children with the combination of severe attention-deficit disorder (ADD) and motor-perception dysfunction (currently recognized as DCD) had marked 'psychotic behaviour'. This latter problem – which was suffered by 1.2% of the general population – was defined as the combination of a triad of social interaction, reciprocal communication and rigid behaviour problems, i.e. the symptom triad now recognized as being at the core of all autism spectrum disorders. Later review of the cases in that study has shown that the vast majority of the group with ADD and DCD (a combination which in Scandinavia is often referred to as deficits in attention, motor control and perception or DAMP) in that study would fall under the DSM-IV diagnostic category of ADHD (Rasmussen & Gillberg, 2000). In summary, then, this study showed that many children with severe ADHD had marked autistic features (including Asperger's syndrome and atypical autism), and that the combination of ADHD, DCD and an autism spectrum disorder occurred in 0.7% (57% of 1.2%) of the general population of Swedish school-age children as early as 30 years ago. This should be contrasted with the reports that, today, 0.6–1.1% of children worldwide are reported to suffer from autism spectrum disorders (Wing & Potter, 2002) and that this prevalence rate has been taken by some as an index of an 'autism epidemic'. The Swedish study performed in the mid 1970s indicated that autism spectrum disorders were just as common then as they appear to be now.

As with Tourette syndrome (see below), the mechanism underlying the empathy problems in ADHD might not always be similar or identical to that encountered in 'autism proper' (whether such a discrete disorder exists or not I am not sure, but let us, for the sake of the present argument, assume that it does). It is possible that, at least in a subgroup, children with ADHD and empathy disorder may be deficient in their ability to empathize with the perspectives of other people because they have attention, hyperactivity and impulsivity problems, hence failing specifically to *attend to* rather than being generally impaired in their understanding of other people's perspectives.

The treatment of ADHD sometimes includes medication with stimulants which have a well-documented beneficial effect in reducing hyperactivity and increasing attentional focusing skills (Greenhill *et al.*, 2002). Occasionally such medication is accompanied by the seeming appearance of autistic/empathy problems in the child. There is now increasing agreement that when such symptoms develop in a child with ADHD treated with a stimulant, this is usually the effect of the 'demasking' of an underlying autism spectrum problem in the child. Reduction of the hyperactivity and inattention 'reveals' the co-existing autistic features/ empathy problems that were previously hidden under the effective mask of extreme behaviour problems associated with ADHD.

7.6 Pervasive developmental disorders not otherwise specified

The DSM category of pervasive developmental disorder not otherwise specified (PDDNOS) is as non-descript as it may appear from the semantic point of view. There are no operationalized criteria and no clear indications as to what degree of clinical impairment is required for the diagnosis to be considered, much less to be made. Many children diagnosed under this umbrella concept will have a disorder which is clearly linked to autism, atypical autism or Asperger's syndrome. However, quite a number probably have problems that are not genetically, neurologically, or clinically linked to autism. Some cases diagnosed under this label would be categorized as suffering from DAMP (in Scandinavia), multiple complex developmental disorder (MCDD) (in parts of the US and in the Netherlands) or atypical autism (in the UK). Many of them would have definite empathy disorders, but, given the lack of clear defining criteria for the PDDNOS category, it is impossible to study its validity and link to empathy problems in the general population.

The overlap of the diagnostic category of PDDNOS with other child neuropsychiatric diagnoses was clearly demonstrated in a recent US study, in which about one in four of children with PDDNOS had combined ADHD and another one in three met criteria for mainly inattentive ADHD (Goldstein & Schwebach, 2004).

7.7 Tourette and other tic disorders

Many individuals with Tourette's syndrome have social interaction problems and empathy deficits (Comings, 1990). The comorbidity of Tourette's syndrome and Asperger's syndrome has been documented in a number of single and multiple case reports (Berthier *et al.*, 2003; Kerbeshian *et al.*, 1995). In a systematic study of a rather larger cohort of individuals with Tourette's disorder, the prevalence of associated autistic features and Asperger's syndrome was very high (Kadesjö & Gillberg, 2000). Conversely, a general population study of Asperger's syndrome (Ehlers & Gillberg, 1993) found a very high rate of associated tics, including full-blown Tourette's syndrome. Thus, whichever perspective is taken, it is clear that empathy deficits, autistic features and Asperger's syndrome are common co-existing problems in people diagnosed as suffering from major tic disorders, including Tourette's syndrome. It is often a matter of the individual clinician's preference or perspective which 'main' diagnosis is portrayed as the clinically most important problem. In my own experience, with a focus in the clinic on autism spectrum disorders (and, hence, empathy problems), tics are often regarded as a second-line or 'comorbid' problem. However, in clinics specializing in Tourette's syndrome and other major tic disorders, empathy problems may well be seen to be a secondary problem, or, indeed, be altogether missed (just as tics are quite often missed by clinicians who have an 'autism perspective').

Some clinical researchers have suggested that early-onset empathy disorders resembling autism (or indeed identical to autism) when associated with early-onset tics/Tourette's syndrome might have a particularly good outcome as regards the autistic type features (Zappella, 2002).

In my clinical practice I have followed a number of children with early-onset (first 4 years of life) major empathy problems that did not amount to full-blown autism or Asperger's syndrome, who later (middle school years) developed severe motor and vocal tics, warranting a diagnosis of Tourette's syndrome. The empathy problems have sometimes been of the autistic type, but on other occasions, characterized more by a common theme of 'meanness' than by a basic failure to cognitively/emotionally take the perspective of other people. Many colleagues have confirmed this clinical impression, but, to my knowledge, no larger scale empirical study has been performed in the field. The empathy problems encountered in these children have often resulted in acts such as being cruel to animals or other children, impulsive lashing out at other people, and physical, sexual, or psychological abuse without remorse. Similar acts are occasionally encountered in children with autism or Asperger's syndrome, though, in my experience, much less often than in Tourette's syndrome. It could be argued that the empathy problems associated with tic disorders may be closely linked to the sometimes extreme degree of impulsivity which is sometimes a clinical hallmark of severe Tourette's syndrome, whereas the empathy problems in autism spectrum disorders are associated with severe cognitive dysfunction in the social-communication domain.

7.8 Obsessive-compulsive disorder (OCD) and obsessive-compulsive personality disorder (OCPD)

Children with severe tic disorders very often have co-existing ADHD and/or OCD (Comings, 1990; Kadesjö & Gilllberg, 2000; Robertson, 2000). In such cases, empathy problems are very common (Kadesjö, 2000). Whether empathy disorders are also over-represented in OCD cases without co-existing tics or ADHD is less well known (Thomsen, 2000).

OCPD according to the DSM-IV is a personality disorder (see below) that cannot be clearly recognized until adolescence or early adult age (APA, 1994). The symptoms of this disorder, however, are present in a proportion of individuals from a much earlier age (Råstam, 1990). There is a striking symptomatic similarity between OCPD as portrayed in the DSM-IV, and the symptoms listed for Asperger's syndrome under the DSM-IV or Gillberg (1991). At least one formal study (Wentz Nilsson *et al.*, 1999) suggests that individuals with autism spectrum disorders in childhood will often meet diagnostic criteria for OCPD at an early adult age. Also, regardless of how these individuals are diagnosed, they usually have severe clinically (reliably) diagnosed 'empathy disorder'.

It is unclear to what extent OCD has anything to do with OCPD (other than the obviously suggestive link at the semantic level).

7.9 Other personality disorders

Most of the personality disorders in clusters A and B of the DSM-IV and (at least) OCPD of cluster C comprise symptoms that have a major bearing on social interaction and intersubjectivity. Schizoid personality disorder is perhaps the most striking of these from the point of view of empathy problems. Several authors (Ssucharewa, 1926; Ssucharewa & Wolff, 1996) have described 'schizoid children' in sufficient detail to suggest the behavioural phenotype of Asperger's syndrome, an autism spectrum disorder diagnosed on the basis of extreme egocentricity and empathy problems (Gillberg, 1991). Follow-up studies of individuals with autism spectrum disorders and follow-back studies of adults with personality disorder diagnoses show clearly that many adult individuals with life-long autism spectrum problems meet criteria for one, two or several of the personality disorders mentioned (Söderström *et al.*, 2005).

7.10 Eating disorders

Several systematic studies by my own group have shown that a considerably sized subgroup of all individuals in the general population suffering from anorexia nervosa also have major problems with empathy (Råstam *et al.*, 2003). In fact, as many as one in six of all cases of teenage-onset anorexia nervosa may have an autism spectrum disorder (Asperger's syndrome, atypical autism and autistic disorder) diagnosable in accordance with DSM criteria for such disorders (or 'pervasive developmental disorders'). Another one in six might have clinically significant empathy problems that are likely to be important when opting for intervention. Individuals with empathy problems will have major difficulty participating in any kind of group (or family) therapy, given the considerably reduced capacity for metarepresentation and interpersonal communication characteristic of such problems. Such therapy is usually regarded as the mainstay of 'treatment' in eating disorders. Those with eating disorders and clinically significant empathy disorders would probably benefit greatly from interventions believed to be effective in autism spectrum disorders, i.e. more concrete, structured and with little, if anything, in the way of symbolic interpretation.

Eating disorders other than anorexia nervosa (including bulimia nervosa) have not been sufficiently studied from the point of view of possible associated empathy problems. Nevertheless, a recent study of adult eating-disordered in-patients (including a number with bulimia nervosa) has demonstrated that a very considerable proportion of all affected have 'comorbid' neuropsychiatric disorders (specifically autism spectrum disorders, Tourette's syndrome and ADHD) (Wentz *et al.*, 2005).

7.11 Selective mutism

Children with refusal to speak in some settings often meet diagnostic criteria for selective mutism. Young children diagnosed with this condition sometimes suffer from an underlying autism spectrum disorder or empathy disorder in which the refusal to speak is but one of a set of problems connected with behavioural rigidity and obsessionality (Kopp & Gillberg, 1997; Kristensen, 2002; Wolff, 1995). Selective mutism is variously conceptualized as an anxiety disorder, a variant of an obsessive-compulsive condition or a social-communication disorder, yet only rarely clinically thought of in the context of disorders of empathy/autism spectrum disorders. Clinicians need to acquaint themselves with the concept of selective mutism being more of a symptom than a syndrome, and that the 'underlying' comorbidity might well be the most important condition from the point of view of intervention and outcome.

7.12 Childhood schizophrenia

Schizophrenia is an extremely rare disorder in childhood (Asarnow & Ben-Meir, 1988), with an increasing number of cases beginning to appear in early adolescence (Coleman & Gillberg, 1996). The diagnosis appears to be somewhat more commonly made in young children in the US than in Europe. I have personally assessed and followed-up thousands of children with neurodevelopmental disorders but have only come across three individuals who met diagnostic criteria for schizophrenia before the age of 8 years. In these cases – and in about one in four of those described in some US cases series with a diagnosis of early-onset childhood schizophrenia – major autistic symptoms were present before the emergence of the clinical picture consistent with a diagnosis of schizophrenia. Studies on adults with schizophrenia have shown the presence of Theory of Mind problems in quite a proportion of affected individuals, indicating a link with empathy problems. Indeed the clinical picture of schizophrenia is often consistent with severe empathy disorder, even though this is not a universal problem in all cases examined. It seems more likely that the Theory of Mind problems documented in some adults with schizophrenia have been present from childhood rather than having occurred for the first time at an adult age. A large body of evidence suggests that schizophrenia is usually a developmental disorder with roots in early childhood (Coleman & Gillberg, 1996; Fish, 1977).

7.13 Bipolar disorder

Several publications have appeared in the recent past documenting the coexistence of autism spectrum disorders and manic-depressive illness/bipolar disorder (deLong & Dwyer, 1988; Gillberg, 1985; Ståhlberg et al., 2004). There have also been reports suggesting that autism and bipolar disorder might be linked at the genetic/familial level (deLong, 1994). Whether bipolar disorder 'in itself' is clearly linked to empathy problems has not been systematically studied as far as I am aware. Clinically, there can be little doubt that manic episodes (and severe episodes of major depression) can comprise extreme degrees of reduced empathy, but it is doubtful whether such empathy problems are also present during 'normothymic' periods.

According to one US group, the autism-bipolar comorbidity is a marker for a fairly homogeneous subgroup within the spectrum of empathy disorders (deLong *et al.*, 2002). Positive response to fluoxetine treatment, family history of major affective disorder (especially bipolar), unusual achievement and hyperlexia in the children appear to define this subgroup. The authors argue that bipolar disorder, unusual intellectual achievement and autism spectrum/empathy disorders cluster strongly in families and may share genetic determinants.

7.14 Conduct disorder and oppositional-defiant disorder (ODD)

ADHD is grouped alongside conduct disorder and ODD as a subcategory of 'disruptive behaviour disorders' in the DSM. Clinically this might have been seen to be appropriate considering the degree of acting-out behaviour often encountered in ADHD, including the common misbehaviour and conduct problems that often ensue in children with early-onset ADHD problems. However, in all those with conduct and oppositional-defiant behaviours unassociated with ADHD, it probably does not make sense to group these two kinds of problems under the same general heading.

We know that ADHD is often associated with autism spectrum and other empathy problems (see above). However, whether conduct disorder/ODD unassociated with ADHD is linked with empathy problems as defined in the present context is not known. Clinically, it would seem clear that many people with criminal behaviours, including a variety of violent activities, may have severe deficits empathizing with the perspectives of other people. However, needless to say, the manipulative abilities of many individuals who exhibit typical problems associated with conduct disorders are no less in doubt. 'Manipulation' does not seem to be a skill that is well developed in autism or any other disorder associated with a deficient ability to take the perspective of other people. Therefore, on balance, in spite of the superficially suggestive link between conduct disorder/ ODD and empathy problems, disruptive behaviour disorders other than those associated with ADHD should probably not be considered to be examples of 'disorders of empathy'. Nevertheless, some authors (e.g. Söderstrom, 2003) seem to argue that 'psychopathy' (which is often construed as the most severe variant of an antisocial personality disorder or conduct disorder) should be interpreted as a disorder of empathy.

On the basis of clinical experience and some small-scale studies it seems likely that conduct disorder/ODD can sometimes be the presenting symptomatic phenotype of a disorder in the autism spectrum (Adams *et al.*, 2002). Therefore, children diagnosed with disruptive behaviour disorders should always be considered from the point of view of possibly suffering from an underlying autistic type symptomatology, including Asperger's syndrome and atypical autism.

7.15 Conclusions

Quite a number of the conditions diagnosed under the childhood section of the DSM-IV and a rather smaller set of those in the adult section are associated with empathy disorders. This association is usually accounted for by a considerable subgroup within the larger group showing severe disorders of empathy, with the remaining group having few or no symptoms of such problems. Empathy disorders with severe problems taking the perspectives of other people have very important implications for understanding the cognitive, social and communicative style of the affected individual and, hence, for intervention. The various diagnostic conditions reviewed in this chapter should be seen as signal markers for the need to evaluate for autistic type empathy problems.

REFERENCES

Adams, C., Green, J., Gilchrist, A., & Cox, A. (2002). Conversational behaviour of children with Asperger Syndrome and conduct disorder. *Journal of Child Psychology and Psychiatry*, **43**(5): 679–690.

Anckarsäter H., Stahlberg, O., Hakansson, C., *et al.* (2005). The impact of ADHD and autism spectrum disorders on temperament, character and personality development. *American Journal of Psychiatry*, 2006; **163**, 1239–44.

American Psychiatric Association (1994). *Diagnostic and Statistical Manual of Mental Disorders* (4th edn.). Washington, DC: American Psychiatric Association Press.

Asarnow, J. R., & Ben-Meir, S. (1988). Children with schizophrenia spectrum and depressive disorders: a comparative study of premorbid adjustment, onset pattern and severity of impairment. *Journal of Child Psychology and Psychiatry*, **29**(4), 477–488.

Asperger, H. (1944). Die autistischen Psychopathen im Kindesalter. *Archiv für Psychiatrie und Nervenkrankheiten*, **117**, 76–136.

Barkley, R. A. (1990). *Hyperactive Children: A Handbook for Diagnosis and Treatment*. New York: Guilford Press.

Berthier, M. L., Kulisevsky, J., Asenjo, B., Aparicio, J., & Lara, D. (2003). Comorbid Asperger and Tourette syndromes with localized mesencephalic, infrathalamic, thalamic, and striatal damage. *Developmental Medicine and Child Neurology*, **45**(3), 207–212.

Carrey, N. J. (1995). Itard's 1828 memoire on 'Mutism caused by a lesion of the intellectual functions': a historical analysis. *Journal of the American Acadademy of Child and Adolescent Psychiatry*, **34**(**12**), 1655–1661.

Cederlund, M., & Gillberg, C. (2004). One hundred males with Asperger Syndrome. A clinical study of background and associated factors. *Developmental Medicine and Child Neurology*, **46**(**10**), 652–660.

Coleman, M., & Gillberg, C. (1996). *The Schizophrenias*. New York: Springer Publishing Company.

Comings, D. E. (1990). *Tourette Syndrome and Human Behaviour*. Duarte, Calif.: Hope Press.

DeLong, G. R., & Dwyer, J. T. (1988). Correlation of family history with specific autistic subgroups: Asperger's syndrome and bipolar affective disease. *Journal of Autism and Developmental Disorders*, **18**(**4**), 593–600.

DeLong, G. R., Ritch, C. R., & Burch, S. (2002). Fluoxetine response in children with autistic spectrum disorders: correlation with familial major affective disorder and intellectual achievement. *Developmental Medicine and Child Neurology*, **44**(**10**), 652–659.

DeLong, R. (1994). Children with autistic spectrum disorder and a family history of affective disorder. *Developmental Medicine and Child*, **36**(**8**), 674–687.

Ehlers, S. & Gillberg, C. (1993). The epidemiology of Asperger syndrome. A total population study. *Journal of Child Psychology and Psychiatry*, **34**(**8**), 1327–1350.

Fish, B. (1977). Neurobiologic antecedents of schizophrenia in children. Evidence for an inherited, congenital neurointegrative defect. *Archives of General Psychiatry*, **34**(**11**), 1297–1313.

Frith, U. (1991). *Autism and Asperger Syndrome*. Cambridge: Cambridge University Press.

Gadow, K. (2005). Pervasive developmental disorders not otherwise specified (PBDNOS). In D. J. Cohen, F. Volkmar (eds.), *Handbook of Autism and Pervasive Developmental Disorders*. New York: John Wiley.

Gillberg, C. (1983). Perceptual, motor and attentional deficits in Swedish primary school children. Some child psychiatric aspects. *Journal of Child Psychology and Psychiatry*, **24**(**3**), 377–403.

Gillberg, C. (1985). Asperger's syndrome and recurrent psychosis – a case study. *Journal of Autism and Developmental Disorders*, **15**, 389–397.

Gillberg, C. (1991). Clinical and neurobiological aspects of Asperger syndrome in six family studies. In U. Frith (ed.), *Autism and Asperger Syndrome* (pp. 122–146). Cambridge: Cambridge University Press.

Gillberg, C. (1992). The Emanuel Miller Memorial Lecture 1991: Autism and autistic-like conditions: subclasses among disorders of empathy. *Journal of Child Psychology and Psychiatry*, **33**, 813–842.

Gillberg, C. (1993). Empatistörningar: grundläggande vid flera psykiatriska handikapp Empathy disorders: basic problems in severe psychiatric handicap conditions. *Läkartidningen*, **90**(**6**), 467–470 (in Swedish).

Gillberg, C. (1995). *Clinical Child Neuropsychiatry*. Cambridge: Cambridge University Press.

Gillberg, C. (1999). Autism and its spectrum disorders. In N. Bouras (ed.), *Psychiatric and Behavioural Disorders in Developmental Disabilites* (pp. 73–95). Cambridge: Cambridge University Press.

Gillberg, C., & Coleman, M. (2000). *The Biology of the Autistic Syndromes*. Cambridge: Cambridge University Press.

Gillberg, C., Santosh, P., & Brown, T. E. (2006). Comorbidity of ADHD with autism, Asperger syndrome, and other autism spectrum disorders. In T. E. Brown (ed.), *American Psychiatric Press Textbook of Attention Deficit Disorders and Comorbidities in Children, Adolescents and Adults*. In press.

Gillberg, I. C., & Gillberg, C. (1989). Asperger syndrome – some epidemiological considerations: a research note. *Journal of Child Psychology and Psychiatry*, **30(4)**, 631–638.

Goldstein, S., & Schwebach, A. J. (2004). The comorbidity of pervasive developmental disorder and attention deficit hyperactivity disorder: results of a retrospective chart review. *Journal of Autism and Developmental Disorders*, **34(3)**, 329–339.

Green, J., Gilchrist, A., Burton, D., & Cox, A. (2000). Social and psychiatric functioning in adolescents with Asperger syndrome compared with conduct disorder. *Journal of Autism and Developmental Disorders*, **30(4)**, 279–293.

Greenhill, L. *et al.* (2002). Guidelines and algorithms for the use of methylphenidate in children with Attention-Deficit/Hyperactivity Disorder. *Journal of Attention Disorders Supplement* **1**: S89–S100.

Kadesjö, B. (2000). Neuropsychiatric and neurodevelopmental disorders in a young school-age population. Epidemiology and comorbidity in a school health perspective, in Department of Child and Adolescent Psychiatry, Institute for the Health of Women and Children (p. 76). Göteborg: Göteborg University.

Kadesjö, B., & Gillberg, C. (1998). Attention deficits and clumsiness in Swedish 7-year-old children. *Developmental Medicine and Child Neurology*, **40(12)**, 796–804.

Kadesjö, B., & Gillberg, C. (1999). Developmental coordination disorder in Swedish 7-year-old children. *Journal of the American Academy of Child and Adolescent Psychiatry*, **38(7)**, 820–828.

Kadesjö, B., & Gillberg, C. (2000). Tourette's disorder: epidemiology and comorbidity in primary school children. *Journal of the American Academy of Child and Adolescent Psychiatry*, **39(5)**, 548–555.

Kadesjö, B., & Gillberg, C. (2001). The comorbidity of ADHD in the general population of Swedish school-age children. *Journal of Child Psychology and Psychiatry*, **42(4)**, 487–492.

Kerbeshian, J., Burd, L., & Klug, M. G. (1995). Comorbid Tourette's disorder and bipolar disorder: an etiologic perspective. *Am J Psychiatry* **152(11)**: 1646–1651.

Kopp, S., & Gillberg, C. (1997). Selective mutism: a population-based study: research note. *Journal of Child Psychology and Psychiatry*, **38(2)**, 257–262.

Kristensen, H. (2002). Selective mutism in children. Comorbidity and clinical characteristics. In *Faculty of Medicine* (p. 652). Oslo: University of Oslo.

Leekam, S., Libby, S., Wing, L., Gould, J., & Gillberg, C. (2000). Comparison of ICD-10 and Gillberg's criteria for Asperger syndrome. *Autism*, **4**, 11–28.

Miller, J. N., & Ozonoff, S. (1997). Did Asperger's cases have Asperger disorders? A research note. *Journal of Child Psychology and Psychiatry*, **38(2)**, 247–251.

Rasmussen, P., & Gillberg, C. (2000). Natural outcome of ADHD with developmental coordination disorder at age 22 years: a controlled, longitudinal, community-based study. *Journal of the American Academy of Child and Adolescent Psychiatry*, **39(11)**, 1424–1431.

Råstam, M. (1990). Anorexia nervosa in Swedish urban teenagers. In *Departments of Pediatrics and Child Psychiatry*. Göteborg: Göteborg.

Rästam, M., Gillberg, C., & Wentz, E. (2003). Outcome of teenage-onset anorexia nervosa in a Swedish community-based sample. *Eur child Adolesc Psychiatry*, **12** suppl 1: 178–90.

Råstam, M., Gillberg, I. C., Gillberg, C., & Johansson, M. (1997). Alexithymia in anorexia nervosa: a controlled study using the 20-item Toronto Alexithymia Scale. *Acta Psychiatrica Scandinavica*, **95**, 385–388.

Robertson, M. M. (2000). Tourette syndrome, associated conditions and the complexities of treatment. *Brain*, **123**(Pt 3), 425–462.

Söderström H. (2003). Psychopathy as a disorder of empathy. *Eur Child Adolesc Psychiatry*, **12**:249–52.

Ssucharewa, G. E. (1926). Die schizoiden Psychopathien im Kindesalter. *Monatsschrift für Psychiatrie und Neurologie*, **60**, 235–261.

Ssucharewa, G. E., & Wolff, S. (1996). The first account of the syndrome Asperger described? Translation of a paper entitled "Die schizoiden Psychopathien im Kindesalter" by Dr. G. E. Ssucharewa; scientific assistant, which appeared in 1926 in the *Monatsschrift für Psychiatrie und Neurologie*, **60**, 235–261. *European Child and Adolescent Psychiatry*, **5**(3), 119–132.

Ståhlberg, O., Soderstrom, H., Rastam, M., & Gillberg, C. (2004). Bipolar disorder, schizophrenia, and other psychotic disorders in adults with childhood onset AD/HD and/or autism spectrum disorders. *Journal of Neural Transmission*, **111**(7), 891–902.

Sturm, H., Fernell, E., & Gillberg, C. (2004). Autism spectrum disorders in children with normal intellectual levels: associated impairments and subgroups. *Developmental Medicine and Child Neurology*, **46**(7), 444–447.

Taylor, E., Dopfner, M., Sergeant, J., *et al.* (2004). European clinical guidelines For hyperkinetic disorder-first upgrade. *Eur Child Adolesc Psychiatry*, **13** Suppl 1, 17–30.

Thomsen, P. H. (2000). Obsessions: the impact and treatment of obsessive-compulsive disorder in children and adolescents. *Journal of Psychopharmacology*, **14**(2 Suppl 1), S31–S37.

Wentz, E., Lacey, J. H., Waller, G., *et al.* (2005). Childhood onset neuropsychiatric disorders in adult eating disorder patients – a controlled pilot study. *European and Child and Adolescent Psychiatry*, **14**, 431–437.

Wentz Nilsson, E., Gillberg, C., Gillberg, I. C., & Råstam, M. (1999). Ten year follow-up of adolescent-onset anorexia nervosa: personality disorders. *Journal of the American Academy of Child and Adolescent Psychiatry*, **38**(11), 1389–1395.

Wing, L., & Potter, D. (2002). The epidemiology of autistic spectrum disorders: is the prevalence rising? *Mental Retardation and Developmental Disabilities Research Reviews*, **8**(3), 151–161.

Wolff, S. (1995). Loners. *The Life Path of Unusual Children*. London: Routledge.

World Health Organization (1993). *The International Classification of Diseases (Classification of Mental and Behavioural Disorders)*. Geneva: World Health Organization.

Zappella, M. (2002). Early-onset Tourette syndrome with reversible autistic behaviour: a dysmaturational disorder. *European Child and Adolescent Psychiatry*, **11**(1), 18–23.

Empathy and autism

Peter Hobson

Developmental Psychopathology Research Unit, Tavistock Clinic and Institute of Child Health

8.1 Introduction

For anyone who needs to be persuaded of the critical role that empathy plays in human interpersonal engagement, or who wants to learn more about the significance of empathy for early human development – or even, perhaps, one who seeks to understand what empathy *is* – there could be few sources of insight more arresting than the phenomenon of early childhood autism. From a complementary perspective, I would contend (against considerable opposition from my fellow researchers in the field) that it is only when one grasps the far-reaching developmental implications of the lack of empathy experienced by children with autism, implications that are serious for cognitive as well as social development, that the pathogenesis of this condition becomes understandable.

These claims exemplify the perspective of developmental psychopathology that I shall be adopting for this chapter. The specialness of the approach is that it involves the coordinated study of typical and atypical development. This allows one to apprehend otherwise obscure processes and mechanisms of typical development on the one hand, and specific forms of derailment in development leading to psychopathology on the other. Just as the study of autism reveals a great deal about empathy, so an appreciation of the developmental role of empathy in typical development promises to deepen our understanding of the pathogenesis of autism.

The best place to start in order to set the scene for the scientific evidence and theoretical discussions that will form the body of this chapter is with Kanner's (1943) account of 11 children whom he described as having 'inborn autistic disturbances of affective contact' (p. 250). It is through clinical descriptions such as these that one grasps what the children are like to observe or to assess, but, more important still, what it *feels like* to be with them and to relate to them. On the one hand, Kanner attempted to capture the children's stance in

Empathy in Mental Illness, eds. Tom F. D. Farrow and Peter W. R. Woodruff. Published by Cambridge University Press. © Cambridge University Press 2007.

relation to others by writing of their 'profound aloneness'; on the other, he conveyed how 'people, so long as they left the child alone, figured in about the same manner as did the desk, the bookshelf, or the filing cabinet' (p. 246). In this latter description, one senses how Kanner felt *himself* to be treated as a piece of furniture. It is this quality of experience that most people find striking about their encounters with children with autism, at least when relating to more severely affected children, and it is through such experience that one begins to grasp how profoundly and disturbingly 'inhuman' it can feel to relate to others without empathy.

What barely needs stating here is that empathy is something that happens *between* people. It is something experienced by one person as a mode of relating to another, part and parcel of what it means to have interpersonal relations, and not merely something that occurs in sporadic bouts of fellow-feeling. 'Affective contact', as Kanner expressed it, is no vague or metaphorical phenomenon: it is a felt and vital part of what makes human interpersonal engagement what it is. So it is that people who relate to children with autism feel the lack of something they expect to be part of their interchange with others; and for children's part, by all appearances, they seem to lack the feel of what personal relatedness really means.

Here is a description of one of Kanner's cases:

Case 9

Charles was brought to the clinic at the age of four and a half years, his mother complaining how 'the thing that upsets me most is that I can't reach my baby'. As a baby, this child would lie in the crib, just staring. When he was one and a half years old, he began to spend hours spinning toys and the lids of bottles and jars. His mother remarked: 'He would pay no attention to me and show no recognition of me if I enter the room. The most impressive thing is his detachment and his inaccessibility. He walks as if he is in a shadow, lives in a world of his own where he cannot be reached. No sense of relationship to persons. He went through a period of quoting another person; never offers anything himself. His entire conversation is a replica of whatever has been said to him. He used to speak of himself in the second person, now he uses the third person at times; he would say, 'He wants' – never 'I want' . . . When he is with other people, he doesn't look up at them. Last July, we had a group of people. When Charles came in, it was just like a foal who'd been let out of an enclosure . . . He has a wonderful memory for words. Vocabulary is good, except for pronouns. He never initiates conversation, and conversation is limited, extensive only as far as objects go'.

In this moving account by a mother who felt she could not reach her baby, we can register the force of Kanner's suggestion that autistic children 'have come into the world with innate inability to form the usual, biologically provided affective contact with people'. Charles was inaccessible to his mother. For his own part, he seemed not to attend to his mother or to other people, nor even to recognize them as beings with whom he could become emotionally engaged: '. . . it was just like a foal who'd been let out of an enclosure'.

In taking an overview of his 11 case descriptions, Kanner listed many other features of the syndrome of autism. Each of these needs to be placed within a developmental account that portrays what is 'basic' to the disorder, and specifies how further impairments arise as developmental sequelae to the primary deficit or deficits. Prominent among the features that Kanner highlighted were the children's failure to assume an anticipatory posture to being picked up; their difficulty in using language to convey meaning to others, even though many could repeat nursery rhymes or even foreign-language lullabies; their tendency to produce sentences that were 'for a long time mostly parrot-like repetitions of heard word combinations', sometimes taking the form of delayed echolalia; their often inflexible (context-insensitive) use of words; their abnormal use of the personal pronouns 'I' and 'you', which might be repeated just as heard, complete with echoed intonation and without adjustment to who was speaking; their unresponsiveness, to the extent that some were considered deaf or hard of hearing; their overriding desire to maintain sameness in their routines and surroundings; and more generally, the lack of variety in their spontaneous activity. Current-day definitions of the syndrome systematize and to some degree extend this description, for example giving prominence to the children's lack of creative symbolic play, but Kanner's characterization still succeeds in conveying the essential features of the syndrome.

Moreover, Kanner stressed how the study of autism might 'help to furnish concrete criteria regarding the still diffuse notions about the constitutional components of emotional reactivity' (p. 150). It is so easy for people who hear talk of autism as an 'interpersonal' disorder, to jump to the mistaken conclusion that this means it is psychogenic, the result of failures in empathy on the part of parents or other caregivers. This is emphatically not the line I am taking in the present chapter. Rather, we need to consider what biological equipment human infants need to bring to the business of social relations, in order to achieve the quality of emotional linkage with others that makes interpersonal involvement and concern what it is. In this chapter I shall not be concerned with the various aetiologies of autism – I believe there are a range of physical disorders that can give rise to the syndrome, and sometimes risk factors such as congenital blindness play a role (e.g. Hobson *et al.*, 1999) – and instead I shall focus on the qualities of social disability that the children share in common.

Before I move on to detail systematic scientific evidence that helps us to characterize the empathy-related impairments associated with autism, I want to cite a final clinical vignette. The reason is that it exemplifies how, once one adopts a developmental perspective on autism and appreciates the knock-on effects of early-arising and continuing disabilities in social engagement – disabilities that entail impoverishment in the children's experience of empathy with and 'personal relatedness' towards other people – then one becomes sensitized to how affected children might lack some of the foundations for constructing *concepts* about people as special kinds of 'thing' with subjective attitudes who have person-specific ways of construing objects and events. Here is what an intelligent young autistic adult said, when interviewed by the psychiatrist Donald Cohen (1980). This man described how the first years of his life were devoid of people:

I really didn't know there were people until I was seven years old. I then suddenly realised that there were people. But not like you do. I still have to remind myself that there are people ... I never could have a friend. I really don't know what to do with other people, really.

So even when the person with autism realizes that there are people, he still finds it difficult to relate to them *as* people. Only slowly does it dawn on him that persons are a special class of things with their own feelings, thoughts and beliefs about the world; and even when he achieves such understanding, insofar as he does, still he lacks the natural ability to engage on a personal level.

In my view (which I have expounded in a recent book, *The Cradle of Thought*, as well as in its dense academic forerunner: Hobson, 1993, 2002/2004), these empathy-related handicaps have repercussions far beyond the domain of inter-personal relations. They affect the development of thinking, self-awareness and reflective action. They are a principal, perhaps *the* principal, reason why the constellation of clinical features we call 'autism' is configured in the way it is. In typical development, at least from the end of the first year of life, human beings are constantly shifted into adopting new ways of relating to and understanding the world and themselves *through* other people; but children impervious to such influences are children unmoved (emotionally *and* intellectually) from a rigid, 'egocentric', single-track apprehension of the things and events that surround them. Moreover they have but a fragile basis for taking an external perspective on themselves and their own actions and mental states. Without the powerful influence of engagement with other people experienced *as* other people – people who are perceived to have attitudes that one responds to, coordinates with and makes one's own – cognitive as well as social development is severely compromised.

All this should suffice to provide the framework for what follows. I shall now select a few areas of research that demonstrate how deficits in empathy are indeed a characteristic feature of autism from the earliest years of life. Although it remains controversial how far such deficits *cause* other features of autism, such as the children's limited joint attention with others or their dearth of symbolic play, I shall stress the potential (and I believe, actual) developmental implications of severe empathic disorder for such domains of psychological functioning. *En passant*, I shall cite some very recent studies of autism that point to an aspect of empathy that is widely underestimated, but developmentally critical: identification with other people.

8.2 Early manifestations of autism

Parental reports (e.g. Dahlgren & Gillberg, 1989; Lord *et al.*, 1993; Stone & Lemanek, 1990; Vostanis *et al.*, 1998; Wing, 1969) provide an important perspective on the early clinical features of autism. In one recent study, for example, Wimpory *et al.* (2000) interviewed parents of very young children who were referred with difficulties in relating to and communicating with others. At the time of interview, the undiagnosed children were between 32 and 48 months old, and it was only subsequently that 10 of these children diagnosed with autism were compared with 10 of the children, matched for age and developmental level, who did not have autism. The parents' reports indicated that as infants, those with autism had a number of abnormalities in the area of person-to-person nonverbal communication and interpersonal contact. Not one of the infants with autism had shown frequent and intense eye contact, engaged in turn-taking with adults, or used noises communicatively, whereas half of the control children were reported to show each of these kinds of behaviour. There were also fewer infants with autism who greeted or waved to their parents, who raised their arms to be picked up, who directed feelings of anger and distress towards people, who were sociable in play, or who enjoyed and participated in lap games. In each of these respects, there were clear limitations in their affective engagement with others.

Such studies provide welcome detail of what one might encompass under the phrase 'lack of empathy', especially concerning attentiveness and mutual relatedness towards other people. But the interviews of Wimpory *et al.* (2000) also highlighted something else, namely what lack of engagement with another person's attitudes might mean for interpersonally coordinated relations *with reference to objects and events in the environment*. For example, not one of the infants with autism but at least half the infants in the control group were reported to offer or give objects to others in the first two years of life. The same was true of pointing at objects or following others' points. Few children with autism were said to show objects to others, and not one was said to have looked between an object of interest and an adult, for example when the infant wanted something out of reach. The evidence suggests that the children's lack of interpersonal engagement extends to circumstances in which they might share experiences of the world with other people. They not only appear to be less empathically connected with other people for their own sake, but also less connected with or able to share others' affective attitudes to a shared world (Kasari *et al.*, 1990).

Retrospective parental reports such as this are complemented by systematic observational and experimental studies. One example is the study by Lord (1995), who assessed 30 two-year-old children referred for possible autism and then reassessed them one year later in order to ascertain which children received a diagnosis of autism at this later stage. On re-examining the data from the earlier assessment, she concluded that the two-year-olds with autism differed from the other children with developmental disorders in specific aspects of: (1) communicative behaviour: their lack of response to another person's voice, absence of pointing, and failure to understand gesture; (2) social reciprocity: lack of seeking to share their enjoyment, failure to greet, unusual use of others' bodies, lack of initiative in directing visual attention, and lack of interest in children; and (3) restricted, repetitive behaviour: hand and finger mannerisms and unusual sensory behaviour. From an early age, therefore, socio-emotional engagement is a distinctive domain of abnormality in children with autism.

Then there are several lines of evidence to suggest that from a young age, the children are abnormal both in expressing and perceiving emotion in others – where to perceive emotion *as* emotion might well entail some emotional experience and/or expression, this being the kind of perception that it is. For example, Snow *et al.* (1987) videotaped matched groups of children with and without autism, aged between 30 months and 4 years, as they interacted with the mother, a child psychiatrist and a nursery school teacher. Across 20 15-s intervals of child interaction with each partner, almost all the positive affect of the non-autistic children was expressed towards the other person. By contrast, the children with autism not only showed less frequent displays of affect, but also these were as likely to occur at seemingly random, self-absorbed moments as in the context of social interaction. Or again, Dawson *et al.* (1990) videotaped 16 autistic children aged 2–6 years and 16 typically developing children matched for receptive language interacting with their mothers. There were no significant differences in the autistic children's frequency or duration of gaze at the mother's face, nor differences in the frequency or duration of smiles in the face-to-face interaction over a snack. However, children with autism were much less likely than typically developing children to combine their smiles with eye contact in a single act that seemed to convey an intent to communicate feelings. Not only this, but very few of the autistic subjects ever smiled in response to their mother's smile. It was also observed that the mothers of the children with autism were less likely to smile in response to their children's smiles, which after all were rarely combined with sustained eye contact. One might question how much sharing or coordination of affective states could take place under these circumstances.

Sigman *et al.* (1992; also Charman *et al.*, 1997) conducted a more direct test of empathic responsiveness. Participants were 30 young autistic children with a mean age of under 4 years, and closely matched non-autistic retarded and typically developing children. The technique was to code these children's behaviour when an adult pretended to hurt herself by hitting her finger with a hammer, simulated fear towards a remote-controlled robot, and pretended to be ill by lying down on a couch for a minute, feigning discomfort. In each of these situations, children with autism were unusual in rarely looking at or relating to the adult. When the adult pretended to be hurt, for example, children with autism often appeared unconcerned and continued to play with toys. When a small remote-controlled robot moved towards the child and stopped about four feet away, the parent and the experimenter, who were both seated nearby, made fearful facial expressions, gestures and vocalizations for 30 s. Almost all the non-autistic children looked at an adult at some point during this period, but fewer than half the children with autism did so, and then only briefly. The children with autism were not only less hesitant than the mentally retarded children in playing with the robot, but they also played with it for substantially longer periods of time. It seemed that they were less influenced by the fearful attitudes of those around them. Here again we find evidence that autistic children are relatively 'unengaged' not only in one-to-one interpersonal-affective transactions, but also with another person's emotional attitudes towards objects and events in the world.

Experimentally structured studies have been important in analysing the nature and specificity of such quasi-naturalistic observations. Ricks (1975, 1979) tape-recorded six 3- and 4-year-old non-verbal children with autism, six non-verbal non-autistic children of the same age who had mental retardation, and six typically developing infants aged between 8 and 11 months, in four situations. The first was a 'request' situation, when the children were hungry and their favourite meals were prepared and shown to them; the second was an occasion of frustration, when the meal was withheld for a few moments; the third was one of greeting, when the children saw their mothers on waking in the morning, or when she returned to the room after an absence; and in the fourth, involving pleased surprise, the children were presented with a novel and interesting stimulus, the blowing up of a balloon or the lighting of a sparkler firework. The recordings of the children's vocalizations in each of these situations were edited, and played back to the mothers of the children. The mother's task was to identify in which context each vocalization had been recorded, to identify her own child, and to identify the non-autistic child. The second set of recordings comprised the request vocalizations of all six autistic children, and the task was for the mother to identify her own child.

The mothers of typically developing infants' vocalizations could easily identify the 'message' of each signal of every infant, but found difficulty in identifying which signals came from their own child. When the tapes of the autistic and non-autistic participants were presented to the autistic children's mothers, these mothers too could recognize the contexts from which their own autistic child's vocalizations had been derived, and they could also identify the signals of the one non-autistic child on tape (often explaining that he 'sounded normal'). What they were unable to do was to recognize the contexts associated with the vocalizations of autistic children other than their own. Each of these children's signals seemed to be idiosyncratic. Correspondingly, and in contrast with the parents of typically developing children, they could readily and unerringly identify their own child from the various vocalizations. Ricks concluded that whereas typically developing infants seem to have an unlearned set of emotionally communicative vocalizations, autistic children either do not develop these signals or, having reached the age of 3–5 years, they no longer use them. On the other hand, their idiosyncratic signals do have emotional meanings. It seems unlikely that such expressions (and see Yirmiya *et al.*, 1989, for a study of the children's atypical facial expressions) could mediate the kind of interpersonal coordination of affect that is the mark of empathy.

8.3 Research with older children and adolescents with autism

It is instructive to trace the evolving patterns of abnormality in social relatedness as the children get older. For example, Lee and Hobson (1998) videotaped children and adolescents greeting an unfamiliar person and later taking their leave. Compared with matched mentally retarded control children, only half as many of the children and adolescents with autism gave spontaneous expressions of greeting, and many failed to respond even after prompting. All the 24 young people without autism made eye contact, but a third of those with autism failed to do so; no fewer than 17 of the former group, but only 6 of those with autism, smiled. In the farewell episode, half the individuals without autism but only three of those with autism made eye contact and said a goodbye. Or again, Attwood *et al.* (1988) observed adolescents with autism and with Down's syndrome interacting with their peers for a total of 20 30-s periods in the playground and at the dinner table. All 15 Down's subjects interacted socially during the period of observation, but only 11 of the 18 autistic children did so. Although the mean number of gestures per interaction did not distinguish the groups, there were differences in the kinds of gesture employed. Both groups used simple pointing gestures and gestures to prompt behaviour, such as those to indicate 'come here' or 'be quiet'; but whereas 10 out of 15 individuals with Down's syndrome used at least one expressive gesture, such as giving a hug of consolation, making a 'thumbs-up' sign, or covering the face in embarrassment, not one such gesture was seen in the autistic group. Here in adolescence, where the picture of social relatedness takes a different form to that of earlier years, individuals with autism were still showing the now-familiar picture of limited empathy.

With such older individuals, too, it is possible to conduct experiments to delineate more specifically which aspects of interpersonal perception and judgement are impaired in autism, and which are relatively spared – yielding insight into the specific aspects of person-perception and responsiveness that are integral to empathy, and those which are probably of peripheral importance. There is now a body of such research suggesting that there are autism-specific deficits in emotion perception and understanding. Most studies have focused upon judgements of emotion in the face (Hobson, 1991 provides an overview of the methodological issues), but here is a study concerning gestural expressions. Moore *et al.* (1997) tested children and adolescents with and without autism, matched for age and verbal ability, and showed them videotape sequences of people's moving bodies depicted merely by dots of light attached to the trunk and limbs. First we presented separate 5-s sequences of the point-light person enacting in turn the gestures of surprise, sadness, fear, anger and happiness (each of which could be recognized with very high reliability among naive raters). In the surprise sequence, for example, the person walked forward and suddenly checked his stride and jerked backward with his arms thrown out to the side; in the sad sequence, the person walked forward with a stooped posture, paused and sighed. The children were told: 'You're going to see some bits of film of a person moving. I want you to tell me about this person. Tell me what's happening'. In response, all but one of the non-autistic children made a spontaneous comment about the person's emotional state for at least one presentation, and most referred to emotions on two or more of the five sequences. In contrast, 10 of the 13 children with autism *never* referred to emotional states, whether correctly or incorrectly. In the case of the children and adolescents with autism, it was the person's movements and actions rather than feelings that were reported. For example, the sad figure was described as 'walking and sitting down on a chair', 'walking and flapping arms and bent down', and 'walking and waving his arms and kneeling down . . . hands to face'. Almost none of the responses were inappropriate, but very few referred to feelings.

A final task was designed to explore how accurately the children and adolescents could name actions and emotions when explicitly asked to do so. We added five new emotionally expressive sequences to the five already described: these showed the point-light person in states of itchiness, boredom, tiredness, cold and hurt. When these sequences were shown, one by one, we said: 'I want you to tell me what the person is feeling'. Alongside this test involving emotions and other attitudes, there was a test for the recognition of non-emotional actions: lifting, chopping, hopping, kicking, jumping, pushing, digging, sitting, climbing and running. Here the instructions were: 'I want you to tell me what the person is doing'. The tasks were adjusted to exclude items on which there were ceiling or floor effects, and to equate tasks for level of difficulty. The participants with autism were not significantly different in their scores on the actions task (mean score 5 out of 8 correct, compared with 6 out of 8 for the control group); but on the emotions task, where once again the control group achieved a mean score of 6 out of 8 correct, the children with autism had a mean score of only 2 out of 8 correct. Here is striking evidence of a *specific* limitation in recognizing emotions in children carefully matched for verbal ability and linguistic productivity.

8.4 Developmental implications

In the introduction to this chapter, I indicated that, in my view, the developmental implications of a lack of empathy in young children with autism are profound for the elaboration of self-awareness, thinking and executive functioning. The studies I have cited are designed to illustrate and illuminate *both* the deficits in empathy-related psychological functions that are characteristic of autism (whether these are manifest in the context of individual testing or interpersonal interactions) *and* how autism may sharpen and clarify our thinking about what constitutes empathy (not only patterns of emotional receptivity and responsiveness, but also the ability to relate to others' attitudes to the world), what is required for empathy (coordination of affect, with the perceptual and expressive propensities this entails), and what is relatively peripheral for empathic involvement, at least in the case of autism (the ability to perceive bodily actions). Although it will not be possible here to argue the case that empathic deficits in autism are a major developmental source of the children's restricted self-awareness, their limited mental state concepts (so-called Theory of Mind), their paucity of symbolic play, their executive dysfunction and their linguistic deficits – in short, that empathic deficits constitute a primary source of the syndrome – I do want to allow myself a few paragraphs to make this sweeping and highly controversial suggestion seem less outrageous than might at first appear.

First, the matter of self-awareness. In a clinical-cum-philosophical approach to autism, Bosch (1970) remarked how the child with autism often seems to lack a sense of self-consciousness and shame, and to be missing something of the ' "self-involvement", the acting with, and the identification with the acting person' (p. 81). In my view, this process of identifying with others is critical in establishing the kinds of inward-facing attitudes that come to be experienced as guilt and other self-conscious emotions such as embarrassment, coyness and shame . . . and also in my view, a process intimately connected with (and perhaps constitutive of) empathy. If guilt requires one to have internalized attitudes to oneself through identifying with the attitudes of others, for example, and if the process of identifying with the attitudes of others is bound up with the propensity to empathize with what others express, then one can see how the emotional implications of empathy are far-reaching. Whatever the validity of this account, it is the case that individuals with autism are not only limited in their awareness of, as well as responsiveness to, the emotional life of others, but they are also restricted in their consciousness of themselves. For instance, Kasari *et al.* (2001) described how high-IQ children with autism could report feeling guilt, but compared with control children they provided fewer self-evaluative statements and were more likely to describe situations in terms of rule-breaking, disruptiveness and damage to property, rather than those of causing physical or emotional harm to others. The researchers concluded that for children with autism, guilt appears to be defined in terms of memorizable rules and actions such as taking toys from school, stealing cookies, running away and so on, rather than in interpersonal, empathic terms. Or again, when Lee and Hobson (1998) conducted 'self-understanding interviews' with groups of children, those with autism were restricted in the feelings they expressed about themselves, and also failed to mention friends or being members of a social group; and Bauminger and Kasari (2000) have described how children with autism speak of loneliness but fail to refer to the more affective dimension of being left out of close intimate relationships.

Second, I want to follow-up my claim that identification may be a process integral to empathy. There is a theoretical reason to suppose that this is likely to be the case, because empathy involves more than responding to someone emotionally: it also means responding to the other person's feelings *as* the other's feelings. In other words, the feelings involved in an empathic response are both one's own, and experienced in relation to the subjective experiences 'felt' as the other's. The important thing about identification is precisely that one feels in accordance with the other, but one does not entirely become the other; and one can then make the other's feelings or attitudes one's own, as it were a part of one's own repertoire, whilst still entertaining those feelings or attitudes as separate from other aspects of the self. One can come to punish oneself, be patient with oneself and so on. Now if human forms of empathy entail identification, in the sense of a specially powerful connectedness through involvement with the other's actions and attitudes that one can transpose to one's own case, then perhaps we should turn to autism to see if there is evidence for weakness in the propensity to identify with others. This issue becomes even more pressing, once one appreciates that it is in being *moved to* the emotional stance of others, and therefore in adopting alternative person-centred perspectives, that children with autism are especially handicapped.

I shall consider a single study from our current programme of research to illustrate the findings that are emerging. Hobson and Lee (1999) tested matched groups of children with and without autism for their ability to imitate a person demonstrating four novel goal-directed actions on objects in two contrasting 'styles', which in most cases meant executing the actions either harshly or gently. The children with autism copied the goal-directed aspect of the actions, but showed marked divergence from the control group insofar as very few adopted the demonstrator's *style* of acting upon the objects involved. We believe that this reveals a distinction between children's ability to observe and copy actions *per se*, relatively intact in autism (and here you may recall autistic children's ability to recognize actions but not attitudes in videotaped point-light displays of humans' gestures), and the propensity to identify with and thereby imitate a *person's* expressive mode of relating to the world, something that is relatively lacking in autism. Consider a further finding of the study. In one condition, the investigator demonstrated strumming a stick against a pipe-rack held against his own shoulder. What happened when the children without autism copied this action is that a substantial majority identified with the demonstrator and positioned the pipe-rack against *their own* shoulders before they strummed it with the stick. By contrast, few of the children with autism made this adjustment: most positioned the pipe-rack on the table directly in front of them. Therefore not only with respect to style, but also with respect to self-orientation, the children with autism did not assume the manner with which the other person executed actions, even though they copied the actions *per se*. We have conducted more recent studies that have confirmed group differences in the imitation of style and self-orientation. It is intriguing that here, in contexts where the emotional quality of the task appears to be minimal, but where identification appears to play a critical role in determining participants' responses, children with autism are distinctive. Perhaps in typical development, identification is a process that is necessary for full empathic engagement, and one that operates in concert with emotional components of interpersonal linkage and differentiation.

Finally, there is the issue of cognitive development. Here I shall make a simple but important point to echo what I wrote in the Introduction. This is that much that is distinctive about the creativity of human cognition depends on symbolizing; and symbolizing depends on taking 'meanings' from one context, and anchoring those meanings in symbols that have an arbitrary form except insofar as they serve as symbolic vehicles. The developmental question is this: how is it that over the first two years of life, young children come to grasp that they have the capacity to decontextualize and represent meanings by way of arbitrary signifiers, such as using a matchbox to represent a car in pretend play? I believe that the answer to this question lies in a form of perspective-taking that is grounded in the children's ability to identify/empathize with the attitudes of others, as these attitudes are directed towards a shared world. In other words, it is empathy-related role-taking that yields children's ability to understand what it means to entertain perspectives and, subsequently, what it means to apply alternative perspectives in communication and in symbolic play. As I have already indicated, similar processes involving the adoption of person-centred perspectives may operate in the development of executive functioning, and in pragmatic aspects of language. If all this is so – and it will require some years of research to determine whether it is – then autism will have led us to see more clearly how far empathy is at the very root of human cognitive as well as social development.

8.5 Autism: a disorder of empathic relatedness?

I need to stress three things by way of concluding this chapter.

First, there is a need to emphasize the *circumscribed* developmental effects of empathic deficits in autism. It is really important that not all aspects of interpersonal relationships require empathic responsiveness, at least not to the same extent. In particular, there are several published studies that indicate how young autistic children *do* respond to separation from and reunion with their caregivers, at least in the short-term (Rogers *et al.*, 1991; Shapiro *et al.*, 1987; Sigman & Mundy, 1989; Sigman & Ungerer, 1984). Many (not all) two- to five-year-old autistic children are like matched non-autistic retarded children in showing somewhat variable reactions to the departure of the caregiver, sometimes showing behavioural and/or mood changes such as fretting, and in responding to reunion by spending more time alongside the caregiver than the stranger. So we must not assume that empathy is needed for all aspects of attachment to others.

Second, I would not want to suggest that children with autism absolutely lack the ability to empathize with others, or even to identify with others. Even a cursory reading of the clinical and experimental literature is enough to dispel this oversimplified view. Yet as Kanner (1943) observed, a lack of affective contact is essential to autism. A complementary point is that we need to entertain the possibility that one can foster or scaffold aspects of empathy in children with autism, at least in some cases. Evidence is now emerging for the effectiveness of interventions that facilitate emotional engagement between children with autism and others (e.g. Bauminger, 2002; Gutstein & Whitney, 2002; Rogers, 2000).

Third, we are on the verge of acquiring new insights from neurofunctional studies of autism. Although it is too soon to derive firm conclusions from functional brain scans about the status and specificity of reported abnormalities in neuronal activity during emotion-related tasks such as those involving the perception of emotion in faces (e.g. Baron-Cohen *et al.*, 1999; Critchley *et al.*, 2000; Schultz *et al.*, 2000), it already seems likely that such investigations will demonstrate how neurological dysfunction underpins and reflects the behavioural and experiential abnormalities of people with autism described in this chapter – and in so doing, highlight afresh the need to derive an adequate developmental story of mind-brain development in autism.

Finally, we should step back and reflect on autism and empathy, and consider how re-shaping our concepts of empathy may help us to understand autism, and how investigations of autism may help us to re-think empathy. There are grounds for concluding that in autism, there is a (if not *the*) critical abnormality in the inter-personal domain, and, more specifically, in empathy and sharing subjective states and coordinating attitudes with other people *vis-a-vis* the world. Probably, children with autism have a range of constitutional abnormalities, but each might operate through a final common pathway that implicates abnormality in the patterned coordination of affectively configured subjective states between the affected child and others. Children with autism appear to have a restricted propensity to empathize and *identify with* other people, to move towards and (in part) assimilate the other person's attitudes and psychological orientations to the world. This impairment has serious implications for the development of their thinking as well as their social relations.

REFERENCES

Attwood, A., Frith, U., & Hermelin, B. (1988). The understanding and use of interpersonal gestures by autistic and Down's syndrome children. *Journal of Autism and Development Disorders*, **18**, 241–257.

Baron-Cohen, S., Ring, H., Wheelwright, S., *et al.* (1999). Social intelligence in the normal and autistic brain: an fMRI study. *European Journal of Neuroscience*, **11**, 1891–1898.

Bauminger, N. (2002). The facilitation of social-emotional understanding and social interaction in high-functioning children with autism: intervention outcomes. *Journal of Autism and Developmental Disorders*, **32**, 283–298.

Bauminger, N., & Kasari, C. (2000). Loneliness and friendship in high-functioning children with autism. *Child Development*, **71**, 447–456.

Bosch, G. (1970). *Infantile Autism* (translated by D. Jordan & I. Jordan). New York: Springer-Verlag.

Charman, T., Swettenham, J., Baron-Cohen, S., *et al.* (1997). Infants with autism: an investigation of empathy, pretend play, joint attention, and imitation. *Developmental Psychology*, **33**, 781–789.

Cohen, D. J. (1980). The pathology of the self in primary childhood autism and Gilles de la Tourette syndrome. *Psychiatric Clinics of North America*, **3**, 383–402.

Critchley, H., Daly, E., Bullmore, E., *et al.* (2000). The functional anatomy of social behavior: changes in cerebral blood flow when people with autistic disorder process facial expression. *Brain*, **123**, 2203–2212.

Dahlgren, S. O., & Gillberg, C. (1989). Symptoms in the first two years of life: a preliminary population study of infantile autism. *European Archives of Psychiatry and Neurological Sciences*, **238**, 169–174.

Dawson, G., Hill, D., Spencer, A., Galpert, L., & Watson, L. (1990). Affective exchanges between young autistic children and their mothers. *Journal of Abnormal Child Psychology*, **18**, 335–345.

Gutstein, S. E., & Whitney, T. (2002). Asperger syndrome and the development of social competence. *Focus on Autism and Other Developmental Disabilities*, **17**, 161–171.

Hobson, R. P. (1991). Methodological issues for experiments on autistic individuals' perception and understanding of emotion. *Journal of Child Psychology and Psychiatry*, **32**, 1135–1158.

Hobson, R. P. (1993). *Autism and the Development of Mind*. Hove: Erlbaum.

Hobson, R. P. (2002/2004). *The Cradle of Thought*. London: Pan Macmillan and New York: Oxford University Press.

Hobson, R. P., & Lee, A. (1999). Imitation and identification in autism. *Journal of Child Psychology and Psychiatry*, **40**, 649–659.

Hobson, R. P., Lee, A., & Brown, R. (1999). Autism and congenital blindness. *Journal of Autism and Developmental Disorders*, **29**, 45–56.

Kanner, L. (1943). Autistic disturbances of affective contact. *Nervous Child*, **2**, 217–250.

Kasari, C., Chamberlain, B., & Bauminger, N. (2001). Social emotions and social relationships: can children with autism compensate? In J. A. Burack, T. Charman, N. Yirmiya, & P. R. Zelazo (eds.), *The Development of Autism* (pp. 309–323). Mahwah, N.J.: Erlbaum.

Kasari, C., Sigman, M., Mundy, P., & Yirmiya, N. (1990). Affective sharing in the context of joint attention interactions of normal, autistic and mentally retarded children. *Journal of Autism and Developmental Disorders*, **20**, 87–100.

Lee, A., & Hobson, R. P. (1998). On developing self-concepts: a controlled study of children and adolescents with autism. *Journal of Child Psychology and Psychiatry*, **39**, 1131–1141.

Lord, C. (1995). Follow-up of two-year-olds referred for possible autism. *Journal of Child Psychology and Psychiatry*, **36**, 1365–1382.

Lord, C., Storoschuk, S., Rutter, M., & Pickles, A. (1993). Using the ADI-R to diagnose autism in preschool children. *Infant Mental Health Journal*, **14**, 234–252.

Moore, D., Hobson, R. P., & Lee, A. (1997). Components of person perception: an investigation with autistic, nonautistic retarded and normal children and adolescents. *British Journal of Developmental Psychology*, **15**, 401–423.

Ricks, D. M. (1975). Vocal communication in pre-verbal normal and autistic children. In N. O'Connor (ed.), *Language, Cognitive Deficits, and Retardation* (pp. 75–80). London: Butterworths.

Ricks, D. M. (1979). Making sense of experience to make sensible sounds. In M. Bullowa (ed.), *Before Speech* (pp. 245–268). Cambridge: Cambridge University Press.

Rogers, S. J. (2000). Interventions that facilitate socialization in children with autism. *Journal of Autism and Developmental Disorders*, **30**, 399–409.

Rogers, S. J., Ozonoff, S., & Maslin-Cole, C. (1991). A comparative study of attachment behaviour in young children with autism or other psychiatric disorders. *Journal of the American Academy of Child and Adolescent Psychiatry*, **30**, 483–488.

Schultz, R., Gauthier, I., Klin, A., *et al.* (2000). Abnormal ventral temporal cortical activity during face discrimination among individuals with autism and Asperger syndrome. *Archives of General Psychiatry*, **57**, 331–340.

Shapiro, T., Sherman, M., Calamari, G., & Koch, D. (1987). Attachment in autism and other developmental disorders. *Journal of the American Academy of Child and Adolescent Psychiatry*, **26**, 485–490.

Sigman, M. D., Kasari, C., Kwon, J. H., & Yirmiya, N. (1992). Responses to the negative emotions of others by autistic, mentally retarded, and normal children. *Child Development*, **63**, 796–807.

Sigman, M., & Mundy, P. (1989). Social attachments in autistic children. *Journal of the American Academy of Child and Adolescent Psychiatry*, **28**, 74–81.

Sigman, M., & Ungerer, J. A. (1984). Attachment behaviors in autistic children. *Journal of Autism and Developmental Disorders*, **14**, 231–243.

Snow, M. E., Hertzig, M. E., & Shapiro, T. (1987). Expression of emotion in autistic children. *Journal of the American Academy of Child and Adolescent Psychiatry*, **26**, 836–838.

Stone, W. L., & Lemanek, K. L. (1990). Parental report of social behaviors in autistic preschoolers. *Journal of Autism and Developmental Disorders*, **20**, 513–522.

Vostanis, P., Smith, B., Corbett, J., *et al.* (1998). Parental concerns of early development in children with autism and related disorders. *Autism*, **2**, 229–242.

Wimpory, D. C., Hobson, R. P., Williams, J. M., & Nash, S. (2000). Are infants with autism socially engaged? A study of recent retrospective parental reports. *Journal of Autism and Developmental Disorders*, **30**, 525–536.

Wing, L. (1969). The handicaps of autistic children – a comparative study. *Journal of Child Psychology and Psychiatry*, **10**, 1–40.

Yirmiya, N., Kasari, C., Sigman, M., & Mundy, P. (1989). Facial expressions of affect in autistic, mentally retarded and normal children. *Journal of Child Psychology and Psychiatry*, **30**, 725–735.

Part II

Empathy and related concepts in health

Neonatal antecedents for empathy

Miguel A. Diego[1] and Nancy Aaron Jones[2]

[1]Department of Pediatrics, University of Miami School of Medicine
[2]Department of Psychology, Florida Atlantic University

9.1 Introduction

To properly address the concept of empathy during infancy, developmental theorists must first define empathy, keeping in mind the resources of infants. Rather most theorists focus on the limitations when referring to empathy during infancy. For example, normal functioning infants have been described as dysregulated, less-than-conscious, egocentric and too immature in their representational and self-other capacities to experience empathy (Eisenberg, 1989; Kiang *et al.*, 2004; Strayer, 1987). It is disheartening to think that newborns must be considered inept, rather than simply developing or evolving. Further these definitions indicate an insufficient understanding of infancy and the way that the brain forms during development.

Intuitively it is assumed that emotions are ubiquitous during infancy (Fox, 1991). While it is obvious that newborns do not have the cognitive and experiential abilities required for fully developed forms of empathy, human beings are equipped to function emotionally from birth and emotionality is a key component of evolving empathy.

Studies have shown that newborns can imitate, discriminate and display many of the primary emotions (Field *et al.*, 1982). Findings from these studies suggest that individuals are born with the dispositional tendency to be alerted by emotion signals and that individual infants differentially respond to these signals (Jones *et al.*, 1997b). Brothers (1989) has even suggested that newborn imitation of emotions is a signal for the capacity for empathy (in some precursor form) in the normal brain, one that is elaborated by cognitive maturation and social experiences. Thus infants are innately endowed, via individual differences in genetic and neurological systems, with the ability to be socially responsive at birth. These systems have the potential to facilitate or attenuate the development of empathy in an adaptive or pathological form.

Empathy in Mental Illness, eds. Tom F. D. Farrow and Peter W. R. Woodruff. Published by Cambridge University Press. © Cambridge University Press 2007.

Ultimately the question is whether empathy can be defined as an evolving capacity during infancy. The answer to this question is yes, as the definition of empathy we adhere to was formed with the recognition of the evolving and coordinated nature of emotions and brain systems in infants. In addition, we recognize individual differences in arousal and regulation, including the genetic, hormonal and neural underpinnings, and we incorporate in our definition of empathy the ability to form ties to another, as in bonding and attachment. In our view, indicators for empathy emerge as early as birth and can be observed in rudimentary emotional expressions, recognition and regulation. Basic processes are then augmented by emerging cognitive and environmental experiences. Ultimately, the functional goal of empathy is to cultivate bonding experiences and social interactions with significant others throughout the lifespan. Only with a unified definition, such as this one, can an understanding of empathy across development progress.

9.2 Models for the development of empathy

Several theoretical models have been proposed to explain the development of empathy from birth to later developmental periods. These models can be classified as: *(1) temperament/newborn arousal and regulation theories; (2) attunement among dyads theories; (3) stage theories; and (4) learning and modelling theories.* While each of these views differs in concentration, each particular model for empathy development includes many overlapping concepts, pointing to the need for a more integrated model. In this section, we present each model individually, yet all have important components for understanding the development of empathy.

The first model focuses on the underlying principle that newborns are endowed with temperamental styles at birth. These temperamental traits are biologically based systems that predispose individual differences in the capacity for emotional and empathic responding. Second is the model that concentrates on the principle that psychobiological attunement between mothers and their infants aligns to form the basis for empathy with underpinnings in the early interaction patterns of the dyad. Third is the model that delineates sequential stages for the development of empathy. In these stage theories, a newborn's distress response to a peer's distress is viewed as the first sign of empathy, one that is elaborated by environmental experience during development to form the basis of empathic responding across the lifespan. Finally, the fourth model is based on learning and modelling principles that suggest family patterns of encouragement and promotion of empathic responding are the basis of empathic capacities. Accordingly, parents who model prosocial and empathic behaviours contribute to their child's learning patterns of behaviours essential for the development of empathy.

9.2.1 Temperament/newborn arousal and regulation theories

Virtually all parents will readily agree that their newborn has their own characteristic style of responding to the world. The construct of temperament has been used to explain these individual differences in dispositions observed by parents and scientists. Though definitions of temperament vary, all theorists agree that newborns exhibit characteristically different patterns of attention/alertness, arousal/reactivity, emotionality, motivational tendencies for approach versus withdrawal and regulatory patterns (Fox *et al.*, 1994). Differing dispositions or patterns of responsiveness and regulation to the environment are thought to be formed from the interaction of genetic, neural, hormonal and physiological systems. Further these systems interact with the environment and are the basis for potential continuity across development (Fox *et al.*, 1994).

A key component of temperament is that individuals differ in tonic arousal patterns that in turn lead to variations in the level of individual reactivity to environmental events. Sensitivity to environmental input, intensity of response patterns and motivational tendencies for approach versus withdrawal are fundamental concepts involved in temperamental reactivity that could affect individual responses to experiences.

Distinct from involuntary responses (e.g. reflexes), infants exert their reactive patterns through the control of their own behaviours and through individual variation in physiological response patterns. Early experiences with emotions are vital to newborns, as the ability to show attentiveness to emotions, to evaluate emotions as salient, and having a motivation to respond to emotions are all an integral part of emotional capacities (Saarni, 1999). Yet, not all infants demonstrate uniform behavioural responses to social events. For example, studies have suggested that newborns of depressed mothers are less likely to orient and also to respond to faces of emotion (Lundy *et al.*, 1996) and we have shown that newborns of depressed mothers are not reactive during cry sounds even though all infants had normal hearing (Jones, 2005).

Further studies using infant participants have also suggested that the physiological reactivity underlying emotions differs for individuals. In a series of studies, researchers (Calkins *et al.*, 1996) have shown that inhibited and socially withdrawn children exhibit a distinct physiological profile as early as infancy. The coordinated behavioural and physiological profiles within individuals can predispose social and psychological disorders, as in the risk for social anxiety noted in these children (Biederman *et al.*, 2001). Similarly, we (Jones *et al.*, 1997a, 1998) have conducted numerous studies that suggest that infants of depressed mothers differ in physiological patterns. As early as birth, investigations demonstrated that newborns and infants of depressed mothers exhibit left frontal hypoactivation in their EEG patterns (Diego *et al.*, 2004; Field *et al.*, 2004; Jones *et al.*, 1997a, 1998), lower vagal tone (Pickens & Field, 1995) and biochemical dysregulation (Field *et al.*, 2004; Lundy *et al.*, 1999), all physiological patterns that have been linked with a disposition for negative affect and depressive tendencies in adults (Davidson, 2004).

Emotion regulation skills are another important component of temperament that has been associated with empathy (Ungerer *et al.*, 1990) and adaptive regulations skills that promote socio-emotional competence (Cole *et al.*, 2004; Saarni, 1999). Although there are various types and definitions of regulation across infancy (Cole *et al.*, 2004), newborn regulatory abilities are simply the behavioural capacity to modulate arousal and reactivity. Newborns modulate arousal through their behaviours (directed gaze, facial expressions, vocalization, gestures, movements, etc.), through their physiological response systems (brain activity patterns, autonomic system activity) and through their somatic responses (e.g. control of respiration, heart rate, vascular and metabolic changes; motor tonicity and signs of state overload, such as hiccoughing, coughing, excessive tongue protrusions, gagging, etc.). Ironically, emotions are both regulators and need to be regulated. Studies have also linked regulatory capacities in infancy to empathy during childhood. For example, researchers have demonstrated that regulatory patterns at 4 months underlie individual differences in empathic responses later in toddlerhood (Ungerer *et al.*, 1990).

What evidence is there that empathy is part of our dispositional characteristics and that this component of temperament has continuity across development? The bulk of evidence for a disposition for empathy has come from empirical investigations using toddlers and preschoolers as participants (Kiang *et al.*, 2004). These studies have concluded that young children have an innate disposition for different arousal patterns that contribute to the development of empathic responses. In one notable study, Miller and Jansen op de Haar (1997) interviewed mothers of high empathy children and found that a large proportion of these mothers reported that their children demonstrated emotionally positive and sociable behaviours and were highly empathic. Correspondence between their emotional and behavioural tendencies was attributed to patterns of temperament observed since birth, specifically their emotional reactivity and self-regulatory skills.

In many of these studies, researchers have also demonstrated connections between empathy and physiological patterns (Liew *et al.*, 2003). Evidence for genetic underpinnings for empathy has also been presented (Zahn-Waxler *et al.*, 1992). However, no studies to date have been conducted to validate the pathway between newborn arousal patterns and the development of empathic capacities.

One significant problem in this area is that there are limits on our understanding of infancy, as there is no evidence for understanding of self and little is known about the emergence of consciousness in infancy (Lewis & Michalson, 1983; Panksepp, 2000). Further our understanding of genetics and the neural bases for empathy is limited, with a possibility of a dissociation between and within physiological and behavioural components, including ones that may assist those who pursue an understanding of empathy (Zahn-Waxler & McBride, 1998).

Ultimately, the conclusions so far suggest that emotional responsiveness is present as early as the newborn period and is a component of individual differences in behavioural and physiological reactivity and regulation, not simply a reflexive response. This argument is important for understanding the development of empathy, as this emotional responsiveness is essential for social interactions and may form the basis for empathy. However, some theorists have contended that infant emotional responsiveness, including newborn facial expression and reactive distress, is reflexive and unreliable. Instead, we contend that reactive distress in newborns is a component of temperament. This is supported by infants' individual differences in overt responses and the observation that infants have the capacity to control and modify their own behavioural response to the environment. As such, incorporating the neonatal period into the study of empathy will logically bolster our understanding of the processes involved in the ontogeny of empathy as well as the central and peripheral nervous system circuits involved during the development of empathy.

9.2.2 Attunement among dyads

Social interactions are an integral part of empathy, and thus it makes sense that empathy would emerge from an emotionally stable relationship. Developmental theorists have argued that attunement is the foundation for emotional stability between mother/infant dyads. Yet the temporal origin in the development of these relationships is unclear. According to some theorists, the attachment relationship is not observed in the newborn, but rather develops over time, with newborn infants unable to form specific attachments due to their inability to discriminate caregivers from other social beings (referred to by John Bowlby as the pre-attachment phase). Others, however, have argued for the capacity to discriminate caregivers as early as birth (referred to as bonding theory), suggesting that neonates have intrinsic ability to form specific attachments. This latter view is supported by research indicating that within the first few hours after birth, newborns can imitate adult-modelled social behaviours (Field *et al.*, 1982), demonstrate a preference for touch (Field, 2000), discriminate their own versus another infants' cry sounds (Dondi *et al.*, 1999), and are able to recognize and show a preference for their mother's voice, face and smell (DeCasper & Fifer, 1980; Porter & Winberg, 1999). These behaviours signal social responsiveness to specific environmental cues that are essential to identify and form relationships between infants and their primary caregiver(s).

Both bonding and attachment theories have been incorporated into the study of empathy, with models suggesting that psychobiological attunement between dyads from the early months of life are precursors for empathic responses (Kestenbaum *et al.*, 1989). Further, it has been suggested that co-regulation, a process that is based in shared neural and biological processes, is the basis upon which parents and their infants form these attunements (Cole *et al.*, 1994).

Several lines of research have contributed to the evidence that processes linked to attunement processes are responsible for the emotionally stable and adaptive relationships between mothers and their infants, ones that contribute to empathic competence. Hofer (1996), for example, has provided data which suggest that the absence or loss of significant others produces negative outcomes while a renewed interactive relationship improved psychobiological adaptation. Further loss and/or prolonged separation have been known to elevate stress hormones and instigate physiological and biochemical dysregulation (Hofer, 1996).

Theorists (Trevarthen & Aitken, 1994) have argued that physiological processes of both mothers and their infants are jointly affected in a positive manner by interactive unity and in a negative way by separation, loss, or neglect. For example, breastfeeding mothers exhibit physiologically beneficial heart rate and skin conductance responses (Wiesenfeld *et al.*, 1985) whereas the heart rates of depressed mothers and their infants are less concordant (Field *et al.*, 1990). This same type of dysregulation is noted in the latter groups' behaviour, with less positive and more negative emotions in dyads enmeshed in dysphoric states (Field *et al.*, 1990). The coordinated physiological and emotional processes between mothers and their infants appear to be necessary for the establishment of the co-regulation processes required for the development of empathic competence.

Neurophysiological and neurobiological processes are also thought to contribute to the interactive harmony of the attuned dyad. While the extent to which neonatal neural systems contribute to the coordinated activity of the dyad during development is unknown, recent theories propose that mirror neurones may be a primary organizing element within developing brains that code the sensations and emotions that form the basis for empathy (Iacoboni & Lenzi, 2002). Even though the data on mirror neurones are preliminary, the adaptive nature of shared physiology and its importance for identifying those with resilience to, or vulnerability for, social and psychological disorders should be probed further.

Enhanced risk for mental health problems is of paramount concern, as those who demonstrate problems with social and emotional dysregulation from infancy are at a severe disadvantage across development. In this regard, two infant groups are particularly noteworthy, those at risk for autistic disorder and those at risk for an array of mental heath problems due to parental depression disorders. While autism is associated with severe emotional dysfunction, identifying the risk factors during the neonatal stage has not been accomplished. Empirical investigations have suggested that infants, later diagnosed as autistic, exhibit uncoordinated interactions with their caregivers, stemming from the inability to regulate and organize emotions (Dawson, 1996). Moreover, the empathy dysfunction observed in autistic children is thought to result from a disrupted prefrontal lobe system (Dawson, 1996). The mechanisms that precipitate this system failure are unknown.

In the second group, newborns of depressed mothers have been shown to exhibit a distinct profile of neurobehavioural dysregulation during pregnancy (Field *et al.*, 2004) and immediately after birth (Field *et al.*, 2004; Jones *et al.*, 1998; Lundy *et al.*, 1999) marked by autonomic nervous system dysregulation in fetuses and neonates, elevated hypothalamic-pituitary-adrenal axis function, and greater left frontal hypoactivation in brain patterns. Disruption in empathic functioning has been linked to similar profiles of neurobehavioural dysregulation in older infants (Jones *et al.*, 2000), suggesting that physiological dysregulation at birth could make the transition into enduring physiology and mental health malfunction within environments where maternal depression remains un-remitted or has limited periods of remission.

Despite these intriguing outcomes, several issues must be addressed by models linking the development of empathy to parental attunement. Most notably research has been unable to separate the individual from their environment. Moreover, there is a natural inclination to view the adult as a greater influence in attunement than the infant. However, this might not be accurate, as attuned adults could be controlling the process of regulation, or the attuned adult could acquiesce to the infant's underlying temperament. Moreover, the study of the shared physiology and potential mirror neurones of attuned dyads may be too difficult or too premature to assess at this point in time. For instance, given the technology currently available, there are limits (in terms of both ethics and feasibility) to studying neural processes in infancy (Davidson & Slagter, 2000). At the same time, it would be naive to exclude newborns and infants from models of empathy, as infancy is an essential period in which emotions and areas of the brain are forming. In addition, the risk for dysfunction is amplified when early dyadic interactive experiences are problematic and dyadic attunement may be the greatest protective factor for mental health problems later in life.

Ultimately, the attunement model posits that adaptive attunement is regulating, that regulation depends on social interactions, and that the emotional life of the child emerges only within the context of interaction with the environment. In essence, infants gain psychological well-being through attuned relationships that serve to regulate their state, their developing mind, and their current and subsequent functioning. Within attuned relationships infants can effortlessly develop emotional competence and empathy, unlike in dysregulated dyads where infants are at risk for unorganized and inflexible regulation or may not develop adaptive emotional competence or competent forms of empathy.

9.2.3 Stage theories

Several stage-type models are prominent when examining the psychological literature that addresses the development of empathy. Among them are the models proposed by Feshbach, Strayer and Hoffman and the empirical studies of Eisenberg and Zahn-Waxler. Several of these models have contributed valuable information to the study of empathy, particularly in regards to the origins of empathy in infancy. Empathy has been viewed by developmental scientists from different levels of analysis, with some models deeming it as primarily affective, primarily cognitive or multidimensional; however, during infancy empathy is most often regarded as an affective process. The accounts of each model will be discussed below, with a special emphasis on the developmental milestones occurring during infancy.

Feshbach views empathy as primarily cognitive and only minimally discusses an affective component. His theory states that children need the ability to differentiate emotions, they need to place themselves in the role of another, and they need to be responsive to emotions to effectively empathize with others. As is common, Feshbach's thinking about empathy focuses mainly on later periods of development (toddler and preschool period) rather than infancy (Feshbach, 1978). Alternatively, Strayer (1987) conceptualized four phases for the development of empathy, the first of which includes a 'less-than-conscious' responsiveness to emotional cues that are then broadened by experience. Her other phases require increasing self-identity and cognitive skills. Notably, her theory also includes shared emotions and emotional resonance that can only be accomplished with increasing cognitive abilities and social experiences. Further, Strayer was the first to discuss the 'avant garde' notion that empathy can emerge without perspective taking, as perspective taking is employed by empathy to facilitate adaptive pro-social behaviours but does not have to precipitate empathy.

Hoffman (2000) outlines five stages in the development of empathy that are experienced across development, with the first stage occurring during the newborn period. To Hoffman, empathy starts at birth. He discusses the reactive cry response, at length, referring to it as an innate precursor to empathic reasoning. Further, he views the reactive cry as an adaptive response originating from human's evolutionary history, one that prepares the infant to signal and alert others in order to promote the survival of the youngest members of the species. He equates reactive cry responses with other forms of unclear or confused behaviours, ones lacking self-other differentiation. Reactive cries are a combination of mimicry, classical conditioning and a circular reaction in which the infant is unable to distinguish between their own cry and that of another's. This latter position has been challenged by the empirical studies by Martin and Clark (1982) and recently by Dondi and his colleagues (1999), who find that infants distinguish between their own cries and that of another infant. Paradoxically, in some of his writings he discounts this newborn cry response as vocal imitation (Sagi & Hoffman, 1976) yet in other writings he argues for imitation and conditioning together accounting for this response during the neonatal period (Hoffman, 2000). Other stages in Hoffman's model (2000) can encompass infants' competencies; however, later stages are more common during childhood. Within subsequent stages the child emerges from an unaware period, to awareness of others as different from themselves, to the awareness of the mind and internal states of others and eventually to the awareness of the entirety of others (including those beyond the immediate context). Although some of Hoffman ideas present a limited perspective of infants and his stages await empirical validation, he added immensely to the field of empathy, as he spearheaded the knowledge that emotional processes influence the development of empathy during infancy.

Two additional developmental scientists have played a pivotal role in our understanding of empathy during development, namely Nancy Eisenberg and Carolyn Zahn-Waxler. Both contend that the interactions of temperament and maternal characteristics are primary factors involved in the development of empathy, yet both also limit the role of infant empathy due to the infant's lack of experience with others in context and their lack of clear self-other differentiation. However, both discuss regulation as a developing, self-organizing skill and that self-development is accomplished through dyads communicating about emotions. Utilizing basic psychophysiological and genetic processes to examine and explain individual differences in personal dispositions and dyadic functioning, these investigations have extended scientific understanding of the origins of infant emotions. For example, Zahn-Waxler's studies demonstrated genetic and psychophysiological underpinnings for empathy, with several studies arguing that the affective component of empathy is inherited (Zahn-Waxler *et al.*, 1992). She recognizes that genes influence biochemistry and the neurohormonal system of individuals to influence empathy by way of attention, emotional discomfort and temperament, but that genes are not directly influential in social behaviours such as empathy. Similarly, many of the studies by Eisenberg and her colleagues (Eisenberg, 1989; Liew *et al.*, 2003) discuss the inherent role of arousal and regulation, uncovering individual differences within autonomic nervous system measures of heart rate and skin conductance, in the formation of empathy. Yet, she also directly discounts newborn's abilities, labelling them as emotional contagion and reflexive. This, we contend, is a limitation of this work, the view that infants are unconscious or unaware processors of information. While this research has contributed greatly to the scientific knowledge linking emotion regulation to the biological processes which are necessary for empathy to occur, these theorists do not discuss the likely influence of neural processes, ones that predispose emotional and empathic capacities. A transactional model would provide an interface between neurophysiological processes and interpersonal processes, both of which are important for the development of empathy, even the antecedent to empathy observed during infancy.

9.2.4 Learning and modelling theories

Behaviourist and social learning models have also attempted to explain the development of empathy. Empirical investigations have demonstrated that parents who model empathic behaviours (e.g. helping, sharing and emotional understanding of another) for their children promote greater empathy in those children. Several types of socialization experiences are thought to correspond to the increased empathic responses in parents, which in turn lead to greater childhood empathy. One factor is the parent's attitudes and beliefs surrounding emotions and empathy (Eisenberg et al., 1991), another is parental discipline practices (Hoffman, 2000), and the third is a parent's own emotionally expressive and affiliative behaviours (Eisenberg et al., 2001).

Although learning and modelling seem to be key factors in socializing more adaptive forms of empathy during childhood, few studies have examined this issue during infancy, as infants do not have extensive experience with parenting behaviours. Yet, antecedents for empathy in childhood are recognized as stemming from infancy. A number of studies, for instance, have reported relationships between children's empathic dispositions and the effects that parental teaching have on subsequent expressions of empathy with others. For example, parents who expressed an attitude that allowed their children to react emotionally (Eisenberg et al., 1991; Saarni, 1999), parents who used inductive discipline techniques (Hoffman, 2000), and parents who demonstrate warm communication patterns had children with greater empathic responses. Conversely those parents that had attitudes discouraging emotional displays, those who used harsh and/or inconsistent discipline, and those parents whose expression of negative affect was pervasive were less likely to have empathic children. One caveat to the latter findings is that parents who restrict their children's expression of emotions that harm another person had children who were empathic, suggesting that not all types of emotional expressions are encouraged by parents of children with empathic tendencies (Eisenberg & McNally, 1993). Further, one longitudinal investigation showed that parents that prioritize their children's emotional needs and well-being grew up in families that stressed sympathy and empathy (Koestner et al., 1990).

Parents influence emotions both positively and negatively. Within the learning and modelling perspective, it is acknowledged that parents teach and model empathy in many ways, demonstrating both direct and indirect behaviours in order to convey empathy to their children. For example, studies have shown that adults directly teach empathy by talking about expressing emotions, a behaviour that encourages the recognition and display of emotions in those children (Dunn *et al.*, 1991). Via a more indirect route, parental arousal and intensity of emotions may promote regulated forms of empathy or in the case of negative arousal and hyper- or hypo-intensity, more dysregulated forms (Liew *et al.*, 2003). Moreover, parents that demonstrate empathy in their disciplinary strategies (and employ inductive strategies) and those with attitudes promoting more positive interactions are both directly teaching and indirectly modelling more adaptive forms of empathy (Hoffman, 2000).

One problem, however, with studies of learning and modelling is that this theoretical perspective limits the type of influences responsible for the development of empathy to the child's environmental input, thereby negating the infant's temperament. The importance of the more subtle communication of emotions, the resilience of children exposed to parental psychopathology and individual differences in biobehavioural and genetic predispositions are ignored in this model, making it less comprehensive and persuasive for our understanding of the development of empathy.

9.3 Overview of associations between newborn distress studies and empathy

Do newborns demonstrate emotional responses that are analogous to empathy? Debate as to whether newborns purposely become distressed in response to the cries of a peer have emerged periodically across the last 30 years. The main issue is whether the reactive cry response is: (1) reflexive (and possibly meaningless), (2) an innate empathic response signalling the tendency for prosocial and altruistic behaviours, (3) an emotional response preparing the infant for social responsiveness, and/or (4) a temperamental tendency predisposing response biases within the individual. Unfortunately, no study has yet uncovered the motivation behind this behaviour. Although numerous theories have speculated as to the motivation for the newborn distress response (Eisenberg, 1989; Hoffman, 2000; Saarni, 1999), to date only a few research reports have been published that reliably demonstrate a capacity to respond emotionally to peer-rendered social signals. These studies and their contribution to understanding the foundations of empathy will be reviewed below.

Simner (1971) conducted one of the first controlled studies of a newborn's responses to cries of another. Across four experiments and nine cohorts, Simner compared newborn responses to a peer-generated cry to five separate stimuli, including: (1) silence, (2) white noise, (3) a synthetic sound, (4) the newborn's own cry and (5) the cry of an older infant. Simner also measured several outcome variables, including the number of infants who responded across conditions, the duration and latency of the response, mouthing behaviours and changes in heart rate compared to prestimulus levels. In the final experiment, Simner also examined the stability of the response for individual infants across a 24-h period. Ultimately Simner determined that a greater proportion of infants cried upon hearing their peer's cries, that the peer-rendered responses were of a shorter latency and a longer duration, and that heart rate patterns changed when infants heard the cries of another. These experiments were not without problems, as there were inconsistencies in some across some of the behavioural and autonomic measures. However, the findings suggest that newborns respond reliably to another infant's cries and thus peer's cries are powerful incentives that produce cries in another newborn. Simner also alluded to the possibility that newborn arousal patterns are innate processes influencing the individual newborn's behavioural responses.

In later work, Sagi and Hoffman (1976) and Martin and Clark (1982) present further evidence that newborn distress responses can be reliably linked to hearing another's distress in babies as young as 18 h old. Adding to Simner's findings, Sagi and Hoffman demonstrated that reactive distress occurs in infants exposed sequentially to the peer cries but not a matched simulated sound, while Martin and Clark showed that reactive cries are specific to others, age-matched peers, and species-specific. The latter study showed that the cries of chimpanzees, older infants, and the infants themselves elicited significantly fewer reactive distress responses than the aforementioned peer cries. Collectively, these researchers contend that the distress vocalizations of newborns upon hearing peer distress can be explained as an innate empathic distress reaction. Further, they suggest that this response is not a conditioned vocal response, as these newborns are too young; nor is it vocal imitation, as it is peer specific and more similar in tone and rhythm to spontaneous distress.

In the most recent study investigating the reactive distress response, Dondi and his colleagues (1999) compared responses elicited as a result of peer cries to the infant's own cries. They measured whether facial distress and non-nutritive sucking are manifested. Instead of using more global measures of distress, Dondi and his colleagues did micro-analytic analyses of facial displays, as the coordinated configuration of facial muscles are thought to convey reliable information about internal states in the infant. Further, non-nutritive sucking and rate of sucking has been used as an indication of self soothing and of auditory discrimination capacities. Dondi and his colleagues demonstrated that newborns react with greater facial distress and a lower sucking rate to another's cries but not to their own cries. These authors further suggest that another's distress produces an innate response in the newborn through physiological arousal, a response that the infant will not habituate to and a response that occurs even during sleep.

We have also completed several studies on the newborn reactive distress response (Jones, 2005). The purpose of our studies was to determine if individual differences in reactive cry responses could be observed in infants of depressed mothers, as these infants are notoriously less responsive to emotion-eliciting events even during the newborn period (Lundy *et al.*, 1996). Our studies have suggested individual differences in newborn distress responses based on personal disposition. Across two studies we have shown that infants of depressed mothers have a delay reactive cry, greater physiological arousal and less ability to regulate that arousal compared to infants of non-depressed mothers. Preliminary heart rate data suggest that these infants demonstrate fewer organized and more stress responses, with less concordance between heart rate and behavioural responses and greater heart rate acceleration compared to infants of non-depressed mothers.

Collectively how do these studies inform us about newborn empathic and emotional responses? The findings of these studies have demonstrated the reliability of the reactive cry response across stimulus conditions, response conditions and cohorts. Moreover, the presence of the neonatal reactive cry response suggests that the neural mechanisms underlying affect are present as early as birth. This is supported by findings indicating that cortical electrical brain activity is present by the beginning of the third trimester (Anand & Hickey, 1987), research indicating that stimuli presented during the third trimester results in cortical activation within the frontal lobes (Moore *et al.*, 2001) and research demonstrating that uterine experiences shape neonatal behaviours (Field *et al.*, 2004).

9.4 Maternal psychological and physiological functioning predict the development of empathy in children

It has become increasingly evident that maternal and infant psychological well-being are intricately interrelated. Further many studies associate maternal psychological distress (i.e. depression, anxiety, stress) with negative effects on psychological well-being in infants and the development of psychopathology in children and adolescents (Allen *et al.*, 1998).

Data from a wide range of studies suggest that the association observed between maternal and infant psychological well-being can in large part be attributed to the influence of a mothers' psychological state during pregnancy on the development of the fetal nervous system. For example, maternal psychological distress during pregnancy is associated with less optimal fetal behaviour and development (Field *et al.*, 2004), and greater risk for fetal growth delay (Diego, 2004), prematurity and low birthweight (Wadhwa, 1998). Infants born to mothers exhibiting psychological distress during pregnancy have smaller head circumferences at birth (Obel *et al.*, 2003), are more likely to exhibit neurobehavioural deficits (Field *et al.*, 2004) and exhibit a profile of physiological dysregulation, marked by elevated cortisol, lower vagal tone and left frontal hypoactivation in EEG patterns, that mimics their distressed mother's physiological profiles (Field *et al.*, 2004; Jones *et al.*, 1998). Furthermore, even after controlling for postnatal maternal distress, children and adolescents of mothers experiencing psychological distress during pregnancy are more likely to exhibit negative affect, unsocial behaviour, hyperactivity, externalizing problems and psychopathology (Van den Bergh & Marcoen, 2004). Ultimately these findings suggest that lack of dyadic attunement across development can adversely affect the foundations of emotional development, including individual differences in empathic processes that lead to socially withdrawn or antisocial disorders.

The effects of maternal psychological state during pregnancy on infant psychological well-being appear to be mediated in large part by maternal neuroendocrine function. Maternal neuroendocrine function during pregnancy is highly dependent on maternal psychological state. For example, maternal stress, depression and anxiety during pregnancy have been associated with elevated glucocorticoid (stress hormones) function (Field *et al.*, 2004; Wadhwa, 1998). These observed alterations in maternal biochemistry are important for fetal development, as maternal glucocorticoids readily cross the placenta and blood–brain barriers (Gitau *et al.*, 1998) and maternal glucocorticoids influence blood flow to the fetus (Glover *et al.*, 1999).

9.5 Dysfunctional socialization experiences influence the development of empathy by disrupting physiological and psychological regulation patterns

Infancy and early childhood are critical periods for the formation of the neural pathways essential for the development of empathy. Even though the vast majority of the neurones in central nervous system are developed by the 20th week of gestation, it is not until infancy and early childhood that most of the synaptic connections between them are formed (Kandel *et al.*, 2000). During the first years of life neural pathways emerge from the rapid formation and pruning of hundreds of trillions of synapses (Kandel *et al.*, 2000). Brain maturation and development is largely a genetically determined process that has evolved from species-typical experiences with the goal of preparing an organism for its species-typical environment. During early development brain maturation is also highly sensitive to environmental factors. Different neural pathways have distinct developmental periods when they are particularly sensitive to environmental factors. This sensitivity to environmental factors results in a high degree of flexibility during early development that ensures that an organism will develop the neural pathways necessary to thrive in a specific environment (Greenough *et al.*, 1987).

Most of the synapses formed in the areas of the brain controlling emotional and memory function occur during the first two years of life (Kandel *et al.*, 2000), a period of time when an infant's environment is primarily mediated by the mother. As such, both functional and dysfunctional socialization experiences can modify brain physiology and behaviours. For example, maternal interaction style can shift brain wave frontal EEG asymmetry patterns during early infancy (Jones *et al.*, 1997a).

Maternal neglect and abuse are dysfunctional socialization experiences that can severely affect the development of the neural pathways necessary for healthy emotional development and functioning. While maternal psychological neglect can lead to the deprivation of the environmental stimulation necessary to maintain experience-based neural pathways, maternal psychological abuse may result in the exposure to non-optimal environmental stimulation that may lead to the formation of aberrant synaptic formation. Both of these experiences have been shown to significantly affect the development of empathy (Glaser, 2000).

9.5.1 Maternal psychological neglect

Maternal psychological neglect during infancy and early childhood has been associated with both short- and long-term cognitive and emotional developmental deficits. For example, maternal psychological neglect has been associated with a cognitive delay during infancy (Egeland & Sroufe, 1981). Emotionally neglected infants are also more likely to develop attachment problems and these infants display greater social withdrawal during childhood (Egeland & Sroufe, 1981). Neglected infants also exhibit problems in emotion regulation and are less able to discriminate emotions (Pollack *et al.*, 2000), antecedents of emotional development that have been linked to problems with empathy. As children, they are more isolated and withdrawn in their social interactions, exhibit low self-esteem and show more negative and less positive affect (Egeland & Sroufe, 1981). It is likely that the absence of adequate social stimulation by a caregiver during infancy results in the weakening of the neural pathways necessary for the development of meaningful relationships with others (Perry, 2001).

It is also likely that maternal psychological neglect during early development results in the aforementioned developmental deficits by limiting the infant's exposure to emotional stimulation and thereby affecting the development and maintenance of experience-based neural pathways. Variations in environmental complexity during early development have been shown to affect brain development. For example, severe neglect observed in children raised in Romanian orphanages has been shown to affect brain growth and healthy psychological progression of emotional responsiveness (Perry, 2001). Deprivation of parental care is associated with social behavioural problems, ones that, to date, have only been altered somewhat by medications containing serotonin (Post & Weiss, 1997), supporting the proposition that brain changes have occurred.

9.5.2 Maternal abuse

As with maternal psychological neglect, maternal abuse during infancy and early childhood has been associated with severe cognitive and emotional deficits. In fact low maternal empathy has been associated with greater risk for child abuse, whereas neglect results in the atrophy of the neural pathways necessary for normal development via the absence of necessary environmental stimulation, and abuse may result in the development of aberrant neural pathways via inappropriate environmental stimulation. Abused children are more likely to be aggressive, lack empathy for others, and exhibit behavioural and attachment problems particularly when they were maltreated during infancy (Manly et al., 2001). Furthermore, maternal maltreatment and abuse has been associated with an increased incidence of psychiatric disorders (Teicher, 2000) and juvenile delinquency and adult criminal behaviour (Widom & Maxfield, 2001).

The negative developmental effects of maternal abuse may stem from its effects on adaptive response patterns resulting from changes to the hypothalamic-pituitary-adrenal (HPA) axis. Maternal abuse (and possibly neglect), endured during early development, may affect the development of the neural pathways underlying the HPA axis and thereby result in long-term effects on the HPA axis. For example, maternal abuse has been associated with both HPA axis dysregulation (Golier & Yehuda, 1998) and reduced hippocampal volume (Bremner and Narayan, 1998), suggesting the potentially permanent effects of abuse especially when intervention is not forthcoming or is substantially delayed.

Ultimately the message garnered from these studies is that the mind and the brain develop in the context of relationships. Maladaptive relationships can lead to dysregulated biobehavioural development. Further the quality of the relationships between a mother and her infant can have permanent effects on development, as the foundation of empathy is within the neurophysiological and neurobiological systems, systems that are intricately linked with significant others. Meaningful alterations in the development of emotional ties between the mother and her infant can results in long-term effects on the development of the brain and the processes by which the brain is modified during development. Lack of maternal responsiveness in the form of neglect and maternal abuse has severe consequences on an infant's physiological and behavioural development. Moreover, the behavioural and emotional concomitants of maltreatment are an alteration of empathic processes across time.

9.6 A new definition and future directions for the study of newborn distress and empathy

The past few decades have produced a wealth of research on newborn and even fetal behaviour and their emotional abilities. The findings suggest that the newborn infant is more than a 'tabula rasa', instead we now view the newborn as a sentient being, equipped to experience their world with highly developed sensory abilities and emotional capacities.

Considering these developments it is only logical to also reconsider our notion of the inept newborn. It is now evident that emotional development commences prenatally, starting with the development of basic perceptual abilities and progressing with the ability of the newborn to sense and discriminate emotional responses in their parents and other social beings. Therefore, we propose a model in which neural underpinnings for emotional processes emerge during the fetal period and can be observed in individual differences in newborn behavioural and affective reactions and ability to regulate those responses. These emotional processes expand in complexity throughout infant and child development and are augmented by adaptive social relationships (as in bonding and attachment) and the preprogrammed maturation of neural systems and cognitive skills. Given this skills-based and dynamic view of the emotional life of the newborn and infant, future research can delve into more promising areas of further inquiry.

9.7 Implications for practice when working with newborns and their mothers

Empathy is an essential component for the development of adaptive social relations and behaviours. As such, any disruption to the development of empathy, particularly during early infancy, is likely to result in adverse outcomes including the development of psychopathology. Research indicates that maternal psychopathology and the neuroendocrine dysregulation associated with it during pregnancy can potentially affect the development of the neural systems that are essential for the development of empathy. As such, it is essential to identify mothers exhibiting these profiles during pregnancy in order to administer early interventions.

While the use of psychotrophic agents during pregnancy is controversial, other interventions such as psychotherapy, feeding interventions (Jones *et al.*, 2004) and touch/massage therapy (Field, 2000) may be used during pregnancy and postnatally to reduce the adverse developmental outcomes exhibited by infants of mothers demonstrating psychopathology/neuroendocrine dysregulation.

By birth, the neonate can discriminate their mother from other women and is able to both discriminate different emotions in others and produce emotional expressions in response to those expressions. This is an adaptive mechanism that allows neonates to efficiently interact with their caregivers and may form the underlying basis for empathic behaviour. While fundamental interaction abilities are exhibited as early as birth, these abilities can be disrupted by a number of internal and external factors. For example, some infants exhibit a profile of neurobehavioural dysregulation as early as birth that affects how those infants respond to their caregivers. Similarly, some mothers exhibit distinct neurobehavioural profiles (intrusive versus withdrawn) that negatively affect how they interact with their infants.

Identifying these dyads is essential for training mothers how to properly interact with their infants. For example, research shows that interaction coaching tailored for a particular mother's interaction style can significantly improve both maternal and infant social behaviours (Malphurs *et al.*, 1996), suggesting that non-invasive or minimally invasive interventions can significantly benefit family relationships if applied early in life.

9.8 Summary

As early as birth, infants are endowed with the neural processes necessary for the perception and expression of emotions required for the establishment and maintenance of the social interactions essential for the infant's survival. These basic affect-processing and expression capacities rapidly develop across infancy and form the bases for higher-order socio-emotional processes including the development of empathy. Individual differences in genetic and neurobehavioural predispositions interact with the exposure to environmental factors early in development to facilitate or attenuate the development of the neurobehavioural pathways necessary for the development of higher-order social interactions, including empathy. As such it is not surprising that the exposure to negative environmental factors such as maltreatment or abuse can hinder the development of empathy and lead to the development of psychopathology. This highlights the need to identify infants at risk for maladaptive development by assessing for both internal and external factors including infant neurobehavioural dysregulation and maternal psychopathology.

REFERENCES

Allen, N. B., Lewinsoln, P. M., & Seeley, J. R. (1998). Prenatal and perinatal influences on risk for psychopathology in childhood and adolescence. *Development and Psychopathology*, **10**, 513–529.

Anand, K. J., & Hickey, P. R. (1987). Pain and its effects in the human neonate and fetus. *New England Journal of Medicine*, **19**, 1321–1329.

Biederman, J., Hirshfeld-Becker, D. R., Rosenbaum, J. F., *et al.* (2001). Further evidence of association between behavioral inhibition and social anxiety in children. *American Journal of Psychiatry*, **158**(10), 1673–1679.

Bremner, J., & Narayan, M. (1998). The effects of stress on memory and the hippocampus throughout the life cycle: implications for childhood development and aging. *Developmental Psychopathology*, **10**, 871–888.

Brothers, L. (1989). A biological perspective on empathy. *American Journal of Psychiatry*, **146**, 10–19.

Calkins, S. D., Fox, N. A., & Marshall, T. R. (1996). Behavioral and physiological antecedents of inhibition in infancy. *Child Development*, **67**, 523–540.

Cole, P. M., Martin, S. E., & Dennis, T. A. (2004). Emotion regulation as a scientific construct: methodological challenges and directions for child development research. *Child Development*, **75**, 317–333.

Cole, P. M., Michel, M. K., & Teti, L. O. (1994). The development of emotion regulation and dysregulation: a clinical perspective. In N. A. Fox (ed.), *The Development of Emotion Regulation: Biological and Behavioral Considerations. Monographs of the Society for Research in Child Development*, **59** (2–3 Serial no. 240), 73–100.

Davidson, R. J. (2004). What does the prefrontal cortex 'do' in affect: perspectives on frontal EEG asymmetry research. *Biological Psychology*, **67**, 219–233.

Davidson, R. J., & Slagter, H. A. (2000). Probing emotion in the developing brain: functional neuroimaging in the assessment of the neural substrates of emotion in normal and disordered children and adolescents. *Mental Retardation and Developmental Disabilities*, **6**, 166–170.

Dawson, G. (1996). Brief report: neuropsychology of autism: a report on the state of the science. *Journal of Autism and Developmental Disorders*, **26**, 179–184.

DeCasper, A. J., & Fifer, W. P. (1980). Of human bonding: newborns prefer their mother's voice. *Science*, **208**, 1174–1176.

Diego, M. A. (2004). Maternal neuroendocrine function and fetal development. Florida Atlantic University. Unpublished Doctoral Dissertation.

Diego, M. A., Field, T., Cullen, C., *et al.* (2004). Prepartum, postpartum and chronic depression effects on infants. *Psychiatry*, **67**, 63–80.

Dondi, M., Simion, F., & Caltran, G. (1999). Can newborns discriminate between their own cry and the cry of another newborn infant? *Developmental Psychology*, **35**, 418–426.

Dunn, J., Brown, J., & Beardsall, L. (1991). Family talk about feeling states and children's later understanding of others' emotions. *Developmental Psychology*, **27**, 448–455.

Egeland, E., & Sroufe, A. (1981). Developmental sequelae of maltreatment in infancy. In R. Rizley, D. Cicchetti (eds.), *New Directions for Child Development: Developmental Perspective on Child Maltreatment* (Vol. 11) (pp. 77–92). San Francisco, Calif.: Jossey-Bass, Inc.

Eisenberg, N. (ed.) (1989). Empathy and related emotional responses. *New Directions for Child Development* (Vol. 44). San Francisco, Calif.: Jossey Bass, Inc.

Eisenberg, N., Fabes, R. A., Schaller, M., Carlo, G., & Miller, P. A. (1991). The relations of parental characteristics and practices to children's vicarious emotional responding. *Child Development*, **62**, 1393–1408.

Eisenberg, N., Gershoff, E. T., Fabes, R. A., *et al.* (2001). Mothers' emotional expressivity and children's behavior problems and social competence mediation through children's regulation. *Developmental Psychology*, **37**(4), 475–490.

Eisenberg, N., & McNally, S. (1993). Socialization and mothers' and adolescents' empathy-related characteristics. *Journal of Research on Adolescence*, **3**, 171–191.

Feshbach, N. D. (1978). Studies of empathic behavior in children. In B. A. Maher (ed.), *Progress in Experimental Personality Research* (Vol. 8) (pp. 1–47). New York: Academic Press.

Field, T. M. (2000). Infant massage therapy. In C. H. Zeanah (ed.), *Handbook of Infant Mental Health*, 2nd edn. (pp. 494–5000). New York: Guilford.

Field, T., Diego, M., Dieter, J., *et al.* (2004). Prenatal depression effects on the fetus and the newborn. *Infant Behavior and Development*, **27**, 216–229.

Field, T., Healy, B., Goldstein, S., & Guthertz, M. (1990). Behavior state matching and synchrony in mother-infant interactions of nondepressed versus 'depressed' dyads. *Developmental Psychology*, **26**, 7–14.

Field, T. M., Woodson, R., Greenberg, R., & Cohen, D. (1982). Discrimination and imitation of facial expressions by neonates. *Science*, **218**, 179–181.

Fox, N. A. (1991). If it's not left, it's right: electroencephalogram asymmetry and the development of emotion. *American Psychologist*, **46**, 863–872.

Fox, N. A., Calkins, S. D., & Bell, M. A. (1994). Neural plasticity and development in the first two years of life: evidence from cognitive and socioemotional domains of research. *Development and Psychopathology*, **6**, 677–696.

Gitau, R., Cameron, A., Fisk, N. M., & Glover, V. (1998). Fetal exposure to maternal cortisol. *Lancet*, **352**, 707–708.

Glaser, D. (2000). Child abuse and neglect and the brain – a review. *Journal of Child Psychology and Psychiatry*, **41**(1), 97–116.

Glover, V., Teixeira, J., Gitau, R., & Fisk, N. M. (1999). Mechanisms by which maternal mood in pregnancy may affect the fetus. *Contemporary Reviews in Obstetrics and Gynecology*, September, pp. 155–160.

Golier, J., & Yehuda, R. (1998). Neuroendocrine activity and memory-related impairments in posttraumatic stress disorder. *Development and Psychopathology*, **10**, 857–869.

Greenough, W. T., Black, J. E., & Wallace, C. S. (1987). Experience and brain development. *Child Development*, **58**, 539–559.

Hofer, M. (1996). On the nature and consequences of early loss. *Psychosomatic Medicine*, **58**, 570–581.

Hoffman, M. L. (2000). *Empathy and Moral Development*. New York: Cambridge University Press.

Iacoboni, M., & Lenzi, G. L. (2002). Mirror neurons, the insula and empathy. *Behavioral and Brain Sciences*, **25**, 39–40.

Jones, N. A. (2005). Heart rate patterns during distress sounds in newborns of depressed mothers. Paper presented at the Society for Research in Child Development, Atlanta, Georgia.

Jones, N. A., Field, T., & Davalos, M. (2000). Right frontal EEG asymmetry and lack of empathy in preschool children of depressed mothers. *Child Psychiatry and Human Development*, **30**, 189–204.

Jones, N. A., Field, T., Fox, N. A., *et al.* (1998). Newborns of mothers with depressive symptoms are physiologically less developed. *Infant Behavior and Development*, **21**, 537–541.

Jones, N. A., Field, T., Fox, N. A., *et al.* (1997a). Infants of intrusive and withdrawn mothers. *Infant Behavior and Development*, **20**, 175–186.

Jones, N. A., Field, T., Fox, N. A., Lundy, B., & Davalos, M. (1997b). EEG activation in one-month-old infants of depressed mothers. *Development and Psychopathology*, **9**, 491–505.

Jones, N. A., McFall, B. A., & Diego, M. A. (2004). Patterns of brain electrical activity in infants of depressed mothers who breastfeed and bottle feed: the mediating role of infant temperament. *Biological Psychology*, **67**, 103–124.

Kandel, E. R., Schwartz, J. H., & Jessel, T. M. (2000). *Principles of Neural Science*, 4th edn. Columbus, Ohio: McGraw Hill.

Kestenbaum, R., Fabes, E. A., & Sroufe, L. A. (1989). Individual differences in empathy among preschoolers: relation to attachment history. In N. Eisenberg (ed.), *Empathy and Related Emotional Responses: New Directions for Child Development* (vol. 44) (pp. 51–64). San Francisco, Calif.: Jossey Bass.

Kiang, L., Moreno, A. J., & Robinson, J. L. (2004). Maternal preconceptions about parenting predict child temperament, maternal sensitivity, and children's empathy. *Developmental Psychology*, **40(6)**, 1081–1092.

Koestner, R., Franz, C., & Weinberger, J. (1990). The family origins of empathic concern: a 26-year longitudinal study. *Journal of Personality and Social Psychology*, **58**, 709–717.

Lewis, M., & Michalson, L. (1983). *Children's Emotions and Moods: Developmental Theory and Measurement*. New York: Plenum Press.

Liew, J., Eisenberg, N., Losoya, S. H., *et al.* (2003). Children's physiological indices of empathy and their socioemotional adjustment: does caregivers' expressivity matter? *Journal of Family Psychology*, **17(4)**, 584–597.

Lundy, B., Field, T., & Pickens, J. (1996). Infants of mothers with depressive symptoms are less expressive. *Infant Behavior and Development*, **19**, 419–424.

Lundy, B., Jones, N. A., Field, T., *et al.* (1999). Prenatal depression effects on neonates. *Infant Behavior and Development*, **22**, 121–137.

Malphurs, J., Larrain, C., Field, T., *et al.* (1996). Altering withdrawn and intrusive interaction behaviors of depressed mothers. *Infant Mental Health Journal*, **17**, 152–160.

Manly, J. T., Kim, J. E., Rogosch, F. A., & Cicchetti, D. (2001). Dimensions of child maltreatment and children's adjustment: contributions of developmental timing and subtype. *Development and Psychopathology*, **13**, 759–782.

Martin, G. B., & Clark, R. D. (1982). Distress crying in neonates: species and peer specificity. *Developmental Psychology*, **18**, 3–9.

Miller, P. A., & Jansen op de Haar, M. A. (1997). Emotional, cognitive, behavioral, and temperament characteristics of high-empathy children. *Motivation and Emotion*, **21**, 109–125.

Moore, R. J., Vadeyar, S., Fulford, J., *et al.* (2001). Antenatal determination of fetal brain activity in response to an acoustic stimulus using functional magnetic resonance imaging. *Human Brain Mapping*, **12(2)**, 94–99.

Obel, C., Hedegaard, M., Henriksen, T. B., Secher, N. J., & Olsen, J. (2003). Stressful life events in pregnancy and head circumference at birth. *Developmental Medicine and Child Neurology*, **45**, 802–806.

Panksepp, J. (2000). Affective consciousness and the instinctual motor system. The neural sources of sadness and joy. In R. Ellis & N. Newton (eds.), *The Caldron of Consciousness: Motivation, Affect and Self-Organization: Advances in Consciousness Research Series* (Vol. 16). Amsterdam: John Benjamins.

Perry, B. D. (2001). The neurodevelopmental impact of violence in childhood. In D. Schetky, E. Benedek (eds.) *Textbook of Child and Adolescent Forensic Psychiatry*. Washington, DC.: American Psychiatric Press, Inc.

Pickens, J., & Field, T. (1995). Facial expressions and vagal tone in infants of depressed and nondepressed mothers. *Early Development and Parenting*, **4**, 83–89.

Pollack, S. D., Cicchetti, D., Hornung, K., & Reed, A. (2000). Recognizing emotion in faces: developmental effects of child abuse and neglect. *Developmental Psychology*, **36**, 679–688.

Porter, R. H., & Winberg, J. (1999). Unique salience of maternal breast odors for newborn infants. *Neuroscience and Biobehavioral Reviews*, **23**, 439–449.

Post, R. M., & Weiss S. R. (1997). Emergent properties of neural systems: how focal molecular neurobiological alterations can affect behavior. *Development and Psychopathology*, **9**, 907–929.

Saarni, C. (1999). *The Development of Emotional Competence*. New York: Guilford Press.

Sagi, A., & Hoffman, M. L. (1976). Empathic distress in the newborn. *Developmental Psychology*, **12**, 175–176.

Simner, M. L. (1971). Newborn's response to the cry of another infant. *Developmental Psychology*, **5**, 136–150.

Strayer, J. (1987). Affective and cognitive perspectives on empathy. In N. Eisenberg & J. Strayers (eds.) *Empathy and its Development* (pp. 218–244). New York: Cambridge University Press.

Teicher, M. D. (2000). Wounds that time won't heal: the neurobiology of child abuse. *Cerebrum: The Dana Forum on Brain Science*, **2(4)**, 50–67.

Trevarthen, C., & Aitken, K. J. (1994). Brain development, infant communication, and empathy disorders: intrinsic factors in child mental health. *Development and Psychopathology*, **6**, 597–633.

Ungerer, J. A., Dolby, R., Waters, B., *et al.* (1990). The early development of empathy: self-regulation and individual differences in the first year. *Motivation and Emotion*, **14**, 93–106.

Van den Bergh, B. R. H., & Marcoen, A. (2004). High antenatal maternal anxiety is related to ADHD symptoms, externalizing problems, and anxiety in 8- and 9-year-olds. *Child Development*, **75**, 1085–1097.

Wadhwa, P. D. (1998). Prenatal stress and life-span development. In H. S. Friedman (ed.), *Encyclopedia of Mental Health* (pp. 265–280). San Diego, Calif.: Academic Press.

Widom, C. S., & Maxfield, M. G. (2001). *An Update on the 'Cycle of Violence.'* Washington, DC: National Institute of Justice.

Wiesenfeld, A. R., Malatesta, C. Z., Whitman, P. B., Granrose, C., & Uili, R. (1985). Psychophysiological response of breast- and bottle-feeding mothers to their infants' signals. *Psychophysiology*, **22**, 79–86.

Zahn-Waxler, C., & McBride, A. (1998). Current perspectives on social and emotional development. In J. G. Adair (ed.), *Advances in Psychological Science* (Vol. 1). *Social, Personal and Cultural Aspects* (pp. 513–546). Hove, England: Taylor and Francis.

Zahn-Waxler, C., Robinson, J. L., & Emde, R. E. (1992). The development of empathy in twins. *Developmental Psychology*, **28**, 1038–1047.

The evolutionary neurobiology, emergence and facilitation of empathy

James Harris

School of Medicine, Johns Hopkins University

10.1 Introduction

Mutual aid between and among members of a species may be the most potent force in evolution. This was the position taken by the Russian evolutionists who proposed that greater emphasis be placed on 'mutual aid' than on 'survival of the fittest' in the struggle for existence (Kropotkin, 1989; Todes, 1989). They noted that those species with the most highly evolved brains having the greatest brain weight and the most complex neocortical development show the greatest social cooperation and are the most sociable.

MacLean's (1990) emphasis on integrated brain function in social adaptation is critical to understanding the evolution of empathy. He and his colleagues provide an ethological perspective on the study of empathy in their paleo-ethological and ethological studies of behaviour. Evolutionary steps toward sociability are highlighted in his studies of audiovocal communication and on the effects of brain lesions on behaviour in lizards (*Anolis carolinensis*), rodents and squirrel monkeys. An increase in social behaviour and social responsiveness accompanies the evolutionary transition from reptiles to mammal-like reptiles to early mammals to primates and humans. Preston and de Waal (2002) suggest that in this evolutionary transition there are proximate and ultimate bases for empathy. Proximately, the perception of an object's state activates the individual's corresponding representations, which activate somatic and autonomic responses. They propose a Perception-Action Model (PAM) that along with experience can predict empathetic behaviour or its absence. They propose that perception-action interacts with prefrontal functioning and that this interaction can explain different levels of empathy across species.

Carter's studies (Carter, 1998, 2003; Carter *et al.*, 1995) of the effects of oxytocin on maternal attachment and pair bonding provide a substrate for the role of

Empathy in Mental Illness, eds. Tom F. D. Farrow and Peter W. R. Woodruff. Published by Cambridge University Press. © Cambridge University Press 2007.

neuroendocrine elements in empathy and understanding the neural circuits that may be involved. Porges' (2001) polyvagal theory emphasizes the evolutionary origins of the autonomic nervous system and the role it plays in affect modulation and social engagement. He emphasizes that there are well-defined neural circuits to support social engagement behaviours and the defensive strategies of fight, flight and freeze behaviours; these neural circuits form a phylogenetically organized hierarchy. Gallese's (2003) and Iacoboni's (Iacoboni *et al.*, 2005) and others' investigations of mirror neurones provide a means for understanding how perception is linked to action, the understanding of intentions of others and emotionality. De Waal's studies (1989) of peacemaking among primates, social grooming and meaningful social support, and Bowlby's (1969) and Ainsworth's (Ainsworth & Bell, 1970) studies of attachment as a motivated human behaviour provide a means to study affective engagement. Lewis' studies (2000) of the self-conscious emotions and other studies that link affect and cognition round out the development processes that will be discussed in this chapter as prerequisites for the emergence of empathy. Empathy is a developmental process whereby individuals come to understand the emotional states of others. The consequences of empathy are compassionate behaviour towards others, moral agency and ethical behaviour based on mercy and justice.

10.2 Mutual aid

Todes (1989) summarizes the work of the Russian evolutionists; he emphasizes that Darwin described natural behaviour in rich tropical settings with abundant resources. These organisms lived in tightly packed, wedgelike, competitive environments, where a small advantage could bring prosperity to one group at the expense of another. Unlike the tropics, Russian natural settings such as Siberia were great and sparsely populated plains. These populations were threatened by physical circumstances, often so severe that one form's slight competitive advantage over another could easily seem insignificant. Todes writes: 'a sudden blizzard or an intense drought might obliterate entire populations of insects, birds, and cattle without regard for difference among them'. The Russian evolutionists proposed 'mutual aid', a driving force in evolution that allowed survival to continue in such physical settings. Although Darwin spoke of both survival of the fittest and mutual aid, his followers placed greater emphasis on the former, yet 'the fittest' may be those whom aid others. MacLean (1985, 1990) and De Waal (1989) provide modern support for the mutual aid hypothesis, especially in regard to empathy. De Waal discusses the work of Trivers (1971) on the evolution of reciprocal altruism and the more controversial topic of group selection for altruism (Wilson & Sober, 1994). However, the study of empathy in development is less controversial than that of altruism and may be the more important factor in understanding mutual aid.

10.3 Neuroethology: the original of parental behaviours

10.3.1 Evolutionary origins of audiovocal communication: the isolation call

Empathy may have entered evolution in the transition from primitive synapsids (mammal-like reptiles) to living mammals. Early mammals were probably nocturnal (hiding from large carnivores) and relied on well-developed senses of smell and hearing. The evolutionary changes critical to the mammalian transition are neuroanatomical changes that facilitate social contact – among them the capacity for audiovocal communication. In mammals, sound in the environment impinges upon the eardrum and is transduced from the eardrum to the inner ear via the small bones in the middle ear known as ossicles. The middle ear of mammals seems to have evolved by adapting bones from the jaw to the middle ear. In non-mammalian vertebrates with jaws, the craniomandibular joint is located between the quadrate region of the palatoquadrate and the articular region of Meckel's cartilage (or its replacement). However, mammals have a dentary-squamosal jaw joint. The mammalian middle ear results from the transference of elements of the accessory jaw, the angular, articular plus prearticular, and quadrate to the cranium to produce the ossicles: the tympanic, malleus and incus. Developmental studies show homologies among jawed vertebrates; however, there had been no fossil evidence to support this hypothesis until the findings of Wang *et al.* (2001). Wang *et al.* found a well-preserved Meckel's cartilage in two Cretaceous mammals from China. This Meckel's cartilage is similar to Meckel's cartilage in the human prenatal period and to that of some extant mammals. This finding points to the relationship of Meckel's cartilage with the middle ear in early mammals. Thus, brain expansion may not be the key element that caused the separation of the post-dentary bones from the dentary as middle ear ossicles during the evolution of mammals. Meckel's cartilage connected the dentary and the ear and probably served as the middle ear in these two mammals. Eventually, these features separated to create two ear ossicles, malleus and incus, in the braincase separated completely from the jaw. The morphology of the two skulls suggests that during the evolution of synapsids (mammal-like reptiles) the dentary enlarged (allowing more muscle attachments) over evolutionary time to enhance mastication while the postdentary unit decreased in size to enhance hearing of high-frequency airborne sounds. Expansion of the brain and changes in the otic capsule may have led to displacement to the location of the ear ossicles distant from the secondary craniomandibular joint in more advanced mammals.

This hypothesis is similar to the detaching mechanism of the ear ossicles in marsupials without requiring brain expansion as the initial trigger. Because all modern mammals – including placentals, marsupials and egg-laying monotremes (such as the platypus) – share the same distinctive middle ear structure, many scientists had assumed that the middle ear evolved just once from the jaw of their common reptilian ancestor. Fossil evidence suggests otherwise. Rich *et al.* (2005) described a well-preserved fossil from an extinct relative of Australia's modern platypus (the earliest known monotreme) that has only one ear bone. Thus, it appears that the middle ear evolved separately and converged in different mammalian lineages. The evolutionary importance of these changes in marsupials is highlighted in that this change evolved independently among the monotreme mammals and the therians (marsupials and placentals). Such independent evolution is referred to as homoplasy. That the angular (homologous with the mammalian ectotympanic) and the articular and prearticular (homologous with the mammalian malleus) bones retained attachment to the lower jaw in a basal monotreme indicates that the definitive mammalian middle ear evolved independently in living monotremes and therians (marsupials and placentals).

In reptiles sound is conducted from the tympanic membrane to the inner ear via a single bone, the stapes. In mammal-like reptiles (subclass Synapsida, order Therapsida) sound is conducted via the stapes, but the articular and quadrate bones also play a role in transmitting sound. In mammals sound is conducted from the tympanic membrane by a series of the three bones previously mentioned: the malleus (formerly the articular bone), the incus (formerly the quadrate) and the stapes. Thus the mammalian stapes is the same as that of their ancestors. But the malleus and incus have moved into the middle ear from their former function as the reptilian jaw joint.

The evolution of the mammalian middle ear enabled low-amplitude, relatively high-frequency airborne sounds (i.e. sounds in the frequency of human voice) to be heard, even when the acoustic environment was dominated by low-frequency sounds. This phylogenetic innovation enabled mammals to communicate in a frequency band that could not be detected by reptiles that were only able to hear lower frequencies due to their dependence on bone conduction to 'hear'. This ability to hear low-amplitude, high-frequency airborne sounds in an acoustic environment dominated by loud low-frequency sounds could only be accomplished when the middle ear muscles were tensed to create a rigidity along the ossicular chain. The tensing of these muscles prevents the low-frequency sounds from being transduced through the middle ear bones from the eardrum to the cochlear and masking the high-frequency sounds associated with human voice.

Thus, a key evolutionary innovation among modern mammals in the establishment of audiovocal communication is the separation of the middle ear bones from the mandible. In mammals, the transformation of jaw bones to ear bones was first documented embryologically, when it was recognized that the reptilian articular bone and the greater part of the mammalian malleus were both formed by ossification of the posterior portion of Meckel's cartilage, the embryonic cartilage of the lower jaw. With the establishment of an embryonic (or neonatal) contact of the mammalian dentary bone with the squamosal of the skull, the middle portion of Meckel's cartilage atrophies, leaving the incus (= reptilian quadrate), malleus (= articular + prearticular) and ectotympanic (= angular) ligamentously attached to the ear region of the skull.

In summary, during the evolutionary transition the dentary bone of the lower jaw developed a neomorphic articulation with the squamosal bone of the skull, thus three of the accessory lower jaw bones were transformed to sound-transmitting units of the middle ear. The articular and prearticular bones became the mammalian malleus, and the angular bone became the ectotympanic (or tympanic ring), which supports the eardrum. An additional synapsid element, the quadrate bone (which, with the articular, forms the primitive synapsid jaw joint), became the mammalian incus. These three delicate bones of the mammalian middle ear – the malleus, incus and stapes – work together to amplify and internally direct sound waves. The development of the ossicles of the middle ear was critical in the evolutionary history of empathy because it allowed the mother to eat, hear and listen at the same time. Thus in early mammalian evolution the ultrasonic isolation call, not audible to predators, could aid the mother in the location of the young.

10.4 Neurophysiology: oxytocin and social behaviour

Neural circuits that support social engagement behaviours and the formation of strong pair bonds are related to oxytocin, a neuropeptide involved in the formation of social bonds. It is now clear that peptides, including oxytocin, are manufactured within the nervous system and released centrally to act upon a variety of central nervous system (CNS) receptors (Carter, 2003). Neuropeptides, including oxytocin and vasopressin, and the adrenal glucocorticoid corticosterone have been implicated in the neural regulation of partner preferences, and in the male, vasopressin has been implicated in the induction of selective aggression toward strangers. Oxytocin has been studied most extensively in the maintenance of social bonds.

Oxytocin is linked to the physiological indexes of empathy and socioemotional adjustment (skin conductance and heart rate variability) in relation to parental care-giving and reciprocal responding. It is the most abundant neuropeptide in the adult hypothalamus and serves integrative functions, coordinating behavioural and physiological processes such as parturition, lactation, maternal behaviour and pair bond formation. It is involved in moderating the behavioural response to stressors and the reactivity of the hypothalamic-pituitary-adrenal (HPA) axis.

The oxytocin system has been systematically studied in prairie voles. Prairie voles spontaneously exhibit several traits found in humans, including the capacity to develop adult heterosexual pair bonds and for both parents and other family members to show parental care. Because prairie voles exhibit social monogamy (formation of pair bonds between adult conspecifics), biparental care and alloparental behaviour, Carter (2003) sought to identify potential neuroendocrine mechanisms involved in this behaviour. These experiments in neonatal prairie voles documented that there are effects of oxytocin and oxytocin receptor antagonists on immediate and lifelong social behaviours. This includes adult pair bonding and parental behaviours and the reactivity of the HPA axis. Thus, the oxytocin system and its targets are sensitive to 'tuning' in early development, with lifelong consequences.

Interactions among oxytocin, vasopressin and glucocorticoids provide substrates for dynamic changes in social and agonistic behaviours, including those required in the development and expression of monogamy (Carter *et al.*, 1995).

Endogenous oxytocin or its receptors and related peptides such as vasopressin may affect and be affected by various social experiences, especially during early life. The neural systems that incorporate oxytocin also are plastic. Oxytocin, acting on its own receptors and through effects on other systems including the HPA axis and the autonomic nervous system, has a powerful capacity to alter physiology and behaviour. Enhanced sociality and parental behaviour follows treatment with oxytocin in adult animals.

Receptors for both oxytocin and vasopressin are localized in areas of the nervous system, especially in the brainstem, which play a role in reproductive, social and adaptive behaviours and the regulation of the autonomic nervous system. Vasopressin and oxytocin may have opposite functions, or may act together. They are capable of acting as antagonists to each other's receptors. Both hormones have been implicated in the control of the autonomic nervous system, with oxytocin having primarily parasympathetic actions and vasopressin serving as a central and peripheral component of the sympathetic nervous system. The behavioural effects of oxytocin and vasopressin correlate with their autonomic actions, supporting the hypothesis that oxytocin and its vagal/parasympathetic activities may integrate a variety of metabolic and behavioural systems. Thus, the release of oxytocin or treatment with this peptide is associated with a reduction in anxiety, obsessiveness and stress reactivity and may serve to counteract the defensive behavioural strategies associated with stressful experiences and the central release of vasopressin and other peptides, such as corticotropin-releasing hormone.

10.5 Evolution of the autonomic nervous system and social engagement

Social approach is initiated after taking into account one's perception of the behaviour of the one who is to be engaged. Does the other elicit feelings of safety and social comfort, discomfort and potential danger or threat to life? Porges (2001,

2003a, 2003b) proposes that the neurobiological underpinnings of social engage-ment are linked to the evolution of the autonomic nervous system and how it relates to emotion. Its evolution provides a means to understand the adaptive significance of mammalian affective processes including courting, sexual arousal, empathy and the establishment of lasting social bonds.

The phylogenic origin of the behaviours associated with the social engagement system is linked to the evolution of the autonomic nervous system. The striated muscles, via special visceral efferent pathways, evolved into a behavioural system that regulated social engagement that involves neural regulation of the auto-nomic nervous system. These changes took place in both somatomotor and visceromotor regulation in the transition from reptiles to mammals. The muscles of the face and head evolved to allow nursing and social engagement. Concurrently a new component of the autonomic nervous system (myelinated vagus) evolved and was regulated by a brainstem nucleus that was involved in the regulation of the striated muscles of the face and head (nucleus ambiguus). This convergence of neural mechanisms established an integrated social engagement system that synergized the behavioural and visceral features of social engage-ment. As a result activation of the somatomotor component would trigger visceral changes that supported social engagement, while modulation of the visceral state either promoted or impeded social engagement behaviours. Stimulation of visceral states would promote behavioural mobilization (i.e. fight or flight behaviours) and impede the expression of social engagement behaviours, while increased activity through the myelinated vagus would pro-mote the social engagement behaviours associated with a calm visceral state. For example, specific neural mechanisms related to feeding and rocking promote calm behavioural and visceral states.

Both the feeding and the passive rocking of an infant promote calmness by their effects on the myelinated vagus. Feeding activates the muscles of mastication via trigeminal efferent pathways, which provide afferent feedback input to the nucleus ambiguus, the source nucleus of the myelinated vagus. Rocking provides direct influence on the vagus by stimulating vagal afferent pathways through the baro-receptors. Activation of the social engagement system dampens the neural circuits including the limbic structures that support fight, flight or freeze behaviours. In mammals the nucleus ambiguus not only coordinates sucking, swallowing and breathing, but it also regulates heart rate and vocalizations in response to stressors. In mammals it is possible, by quantifying the amplitude of respiratory sinus arrhythmia, to assess the tonic and phasic regulation of the vagal pathways originating in the nucleus ambiguus.

Overall Porges' Polyvagal Theory proposes that there is a phylogenetic shift in the neural regulation of the autonomic nervous system that passes through three stages, each with an associated behavioural strategy. There are three components to the autonomic nervous system (visceral afferents, sympathethic nervous system and parasympathetic nervous system) that may be linked to affective experience. The theory is based on an understanding that adaptive behaviours are supported by three neural circuits linked to the autonomic nervous system. Each circuit represents a different phylogenetic stage of the vertebrate autonomic nervous system. These three distinct autonomic subsystems are phylogenetically ordered and behaviourally linked. The first stage is represented by the unmyelinated visceral vagus nerve that facilitates digestion and responds to environmental threat by reducing metabolic activity. Its visceral afferents play a role in determining feelings. For example, they provide knowledge of hunger but also may convey the sense of nausea associated with social distress ('sick to their stomach') or breathlessness, the feeling that the heart has stopped, or terror. Behaviourally, its activation leads to behavioural immobilization (e.g. feigning death in animals, vasovagal syncope and behavioural shutdown, dissociation in humans).

The second stage involves the sympathetic nervous system that increases metabolic output and inhibits the visceral vagus resulting in behavioural mobilization, providing the energy for motor activity, to fight or to flee. Intense feelings of anger or anxiety might be associated with its activation. It increases cardiac output and inhibits gastric motility.

The third stage, involving the parasympathetic nervous system, is characteristic of mammals and involves the myelinated vagus nerve that rapidly regulates cardiac output to facilitate social engagement or disengagement. It is linked to affect and affective regulation in adaptive social behaviour. It is involved in growth and restoration of activity after stress and a sense of social safety.

In mammals the vagus nerve has two branches: one of these originates in dorsal motor nucleus of the vagus and regulates subdiaphragmatic organs, e.g. the digestive tract; the other regulates the heart. The branch that regulates the heart evolved, during mammalian embryology, from cells from the dorsal vagus that migrated to form the nucleus ambiguus. There, cell bodies were formed for visceromotor myelinated axons that inhibit the sinoatrial node, the cardiac pacemaker. Through downregulation of cardioinhibitory vagal tone to the heart, a 'vagal brake' regulates heart rate and maintains it. However, rapid increases in cardiac output may occur with activation of the sympathetic adrenal system. If stress persists the heart rate may be increased via the sympathetic nervous system. Engaging the vagal brake results in sympathetic inhibition, slowing of the heart rate, decreased metabolic activity, self-soothing and calm. When demands are placed, the autonomic nervous system follows a phylogenetic strategy in response, starting with the newest system, and if it fails then reverting to more primitive autonomic responses.

The mammalian vagus that regulates the heart is neuroanatomically linked to the cranial nerves that regulate social engagement through facial expression, vocalization and listening. In humans the neural regulation of middle ear muscles, a necessary mechanism to extract the soft sounds of human voice from the loud sounds of low-frequency background noise, involves this system. Thus, Polyvagal Theory links the evolution of the autonomic nervous system to affective experience, emotional expression, facial gestures, vocal communication and contingent social behaviour. Deficits in the social engagement system compromise spontaneous social behaviour, social awareness, affect expressivity, prosody and language development. The detection of safe and trustworthy facial features from facial expression, voice and movement activates a neural circuit that projects from the temporal cortex (fusiform gyrus, superior temporal sulcus) to the central nucleus of the amygdala to inhibit defensive limbic functions; this system disables limbic systems associated with fight, flight and freeze behaviours.

Empathy involves activation of this vagal social engagement system, which is composed of a somatomotor component (pathways that regulate the muscles of the head and face) and a visceromotor component (the myelinated vagus that regulates the heart and bronchi). The social engagement system regulates the eyelids (social gaze and social recognition or greeting gesture), facial muscles (emotional expression), middle ear muscles (extracting human voice spectrum from background sounds), muscles of mastication (ingestion), laryngeal and pharyngeal muscles (sucking, swallowing, vocalizing, breathing), and muscles of head turning and tilting (social gesture and orientation). The patterns of motor response determine the extent of social engagement. Moreover, the phylogenetic development of the mammalian vagus is paralleled by specialized communication described in Section 10.4, via oxytocin and vasopressin, between the hypothalamus and the medullary source nuclei of the visceral vagus, which facilitates sexual arousal and the development of enduring pair bonds. The establishment of enduring pair bonds depends on co-opting the visceral vagus from an immobilization system associated with fear and avoidance to an immobilization system associated with safety and trust. Social behaviours associated with nursing, reproduction and the formation of strong pair bonds require immobilization without fear.

10.6 Mirror neurones

A sense of social safety may be necessary for empathetic responding. Section 10.5 describes autonomic activity and links it to emotional engagement. This section will address motor behaviour and its links to intentionality and emotions. Understanding the intentions of others while watching their actions is a fundamental aspect of social behaviour. Although the neural and functional mechanisms that underlie this ability are poorly understood, studies of mirror neurones are providing new insights. The neuronal capacity to code a 'like me' analogy between self and others is a basic prerequisite for social cognition. The 'like me' analogy may rest upon a series of 'mirror-matching' mechanisms (Gallese, 2003). These mechanisms provide a unifying perspective for the neural basis of social cognition. Mirror neurones may provide biological continuity to understanding the evolution of empathy.

10.6.1 Role in understanding intentions

William James (James, 1890) proposed that actions are intrinsically linked to perception and wrote that 'every mental representation of a movement awakens to some degree the actual movement which is its object'. Thus, observing, imagining or preparing to act might activate the motor programmes necessary to carry out that action. The discovery of mirror neurones in the monkey ventral premotor cortex provides some support for the hypothesis that there is a common code that involves perception and action. In the monkey such neurones discharge both when the monkey performs certain hand movements and when it observes another monkey or a human performing similar hand movements. The brain cells fire equally when performing an action or perceiving the same action performed. However, mirror neurones respond only to the sight of goal-directed actions; they respond only when the monkey observes a hand grasping an object, and not at the sight of the hand or the object alone. Moreover, mirror neurones also appear to distinguish between biological and non-biological motion; they respond only to the observation of hand–object interactions but not to the same action performed by a mechanical tool (Rizzolatti & Craighero, 2004). Thus, the meaning of a gesture is understood as it is reproduced within the observer.

Regarding the brain systems involved in mirror neurone activity, the monkey ventral premotor cortex (area F5) receives information about an observed action involving biological motion from the superior temporal sulcus (STS). Single cell studies in the macaque monkey show that STSa cells selectively respond to depictions of the face and the body, either in action or represented by a static image (Oram & Perrett, 1996). Such response properties of neurones in STSa are consistent with involvement of the STS in the visual recognition of others' actions (Jellema et al., 2000). The parietal cortex may also contain neurones with mirror properties, responding to both the execution of a movement and observation of a movement. Recognizing the movements of other animate objects allows them to be categorized as threatening or engaging and may allow prediction of future actions and preparation for an appropriate response.

This research in rhesus monkeys has stimulated research in humans. Iacoboni et al. (2005) used functional magnetic resonance imaging (fMRI) to study intentionality in humans. Twenty-three individuals observed three kinds of stimuli: grasping hand actions without a specific context, context only (scenes containing objects) and grasping hand actions performed in two different contexts. In the last condition the context suggested the intention associated with the grasping action (either drinking or cleaning). When actions were embedded in contexts, compared with the other two conditions, there was a significant signal increase in the posterior part of the inferior frontal gyrus and the adjacent sector of the ventral premotor cortex where hand actions were observed. They concluded that premotor mirror neurone areas (active during the execution and the observation of an action) previously thought to be involved only in action recognition are also involved in making sense of the intentions of others. Thus, to suggest intention is to infer a subsequent goal: this is an operation that can be carried out automatically by the motor system.

10.6.2 Role in understanding emotional states

Thus, there appears to be a direct, motor-mediated type of action understanding, and a cognitive type of understanding based on the interpretation of visual representations. There is evidence that this is also true for emotion understanding. When the concept of empathy (Einfühlung) was originally introduced, a critical role for *inner imitation* of the actions of others in generating empathy was considered. It was proposed that, outside of conscious awareness, empathic individuals would mimic the postures, mannerisms and facial expressions of others. In keeping with this idea, in addition to understanding actions through mirror neurones, a similar mechanism may be involved in *understanding* and *experiencing* the emotional states of others.

In regard to understanding emotional states, in the primate brain, the limbic system is critical for emotional processing and behaviour. Anatomical data suggest that a part of the insular lobe is connected with the limbic system and with posterior parietal, inferior frontal and superior temporal cortex. This pattern of connectivity makes the insula a likely candidate for relaying action representations to limbic areas processing emotional content. The insula is involved in the perception and experience of the affect termed disgust. Current evidence suggests that the visual sectors of the amygdala are *primarily* linked to the experience and perception of fear; however, the anterior sector of the insula is linked to the experience and perception of disgust. In the anterior insula, visual information about the emotions of others is directly mapped onto the same viscero-motor neural structures that underlie the experience of that emotion in the observer. Although direct mapping can occur, this may be one way in which the emotions of others can be understood. Others' emotions can be also understood on the basis of the cognitive elaboration of the observed expressions. These two possibilities are not mutually exclusive. The first, the earliest in evolutionary terms, is experience-based, whereas the second is a cognitive elaboration of observations. The earlier direct viscero-motor mechanism may scaffold the cognitive description.

Wicker *et al.* (2003) conducted an fMRI study to assess insula functioning. The participants inhaled odorants that produced a strong feeling of disgust. The same individuals observed video clips showing the facial emotional expression of disgust. Observation of such faces and actually feeling disgust activated the same regions in the anterior insula and to a lesser extent in the anterior cingulate cortex. Just as observing hand actions activates the observer's motor representation of that action, so also in this study observing an emotion activated the neural representation of that emotion.

Carr *et al.* (2003) used fMRI to investigate how action representation modulates emotional activity. Eleven healthy, right-handed subjects (seven males and four females) either observed or imitated emotional facial expressions. The authors hypothesized that if action representation mediation is essential to empathy and the understanding of the emotions of others, observation of emotional facial expression should activate the same brain motor regions that are activated during the imitation of the emotional face expressions. In addition, modulation of the action representation circuit onto limbic areas through the insula would predict greater activity during imitation compared with observation of emotion. They found that the observation of emotional expressions activated premotor areas. Moreover, fronto-temporal areas relevant to action representation, the amygdala, and the anterior insula had significant signal increase during imitation when compared with observation of facial emotional expression. The authors conclude that we understand the feelings of others via a mechanism of action representation that shapes emotional content and that our empathic resonance is grounded in the experience of our bodies in action and the emotions associated with specific bodily movements. Thus, an empathic action elicits the representation of the actions associated with the emotions that are observed. This empathic resonance takes place through communication between action representation networks and limbic areas via the insula.

Neuroimaging is being used to understand other aspects of emotion processing, In another study (Leslie *et al.*, 2004) 15 individuals (8 men, 7 women) watched films of facial expressions (smile or frown) and hand movements (move index or middle finger) while their brain activity was studied using fMRI. They watched the films under three different conditions: passive viewing, active imitation and an active motor control. They also carried out a verb generation task to identify language-processing areas. Evidence for a common cortical imitation circuit for both face and hand imitation, involving Broca's area, bilateral dorsal and ventral premotor areas, right superior temporal gyrus supplementary motor area, posterior temporo-occipital cortex and cerebellar areas, was reported. For faces, passive viewing resulted in significant activation in the right ventral premotor area, whereas imitation produced bilateral activation. These results are consistent with right hemisphere dominance for emotional processing. There also may be a right hemisphere mirroring system that could provide a neural substrate for empathy.

10.7 Social bonding and attachment

The steps in the establishment of social life linked to the separation cry, affective attunement, attachment behaviours, maternal care and play may all be linked to empathy. Attachment, the emergence of hierarchical relationships, affective modulation and working models of relationships involve affective engagement. The emergence of mother/infant attunement and attachment, the physiology of the separation response and grief, play and the role of rapid eye movement (REM) sleep in the consolidation of memory and in subsequent adaptive responses are legitimate areas of study in regard to empathy. Most striking are evolutionary changes that lead to social bonding and attachment. Consciousness may have its rudimentary beginnings with affective arousal directed toward the feeding of the young (Harris, 1998). Sociability may emerge as the mother develops the capacity to attend to the infant's cry, nurse her infant and provide a safe environment for mastery play. In primates eye to eye contact with the young and the capacity to grieve the loss of conspecifics is found in chimpanzees, especially bonobos. In *Homo sapiens*, not only grief, but also expressive gestures of comfort toward the bereaved make their appearance.

10.8 Development of empathy in childhood

Empathy is viewed as both cognitive and emotional. Cognitive empathy (Theory of Mind) refers to the intellectual/imaginative appreciation of the mental state of another while emotional or affective empathy refers to an emotional response toward others' emotional responses. An empathic, emotional response must be appropriate to the observed mental state. It may occur to match the others' feeling, for example feeling fear when another is frightened, or go beyond matching the affect and be responsive to it, for example showing sympathy or compassion. To be empathic the response is directed towards the other and not toward oneself; happiness at another's misfortune is not empathy (Lawrence *et al.*, 2004). The term moral agency is used to describe both the ability to refrain from inhumane behaviour and the capacity to behave humanely. With the development of the self, self-organization, self-reflection and the capacity for self-regulation are established. In the process empathy may mature and be an underlying factor in the establishment of moral agency.

Empathy is a developmental process whereby individuals come to understand the emotional states of others. The perception of facial expressions in primates and humans evolves and leads to a basic understanding of their emotional significance (Ekman, 1972; Parr, 2003). Physiological responses to the perception of pleasure and distress in monkeys and apes are demonstrable (Parr, 2003). In primates changes in peripheral skin temperature differ based on the emotional valence of video scenes. Skin temperature increases in response to positive scenes, such as play or greeting rituals, and decreases in response to negative scenes, such as aggression and threats. Understanding the extent to which non-human animals resonate to the perceived emotion of conspecifics may be an important starting point for comparative studies of empathy. This idea is consistent with there being an evolutionary continuity in the emergence of empathic feelings.

Developmental studies have long focused on empathy. Infant and child development researchers were investigating visual perception (Gibson & Pick, 2000), emotions (Levenson, 1996), early imitation (Meltzoff, 1990) and the origins of social cognition and intersubjectivity (Gergely & Watson, 1999; Rochat et al., 1999, Rochat, 2001) before mirror neurones that may link perception and action were discovered.

What do these studies contribute to our understanding of how infants, children and adolescents develop in relation to others as they vicariously experience and understand others' feelings, thoughts and attitudes through sensory, perceptual and cognitive experiences. Rochat (2002) summarizes the developmental literature and lists six levels of empathy in the first 5 years of life as follows:

1. At birth, infants manifest passive emotional resonance that is automatically triggered and biologically determined.

2. By the second month, there is the emergence of active reciprocation through social smiling and complex engagement and regulation of face-to-face exchanges with caretakers. Besides emotional contagion, infants begin to manifest a new conversational posture towards others; they actively co-construct shared experience through imitation and reciprocal games (Rochat et al., 1999). They smile more toward people than objects and react reflexively to movement of gaze that primes one's own eye movements (Frith & Frith, 2003).

3. By 6 months infants are surprised if an object moves on its own but not if a person does. At about 9 months of age, infants attempt to share their attention with others in regard to objects and events in the environment. They are actively involved in developing 'so-called secondary intersubjectivity' (Carpenter et al., 1998). Now the infants' context of empathy moves beyond beyond face-to-face exchanges. They can separately represent goals of agents and the means used to reach the goal.

4. By 12 months infants can respond to an object as an intentional agent. By about 14 months, infants can identify themselves as unique and recognize themselves in mirrors. Now they can begin to identify with or project themselves into others (projective empathy). At around this age children start discriminating others as partners who are imitating them (Agnetta & Rochat, 2004). By 18 months joint attention emerges as the infant and adult look together at a third object; this is the beginning of mentalizing with deliberate imitation and the ability to track the speaker's intention when learning words.

Distress expressions and motor actions that alleviate the stress of another seem to become coordinated only following the emergence of mirror self-recognition. Rather than two processes, for example a vicarious emotional sharing process and a cognitive process of perspective taking or Theory of Mind, Bischof-Kohler (1994) proposes that insight is mediated by the empathic response itself and that such self-objectification is the only essential precondition of empathy: it draws a clearcut distinction between self and others. (Bischof-Kohler, 1994). This was tested in an investigation involving 36 girls and boys aged 14–22 months. In two separate sessions the individuals carried out a 'rouge test' for self-recognition and were confronted with a person in need, who demonstrated grief. In both experiments, only those individuals who recognized themselves tried to help others, whereas non-recognizers were indifferent.

5. By 24 months of age, children start to manifest self-conscious emotions including embarrassment (Lewis, 2000). Also at this age, children begin to engage in systematic comparisons, categorization, and ultimately conceptualization of the self in relation to other people. They begin to construe how they should feel based on how others might feel about them. Other self-conscious emotions such as pride and shame begin to emerge.

6. Between the ages of 4 and 6 years normally children develop full awareness of mental states and their role in the explanation and prediction of others' behaviour. There is the unambiguous ability to theorize about others' minds, the capability to recognize false beliefs and the beginning of distinguishing objective from subjective thoughts. Also there is the ability to construe feelings and emotions held by the self and by others that are more or less congruent (Perner, 1991). From this point on, children become capable of adopting a theoretical stance towards others, able to conjecture about the emotional state of others in relation to their own.

This emergence allows over time for cognitions such as, the child 'knows it knows'. Toward the third year, meta-representation leads to knowledge that they 'know something that another does not know'. The emergence of self also allows for further development of the self-conscious emotions. Self-conscious, moral or social emotions, such as shame, guilt and pride, emerge that are basic to forming relationships with others.

The sense of we-ness expands. Self meta-representation is gradually linked to cognitive and social emotional behaviours (Lewis, 1992, 2002). Thus the empathic response necessitates the cognitive representation of myself, self-representation. Lewis suggests that any theory of the development of empathy needs to incorporate the emergence of a self-representation. By age 8 affect is increasingly linked to cognition as moral responses begin to develop and it is increasingly possible, in one's imagination, to consider how the other might feel. With the onset of adolescence there is an intensification of emotions and a deepening of friendships. Now hypotheses are generated about why people are treated as they are and ideal goals for human interactions are discussed. With continuing maturation empathy plays a central role in moral development as social justice and mercy towards those in distress are seen as critical for continued social evolution.

With the growing interest in empathy there is increasing interest in objectively measuring it. Measures for young children, adolescent and young adults have been described. For younger children there is the The Young Children's Empathy Measure. This is a brief measure of pre-schoolchildren's cognitive and affective perspective taking developed to assess children's empathy. The children's empathy scores were correlated with their chronological ages and social development, but not with their IQs. Of intererest, empathy toward children was correlated with empathy for pets. Those children with a strong bond to a pet had higher scores on empathy than children without pets (Poresky, 1990).

Bandura *et al.* (2003) carried out a prospective study in 464 adolescents, aged 14–19 at first assessment, and aged 16–21 years at second assessment. They tested the paths through which perceived self-efficacy for affect regulation is linked to perceived behavioural efficacy in mastery of psychosocial functioning. Self-efficacy in regulating positive and negative affect is accompanied by greater efficacy in managing one's academic achievement, resisting social pressures for antisocial activities and demonstrating empathy towards others' emotional experiences. Overall, perceived empathic self-efficacy contributed to psychosocial functioning and was accompanied by prosocial behaviour.

Eisenberg *et al.* (2002) measured prosocial personality and prosocial moral judgement in young adults and the interrelations among them were evaluated. Reports of prosocial characteristics were obtained at ages 21–22, 23–24 and 25–26 years and prosocial judgement was assessed using interviews producing an objective measure of prosocial moral reasoning at several ages. Prosocial behaviour and empathic responding in childhood and observations of prosocial behaviour in preschool children also were ascertained. There was interindividual continuity in prosocial disposition. Prosocial dispositions in adulthood were found to relate to empathy/sympathy and prosocial behaviour at the younger ages. Moreover, both interview and objective measures of moral reasoning were interrelated in late adolescence/early adulthood and found to correlate with participants' and friends' reports of a prosocial disposition.

10.9 Summary

There is evolutionary continuity in neural systems that provide the basis for empathy and the emergence of mutal aid among members of a species. Developments that make empathy possible include: changes in middle ear structure to allow the mother to hear the young while eating, linking infant vocalization to oxytocin release and enhanced social bonding, autonomic regulation of emotional arousal, mirror neurones attuned to intentionality of others, affect attunement and attachment, self-awareness, self-conscious emotions, role play, mental flexibility and the capacity to link affect and cognition and establish a sense of moral agency. Each of these processes is linked to specific neural systems. Studies of empathy in humans are advancing with the introduction of neuroimaging techniques and new approaches identify empathy as an important area for study. Empathy and trust are being investigated in multiple ways ranging from economic exchange (trust game) to neuroethics and moral agency. Perhaps the renewal of interest in empathy will eventually confirm that mutual aid is indeed the most potent force in evolution.

REFERENCES

Agnetta, B. & Rochat, P. (2004). Imitative games by 9-, 14-, and 18-month-olds. *Infancy*, **6**, 1–36.

Ainsworth, M. D., & Bell, S. M. (1970). Attachment, exploration, and separation: illustrated by the behavior of one-year-olds in a strange situation. *Child Development*, **41**, 49–67.

Bandura, A., Caprara, G. V., Barbaranelli, C., Gerbino, M., & Pastorelli, C. (2003). Role of affective self-regulatory efficacy in diverse spheres of psychosocial functioning. *Child Development*, **74**, 769–782.

Bischof-Kohler, D. (1994). [Self object and interpersonal emotions. Identification of own mirror image, empathy and prosocial behavior in the 2nd year of life.] *Zeitschrift für Psychologie mit Zeitschrift für angewandte Psychologie*, **202**, 349–377.

Bowlby, J. (1969) *Attachment*. New York: Basic Books.

Carpenter, M., Nagell, K., & Tomasello, M. (1998). Social cognition, joint attention, and communicative competence from 9 to 15 months of age. *Monographs of the Society for Research in Child Development*, **63**, i–vi, 1–143.

Carr, L., Iacoboni, M., Dubeau, M. C., Mazziotta, J. C., & Lenzi, G. L. (2003). Neural mechanisms of empathy in humans: a relay from neural systems for imitation to limbic areas.

Proceedings of the National Academy of Sciences of the United States of America, **100**, 5497–5502.

Carter, C. S. (1998). Neuroendocrine perspectives on social attachment and love. *Psychoneuroendocrinology*, **23**, 779–818.

Carter, C. S. (2003). Developmental consequences of oxytocin. *Physiology & Behavior*, **79**, 383–397.

Carter, C. S., DeVries, A. C., & Getz, L. L. (1995). Physiological substrates of mammalian monogamy: the prairie vole model. *Neuroscience and Biobehavioral Reviews, Summer*, **19**(2), 303–314.

De Waal, F. (1989). *Peacemaking Among Primates*. Cambridge, Mass.: Harvard University Press.

Eisenberg, N., Guthrie, I. K., Cumberland, A., *et al.* (2002). Prosocial development in early adulthood: a longitudinal study. *Journal of Personality and Social Psychology*, **82**, 993–1006.

Ekman, P. (1972). *Emotions in the Human Face*. Cambridge: Cambridge University Press.

Frith, U., & Frith, C. D. (2003). Development and neurophysiology of mentalizing. *Philosophical Transactions of the Royal Society of London. Series B, Biological Sciences*, **358**, 459–473.

Gallese, V. (2003). The roots of empathy: the shared manifold hypothesis and the neural basis of intersubjectivity. *Psychopathology*, **36**, 171–180.

Gergely, G., & Watson, J. S. (1999). Early social-emotional development: contingency perception and the social-feedback model. In P. Rochat (ed.), *Early Social Cognition*. Mahwah, N.J.: Erlbaum.

Gibson, E. J., & Pick, A. D. (2000). *An Ecological Approach to Perceptual Learning and Develolpment*. New York: Oxford University Press.

Harris, J. C. (1998). *Developmental Neuropsychiatry*. New York: Oxford University Press.

Iacoboni, M., Molnar-Szakacs, I., Gallese, V., *et al.* (2005). Grasping the intentions of others with one's own mirror neuron system. *Public Library of Science Biology*, March, **3**(3), e79.

James, W. (1890). *The Principles of Psychology*. New York: Holt.

Jellema, T., Baker, C. I., Wicker, B., & Perrett, D. I. (2000). Neural representation for the perception of the intentionality of actions. *Brain and Cognition*, **44**, 280–302.

Kropotkin, P. I. (1989). *Mutual Aid: A Factor in Evolution*. Montreal: Black Rose.

Lawrence, E. J., Shaw, P., Baker, D., Baron-Cohen, S., & David, A. S. (2004). Measuring empathy: reliability and validity of the Empathy Quotient. *Psychological Medicine*, **34**, 911.

Leslie, K. R., Johnson-Frey, S. H., & Grafton, S. T. (2004). Functional imaging of face and hand imitation: towards a motor theory of empathy. *Neuroimage*, **21**, 601–607.

Levenson, R. W. (1996). Biological substrates of empathy and facial modulation of emotion: two facets of the scientific legacy of John Lanzetta. *Motivation and Emotion*, **20**, 185–204.

Lewis, M. (1992). *Shame. The Exposed Self*. New York: The Free Press.

Lewis, M. (2000). Self Conscious emotions: Embarrassment, pride, shame, and guilt. In M. Lewis & J. Haviland-Jones (eds.) *Handbook of Emotions*. New York: Guilford Press.

Lewis, M. (2002). Empathy requires the development of the self. *The Behavioral and Brain Sciences*, **25**, 42.

MacLean, P. D. (1985). Brain evolution relating to family, play, and the separation call. *Archives of General Psychiatry*, **42**, 404–417.

MacLean, P. D. (1990). *The Triune Brain in Evolution: Role in Paleocerebral Functions*. New York: Plenum Press.

Meltzoff, A. N. (1990). Foundations of developing a concept of self: the role of imitation in relating self to other and the value of social mirroring, social modeling, and self practice in infancy. In D. B. M. Cicchetti (ed.), *The Self in Transition: Infancy to Childhood*. Chicago, IU.: Chicago University Press.

Oram, M. W., & Perrett, D. I. (1996). Integration of form and motion in the anterior superior temporal polysensory area (STPa) of the macaque monkey. *Journal of Neurophysiology*, **76**, 109–129.

Parr, L. A. (2003). The discrimination of faces and their emotional content by chimpanzees (Pan troglodytes). *Annals of the New York Academy of Science*, **1000**, 56–78.

Perner, J. (1991). *Understanding the Representational Mind*. Boston: MIT Press.

Poresky, R. H. (1990). The Young Children's Empathy Measure: reliability, validity and effects of companion animal bonding. *Psychological Reports*, **66**(3 Pt 1), 931–936.

Porges, S. W. (2001). The polyvagal theory: phylogenetic substrates of a social nervous system. *International Journal of Psychophysiology*, **42**, 123–146.

Porges, S. W. (2003a). Social engagement and attachment: a phylogenetic perspective. *Annals of the New York Academy of Science*, **1008**, 31–47.

Porges, S. W. (2003b). The Polyvagal Theory: phylogenetic contributions to social behavior. *Physiology & Behavior*, **79**, 503–513.

Preston, S. D., & de Waal, F. B. (2002). Empathy: its ultimate and proximate bases. *The Behavioral and Brain Sciences*, **25**(1), 1–20; discussion 20–71.

Rich, T. H., Hopson, J. A., Musser, A. M., Flannery, T. F., & Vickers-Rich, P. (2005). Independent origins of middle ear bones in monotremes and therians. *Science*, **307**, 910–914.

Rizzolatti, G., & Craighero, L. (2004). The mirror-neuron system. *Annual Review of Neuroscience*, **27**, 169–192.

Rochat, P. R. (2001). Social contingency detection and infant development. *Bulletin of the Menninger Clinic*, **65**, 347–360.

Rochat, P. (2002). Various kinds of empathy as revealed by the developing child, not the monkey's brain. *The Behavioral and Brain Sciences*, **25**, 45–46.

Rochat, P., Querido, J. G., & Striano, T. (1999). Emerging sensitivity to the timing and structure of protoconversation in early infancy. *Developmental Psychology*, **35**, 950–957.

Todes, D. P. (1989). *Darwin Without Malthus: The Struggle for Existence in Russian Evolutionary Thought*. New York: Oxford University Press.

Trivers, R. (1971). The evolution of reciprocal altruism. *Quarterly Review of Biology*, **46**, 35–57.

Wang, Y., Hu, Y., & Meng, J., & Li, C. (2001). An ossified Meckel's cartilage in two Cretaceous mammals and origin of the mammalian middle ear. *Science*, **294**, 357–361.

Wicker, B., Keysers, C., Plailly, J., *et al.* (2003). Both of us disgusted in My insula: the common neural basis of seeing and feeling disgust. *Neuron*, **30;40**(3), 655–664.

Wilson, D. S., & Sober, E. (1994). Reintroducing group selection to the human behavioral sciences. *The Behavioral and Brain Sciences*, **17**, 585–654.

Naturally occurring variability in state empathy

John B. Nezlek[1], Astrid Schütz[2], Paulo Lopes[3] and
C. Veronica Smith[4]

[1]Department of Psychology, College of William & Mary
[2]Department of Psychology, Chemnitz University of Technology
[3]Department of Psychology, University of Surrey
[4]Department of Psychology, University of Delaware

11.1 Introduction

A traditional and important distinction in the study of most individual differences is that between a trait and a state. For psychologists, traits are relatively stable and enduring characteristics that tend to be considered more as causes of behaviours (including the selection of situations) than as outcomes. The adverb 'relatively' is included as a qualifier because traits may change over an extended period of time (e.g. over a decade or a lifetime), but for most intents and purposes, it is assumed that traits do not change. In contrast, states are presumed to change and are more often thought of as outcomes or reactions to circumstances, although it is entirely possible to think of states as causes of behaviours including the selection of situations and circumstances. There is no fixed time period over which a state must or should exist – the length of a state can vary from minutes to hours, perhaps encompassing an entire day. Regardless, the assumption is that states change, and such changes are meaningful and represent something other than random fluctuation.

The state–trait distinction is particularly important because it cannot be assumed that constructs at the two levels of analysis function in the same ways. That is, state- and trait-level phenomena may be governed by, or reflect, different psychological processes (e.g. Tennen *et al.*, 2005). Consistent with this distinction, state- and trait-level relationships are mathematically independent (e.g. Nezlek, 2001). Any type of relationship at one level of analysis can co-exist with any type of relationship at another level of analysis. For example, trait empathy may be

Empathy in Mental Illness, eds. Tom F. D. Farrow and Peter W. R. Woodruff. Published by Cambridge University Press. © Cambridge University Press 2007.

positively related to trait self-esteem, whereas state empathy may be unrelated or negatively related to state self-esteem.

It is important to note that differences in relationships across levels of analysis do not create paradoxes or require decisions about which level of analysis is correct. Both are correct and neither is incorrect. Determining which is correct needs to be based on the question at hand. If one is interested in trait-level phenomena, then trait-level analyses and relationships are correct, whereas if one is interested in state-level phenomena, then state-level analyses and relationships are correct.

In addition to questions about level of analysis, when considering empathy one must consider how empathy is defined. Although there is no agreement about a single definition of empathy, there appears to be some agreement about different definitions of empathy, or at least some similarity across researchers in how empathy has been defined. In their review of empathy research, Duan and Hill (1996) discussed various different definitions of empathy, two of the more prominent of which we describe here.

1. A cognitively focused definition emphasizing that empathy is the understanding of another person's thoughts and feelings. Duan and Hill labelled this as intellectual empathy.

2. An affectively focused definition emphasizing how people react to others' emotional experiences. Duan and Hill labeled this as empathic emotions.

In addition, we think it is useful to consider a third definition combining these two, which emphasizes people's ability to infer another's thoughts and feelings and to experience those feelings. Duan and Hill discussed this matter but did not apply a label per se. This third dimension, representing the interaction of the cognitive and affective dimensions, might shed light on the relationship between empathy and social interaction. In relevant contexts, someone who is both cognitively and affectively empathic might relate to others in qualitatively different ways than those who are empathic in only one domain.

Empathy, in its various manifestations, has been studied as both a state and a trait. We will not attempt to summarize the vast literature on empathy other than to note that studies of trait empathy are fairly similar in structure, design and focus to studies of other traits. The research has examined how empathy is related to other traits, how trait empathy is related to various behaviours, and so forth. Moreover, an emphasis on trait empathy seems to dominate research on empathy within the context of therapy. Due to inconsistencies in how researchers have examined empathy, Duan and Hill (1996) could not offer any firm conclusions about the role empathy plays in the therapeutic process. They did, however, note the following, 'In addition to measurement problems, research in this area is limited by the seemingly fixed assumption of individual differences and the lack of attention to intraindividual differences' (p. 266). Intraindividual differences is another term for within-person state variability.

To the extent that it has been studied, state empathy has been studied primarily in laboratory-based experiments. Laboratory studies of empathy have focused on empathy as an outcome, a result of situational factors such as motivation (e.g. Ickes *et al.*, 1990; Simpson *et al.*, 1995), taking another's perspective (e.g. Batson *et al.*, 2002) and similarity (e.g., Batson *et al.*, 1995) to mention a few. This research covers a wide range of topics and suggests that situational factors influence empathic responses in complex ways. For example, Ickes *et al.* (1990) found that increased motivation (greater interest in an interaction partner) led to greater empathy. In contrast, Simpson *et al.* (1995) found that under some circumstances (e.g. when the emotions another person might be experiencing might be threatening) empathic accuracy can be negatively related to motivation.

What is absent from the present body of research (regardless of its focus) is research on naturally occurring state empathy. Naturally occurring in this instance does not refer to changes brought about by therapeutic interventions or the artificial intervention of a social scientist conducting a study; rather it refers to changes that occur in people's everyday lives. In this chapter we describe the results of two studies of naturally occurring state empathy. In one study, participants described how empathic they felt each day, and in the other study, participants described how empathic they felt during the individual social interactions they had each day.

11.2 Issues in studying states

As mentioned earlier, the term 'psychological state' has been applied to various time periods, and so when studying psychological states, it is critical to define to what or over what time period a state is meant to exist. In terms of studying naturally occurring variability in states, as discussed by Wheeler and Reis (1991), most studies of everyday life can be classified as a function of the basis on which data are collected. State-level observations may be linked to specific events or may be collected following the passage of a certain period of time, what Wheeler and Reis (1991) described respectively as event- or interval-contingent data collection. In this chapter, we describe the results of two studies, one that used event-contingent data collection and another that used interval contingent collection.

The collection of multiple state observations (a strategy sometimes described as intensive repeated measures) provides the opportunity to investigate various relationships, including state-level relationships per se. For example, if two constructs such as empathy and anxiety are measured at the state level, the relationship between these states can be examined. If other data besides psychological states themselves are collected (e.g. situational variables such as the presence of a close friend), the relationships between psychological states and situational variables can be examined. Moreover, individual differences in such within-person relationships can also be examined. For example, the association between empathy and anxiety may be stronger for some than for others, or the presence of a close friend may be associated with greater increases in empathy for some people than for others.

When thinking of state empathy, or any other psychological state, one of the first considerations for many psychologists is the relationship between states and traits. For most, this relationship is captured by how closely state manifestations of a trait correspond to that trait. For example, are highly empathic people always more empathic than less empathic people? As sensible as such a criterion may appear, the study of individual differences is littered with failures to find such correspondence. These failures led Mischel and associates to, more or less, dispense with the idea of a trait, and emphasize how people differ across situations.

In recent descriptions of this approach (e.g. Mischel & Shoda, 1999), personality is defined in terms of people's patterns of responses to situations. People can be inconsistent in how they feel, think and behave in different situations, but they are consistent in these differences. For example, Person A might be empathic with close friends but not with business associates, whereas Person B might be empathic with business associates but not with close friends. The type of data described in this chapter allow for the investigation of such possibilities, and discussions of frameworks for such analyses are presented in Nezlek (2001, 2003).

Although we do not believe as strongly as Mischel and colleagues that the psychological trait is not a useful construct, we think that it is unwise to assume that any characteristic will be expressed without variation across time and space. Our position corresponds to what is often referred to as an 'interactionist' approach. Our thinking is that the existence of situational or temporal variability in a psychological construct does not mean that a trait does not exist; rather, we believe that constructs exist as both states and traits. We focus on state empathy in this chapter as an alternative to the emphasis on traits that characterizes much of the existing research on empathy.

11.3 Daily variability in state empathy

The first (and only to our knowledge) study of naturally occurring variability in state empathy of which we are aware is by Nezlek *et al.* (2001). This study is structurally similar to a number of studies that have examined the variability of various psychological states. On a regular basis over some fixed period of time, individuals provide state-level measures, and analyses focus on the within-person relationships among these measures. Much of the research on state variability has focused on the within-person covariation between psychological states and events in people's day-to-day lives, and the Nezlek *et al.* study examined within-person relationships between daily events and daily reports of empathy.

Although much of the research on within-person variability has concerned the state variability of mood, it is clear that various psychological states vary independently of mood (e.g. Nezlek, 2005), and the Nezlek *et al.* (2001) study examined the within-person covariation between empathy and mood and between empathy and other psychological states. Various aspects of this study are not described in detail in this chapter; detailed descriptions of all procedures and analyses can be found in the published article.

Participants in the Nezlek *et al.* study were undergraduates who provided data twice a week for up to 10 weeks. The twice-weekly schedule was used to avoid possible problems (e.g. boredom) that might occur if participants provided data on consecutive days. As it turned out, participants' responses in this study were comparable to the responses of participants who provided data on consecutive days, suggesting that the interval over which data were collected was not important.

Each day, participants described how empathic they felt they had been by responding to four questions taken from the Balanced Emotional Empathy Scale (BEES; Mehrabian, 1996). The BEES is a widely used pencil and paper measure of what is called empathic emotions: the extent to which a person is moved by the emotions of others. Daily empathy was measured with the following four items taken from the BEES reworded for daily administration: 'The sadness of a close one easily rubs off on me', 'I don't get overly involved with friends' problems', 'I am not affected easily by the strong emotions of people around me', and 'Another's happiness can be very uplifting for me'. Following the scoring used for the BEES, daily empathy was defined as the sum of the responses to these items, with the second and third items being reversed scored. Responses were made using scales of 1–7 with the endpoints labelled 'strongly disagree' and 'strongly agree'.

Participants also provided various other daily measures. One was self-esteem, using four items based on Rosenberg (1965), a widely used trait measure of self-esteem. Another was a daily measure of depressogenic adjustment consisting of three items based on Beck's (1967) triad, which concerned feelings about one's self, one's life in general and optimism about the future. The validity and reliability of these two measures are discussed in Nezlek and Gable (2001). Participants also described their daily mood using the state version of the PANAS (Watson *et al.*, 1988), which measures positive active mood (e.g. happy, excited) and negative active mood (e.g. anxious, nervous), and they provided a daily measure of need for cognition based on Cacioppo and Petty's (1982) trait measure. Finally, they described the events that occurred each day, using a measure based on Butler *et al.* (1994). Daily events were classified into four types: positive social, negative social, positive achievement and negative achievement.

The self-esteem and depressogenic adjustment measures were included to examine within-person relationships between psychological well-being and empathic emotions. That is, how much does an individual's well-being fluctuate with his or her sensitivity to other's emotions? Daily mood was included because we were interested in knowing how being sensitive to others' emotions was related to one's own feelings. Within a cognitive framework, empathy is conceptualized in terms of how people imagine what another person is experiencing. This suggests that individual differences in empathy may reflect individual differences in how cognitively active people are. People who are less cognitively active may be less empathic because they think less about other people, which may reflect the fact that they think less about things in general. Daily (state) need for cognition was included to examine this possibility.

Finally, we measured daily events to examine the covariation between empathy and daily events under the assumption that events represent a necessary but not sufficient condition for the experience of empathy. Empathy requires some sort of target, and people are more empathic when the feelings of others are more salient. On the other hand, people are not empathic simply because they are with others or something is happening. This highlights the importance of distinguishing trait from state empathy. As a trait, empathy is some sort of cross-situational ability or potential to recognize or react to the emotions of others, whereas as a state, it is the extent to which people actually recognize or react to others' emotions at specific points in time.

Daily events were differentiated on the basis of whether they were social or achievement related. This distinction not only recalls such classic dichotomies as Freud's 'Arbeit und Liebe' (Work and Love), it also distinguishes events that are more likely to provide a basis for experiencing empathy (social events) from those that are less likely to provide such a basis (achievement events).

These daily measures were analysed with a series of multilevel random coefficient models. This technique estimated mean state empathy and divided the total variance of empathy into between- and within-person components (i.e. trait and state variability). Across all participants and all days, mean state empathy was 16.0, corresponding to a point just above the midpoint of the scale, an average response of 4 on the scale of 1–7. So, in their daily lives, people felt that the emotions of others affected them, but did not on average affect them very strongly. Consistent with many conceptualizations of the relationships between states and traits, mean daily empathy was positively related ($r = 0.7$) to trait empathy, (i.e. scores on the BEES.)

For the daily measure of empathy, approximately half the variance was within-persons (10.7) and half (9.3) was between-persons (i.e. state and trait). Over the course of the study, intraindividual variability in daily empathy was as great as the interindividual variability in mean empathy (aggregated across the days of the study). As indicated by the relationship between trait empathy and mean state empathy, people who had greater trait empathy also reported greater state empathy. Nevertheless, this relationship was far from perfect. These findings are prima facie evidence for considering empathy as both a trait and a state. If we want to know how empathic a person feels on any given day, we need to know that individual's trait empathy and we need to know something about the type of day a person is having – the focus of the next set of analyses.

The analyses also examined within-person (i.e. state or daily level) relationships between daily empathy and daily self-esteem, depressogenic adjustment, mood, need for cognition and events. For each person, a set of within-person relationships was estimated. The analyses found that mean state-level relationships between empathy and self-esteem, between empathy and depressogenic adjustment, and between empathy and the need for cognition were not significantly different from zero. On average, people's daily empathic feelings were unrelated to their self-evaluation, their psychological well-being and to how cognitively active they felt. Although null results are not always informative, the lack of such relationships suggests that reports of daily empathy did not simply reflect how well people were feeling about themselves and their lives or how much they were thinking in general. Moreover, these null results also strongly suggest that relationships between empathy and other measures are not simply due to response bias, (i.e. extreme responding on all scales.)

As expected, daily empathy was related to both daily positive and daily negative affect. (Research on trait empathy has found both types of relationships.) Stronger daily emotions, both positive (PA) and negative (NA), were associated with greater empathy. The mean within-person coefficients were 0.66 ($p < 0.01$) for PA and 0.33 ($p < 0.05$) for NA. On average, an increase of 1.0 in PA was associated with an increase of 0.66 in empathy scores, and a 1.0 increase in NA was associated with a 0.33 increase in empathy scores. The causal relationships among these measures are not clear from these results. It is possible that stronger emotions lead to stronger empathy; it is also possible that greater empathy (defined as being sensitive to the emotions of others) leads to stronger emotions, or both causal relationships are possible.

Also as expected, daily empathy was related to both positive and negative social events but was not related to either positive or negative achievement events. The more social events people had, the more empathic they felt. The mean within-person coefficients were 1.18 for positive social events ($p < 0.01$) and 0.51 for negative social events ($p < 0.05$). Social contact is a necessary, but not sufficient, condition for empathy. So, achievement contexts in which social contact is either absent or relatively unimportant are not contexts in which empathy is particularly salient. What is particularly interesting about these results is that greater empathy was associated with increased negative social activity (e.g. conflict, disappointment, etc.). These relationships between events and empathy and mood and empathy suggest that people are empathic even when being empathic may entail experiencing negative emotions.

Given these relationships, additional analyses were done examining the joint relationships among empathy, social events and mood. Different analyses were conducted involving different combinations of PA, NA and positive and negative social events as predictors of daily empathy. These analyses found that when NA and negative social events were included together, negative social events were not significantly related to daily empathy. These results suggest that that daily NA mediated relationships between daily empathy and daily negative social events. Negative events lead to increased NA, which in turn leads to increased empathy. Such a pattern makes sense given that it is likely that the other people present during these negative social events were also experiencing negative feelings. No such mediational relationship was found between PA and positive social events.

One of the advantages of the data structure and analyses used for this study is the ability to examine individual differences in the within-person relationships between daily empathy and other daily measures. A series of analyses examining such individual differences in terms of various trait-level characteristics (empathy, PA and NA, depressive symptoms, need for cognition, trait self-esteem) found no relationships between these trait-level characteristics and within-person relationships between daily empathy and other daily measures.

11.4 Empathy in naturally occurring social interaction

The second study we will discuss is a social interaction diary study conducted in Chemnitz, Germany. Participants in this study, 100 undergraduates at Chemnitz Technical University, maintained a variant of the Rochester Interaction Record (Wheeler & Nezlek, 1977) for two weeks. Using a standardized form and a website, they described all the social contacts they had each day, typically at the end of the day. These descriptions included the other people who were present during the interaction, what they were doing during the interaction and how they felt about the interaction. Participants described 4587 interactions, across an average of 12 days, and the average number of interactions recorded per day was 3.9.

This method represents what Wheeler and Reis described as event-contingent data collection because data collection was triggered by the occurrence of an event, a social interaction. A detailed description of this study can be found in Lopes *et al.* (2004). Particularly relevant to our concerns, participants also indicated, using a scale of 1–9, how well they felt they understood the emotions of the people with whom they were interacting. This corresponds to what is often described as intellectual empathy.

The data were analysed with a series of multilevel random coefficient models (Nezlek, 2003), which estimated mean state empathy and divided the total variance of empathy into between- and within-person components (i.e. trait and state/interaction variability). Across all participants and all interactions, mean state empathy was 6.1, corresponding to a point somewhere between the midpoint of the scale and the maximum value. In everyday interaction, people felt that they understood the emotions of others well but not, on average, very well. Participants also completed the MSCEIT, an ability measure of emotional intelligence (Mayer *et al.*, 2002). One of the subscales of the MSCEIT measures understanding emotions, and scores on this subscale were positively related ($p < 0.05$) to participants' self-reports of how well they understood the emotions of their co-interactants, supporting the validity of these self-reports.

For the interaction-level measure of empathy, approximately two-thirds of the variance was within-persons at the interaction level (2.7) and one-third (1.4) was between-persons. That is, the variability in empathy across interactions was greater than the variability across people in mean empathy (aggregated across each person's interactions). As indicated by the relationship between MSCEIT scores and mean interaction (state) empathy, people who could understand others' emotions also reported greater understanding during interactions. Nevertheless, this relationship was far from perfect. Similar to the previous study, these findings are prima facie evidence for considering empathy as both a trait and a state.

If we want to know how empathic a person feels during a particular social interaction, we need to know that individual's trait empathy and we need to know something about the interaction. Moreover, as suggested by the distribution of variance for interaction empathy (twice as much at the interaction level than at the person level) and by the fact that in the daily study, empathy covaried with only social and not achievement events, the nature of social encounters seems to be critical in understanding how empathic people feel. There are numerous ways to classify interactions, and for present purposes we examined differences in empathy as a function of size (dyads versus non-dyads), activity and the relationships participants had with the others who were present.

The analyses comparing dyads found that people felt less able to read others' emotions in non-dyads ($M = 5.8$) than in either same-sex or opposite-sex dyads

Table 11.1: Empathy and nature of social interaction

Activity	Empathy
Eating	6.4[b]
Going out	5.9[c]
Working	5.6[d]
Hobbies/relaxation	6.3[b]
Exchange affection	7.4[a]
Other	6.0[c]

Note: Means sharing a subscript were not significantly different at $p < 0.05$.

($Ms = 6.2$, 6.4 respectively, $p < 0.01$). This makes sense given that, in dyads, there is only one person to whom one needs to attend, and people can devote more cognitive resources to understanding a single person than when they need to understand the feelings of more than one. This reasoning is consistent with the results of a study by Davis *et al.* (1996), who found that a competing task (a distracting memory task) diminished people's perspective-taking abilities. To some extent, an individual's cognitive resources are fixed, and the more tasks individuals face (i.e. the more people they need to read) the fewer resources they can allocate to any single task.

The results of analyses comparing cognitive empathy across interactions involving different activities were quite clear. These results are summarized in Table 11.1. When people exchanged physical affection (which was broadly defined to include different levels of intimacy), they felt they could understand others' emotions very clearly ($M = 7.3$). This was no doubt due in part to the fact that such interactions were invariably dyads and that emotional feelings were probably uniformly positive and strong and relatively unambiguous. During normal everyday events with smaller numbers of their social groups (eating and hobbies/relaxation), people felt that they could understand the emotions of others pretty well ($Ms = 6.4$). In contrast, when going out (parties, pub-crawling, etc.) and probably surrounded by people, they felt less able to understand the emotions of others. Finally, and in agreement with the results of the first study, people felt the least able to understand the emotions of others during work ($M = 5.6$).

The results of analyses that examined the influence of the presence or absence of certain types of relational partners were also quite clear. Consistent with the previous results on exchanging physical affection, the presence of a romantic partner was associated with greater empathy, a difference of 0.4. In contrast, the presence of acquaintances (those whom people knew but who were not close friends) and of strangers was associated with decreases in empathy, differences of 0.66 and 1.16 respectively.

11.5 Implications for mental health

The studies described in this chapter have implications for our understanding of the roles empathy may play in establishing and maintaining mental health and for our understanding of how to study such roles. Most important, these two studies on naturally occurring empathy in combination with the extensive body of laboratory-based studies suggest that we need to think of empathy as both a trait and a state. That is, people may have some sort of dispositional ability to perceive and experience the emotions of others, but it appears that situational factors can influence if not overwhelm the expression of such abilities.

At least at the within-person level of analysis, it appears that empathy, defined in terms of people's sensitivity to the emotions of others, is not related to psychological well-being. In the first study, daily empathy was not related to daily self-esteem or daily feelings of depression. Although at first this finding may seem to contradict existing research, which more or less has discussed empathy as a component of mental health, it really does not. Emotional empathy (or empathic emotions as labelled by Duan & Hill, 1996) may or may not be adaptive. Simply feeling stronger emotions when those around you are feeling stronger emotions may or may not lead to increased well-being. There may be times when it does (e.g. being able to share someone else's happiness), and there may be times when it does not (e.g. becoming anxious when others are anxious). To the extent that empathy can amplify the experience of emotions in social interaction, it might contribute to affect intensity or volatility without influencing the mean balance of positive and negative affect, which is considered an indicator of well-being.

As is the case with so many processes, whether or not empathy (or empathic emotions) is adaptive probably depends on the situation. In this regard, the capacity to experience empathy in the right contexts can be viewed as a skill or ability rather than as an automatic, dispositionally driven process. Similar to the conceptualization of emotional intelligence as a trainable ability underlying the MSCEIT, it would seem that it would be most adaptive to know when to be empathic and when not to be. Such an ability is likely related to people's ability to regulate their emotions.

Nevertheless, although control over one's emotions may be desirable, empathy may be difficult to inhibit. For example, numerous studies have found that people tend to feel and express the same affective states that others are experiencing and expressing, and there is evidence that, to some degree, such emotional contagion is not governed by conscious processes (e.g. Hatfield *et al.*, 1994). The possibility that empathic emotions may not be controllable was also suggested by the lack of individual differences in within-person relationships between daily empathy and daily social events, particularly negative social events. Although these relationships varied across participants, this variability did not correspond to various trait measures of well-being such as depression, self-esteem and anxiety. How strongly people reacted empathically was not related to their psychological adjustment.

Recognizing the state component of empathy may have implications for therapeutic interventions. Assuming that empathy is positively related to well-being begs the question of what type of empathy under what circumstances? The present discussion was not intended to address the former question but does provide some guidance for addressing the latter. Both studies of naturally occurring variability in empathy suggest that empathy is not particularly salient during work- or task-focused interactions. Of course, if someone is having trouble with work-related issues, it may be important to address these issues, but, by and large, it appears that empathy is most salient in socially focused situations. In some ways, this point is patently obvious – empathy is defined in terms of others' emotions.

Nevertheless, when thinking of empathy as an aspect of mental health, it is probably best to think more about specific types of empathy under specific circumstances than to think globally about some sort of general (or 'g') factor. That is, at the trait level, most conceptualizations of empathy have emphasized a global characteristic or skill. If you are empathic in one setting or in one way, you are likely to be empathic in another. The present results suggest however that empathy may be a multifaceted construct, a collection of specific 's' factors, albeit with the possibility of some sort of general ability.

The need to think more specifically about how and when people are empathic should inform studies of empathy. More context-specific research might help us understand the costs and benefits of dispositional empathy, and how the flexible activation and deactivation of state empathy contributes to social interaction and resilience. Although trait-level studies have been and will continue to be valuable, they need to be complemented by studies that incorporate the important within-person variability in empathy. We hope this chapter has highlighted the importance of modelling this variability and provided some guidance for doing this.

REFERENCES

Batson, C. D., Turk, C. L., Shaw, L. L., & Klein, T. R. (1995). Information function of empathic emotion: learning that we value the other's welfare. *Journal of Personality and Social Psychology*, **68**, 300–313.

Batson, C. D., Chang, J., Orr, R., & Rowland, J. (2002). Empathy, attitudes, and action: can feeling for a member of a stigmatized group motivate one to help the group. *Personality and Social Psychology Bulletin*, **28**, 1656–1666.

Beck, A. T. (1967). *Depression: Clinical, Experimental, and Theoretical Aspects*. New York: Harper & Row.

Butler, A. C., Hokanson, J. E., & Flynn, H. A. (1994). A comparison of self-esteem lability and low trait self-esteem as vulnerability factors for depression. *Journal of Personality and Social Psychology*, **66**, 166–177.

Cacioppo, J. T., & Petty, R. E. (1982). The need for cognition. *Journal of Personality and Social Psychology*, **42**, 116–131.

Davis, M. H., Conklin, L., Smith, A., & Luce, C. (1996). Effect of perspective taking on the cognitive representation of persons: a merging of self and other. *Journal of Personality and Social Psychology*, **70**, 713–726.

Duan, C., & Hill, C. E. (1996). The current state of empathy research. *Journal of Counseling Psychology*, **43**, 261–274.

Hatfield, E., Cacioppo, J. T., & Rapson, R. L. (1994). *Emotional Contagion*. New York: Cambridge University Press.

Ickes, W., Stinson, L., Bissonnette, V., & Garcia, S. (1990). Naturalistic social cognition: empathic accuracy in mixed-sex dyads. *Journal of Personality and Social Psychology*, **59**, 730–742.

Lopes, P. N., Brackett, M. A., Nezlek, J. B., *et al.* (2004). Emotional intelligence and social interaction. *Personality and Social Psychology Bulletin*, **30**, 1018–1034.

Mayer, J. D., Salovey, P., & Caruso, D. (2002). *Mayer-Salovey-Caruso Emotional Intelligence Test (MSCEIT): User's Manual*. Toronto: Multi-Health Systems, Inc.

Mehrabian, A. (1996). *Manual for the Balanced Emotional Empathy Scale (BEES)*. (Available from Albert Mehrabian, 1130 Alta Mesa Road, Monterey, CA 93940).

Mischel, W., & Shoda, Y. (1999). Integrating dispositions and processing dynamics within a unified theory of personality: The Cognitive-Affective Personality System. In L. A. Pervin & O. P. John (eds.), *Handbook of Personality Theory and Research* (pp. 197–218). New York: Guilford Press.

Nezlek, J. B. (2001). Multilevel random coefficient analyses of event and interval contingent data in social and personality psychology research. *Personality and Social Psychology Bulletin*, **27**, 771–785.

Nezlek, J. B. (2003). Using multilevel random coefficient modeling to analyze social interaction diary data. *Journal of Social and Personal Relationships*, **20**, 437–469.

Nezlek, J. B. (2005). Distinguishing affective and non-affective reactions to daily events. *Journal of Personality*, **73(6)**, 1539–1568.

Nezlek, J. B., Feist, G. J., Wilson, F. C., & Plesko, R. M. (2001). Day-to-day variability in empathy as a function of daily events and mood. *Journal of Research in Personality*, **35**, 401–423.

Nezlek, J. B., & Gable, S. L. (2001). Depression as a moderator of relationships between positive daily events and day-to-day psychological adjustment. *Personality and Social Psychology Bulletin*, **27**, 1692–1704.

Rosenberg, M. (1965). *Society and the Adolescent Self-Image*. Princeton, N.J.: Princeton University Press.

Simpson, J. A., Ickes, W., & Blackstone, T. (1995). When the head protects the heart: empathic accuracy in dating relationships. *Journal of Personality and Social Psychology*, **69**, 629–641.

Tennen, H., Affleck, G., & Armeli, S. (2005). Personality and daily experience revisited. *Journal of Personality*, **73(6)**, 1465–1483.

Watson, D., Clark, L. A., & Tellegen, A. (1988). Development and validation of brief measures of positive and negative affect: the PANAS scales. *Journal of Personality and Social Psychology*, **54**, 1063–1070.

Wheeler, L., & Nezlek, J. (1977). Sex differences in social participation. *Journal of Personality and Social Psychology*, **35**, 742–754.

Wheeler, L., & Reis, H. (1991). Self-recording of everyday life events: origins, types, and uses. *Journal of Personality*, **59**, 339–354.

Neuroimaging of empathy

Tom F. D. Farrow

Academic Clinical Psychiatry, University of Sheffield

12.1 Introduction

Empathy, the ability or process 'to identify with and understand another's situation, feelings and motives' would initially appear an unlikely candidate for neuroimaging research. Being aware of, and interpreting, other's behaviour on an emotional level is likely to be recently evolved and hence a 'high-level' cognitive process. Such complex brain processes are generally considered as unlikely to have a dedicated brain region serving them, or to be easy to isolate for examination.

  This chapter will describe how empathy has been dissected into a set of component cognitive processes, how brain imaging researchers have designed experiments to examine various combinations of these components, and what these finding may tell us about empathy's neurophysiological basis.

12.2 A neuroimaging primer

It may be useful to begin by summarizing the field of neuroimaging, and highlighting which aspects may be of relevance. Structural neuroimaging concerns the physical size and integrity of brain tissue, and in as much as there may be a relationship between size and function, if we could identify brain regions which were part of an empathy system or circuit, then investigating their size or integrity may be informative (presuming that we can objectively measure subjects' behavioural empathic levels). Functional neuroimaging utilizes surrogate markers (normally regional blood flow) to infer which parts of the brain are 'active' whilst a specific task or mental process is undertaken. It is assumed that increases in blood flow are associated with increased functional activity, though such activity may represent the firing of either excitatory or inhibitory neurones. Positron emission tomography (PET; a type of functional neuroimaging) utilizes a fast decaying

Empathy in Mental Illness, eds. Tom F. D. Farrow and Peter W. R. Woodruff. Published by Cambridge University Press. © Cambridge University Press 2007.

radioactive dye (often oxygen-15) injected into the body to track the brain's regional blood supply. By repetitively performing a single task over a relatively long time (3–5 min) it is possible to see where the blood is directed and hence, by inference, where the brain is activated. Functional magnetic resonance imaging (fMRI) is a non-invasive neuroimaging technique that relies on the differing properties of oxy-haemoglobin and deoxy-haemoglobin (oxygenated and deoxygenated blood) in a magnetic field. This allows mapping of the distribution of oxygenated blood (and by inference neuronal activity) in response to a particular task. fMRI scans are designed such that subjects perform contrasting tasks, the demands of which are matched as far as possible, so as only to differ by the specific cognitive process of interest. By subtracting the 'baseline' task from the 'active' task, many of the background and other processes unrelated to the cognitive process of interest (e.g. perceiving the noise of the scanner) are excluded. Tasks in an fMRI scanner are typically performed in an alternating fashion with each block lasting 10–20 s, or as an 'event-related' design where neural responses to single tasks (each typically <3 s duration) are recorded and summated (c.f. PET imaging). In fMRI, brain activations to complex psychological paradigms such as empathy (as opposed to, say, visual cortex activation when viewing a flashing chequerboard pattern) are rarely strong enough for reliable and meaningful areas to be identified in single subjects. It is therefore more common for reported activations to be group-averaged. The error inherent in the reported neuroanatomical location of activations is therefore heavily influenced by inter-subject variability in brain anatomy (commonly quoted to be in the order of 8–12 mm). Areas of activation or structural change are reported by two methods – neuroanatomical name (i.e. brain region) and Brodmann's Area (BA; a functional and cytoarchitectonic parcellation of brain grey matter, similar but not identical to the brain's gyral folds). For the non-specialist reader, areas relevant to this chapter are shown in Figure 12.1.

Functional neuroimaging techniques such as PET and fMRI also allow examination of brain changes within a group over time, such as those changes induced by psychotherapeutic or pharmacological intervention and accompanying symptom resolution. Ultimately, successful functional neuroimaging of complex psychological brain processes is almost entirely reliant on the ability of the task performed in the scanner to engage the cognitive process of interest.

12.3 Component cognitive processes relevant to empathy

For the purposes of designing functional neuroimaging paradigms to tap empathy, proposed component cognitive processes need to be elucidated. Therefore, any

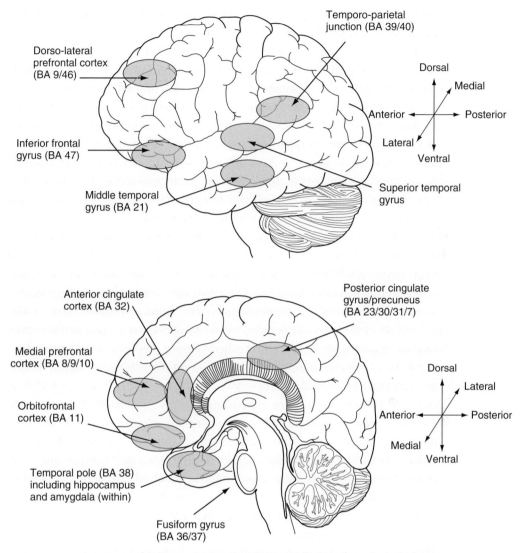

Figure 12.1. View of the brain from the left showing lateral (top picture) and midline (bottom picture) surfaces. Areas relevant to this chapter are identified. These are identified for the non-specialist reader and do not represent the shape or extent of each region

neuroimaging study which has examined any of these component cognitive processes (in isolation or in groups) will also be of interest in understanding empathy's neurophysiological basis. These component processes and areas of interest include:

1. Attending to socially relevant stimuli including facial (expression) and body (posture, movements) perception. This perceptual ability is central to social

cognition – 'the mental processes underlying social perception and social judgements'. Empathy is an aspect of social cognition and dependent on our interaction with, and perception of, the people around us. When based on deliberation and intent (and thereby requiring motivational and attentional systems), empathic judgements may also revolve around such issues as the morality of the situation in question.

2. Theory of Mind (ToM) – 'the attribution of independent mental states to self and others in order to explain and predict others' behaviour'. This capacity is often described as seeing the world from someone else's point of view or perspective. A common task in ToM-based paradigms is the 'false belief task'. This is often classified according to whether the ToM attribution is first order ('A thinks X') or second order ('A thinks B thinks X').

3. Self-awareness or the ability to self-reflect is required to understand and project emotions onto others.

4. Mirror neurones. These specialist cells are activated in association with, for example, moving one's hand but also when watching another's hand movements. The discovery that certain regions of the brain activate in response not only to performing a task, but also to watching another person perform that task, suggests that we may interpret others' actions (and emotions) by simulating them in our own brains (see Chapter 23 on the perception-action model and Chapter 24 on simulation theory).

5. Emotion processing and emotional and affective intuition. Empathy can also be a more automatic, subconscious response and involve little if any deliberate reasoning. This automatic cognitive response, which is often associated with a measurable autonomic (bodily, visceral) component, may involve separate brain structures to those involved in more 'conscious' empathic cognitions.

Any attempt to use neuroimaging to investigate empathy as a whole should take the following points into consideration:

1. There is almost certainly no 'empathy centre', but rather integrated activity in groups or networks of interconnected brain regions.

2. Empathy is not a unitary concept and can probably be elicited by a number of methods (e.g. with or without a face-processing component). A 'definitive' empathy paradigm therefore does not exist. This is likely to lead to different brain activations to empathy paradigms, dependent on which component processes are evoked.

3. An MRI scanner is a hostile and 'ecologically invalid' environment. Even if paradigms are capable of evoking 'active empathy', the real-world transferability of this is debatable. The subtle distinctions between empathy, sympathy and 'detached concern', and the possibility that the cognitive and affective

components of empathy are dissociable mean that results should be treated with caution and interpreted in the context of the cognitive paradigm that was used to evoke them.

Results of functional neuroimaging of empathy paradigms can be interpreted in the light of hypothesized regions (see Section 12.4), but due to the preliminary nature of research in this field, post hoc interpretation of non-hypothesized regions may also shed light on understanding empathy's neurophysiological basis.

12.4 Neuroimaging studies of component parts of empathy

12.4.1 Socially relevant stimuli

Perception of socially relevant stimuli has been mainly localized to the temporal lobes (Adolphs, 2001). Areas within the posterior superior temporal sulcus [Brodmann's Area (BA) 39] are activated in response to biologically and socially salient visual motion stimuli (Allison *et al.*, 2000). However, face perception, as possibly the most important flag of social relevance, has been reported to be divided between the fusiform gyrus (BA 36/37; invariant features, e.g. identity) and the posterior superior temporal gyrus (BA 39/40; expression and gaze; Haxby *et al.*, 2000).

Empathy may involve little if any deliberate reasoning (Greene & Haidt, 2002) or may be a conscious cognitive choice. The decision as whether to empathize (when empathy is based upon deliberation and intent) may be heavily dependent on the perceived morality (reason, emotion and affective intuition) of the situation. Greene and colleagues in an fMRI study (Greene *et al.*, 2001) used moral dilemmas as probes, and identified three regions: medial frontal gyrus (BA 9/10), posterior cingulate gyrus (BA 31) and bilateral angular gyrus (BA 39; in the temporo-parietal junction area) as differentiating moral from non-moral judgements. Another study of the neural basis of moral emotions (Moll *et al.*, 2002) replicated (amongst other regions) medial prefrontal cortex (BA 10/46 and 9) activation, further associating this region with social behaviours.

12.4.2 Theory of Mind and social cognition

Functional imaging studies of healthy volunteers performing Theory of Mind (ToM) tasks (Fletcher *et al.*, 1995; Gallagher *et al.*, 2000; Goel *et al.*, 1995) have all implicated a specific region of left prefrontal cortex (BA 8/9/10). Goel and colleagues in a PET study had subjects deciding whether Christopher Columbus (the fifteenth century European explorer) could infer the function of an object from a picture (i.e. seeing the world from Christopher Columbus' perspective). Fletcher and colleagues in another PET study had subjects reading, and answering questions about, short stories, half of which required ToM to correctly respond. Gallagher and colleagues in an fMRI study repeated the paradigm used by Fletcher and colleagues and additionally had subjects viewing cartoons which required ToM to interpret. The consistency of left prefrontal cortex activation in response to these radically different paradigms and across imaging modalities is striking. While dorso-medial prefrontal cortex (DMPFC) is associated with tasks emphasizing self reference and ToM tasks (Fletcher *et al.*, 1995; Gallagher & Frith, 2003; Goel *et al.*, 1995), dorso-lateral prefrontal cortex (DLPFC) is associated with working memory and executive functions. Other areas activated by these paradigms included posterior cingulate cortex [BA 31; associated with internal (visceral) state monitoring and self behaviour evaluation], precuneus (BA 7; associated with episodic memory retrieval and mental imagery), left temporal lobe (BA 21, 38) and temporo-parietal junction/posterior superior temporal gyrus/angular gyrus (BA 39/40). A PET study repetition of Fletcher and colleagues' 1995 study (Happé *et al.*, 1996) in patients with Asperger's syndrome (who show ToM deficits) found no activity in the previously reported left prefrontal region with, rather, an adjacent, more ventral area of medial prefrontal cortex (BA 9/10) being activated.

ToM has been further subdivided into 'hot' and 'cold' cognition or reasoning (Goel & Dolan, 2003) differentiating the inference of others' epistemic states (beliefs, knowledge, focus of attention) from that of others' affective states (emotions, preferences, beneficent or hostile intentions). Goel and Dolan (2003) reported that a reciprocal prefrontal activation pattern exists as a function of emotional saliency. Specifically, whereas 'cold' reasoning activated DLPFC and suppressed ventro-medial prefrontal cortex (VMPFC), the reverse occurred in response to 'hot' cognition. It is noteworthy however in this study, that whilst the DLPFC activations were left lateralized, the VMPFC activations were midline or bilateral. A review of functional neuroimaging of ToM (Gallagher & Frith, 2003) identified a set of three areas which are repeatedly activated by, and associated with, ToM paradigms; namely, the anterior paracingulate cortex (a division of medial prefrontal cortex approximately corresponding to BA 9/32), the superior temporal sulcus (STS; BA 39/40) and the temporal poles bilaterally (BA 38). Gallagher and Frith (2003) argue that the anterior paracingulate cortex is involved in 'mentalizing' or is 'the location of the cognitive mechanism underpinning the ability to represent mental states "decoupled" from reality', whereas the STS and temporal poles are involved in abilities that aid mentalizing. While the STS may be involved in the perception of intentional behaviour [biological motion or stimuli which signal the actions and intentions of another individual (Allison *et al.*, 2000)], the temporal poles are involved in the retrieval from memory of personal (semantic and episodic) experiences. Other possibly relevant cognitive paradigms which have activated the STS include being the target of another's emotions (Wicker *et al.*, 2003a). The temporo-parietal junction (BA 39/40; an area of posterior STS) has been reported to be specific to reasoning about the content of others' mental states (as opposed to another's simple physical presence; Saxe & Kanwisher, 2003). Other regions which may be more related to social tasks in general rather than being prerequisites for ToM (but are sometimes activated in response to ToM paradigms) include the amygdala and orbitofrontal cortex. The amygdala (particularly left) is most frequently associated with fear perception and conditioning, and memory modulation central to emotional processing, whilst the orbitofrontal cortex is associated with reward and decision-making in the context of emotional situations. Lesions of the orbitofrontal cortex may lead to ToM deficits (Stone *et al.*, 1998).

Some lesional data on the role of the amygdala (Fine *et al.*, 2001) and frontal cortex (Rowe *et al.*, 2001) in ToM, and research on whether ToM and general executive functions are interdependent are slightly contradictory however to the previously reported functional neuroimaging findings. Fine and colleagues (2001) report a case study of a 32-year-old patient with a congenital or early-onset left amygdala lesion. Despite being severely impaired in their ability to represent mental states, the patient was unimpaired on a wide range of general executive functioning tests. This appears to contradict the interpretive assumptions of many ToM neuroimaging studies which suggest that ToM is mediated by general executive functioning. Rowe and colleagues (2001) studied 31 patients with unilateral frontal lobe lesions following neurosurgery. All patients exhibited significant impairment on both first- and second-order ToM false belief tests, and on a range of executive functioning tests. However again, as in the study by Fine and colleagues (2001), the executive functioning deficits appeared to be independent of the ToM impairments. This may highlight a possible distinction between what is essential for ToM attributions (as revealed by lesional studies) and brain regions involved in ToM attributions in an 'optimal system' (as revealed by neuroimaging in healthy subjects). A further lesional study examining five patients with bilateral orbitofrontal damage and five patients with left DLPFC damage (Stone *et al.*, 1998) showed that orbitofrontal lesion patients performed similarly to those with Asperger's syndrome (i.e. performing poorly on second-order ToM tasks), but that the DLPFC patients showed no such deficits. As well as a 'false belief' task the authors had a 'faux pas' task, again on which patients with bilateral orbitofrontal damage performed poorly. Faux pas tasks include an element of empathy as they require both an understanding of a false or mistaken belief and an empathic inference of the effect that it has on another person.

12.4.3 Self-awareness

Empathy may also be reliant on self-awareness and the ability to consciously reflect on one's sense of self, as this ability guides our social interactions. An fMRI study (Johnson *et al.*, 2002) had 11 volunteers consciously reflecting on their own traits, abilities and attitudes (e.g. 'I'd rather be alone', 'I have a quick temper') contrasted with factual knowledge judgements (e.g. 'You need water to live', 'Ten seconds is more than a minute'). All 11 subjects individually (as well as in a group activation analysis) activated anterior medial prefrontal cortex (BA 9/10; right lateralized in 5, left lateralized in 3 and midline in 3) and posterior cingulate cortex (BA 23/30/31). The posterior cingulate cortex is often associated with retrieval of episodic autobiographical memories, but in this context its role in the evaluation of emotional salience of stimuli or mediating an interaction between memory retrieval and emotion (Maddock, 1999) may be more relevant. A posterior cingulate/precuneus (BA 7/31) activation was reported in another study to dissociate between interacting with a human or computer partner and 'inferring the intentions of real social partners with whom they are directly interacting and whose behaviour has consequences for their material well-being' (Rilling *et al.*, 2004).

12.4.4 Mirror neurones

Some groups of neurones are called 'mirroring neurones' or 'mirror neurones' because they are activated both by performing and observing an intentional action (Gallese & Goldman, 1998; see also Schulkin, 2000). Neurophysiological evidence would further suggest that these mirror neurones may be active even when crucial parts of the actions are obscured and can only be inferred (Umiltà *et al.*, 2001). Mirror neurones are pertinent to empathy, in the debate as to whether empathy is underpinned by 'simulation theory' or 'theory-theory' (Preston & de Waal, 2002). While simulation theory states that our ability to recognize and reason about other people's states of mind is an example of experience projection, i.e. we know others' minds by simulation, theory-theory states that we employ a theory to make attributions of mental states of others, i.e. our understanding of mind is a framework or a theory analogous to scientific theories. Simulation theory may be particularly relevant in understanding situations which are not easily encoded into language (e.g. emotionally salient ones), thereby suggesting a role for conscious experience in social cognition. Mirror neurones would support simulation theory rather than theory-theory as a mechanism for individuals to detect and interpret conspecifics' mental states and to facilitate a more general mind-reading ability. Mirror neurones are relevant to empathy because they would enable an organism to detect certain mental states of observed conspecifics, possibly a precursor to, or component of, a more general mind-reading ability.

12.4.5 General emotional processing

Individual neuroimaging studies of general emotion have activated a very wide range of areas, probably partly due to heterogeneity in task design, imaging methods and analysis. Meta-analytic reviews (e.g. Phan *et al.*, 2002) have sought to report consistent inter-study findings. The role of medial prefrontal cortex (MPFC; BA 9) in general emotional processing and the anterior cingulate cortex in imagery and emotional tasks requiring cognitive demand are probably the two most robust and reproducible finds with relevance to empathy. A more specific role for the MPFC in internally attended emotional states and the cognitive aspects (e.g. identification and appraisal) of emotional processing is now beginning to emerge. As emotion and social cognition appear to depend on some of the same brain regions, this may explain why social cognition and empathy deficits often coexist in disorders such as autism, schizophrenia, depression and post-traumatic stress disorder (PTSD; Grady & Keightley, 2002).

12.5 Studies of empathy itself

It should initially be re-iterated that a definitive empathy paradigm almost certainly does not exist, due partly to the wide-ranging definition and partly to the fact that different stimuli may evoke empathic responses, but that these may not be identical neurophysiologically. To date there have been few studies which have attempted to neuroimage empathy as a unitary concept, and all have approached the 'challenge' in individual ways. At this early stage of research in the 'field' it is therefore preferable to look for overlaps in findings rather than a consensus.

12.5.1 Emotional mimicry studies

In a hypothesis encompassing a 'seamless integration among perception, socially relevant mimicry [the "chameleon effect"], emotional experience and empathy', one study investigated the existence of a human mirroring system for affective facial expressions, and how this underpins empathy (Leslie *et al.*, 2004). Subjects underwent fMRI whilst passively viewing, actively imitating or independently generating facial expressions. Results suggested that conscious imitation of facial expression is dissociable from unconscious mimicry (hypothesized to underlie empathy) when passively viewing faces and that this latter ability is localized to right ventral premotor cortex [BA 6 (immediately posterior to Broca's area)], thereby providing evidence for a motor theory of empathy.

A very similar paradigm to that used by Leslie and colleagues was used by a different group (Carr *et al.*, 2003), but was approached from a different perspective and thus interpreted in a different light. The only substantive difference between the two studies was that Carr and colleagues used still pictures of faces (or parts thereof) whereas Leslie and colleagues used short (2-s) video clips. Carr and colleagues' paper postulates a fronto-temporal circuit connected via the insula to the limbic system, thereby characterizing empathy as a process by which action representation modulates emotional activity. The structural neuroanatomical basis and flow of information of the 'action representation' part of this model is explicitly hypothesized as follows:

... the circuit of frontoparietal networks interacting with the superior temporal cortex is critical for action representation. This ... circuit is composed of inferior frontal and posterior parietal neurons that discharge during the execution and also the observation of an action (mirror neurons), and of superior temporal neurons that discharge only during the observation of an action. ... [T]his circuit is critical for imitation and ... within this circuit, information processing ... flow[s] as follows. (i) The superior temporal cortex codes an early visual description of the action and sends this information to posterior parietal mirror neurons ... (ii) The posterior parietal cortex codes the precise kinesthetic aspect of the movement and sends this information to inferior frontal mirror neurons ... (iii) The inferior frontal cortex codes the goal of the action ... (iv) Efferent copies of motor plans are sent from parietal and frontal mirror areas back to the superior temporal cortex, such that a matching mechanism between the visual description of the observed action and the predicted sensory consequences of the planned imitative action can occur. (v) Once the visual description of the observed action and the predicted sensory consequences of the planned imitative action are matched, imitation can be initiated.

A largely overlapping network including the premotor face area, dorsal inferior frontal gyrus (BA 44/45), superior temporal sulcus, insula and amygdala was activated by both observing and imitating emotional facial expressions, with the fronto-temporal network being significantly more activated by imitation than observation.

12.5.2 Disgust

Another study investigating whether there is a common neural basis to understanding and experiencing an emotion (Wicker *et al.*, 2003b) used fMRI to examine subjects' neural response to odorant-induced disgust and viewing faces expressing disgust. Both tasks activated right anterior insula and inferior frontal gyrus. In a similar way therefore to motor mirror neurones, observing an emotion appears to activate a neural representation of experiencing an emotion, thereby providing a mechanism for understanding others' behaviour.

12.5.3 Pain

In a further fMRI study of an understanding/experiencing neural overlap (Singer *et al.*, 2004), pain (self experienced and observing a loved one receiving) was examined. While bilateral anterior insula and rostral anterior cingulate cortex were common to both tasks, additional areas (sensorimotor cortex, somatosensory cortex and caudal anterior cingulate cortex) were activated exclusively in the experiencing pain condition. The authors conclude that 'only that part of the pain network associated with its affective qualities, but not its sensory qualities, mediates empathy'. Interestingly, the anterior insula and anterior cingulate cortex activations correlated with subjects' individual empathy scores. These findings again suggest that our ability to empathize has evolved from a system for representing our internal bodily states and subjective feeling states. Another study used perceiving other's pain to investigate a central component of empathy, the 'interpersonal sharing of affect' (Jackson *et al.*, 2005). Perceiving and rating other's pain was associated with activation of regions including anterior cingulate cortex (ACC) and insula. Furthermore the change in ACC activity (between viewing painful and non-painful scenarios) was positively correlated with subjects' ratings of others' pain, a possible surrogate measure of the extent of interpersonal empathic engagement. The specific area of ACC activated was the rostro-dorsal region (sometimes referred to as the 'cognitive cingulate' and associated with error monitoring and selecting among competing responses) as opposed to the caudo-ventral anterior cingulate, more associated with autonomic responses. This may be relevant when distinguishing whether an affective (bodily sensation) empathic engagement has occurred.

12.5.4 Empathy and sympathy

In contrast to empathy, sympathy might be defined as 'The affinity, association or relationship between persons wherein whatever affects one similarly affects the other', possibly distinguishing it as an 'intellectual understanding' of another person compared with empathy's 'emotional knowing'. These two concepts have a large overlap however, and differentiating them for the purposes of neuroimaging is extremely challenging. A PET study of a combination of sympathy and empathy, with concomitant skin conductance response (SCR; i.e. affective, bodily arousal) recording (Decety & Chaminade, 2003) had subjects watching individuals recounting sad or neutral stories with congruent or incongruent affect (neutral, happy or sad facial expression). Decety and colleagues reported right inferior parietal lobule (BA 39/40) activation to be associated with 'shared representations' or 'concern for others ... [simulating] the affective experiences of others ... the self [taking] the perspective of others', while general emotional content activated left inferior frontal gyrus and bilateral temporal poles. VMPFC (BA 32) activation and the largest SCR response were associated in this study with social conflict arising from the mismatched story content and facial expression condition. This latter finding may have resonance with the idea that the strength of empathic response is to some degree modulated by the difference in affect between the 'empathizer' and the subject of their empathy.

12.5.5 Empathy and forgiveness

In an fMRI study of empathy and forgivability (Farrow *et al.*, 2001), healthy subjects were required to make judgements from the perspective of another person as to what would be the most likely explanation for their affective state, or which of two crimes was more forgivable. Forgivability comprises multiple cognitive components, one of which may be the ability to empathize with others, including an aggressor (Denton & Martin, 1998). Empathic judgements activated left medial frontal gyrus (BA 9), left inferior frontal gyrus (BA 47), posterior cingulate/precuneus (BA 31/7) and left middle temporal gyrus (BA 21) whilst forgivability judgements activated left medial frontal gyrus (BA 9/10) and posterior cingulate cortex (BA 31). Both paradigms also activated orbitofrontal cortex (BA 11), possibly due to this region's role in evaluating the relative merits of two options. The most striking difference between the activations to empathic and forgivability judgements was the left middle temporal gyrus activation. While suggesting that attempting to understand others is physiologically distinct from determining the forgivability of their actions, the difference may also be due to the fact that the forgivability scenarios were based around unknown individuals, while the empathic scenarios were based on personal acquaintances. This difference in the paradigm design may highlight an important distinction of whether empathy is differentially applied to known or unknown (simulated) individuals and whether these are associated with different brain substrates.

These empathy and forgivability judgement paradigms have been repeated in patients with PTSD (Farrow *et al.*, 2005) and schizophrenia (Lee *et al.*, 2003). Both studies involved scanning patients on two occasions, 3 to 5 months apart, during which time PTSD patients received a course of cognitive behavioural therapy (CBT) and patients with schizophrenia received 'treatment as usual' (anti-psychotic medication). The latter (Lee *et al.*, 2003) study also conducted the empathy and forgivability paradigms on a new group of 14 healthy subjects on two occasions. Whereas the patients with PTSD and schizophrenia showed increased activation in task-relevant regions (e.g. left medial prefrontal cortex, posterior cingulate gyrus) at the second scan, healthy subjects revealed a *reduced* amount. These early data illustrate the potential for mapping the brain's response to treatment interventions in a systematic manner, in this case using an empathy paradigm, a central component of which (social cognition) is known to be abnormal in both patients with PTSD and schizophrenia (Grady & Keightley, 2002).

12.6 Other relevant neuroimaging studies

Two further neuroimaging studies which may inform our understanding of the neurophysiology of empathy examined social exclusion (Eisenberger *et al.*, 2003) and aggressive behaviour (Pietrini *et al.*, 2000). Social exclusion involves distress at being 'left out' and a lack of the soothing feeling of being in the presence of others. This could be reframed (though the authors of the article in question do not) as a feeling that others are not empathizing with you. In line with results from neuroimaging studies of pain, ACC was activated, and correlated with levels of self-reported distress. ACC activity and its role in conflict monitoring were modulated by right ventral prefrontal cortex, a brain region associated with inhibition of negative affect (Hariri *et al.*, 2000).

The presence of empathy acts as a mitigator of aggressive behaviour (Björkqvist & Österman, 2000), possibly particularly physical aggression. In a PET study of imaginal aggressive behaviour (Pietrini *et al.*, 2000), healthy subjects had associated *decreased* activity (functional deactivation) in VMPFC and orbitofrontal cortex. The possible interpretation of these results as inhibition of empathy towards someone that you are about to hurt is compelling. As further supporting evidence, patients with personality disorders and a history of aggressive behaviour are reported to have reduced ventral prefrontal cortex glucose utilization (Goyer *et al.*, 1994) and grey-matter volumes (Raine *et al.*, 2000).

Finally, lesional data have suggested that right ventro-medial cortex is most consistently associated with empathic deficits (Shamay-Tsoory *et al.*, 2003), but that other neuropsychological functions (such as ToM and cognitive flexibility) and related deficits (e.g. understanding sarcasm; Shamay *et al.*, 2002) are so intimately related that disentangling them is extremely complex.

12.7 Conclusions

Ten years of neuroimaging of the postulated component parts of empathy and five years of increasingly sophisticated 'full' empathy paradigms have begun to provide a consensus as to which brain regions form a core network and which regions may be specific to the subtleties of the individual cognitive probes used. The 'empathic experience' may ultimately be shown to be irreducible, but until we are able to convincingly elicit 'true' empathy in the scanner, the investigation of component parts is a good foundation on which to base further work. Medial prefrontal cortex, posterior cingulate and various temporal lobe regions (superior temporal sulcus/temporo-parietal junction/temporal pole) have all been so frequently and consistently reported as to be considered as 'core'. The roles of (mainly subregions such as) ACC, orbitofrontal cortex, amygdala, insula and precuneus are associated with specific components or aspects which differentiate between the various interpretations of how to design a paradigm to tap empathy. The connection of superior temporal regions and inferior frontal cortices to the limbic system via the insula [a critical relay from action representation to emotion (Carr *et al.*, 2003)] may prove to be an important pathway in the neuropathology of many neuropsychiatric disorders with dysempathy as a central feature. Furthermore, studies of ToM in Asperger's syndrome (Happé *et al.*, 1996) and empathy and forgivability in PTSD (Farrow *et al.*, 2005) and schizophrenia (Lee *et al.*, 2003) would suggest that alterations to the location and extent of activations are present in certain disorders. As stated previously, detailed interpretation of brain activations to empathy paradigms is only meaningful in the context of exactly which task was performed and cannot presently be considered generalizable to empathy as a whole. The concurrent recording of the skin-conductance response and brain activation has recently begun (e.g. Decety & Chaminade, 2003) and may significantly enhance our understanding of how the affective and cognitive components of empathy interact.

REFERENCES

Adolphs, R. (2001). The neurobiology of social cognition. *Current Opinion in Neurobiology*, **11**, 231–239.

Allison, T., Puce, A., & McCarthy, G. (2000). Social perception from visual cues: role of the STS region. *Trends in Cognitive Sciences*, **4**, 267–278.

Björkqvist, K., & Österman, K. (2000). Social intelligence – empathy = aggression? *Aggression and Violent Behavior*, **5**, 191–200.

Carr, L., Iacoboni, M., Dubeau, M.-C., Mazziotta, J. C., & Lenzi, G. L. (2003). Neural mechanisms of empathy in humans: a relay from neural systems for imitation to limbic areas. *Proceedings of the National Academy of Sciences of the United States of America*, **100**, 5497–5502.

Decety, J., & Chaminade, T. (2003). Neural correlates of feeling sympathy. *Neuropsychologia*, **41**, 127–138.

Denton, R. T., & Martin M. T. (1998). Defining forgiveness: an empirical exploration of process and role. *The American Journal of Family Therapy*, **26**, 281–292.

Eisenberger, N. I., Lieberman, M. D., & Williams, K. D. (2003). Does rejection hurt? An fMRI study of social exclusion. *Science*, **302**, 290–292.

Farrow, T. F. D., Hunter, M. D., Wilkinson, I. D., *et al.* (2005). Quantifiable change in functional brain response to empathic and forgivability judgments with resolution of posttraumatic stress disorder. *Psychiatry Research – Neuroimaging*, **140(1)**, 45–53.

Farrow, T. F. D., Zheng, Y., Wilkinson, I. D., *et al.* (2001). Investigating the functional anatomy of empathy and forgiveness. *NeuroReport*, **12**, 2433–2438.

Fine, C., Lumsden, J., & Blair, R. J. R. (2001). Dissociation between 'theory of mind' and executive functions in a patient with early left amygdala damage. *Brain*, **124**, 287–298.

Fletcher, P. C., Happé F., Frith, U., *et al.* (1995). Other minds in the brain: a functional imaging study of 'theory of mind' in story comprehension. *Cognition*, **57**, 109–128.

Gallagher, H. L., & Frith, C. D. (2003). Functional imaging of 'theory of mind'. *Trends in Cognitive Sciences*, **7**, 77–83.

Gallagher, H. L., Happé, F., Brunswick, N., *et al.* (2000). Reading the mind in cartoons and stories: an fMRI study of 'theory of mind' in verbal and nonverbal tasks. *Neuropsychologia*, **38**, 11–21.

Gallese, V., & Goldman, A. (1998). Mirror neurons and the simulation theory of mind-reading. *Trends in Cognitive Sciences*, **2**, 493–501.

Goel, V., & Dolan, R. J. (2003). Reciprocal neural response within lateral and ventral medial prefrontal cortex during hot and cold reasoning. *NeuroImage*, **20**, 2314–2321.

Goel, V., Grafman, J., Sadato, N., & Hallet, M. (1995). Modeling other minds. *NeuroReport*, **6**, 1741–1746.

Goyer, P. F., Andreason, P. J., Semple, W. E., *et al.* (1994). Positron-emission tomography and personality disorders. *Neuropsychopharmacology*, **10**, 21–28.

Grady, C. L., & Keightley, M. L. (2002). Studies of altered social cognition in neuropsychiatric disorders using functional neuroimaging. *Canadian Journal of Psychiatry*, **47**, 327–336.

Greene, J., & Haidt, J. (2002). How (and where) does moral judgment work? *Trends in Cognitive Sciences*, **6**, 517–523.

Greene, J. D., Sommerville, R. B., Nystrom, L. E., Darley, J. M., & Cohen, J. D. (2001). An fMRI investigation of emotional engagement in moral judgement. *Science*, **293**, 2105–2108.

Happé, F., Ehlers, S., Fletcher, P., *et al.* (1996). 'Theory of mind' in the brain. Evidence from a PET scan study of Asperger Syndrome. *NeuroReport*, **8**, 197–201.

Hariri, A. R., Bookheimer, S. Y., & Mazziotta, J. C. (2000). Modulating emotional responses: effects of a neocortical network on the limbic system. *NeuroReport*, **11(1)**, 43–48.

Haxby, J. V., Hoffman, E. A., & Gobbini, M. I. (2000). The distributed human neural system for face perception. *Trends in Cognitive Sciences*, **4**, 223–233.

Jackson, P. L., Meltzoff, A. N., & Decety, J. (2005). How do we perceive the pain of others? A window into the neural processes involved in empathy. *NeuroImage*, **24**, 771–779.

Johnson, S. C., Baxter, L. C., Wilder, L. S., *et al.* (2002). Neural correlates of self reflection. *Brain*, **125**, 1808–1814.

Lee, K. H., Egleston, P. N., Brown, W. H., *et al.* (2003). Treatment induced changes in brain activation in empathy in people with schizophrenia. *NeuroImage*, **19**, 117.

Leslie, K. R., Johnson-Frey, S. H., & Grafton, S. T. (2004). Functional imaging of face and hand imitation: towards a motor theory of empathy. *NeuroImage*, **21**, 601–607.

Maddock, R. J. (1999). The retrosplenial cortex and emotion: new insights from functional neuroimaging of the human brain. *Trends in Neurosciences*, **22**, 310–316.

Moll, J., de Oliveira-Souza, R., Eslinger, P. J., *et al.* (2002). The neural correlates of moral sensitivity: a functional magnetic resonance investigation of basic and moral emotions. *The Journal of Neuroscience*, **22**, 2730–2736.

Phan, K. L., Wager, T., Taylor, S. F., & Liberzon, I. (2002). Functional neuroanatomy of emotion: a meta-analysis of emotion activation studies in PET and fMRI. *NeuroImage*, **16**, 331–348.

Pietrini, P., Guazzelli, M., Basso, G., Jaffe, K., & Grafman, J. (2000). Neural correlates of imaginal aggressive behavior assessed by positron emission tomography in healthy subjects. *American Journal of Psychiatry*, **157**, 1772–1781.

Preston, S. D., & de Waal, F. B. M. (2002). Empathy: its ultimate and proximate bases. *Behavioral and Brain Sciences*, **25**, 1–72.

Raine, A., Lencz, T., Bihrle, S., LaCasse, L., & Colletti, P. (2000). Reduced prefrontal gray matter volume and reduced autonomic activity in antisocial personality disorder. *Archives of General Psychiatry*, **57**, 119–127.

Rilling, J. K., Sanfey, A. G., Aronson, J. A., Nystrom, L. E., & Cohen, J. D. (2004). The neural correlates of theory of mind within interpersonal interactions. *NeuroImage*, **22**, 1694–1703.

Rowe, A. D., Bullock, P. R., Polkey, C. E., & Morris, R. G. (2001). 'Theory of mind' impairments and their relationship to executive functioning following frontal lobe excisions. *Brain*, **124**, 600–616.

Saxe, R., & Kanwisher, N. (2003). People thinking about thinking people. The role of the temporo-parietal junction in 'theory of mind'. *NeuroImage*, **19**, 1835–1842.

Schulkin, J. (2000). Theory of mind and mirroring neurons. *Trends in Cognitive Sciences*, **4**, 252–256.

Shamay, S. G., Tomer, R., & Aharon-Peretz, J. (2002). Deficits in understanding sarcasm in patients with prefrontal lesion is related to impaired empathic ability. *Brain and Cognition*, **48**, 558–563.

Shamay-Tsoory, S. G., Tomer, R., Berger, B. D., & Aharon-Peretz, J. (2003). Characterization of empathy deficits following prefrontal brain damage: the role of the right ventromedial prefrontal cortex. *Journal of Cognitive Neuroscience*, **15**, 324–337.

Singer, T., Seymour, B., O'Doherty, J., *et al.* (2004). Empathy for pain involves the affective but not sensory components of pain. *Science*, **303**, 1157–1162.

Stone, V. E., Baron-Cohen, S., & Knight, R. T. (1998). Frontal lobe contributions to theory of mind. *Journal of Cognitive Neuroscience*, **10**, 640–656.

Umiltà, M. A., Kohler, E., Gallese, V., *et al.* (2001). I know what you are doing: a neurophysiological study. *Neuron*, **31**, 155–165.

Wicker, B., Keysers, C., Plailly, J., *et al.* (2003b). Both of us disgusted in my insula: the common neural basis of seeing and feeling disgust. *Neuron*, **40**, 655–664.

Wicker, B., Perrett, D. I., Baron-Cohen, S., & Decety, J. (2003a). Being the target of another's emotion: a PET study. *Neuropsychologia*, **41**, 139–146.

The neurophysiology of empathy

Nancy Aaron Jones and Chantal M. Gagnon

Department of Psychology, Florida Atlantic University

13.1 Theories of empathy

13.1.1 Evolutionary theories of empathy

Darwin (1872) contended that emotions are primary regulators of social inter-action and that interspecies communication of emotion is innate and has adaptive value. Within this framework, empathy, which involves recognizing emotions and adjusting social interactions accordingly, would provide individuals and groups who possess this ability with an evolutionary advantage.

Several contemporary theoretical papers have also emerged in the psychological literature that discuss the evolution of empathy and its neural substrates. For example, Brothers (1989) introduced an evolutionary theory of empathy, defining the concept of empathy across maturational levels. He and others (Hoffman, 2000; Trevarthen & Aitken, 1994) argue that empathy is an innate biologically based process in more evolved species. Empathy's evolution in phylogeny and ontogeny is based on the need for more evolved species to be able to communicate with important others, such as caretakers and attachment figures. While the theoretical models proposed differ in the exact mechanism impelling the development of empathy, they agree that variation between individuals in levels of empathic processing derives from evolved variation in genetic endowments and is modified by environmental experiences. Ultimately these theories recognize that empathy, a key component of social communication during development, is adaptive, promotes survival and has a neurological basis.

13.1.2 Somatic theories of empathy

The somatic theories have their origins in the writings of William James (1884) and Walter Cannon (1927), with James arguing that emotions were intertwined with bodily sensations and Cannon focusing on the brain's role in emotion.

Empathy in Mental Illness, eds. Tom F. D. Farrow and Peter W. R. Woodruff. Published by Cambridge University Press. © Cambridge University Press 2007.

Contemporary theories, such as Damasio's Somatic Marker Hypothesis (Damasio, 2000) and Porges' Polyvagal Theory (Porges, 2003), rely heavily on the workings of neurological systems to explain the progression of emotions and the associated bodily changes in response to environmental events. Employing a brain–body connection to investigate individual differences in emotional reactivity and regulation (Doussard-Roosevelt *et al.*, 2001), these theories are important because they contribute to our understanding of how entire systems can be involved in coordinated functioning for empathy.

13.1.3 Individual differences theories of empathy

A final group of theories converge on the issue of individual differences in reactivity and arousal. Historically individual differences were examined when potential risk for physical or psychological impairments, as a result of neurophysiological injury or socially mediated dysfunction, were uncovered. The most well-known case of injury to the brain is the case of Phineas Gage (Harlow, 1868), which documented dramatic changes in personality, including decreased ability to display empathic responses. Similarly, individual differences in dysfunctional emotional processes also stemmed from socially mediated syndromes/illnesses, as reported by the clinical case studies of Freud (Freud & Breuer, 1895). However, scientific investigation of the connection between emotions and neural systems was not undertaken because neurones were not well understood and there were methodological constraints in studying brain function at the time.

More recently, scientists (Gainotti, 1989) provided empirically based descriptions of differences in brain dysfunction and the associated emotional consequences, describing 'catastrophic reactions' in left-hemisphere-lesioned patients and reactions of indifference in right-hemisphere-lesioned patients. Moreover, Robinson and his colleagues (1984) demonstrated that there was localization of emotional responses to the anterior regions of the brain, impelling further theoretical interest and empirical studies on the specialization of the two hemispheres as well as specialization of the anterior region for the processing of emotionally relevant stimulus events.

Developmental studies have investigated these models. For example, Fox and his colleagues (Fox, 1991; Fox *et al.*, 1994) contend that individual differences in emotional reactivity are innate, neurophysiological processes, stemming from the motivational tendencies for approach versus withdrawal, a continuum that has both behavioural (Carver, 2001) and physiological (Fox *et al.*, 1994) sources of verification. As such, an individual's emotional experience is the result of two differing systems in the organism: the motivational tendency for approaching novel and interesting events or situations in order to explore and learn, versus the tendency for withdrawing or escaping from repugnant and potentially damaging events or environments. Neurophysiological correlates of the approach–withdrawal continuum have also been documented by Fox and his colleagues (Fox *et al.*, 1994), with the approach system associated with the development of left frontal brain activity patterns and the withdrawal system associated with right frontal brain activity patterns.

Empathy is conceptualized in this model as a complex emotion emerging and unfolding from the approach system. For instance, the approach motivation system undergirds infants' and children's interest in novel and social events and enables the subsequent development of concern and responsibility (Fox, 1991). Empirical studies have focused on delineating individual differences in innate dispositions, the associated involvement of neural systems, and the role of environmental modifiers affecting the dispositions during normal development (Fox *et al.*, 1994). Fox example, Young *et al.* (1999) demonstrated that individual infants with lower arousal patterns showed less empathy during toddlerhood than infants demonstrating higher arousal patterns. Further, children who were labelled as behaviourally inhibited (a withdrawing tendency) were less empathic with an unfamiliar adult than children not prone to inhibited behaviours. While somewhat limited, these data suggest that specific patterns of temperamental reactivity can be predictive of empathic responding and patterns of risk for empathic dysregulation.

In a complementary series of theoretical and empirical papers based in individual differences theories, Davidson (Davidson, 2004; Tomarken *et al.*, 1990) have focused their efforts on outlining the association between brain functioning and socioemotional risk factors for psychopathology. In their view individual differences in genetic and neurophysiological processes form a potential diathesis and specific environmental stressors experienced by individuals with this diathesis may have an increased risk for psychopathology. Davidson's theories, primarily focusing on delineating the basis for depression, have expanded the scientific understanding of the lateralization and specialization of brain regions for understanding individually based predispositions for psychopathology. Empirical work by Davidson and his colleagues has associated EEG asymmetries with: (1) positive and negative emotional experiences (Tomarken *et al.*, 1990); (2) individual differences in risk for psychopathology (Davidson, 2004); and (3) potential mechanisms responsible for psychological well-being (Urry *et al.*, 2004).

In summary, individual differences theories attempt to elucidate risk and protective factors that contribute to adaptive versus maladaptive emotional processes. Using this theory to understand individual differences in empathic reactivity and neurophysiological correlates associated with changes in empathic processes across development will provide essential information to understand the nature of empathy in humans.

13.2 EEG activity – a method of measuring brain–behaviour relations

Multiple methods have been used to study brain functioning, among them the patterns of electrical activity recorded by an electroencephalogram (EEG). The electrical activity present at the scalp that is measured by the EEG represents the fluctuation of excitatory and inhibitory postsynaptic potentials across time. During the last 75 years, much progress has been made in understanding the genesis and dynamics of the human EEG (Fox *et al.*, 2000). Neuropsychological reports suggest that cortical pyramidal neurones are responsible for the electrical activity recorded from the surface of the scalp (Thatcher & John, 1977).

In addition, recent reports suggest that the activity of cortical pyramidal neurones could be regulated, in part, by subcortical inputs including the limbic circuits that may indirectly generate electrical activity at the scalp (Davidson, 2004). Thus the electrical activity recorded by the EEG reflects the extracellular potentials of nearby cortical neurones, whose activity is modulated by a wide range of cortical and subcortical inputs. As such, mental states including cognitive processing, affective states and arousal levels will alter the activity and synchronization of underlying cortical neuronal networks, resulting in electrical potentials with distinct characteristics.

Several different measurement properties of the EEG have been viewed as useful for investigating brain and behaviour relations, among them are: (1) the frequency components, (2) the power spectra at different points in development and (3) the specialization of different hemispheres within various regions of the brain (also referred to as EEG asymmetry or hemispheric lateralization). The frequency composition of scalp electrical activity remains the most widely studied component of the EEG signal. Even though the frequency range for the human EEG ranges from very low to very high frequencies, the vast majority of research conducted on EEG and emotions, however, has focused exclusively on activity within the alpha frequency band (traditionally defined at 8–13 hertz in adults). Alpha activity is mostly sinusoidal in form and can be recorded over widespread scalp regions and it shows a linear increase in amplitude from anterior to posterior regions (Nunez *et al.*, 2001). Alpha activity is reciprocally associated with cortical activation inasmuch as amplitude and synchronized rhythmic frequencies in the alpha band activity are attenuated during mental activity (Nunez *et al.*, 2001).

During development dynamic changes in the brain (i.e. synaptogenesis, mylenation of the axons, and hemispheric integration across the corpus collosum) present simultaneously challenging and intriguing problems. Both measurement issues and functionality questions arise. Increases in EEG power, magnitude and peak frequency signal maturation of the brain, making the spectral properties of the human EEG important measures of development. However, the spectral properties differ within specific regions of the cortex across development. Studies have reported a shift downward in the spectral properties of the EEG during infancy and childhood, suggesting that it would not be meaningful to use the adult frequency band definitions to study infant and child EEG patterns (Pivik *et al.*, 1993). During the first year of life the majority of EEG activity occurs within the 3- to 12-Hz frequency band (Jones *et al.*, 1998) showing a peak of 6–9 Hz at around six months of age (Bell, 1998; Bell & Fox, 1994). Using a wider frequency band that encompasses all frequencies in which there is a substantial amount of power (i.e. 3–12 Hz) or using a narrow frequency band centred around the peaks in the spectrum (i.e. 6–9 Hz) (Pivik *et al.*, 1993) is still being debated. In addition, the functional abilities of the different regions of the cortex during infancy and childhood have been under question. Specifically, the frontal lobes have been ignored by some researchers, as they have a more protracted course. However, neuroimaging and neurophysiological studies (Chugani, 1994; Fox *et al.*, 2000) have shown that the frontal cortex is not inactive during development and may in fact provide the more intriguing functional information during the process of maturation. Studies have demonstrated important associations between emotions and frontal EEG activity in infant participants (Jones *et al.*, 1997, 1998).

With increasing intercommunication between hemispheres (Fox *et al.*, 1994), computation of EEG asymmetry values have also been utilized extensively in adult and developmental research paradigms. EEG asymmetries are comparisons between relative power scores within the left compared to the right (or the right compared to the left) hemispheres. These measures of the relative power in the brain's electrical activity have been associated empirically with several processes including the current emotional processing of various states (Tomarken *et al.*, 1990), the regulation and modulation of emotion (Fox *et al.*, 1994) and/or the predisposition for certain traits, personal styles and potentially for psychopathology (Davidson, 2004; Jones *et al.*, 1998, 2000).

In summary, the electrical activity of the brain can be measured by an EEG, a measurement of cortical pyramidal neurones influenced by cortical and subcortical inputs. During development the spectral properties of the EEG change yet these properties and their relation to affective processes have provided information important to the understanding of the neural basis of temperament and potential risk for psychopathology. Compared to other measures of neural–behaviour investigations, the advantage of measuring EEG activity is its superior temporal resolution, making it ideal for studying rapidly changing physiological processes such as empathy and for studying the development of emotions including empathy. The primary disadvantage is its poor spatial resolution, a problem that can be remedied by studying measures of EEG activation in corroboration with other measures of neural functioning that have good spatial resolution such as PET scans and fMRI (Davidson, 2004).

13.3 Overview of associations between brain regions and empathy

Multiple systems in the subcortical and cortical regions of the brain control nearly all types of human behaviours including the emotional and representational processes associated with empathy. In this section the neural circuitry implicated in empathic processes will be reviewed. In order to understand the neurophysiology of empathy, it is necessary to grasp the complexity and interdependence of the multiple structures and hierarchies of the neural systems involved. It is equally important to comprehend the interdependence of the motivational and emotional processes initiated and maintained during the experience of empathy. This includes understanding the subprocesses involved in empathy, such as perception, bodily sensations, attention, memories, motor programs, as well as the mental representations of the self, others and the social environment. Although a number of subcortical regions are involved in these processes at a microanalytic level (e.g. the cerebellum's role in attention shifts and the hypothalamus' role in maintaining homeostasis) the focus of this section will be on the higher neural systems implicated during the processing of empathy. From a physiological perspective, the processes of empathy include: (1) the limbic circuitry (subcortical areas with elaborate interconnections to the cortical region); (2) the temporal cortex (implicated in processing emotional memories); (3) the frontal cortex (especially the hemispheric specialization of the prefrontal cortex which has been identified as a source for the regulation of emotions); and (4) the autonomic nervous system (a system that activates the action sequence for the response).

13.3.1 The limbic circuitry

While some have argued that delineation of the structures within the 'limbic system' is arbitrary (LeDoux, 1996), studies of the limbic circuit's role in emotion-related processes have continued. Neuroscientists conceptualize the limbic circuitry as an interacting network of structures (Trevarthen & Aitken, 1994). Major connections of limbic circuits include the prefrontal and sensory association cortexes that connect with the cingulate cortex, the hippocampal formation and the amygdala, with these last two structures connecting to different regions of the hypothalamus, which in turn connect to the cingulate cortex through the anterior thalamus (Kandel *et al.*, 2000).

Although much is known about the anatomy of the limbic structures and the pathways that connect them to each other and to other parts of the brain, exactly how they function in emotion and empathy is still largely conjecture. How are structures in this system implicated in emotional and empathic processes? The answer to this question depends on the type of process within empathy that is being assessed. For example, the amygdala responds fast (as in emotions such as fear) and has ascending projections to the cortex. Researchers have suggested that this pathway may allow the amygdala to modulate and/or regulate the cognitive processes transferred to the cortex (LeDoux, 1996). Thus during emotional processes such as empathy, the amygdala may function by helping to associate external information (e.g. another person's emotion) with internal representations (e.g. one's own episodic memories of that emotion) and the associations that include incentive for rewards to motivate helping or alternatively punishments that inhibit helping. In other words, the amygdala-to-temporal-to-frontal cortex connection may function to assist in memory consolidation or matching memories of moods to current emotional states, via the hippocampus and temporal lobe, and then regulating emotional content during empathy-eliciting situations via the prefrontal cortex. Moreover, Panksepp (2000) has proposed that the anterior thalamic to cingulate system, including the septal areas and the hypothalamus, is involved in attachment and affiliative behaviours. Another structure in the limbic system that plays a significant role is the sensory association cortex, an area that is thought to integrate sensations in the self and those involved when observing another's emotional state. Additionally, the limbic circuit has numerous projections to the cingulate and frontal cortexes, areas that are implicated in the perception and regulation of emotions. In sum, while the limbic circuitry plays an important role sensing, perceiving and relaying empathy-based information, the control and regulation of empathy are accomplished by the interaction of limbic circuits with higher cortical areas.

13.3.2 The temporal lobes

The position of the temporal lobe in relation to the prefrontal lobes (especially the dorsolateral and ortibal areas) and the limbic system makes it an essential cortical structure for empathy, as the temporal lobe is below the Sylvian fissure and directly anterior to the parietal and occipital lobes. Further, the subcortical temporal structures include the limbic circuitry, the amygdala and the hippocampal formation.

The temporal lobe is involved in multimodal matching of sensory information, facial expressions (primarily the right temporal lobe), memories (primarily the left temporal lobe), content evaluation of sensory stimuli and spatial navigation, all of which are important processes related to empathy (Kandel *et al.*, 2000). Emotion requires perception of the stimulus with subsequent communication to areas of the brain that are responsible for the production of emotions; empathy requires an additional component of imitating the production of the emotional event. In a model proposed by Iacoboni and Lenzi (2002), the temporal region functions in an essential way to relay and coordinate the frontal to parietal lobes and the associated limbic circuitry to produce the experience empathy. Specifically their model focuses on the insular to frontal connections, which are believed to be the circuitry involved in communication of the feeling tone in empathy. Using fMRI, Iacoboni and Lenzi (2002) have provided some support for their model in human imitation studies of facial expression; however, active imitation did not show any more insular activity than passive viewing of facial displays while the insular to frontal connections demonstrated more fMRI activity during imitation, suggesting that frontal lobe involvement may be more important for processing empathy.

13.3.3 The frontal lobes

The frontal region of the brain includes: (1) the motor cortex, which is responsible for movements; (2) the premotor cortex, which is responsible for selecting movements (including planning, sequencing and preparations for executing motor actions); and (3) the prefrontal cortex, which is responsible for the integration of cognitive and emotional processes inasmuch as appropriate movements are selected for specific environmental contexts (Kandel *et al.*, 2000). While the prefrontal cortex is functionally heterogeneous, much of this area has been shown to be fundamentally related to processes that are necessary for emotional and empathic responses. Three sectors of the prefrontal cortex implicated in empathic processes are the dorsolateral, ventromedial and orbital areas. The dorsolateral region is believed to maintain, manipulate and select working memories (Bell, 1998; Davidson, 2004), in as much as the memories deemed important are maintained within the mind and alternative responses are considered, a process in which other sensory, limbic and motor areas are activated to guide behaviour (Davidson, 2004). In addition, evidence suggests that the dorsolateral sector of the prefrontal cortex is mainly involved in representational processes while the ventromedial area maintains memories and combines both short- and long-term goals into a behavioural response. Further, associations between ventromedial prefrontal cortex asymmetries and behavioural responses may include the ability to inhibit a response in order to obtain a selected goal (Tranel *et al.*, 2002). For example, response inhibition would be important for empathy, as the emotion must be felt for another to maintain the relationship (the goal) whereas if the emotion is felt directly for oneself then it does nothing for the relationship with another. Finally, the orbital areas, both frontal and lateral, are thought to be involved in assigning affective significance to contexts or events (Hornak *et al.*, 2003).

That the two hemispheres of the frontal region of the brain may have unique and increasing involvement in the processing of emotions associated with empathy has only begun to be investigated empirically (Davidson, 2004; Fox *et al.*, 1994). As the brain becomes more integrated across development both regions appear to play a role in emotional processes. Further each hemisphere has been shown to have a specialized role. As reviewed previously, the left frontal region has been shown to be specialized for the processing of positive, approach-related emotions whereas the right frontal region processes negative, withdrawal-related emotions (Davidson, 2004; Fox, 1991). This would imply that both hemispheres are involved at different stages in the processing of empathy; however, it suggests that the left hemisphere regulates the experience of empathy, as empathy is an approach-related response (Jones *et al.*, 2000). Much more work on these specializations of the two hemispheres needs to be accomplished before definitive conclusions can be drawn. Moreover, the relationship between hemispheric specializations and the development of emotions in general needs further support and delineation.

13.3.4 The autonomic nervous system

Finally, previous studies have demonstrated that there are important autonomic nervous system (ANS) correlates of empathy (Zahn-Waxler *et al.*, 1995), correlates that are integrated with cortical functioning (Fox, 1991; Porges, 2003). Much of the workings of the brain are through its control of the bodily systems, making the study of ANS processes central to the study of empathy. From a physiological perspective, the ANS includes the sympathetic and parasympathetic branches, each working together but performing antagonistic functions. Simply stated, the sympathetic system activates the bodily energies and the parasympathetic system conserves energy and resources. Thus one could argue that the ANS implements the intensity of the emotional response through its control of bodily processes.

During the process of empathy, the sympathetic system is believed to be associated with the initial response of alert to another's distress while the parasympathetic system enables the observer to regulate their own emotional arousal to facilitate helping and prosocial behaviours. Although scientists have recognized the ultimate control of the neural circuits, the preponderance of developmental studies, to date, have been on the relationship between autonomic measures and empathic responses (Zahn-Waxler *et al.*, 1995).

13.4 Empirical studies of the neurophysiological substrates of empathy

13.4.1 In development

While there is a plethora of empirical evidence that supports the anterior region's involvement in adult cognitive abilities, moods and emotional disorders

(Davidson, 2004), relatively fewer studies have investigated the child's developing empathic skills and the associated higher cortical functioning. Part of the reason is simply that brain processes during development are not well understood and are challenging to measure. For instance, EEG interpretation guidelines used in adults are not applicable to children and hemispheric specialization in emotional reactivity has only recently been uncovered (Fox *et al.*, 2000; Pivik *et al.*, 1993). Additionally, the right and left hemispheres of the frontal lobes appear to mature at different rates. Further the left frontal region, the region most implicated in empathy, shows a slow and multifaceted developmental course (Bell, 1998; Bell & Fox, 1994; Chugani, 1994). In short, while brain function in children appears to be different than brain function in adults, little is known about the meaning of those differences. Are certain parts of children's brains underdeveloped or do they simply function in a qualitatively different way at this age? That question remains unanswered; however, developmental neurophysiological studies are the most promising area of investigation for uncovering risk and protective factors during the development of social emotions.

While this area of research is still relatively new, a number of associations between physiology and empathy have nonetheless been investigated. Three very diverse and sometimes disparate lines of research have implicated the cortex, specifically the frontal region, in the development of empathy. These three theoretical approaches are reviewed below.

13.4.2 Biobehavioural preparedness

Several researchers have posited the theory that humans are born with, to varying degrees, a biological preparedness for social interaction (Brothers, 1989; Hoffman, 2000; Trevarthen & Aitken, 1994). Studies designed to investigate this ability have shown that newborn facial expressions can be reliably measured and are accompanied by a physiological and measurable response (Field, 1989). This has been interpreted to indicate an innate capacity for responding emotionally to social information from others. That infants model fear, distress, disgust and surprise, and attend to happiness, sadness and surprise underscores the importance of the communication of emotions (Field, 1989).

Notably, early studies of newborn facial expressivity merely argued that newborns reflexively copied faces that were observed, suggesting that newborns neither felt the emotion nor did they have their own characteristic style of responding. Most developmental scientists, today, believe differently, as current studies have linked the production of facial displays with simultaneous changes in autonomic and neural processes, which is an indicator of individual differences in response styles (Field, 1989). For example, studies by Field and her colleagues (Field, 1989) have demonstrated that those newborns with high emotional expressivity exhibited low heart rate variability and low heart period (higher heart rate) whereas those with low emotional expressivity exhibited high heart rate variability and high heart period (lower heart rate). Additionally, we (Jones *et al.*, 1997) demonstrated that right frontal EEG asymmetry was related to more distress expressions in infants. Further, individual differences in emotional reactivity and physiological regulation were present from birth, with infants of depressed mothers showing less emotional responsiveness at birth, greater physiological dysregulation and less empathy later in childhood (Jones *et al.*, 1998, 2000).

Research has also shown that newborns respond with distinct behavioural patterns to the distress of another (Dondi *et al.*, 1999; Hoffman, 2000). For example, Dondi and his colleagues (1999) showed that newborns cry to the distress sounds of another infant yet they do not cry while listening to their own cries. Findings like these have led researchers to propose an evolutionary basis for empathy (Hoffman, 2000). Detecting an emotion in a peer, and the autonomic and neurophysiological responses that seem to mimic the physiology of the distressed object are speculated to signal a biological preparedness for emotions and ultimately a physiological substrate for empathy.

13.4.3 Heritability

Some investigators have demonstrated a potential genetic basis for empathy (Hoffman, 2000). For example, Zahn-Waxler *et al.* (1992) found modest evidence for heritability of empathy and prosocial behaviours in 14- to 20-month-old monozygotic and dizygotic twins.

Further, empathic reasoning was associated with fewer behavioural problems in twin studies, suggesting a possible genetic basis for risk and resilience for psychopathology (Zahn-Waxler *et al.*, 1996). Ultimately, these findings have been used to suggest that empathy has genetic influences as well as environmental ones (due to the modest heritability factor) during normal and problematic development.

13.4.4 Individual contributions and temperament

Autonomic and neural functioning have been linked to the development of empathy, thus it is highly plausible that individual differences in neural system function support or inhibit its development (Jones *et al.*, 1998, 2000). As we will see more in depth in the next section, coordinated activity between a caregiver and an infant is required for adaptive regulation of emotions, a process that leads to empathic competence across the lifespan. As with any relationship, both individuals bring their unique temperament and biological inclinations to the equation. Thus individual contributions can set the tone for future interactions in that relationship.

One method of evaluating individual differences in social interactions and response styles to social events is with the use of autonomic nervous system measures, which have been associated with neurological development and empathy. Moreover, developmental studies have shown consistent patterns of heart rate responding related to empathic behaviours. In a number of studies (Zahn-Waxler *et al.*, 1995), a link between heart rate deceleration and empathy has been supported. The data suggest that heart rate deceleration may be an index of other-oriented attention and thus an index of empathy, whereas heart rate acceleration may be an index of self-oriented attention and thus an index of anxiety or fear. For instance, Zahn-Waxler and her colleagues (1995) tested children at risk for externalizing problems and determined that heart rate deceleration during an empathy-inducing stimulus (and higher heart rate at baseline) predicted empathic concern and prosocial behaviours. In addition, lower tonic heart rate (i.e. baseline) was associated with aggression and avoidance, behaviours that inhibit empathic responding.

Although studies have established a link between individual differences in hemispheric specialization and emotional responsiveness (Davidson, 2004; Fox, 1991), in only a few studies have we examined the relationship between empathy and brain electrical activity patterns in: (1) children of depressed mothers compared to psychologically healthy controls and (2) children who were prenatally exposed to cocaine compared to an unexposed, demographically matched control group (Jones *et al.*, 1998, 2000). Across several studies, our findings suggest that greater relative right frontal asymmetry and lack of empathic behaviours are present in children of depressed mothers and children prenatally exposed to cocaine, with both groups showing greater right and left hemispheric activity (with the right hemisphere activity more pronounced) in the frontal region. Right frontal asymmetry has been implicated in negative moods and inhibited temperament, suggesting individual differences in biobehavioural risk factors for these children. Lack of empathy was associated with maternal-reported anxiety, conduct problems, hyperactivity and impulsive behaviours in children of depressed mothers and in children who were cocaine-exposed during gestation. These later findings, although based on a potentially biased maternal report, could affect caregiver–child interactions across development and could have an effect on the development of neural processes. Although inconclusive, these data should be used to provide a spring board for further studies on the development of empathy, cognitive abilities, social skillfulness, and neurophysiological changes, as these areas are most influenced by neural plasticity during development.

13.4.5 In adults

Studies examining the neurophysiology of empathy in healthy adults are scarce, as most studies focus on understanding simple emotions or emotion-linked traits in adults (Davidson, 2004; Tomarken *et al.*, 1990). Nonetheless, the research in existence, to date, indicates that empathy may be a personality trait that has a neurophysiological basis. For example, Levenson and Ruef (1992) examined the physiological responses of adults watching a marital interaction and found that perceptions of another's emotions were most accurate when the observer matched the object's physiological state for negative emotions. For positive emotions, accuracy was correlated to lower cardiovascular arousal in the observer. This finding lends some support to the theories of 'mirror neurones' through which individual's matched physiology supports the ability to subjectively represent what another is feeling (Gallese, 2003). These theories are intriguing, albeit in need of further elucidation with empirical evidence.

Neurophysiological studies of emotions suggest that positive, approach-oriented emotions and individual differences in personality traits are related to neurophysiological activity in consistent ways (Tomarken et al., 1990). Specifically approach-related emotions and tendencies are associated with the left frontal regions of the brain. Recently, studies (Urry et al., 2004) have even demonstrated that eudemonic emotions (i.e. those emotions related to feelings of well-being stemming from an orientation toward inner happiness and life-purpose) are associated with left frontal EEG asymmetry. Similarly other studies have suggested that depressive symptoms are associated with right frontal EEG asymmetry due to left frontal hypoactivation.

In summary, human infant, child and adult studies have associated the neuro-physiological activation of brain areas with emotions, yet these associations with empathy are an understudied area of research. Only a handful of studies have suggested that empathy may be a process carried out by the left frontal regions of the brain. Understanding the progression of empathy in the brain would inform both scientific and clinical endeavours. Thus, future research should investigate these issues more fully, especially during the stages of plasticity in development.

13.5 Dysfunctional socialization experiences and changes in brain activation and empathic responding

It is now well established in the literature that personality traits are most often the result of the interplay between genetic endowment and developmental milieu. Cerebral functioning has a much greater impact on adaptive socioemotional functioning than previously thought and, conversely, the socioemotional environment has a determinative effect on the development and proper functioning of the human brain. In other words, sequential, normal neurodevelopment is dependent on the environmental conditions and circumstances of each child (Glaser, 2000) particularly in utero and during the formative first few years of life.

During the first few years of life, the infant's neural network is more malleable than at any other time during the lifespan (Bell, 1998). Accordingly, this critical period of brain development provides tremendous opportunity for the development of adaptive functions while at the same time making the infant enormously vulnerable to the impact of environments that either inhibit growth or fail to provide the input needed for optimal growth. The frontal lobes' period of plasticity specifically extends into the second year of life (Fox *et al.*, 1994). Thus, if appropriate environmental input is not provided, or, if inappropriate stimuli are introduced in early childhood, executive functions under frontal lobe control, such as emotion regulation and empathy, will miss their opportunity for normal development, leaving the growing child with a functional deficit that will not easily be ameliorated later.

There are two general ways in which environment affects brain development. Some growth is experience-expectant, meaning that pre-programmed neuro-developmental sequences are triggered by experiences that are reasonably expected to happen during the course of normal development. Other processes of brain development are referred to as experience-dependent, in that neural structures are not necessarily anticipating certain experiences, but are highly receptive to them (Greenough & Black, 1992). Unlike experience-expectant development, which sets off genetically predetermined synaptic growth, experience-dependent development provides the opportunity for creation of new synaptic connections as a response and consequence of environmentally based experiences (Bell & Fox, 1994; Glaser, 2000). The maturation of the orbito-frontal system is primarily experience-dependent, with empathic ability developing only if it is adaptive within the context of the young child's limited environment, which often consists primarily of the attachment figures. The absence of appropriate learning experiences can lead to changes in the functional organization of the brain; synaptic connections will form (or fail to form) in accordance with the information the child receives from his/her environment (Bell & Fox, 1994). The neural pathways that remain, for better or for worse, will become the foundation of the child's emotional capabilities (Courchesne *et al.*, 1994).

Responsive, affectionate caregiving facilitates bonding and attachment, and it is within that context that the infant's brain develops the capacity for more elaborated emotional regulation and empathic social interactions. The sight of a responsive mother's face triggers the release of high levels of endogenous opiates in the child (Hofer, 1994), thus forming an association between social reciprocity and pleasure. Furthermore, an attuned mother–child dyad will develop an emotional transaction 'rhythm' (Jaffe *et al.*, 2001) that fosters the growth of neural pathways for emotion regulation in the child (Fox *et al.*, 1994).

Human offspring are instinctively drawn to their social environment and to their caregivers to reduce emotional discomfort and to be restored to a more balanced state. Then, based on the caregiver's pattern of responses, the child develops a working model of the world. Stated differently, not only does the attuned, attentive caregiver provide the child with the building blocks of affect regulation, but also teaches the child that he/she can expect affectionate treatment from others. Attuned mother–infant dyads are engaged in a dance, a form of non-verbal rhythmic communication in which each partner both affects and reflects the emotional state of the other (Fogel & Bramco, 1997). During this physiological and behavioural dance, the partners synchronize and mirror each other's psychophysiology and amplify each other's positive affective states creating a synergistic effect. It is within these types of interactions that the capacity for empathy develops.

As such, a caregiving relationship that is characterized by abuse or neglect impedes the development of empathy (Glaser, 2000). Harmful or neglectful caregiving leads to an alteration of the neural system, hence a disruption of proper emotion-processing functions (Schore, 1996) that perpetuates into adulthood (Glaser, 2000). Studies have revealed left fronto-temporal EEG abnormalities in paediatric psychiatric inpatients (Ito et al., 1998) and limbic system dysfunctions in adult psychiatric outpatients with histories of abuse (Teicher et al., 1993).

In the context of abuse, empathy is not adaptive so the abused child develops only a limited capacity for it. Caregiving by an abusive mother encourages a dissociative response in the child (Schore, 1996). The unregulated affect of the mother (in addition to the infant's own unregulated affect) overwhelms the child's capacity to cope, and the infant defensively disconnects from interaction. In the case of a non-attentive mother, the child disconnects from the interaction to reciprocate the mother's state. For instance in laboratory experiments, children of depressed mothers, which often translates into emotional deprivation or insensitive-intrusive caregiving, responded less empathically than normal controls (Jones et al., 1997, 2000).

Animal studies shed additional light on the effects of early maternal deprivation on brain development. In experiments, animal infants deprived of normal maternal interaction have stress reactions resulting in cerebral cell death (Plotsky & Meaney, 1993). In humans, stress enhances the release of dopamine in the prefrontal cortex, which, along with noradrenaline (Charney et al., 1993) and elevated cortisol levels (Gunnar, 1998), is associated with dysfunction of the frontal regions of the brain (Arnsten, 1999). In fact, our own studies have shown that maternal biochemical stress levels can negatively affect the growth and psychobiological development of neonates (Lundy et al., 1999).

In sum, early environmental experiences have lasting socioemotional consequences and may alter an individual's developmental path altogether. While
neuropsychobiological studies on traumatized infants and young children are
scarce (with no psychophysiological studies on this topic that we know of), and
may not yet account for individual variation in adaptation among abused and
neglected children, the totality of the evidence thus far points us in the direction
that early socialization is critical to the development of empathy and much of this
process involves shared and changed physiology.

13.6 Frontal lobe dysfunction and consequences for empathic responding

Thus far, research on the physiology of emotions leads us to conclude that
empathy is mostly a function of the fronto-orbital cortexes and the limbic system.
It follows then, that disruption of frontal lobe functioning would impair an
individual's ability to be socially adaptive. Indeed, the literature supports that
assumption. In this section, we will examine how dysfunction in the frontal lobes,
whether from developmental abnormality, traumatic injury, or disease, can result
in lack of empathic abilities and psychopathology.

A handful of DSM-IV (American Psychiatric Association, 1994) disorders are
characterized by empathy deficits. In children, they include autism spectrum
disorders (autistic disorder, Asperger's disorder, and other pervasive developmental disorders) and disruptive behaviour disorders (attention deficit-hyperactivity
disorder, conduct disorder and oppositional defiant disorder). In adults, these
include antisocial personality disorder, borderline personality disorder, schizophrenia and factitious disorder by proxy (Appendix B: Criteria Sets and Axes for
Further Study). This last disorder however is controversial and both its aetiology
and neurophysiological correlates are in need of further scientific inquiry.

The disorder most often linked by the literature to frontal lobe dysfunction is
antisocial personality disorder (ASPD) (Damasio et al., 1990). A number of studies
have evaluated post-morbid behaviour in individuals who sustained damage to the
frontal lobes from traumatic injury and/or brain disease (Grattan & Eslinger, 1989;
Shamay-Tsoory et al., 2003). Collectively, these studies have found that previously
high functioning, sociable individuals now exhibited enough psychosocial mal-
adaption to meet diagnosis criteria for ASPD. Physiologically, these individuals
exhibited hypoactivation of somatic states, as indicated by attenuated skin conductance responses when presented with socially meaningful, empathy-inducing
stimuli (Damasio et al., 1990).

In addition to ASPD, frontal lobe dysfunction may play a role in the development of borderline personality disorder (BPD). In support of this hypothesis,
Völlm and his colleagues (2004) found that both ASPD and BPD patients activated

more widespread prefrontal and temporal areas than healthy controls in a response inhibition task. This result can be interpreted as indicating that ASPD and BPD patients need to recruit additional resources to compensate for frontal lobe dysfunction. This interpretation is consistent with Raine's (Raine *et al.*, 2000) finding that individuals with ASPD have 11% less prefrontal grey matter than healthy controls, and with other findings that individuals with BPD have smaller frontal lobe volumes (Lyoo *et al.*, 1998).

Similarly, with childhood disorders, specifically with autistic disorder 'often an individual's awareness of others is markedly impaired. Individuals with this disorder may be oblivious to other children [...], may have no concept of the needs of others, or may not notice another person's distress' (DSM-IV, p. 66). This latter feature describes the observed lack of empathy in autistic children. In fact, Blair (1999) found that when children with autism are encouraged to focus their attention on another person's distress they simultaneously exhibit greater skin conductance responses. Yet, despite this autonomic arousal, they fail to respond behaviourally. A likely explanation is that individuals with autism have difficulty with the cognitive appraisal of what they are witnessing, fail to understand its social meaning, and thus fail to respond behaviourally. Researchers have speculated that the cerebello-frontal pathway may be involved in autism (Dawson, 1996). It is likely that a disruption in frontal lobe functioning accounts for the observed empathy deficits in this disorder.

Research on frontal lobe involvement in empathy deficits of children with disruptive behaviour disorders, on the other hand, is much more inconclusive, and even sometimes contradictory. For instance, while PET studies found reduced metabolism in frontal regions of ADHD children (Amen & Carmichael, 1997), other studies found no clear differences between ADHD and control children in heart rate and skin conductance (Zahn-Waxler *et al.*, 1995).

In summary, while frontal lobe dysfunction appears to play a critical role in the development of certain psychopathologies, much of the evidence is inconclusive and in need of both replication and novel research designs. Additionally, it may be useful, as we move forward with the exploration of disorders associated with empathy deficits, to distinguish between those that also involve malevolence, such as psychopathy, and those that are of a more benign (although important) quality, such as autism. While they may both have neurophysiological substrates in common, they are indeed qualitatively different. At this point in time, however, the exact neurophysiology of any empathy deficits remains a mystery. Nonetheless, the technological advances in brain mapping and the re-emergence of data and research interest in the phenomenon of empathy are promising.

13.7 Summary

Empathy is a necessary component of positive human social relationships, which, in turn, undergird mental health. As methods of scientific inquiry improve and technology provides us with increasingly useful tools, our knowledge and understanding of human social emotions expand. Evolving understanding of the neurophysiological systems has supported the association between frontal lobe functioning and empathy. Specifically frontal areas have been shown to have a prominent role in influencing empathic responding. Additionally, multiple areas of the brain are involved in empathy at different levels of processing, including limbic and temporal, as well as autonomic nervous system functions. The plasticity of the human brain, particularly the frontal lobes, in the early years of life provides if not a blank slate, an easily modifiable slate for environment to write on. Thus, an individual's experiences within their environment provide the conditions for neural predispositions to express themselves. During this sensitive period, the growing child's world consists almost entirely of the primary caregiver. This relationship teaches the child about human social interaction (via maternal behaviour) and self-regulation of emotional arousal (via psychobiological attunement). Healthy early relationships are essential to optimal neural development, which in turn is critical for the development of empathy. In sum, it appears that empathy involves multiple brain regions and that individual variation in environmental experiences can modify neurophysiology, resulting potentially in deficits in empathic processes.

Dysfunctions in the fronto-orbital cortex and the limbic system are believed to reduce the individual's capacity for empathic responding and can lead to social impairment and psychopathology. Individuals with psychological and neurological disorders that are characterized by empathy deficits have neuroimaging patterns and physiological responses that differ from those of healthy individuals. While research on frontal lobe functioning in the context of empathic abilities is still in its infancy, the findings to date suggest this will likely be a fruitful avenue for expanding our knowledge of the neurophysiological substrates of empathy.

REFERENCES

Amen, D., & Carmichael, B. (1997). High-resolution brain SPECT imaging in ADHD. *Annals of Clinical Psychiatry*, **9**, 81–86.

American Psychiatric Association. (1994). *Diagnostic and Statistical Manual of Mental Disorders* (4th edn.). Washington, DC: American Psychiatric Association Press.

Arnsten, A. (1999). Development of the cerebral cortex: XIV. Stress impairs prefrontal cortical function. *Journal of the American Academy of Child and Adolescent Psychiatry*, **38**, 220–222.

Bell, M. A. (1998). The ontogeny of the EEG during infancy and childhood: implications for cognitive development. In B. Garreau (ed.), *Neuroimaging in Child Neuropsychiatric Disorders* (pp. 97–111). Berlin: Springer-Verlag.

Bell, M. A., & Fox, N. A. (1994). Brain development over the first year of life: relations between electroencephalographic frequency and coherence and cognitive and affective behaviors. In G. Dawson, & K. W. Fischer (eds.), *Human Behavior and the Developing Brain* (pp. 314–345). New York: Guilford Press.

Blair, R. J. (1999). Psychophysiological responsiveness to the distress of others in children with autism. *Personality and Individual Differences*, **26**, 477–485.

Brothers, L. (1989). A biological perspective on empathy. *American Journal of Psychiatry*, **146**, 10–19.

Cannon, W. B. (1927). The James–Lange theory of emotion: a critical examination and an alternative theory. *American Journal of Psychology*, **39**, 106–124.

Carver, C. S. (2001). Affect and the functional bases of behavior: on the dimensional structure of affective experience. *Personality and Social Psychology Review*, **5**, 345–356.

Charney, D., Deutch, A., Krystal, J., Southwick, S., & Davis, M. (1993). Psychobiological mechanisms of post traumatic stress disorder. *Archives of General Psychiatry*, **50**, 294–305.

Chugani, H. T. (1994). Development of regional brain glucose metabolism in relation to behavior and plasticity. In G. Dawson, & K. W. Fischer (eds.), *Human Behavior and the Developing Brain* (pp. 153–175.). New York: Guilford Press.

Courchesne, E., Chisum, H., & Townsend, J. (1994). Neural activity-dependent brain changes in development: implications for psychopathology. *Development and Psychopathology*, **6**, 697–722.

Damasio, A. R. (2000). A second chance for emotion. In R. D. Lane, & L. Nadel (eds.), *Cognitive Neurosciences of Emotion* (pp. 12–23). New York: Oxford University Press.

Damasio, A. R., Tranel, D., & Damasio, H. (1990). Individuals with sociopathic behavior caused by frontal damage fail to respond autonomically to social stimuli. *Behavioural Brain Research*, **41**(2), 81–94.

Darwin, C. (1872). *The Expression of the Emotions in Man and Animals*. Oxford: Oxford University Press.

Davidson, R. J. (2004). What does the prefrontal cortex 'do' in affect: perspectives on frontal EEG asymmetry research. *Biological Psychology*, **67**, 219–233.

Dawson, G. (1996). Brief report: neuropsychology of autism: a report on the state of the science. *Journal of Autism and Developmental Disorders*, **26**, 179–184.

Dondi, M., Simion, F., & Caltran, G. (1999). Can newborns discriminate between their own cry and the cry of another newborn infant? *Developmental Psychology*, **35**, 418–426.

Doussard-Roosevelt, J. A., McClenny, B. D., & Porges, S. W. (2001). Neonatal cardiac vagal tone and school-age developmental outcome in very low birth weight infants. *Developmental Psychobiology*, **38**, 56–66.

Field, T. (1989). Individual and maturational differences in infant expressivity. In N. Eisenberg (ed.), *New Directions for Child Development* (Vol. 44). *Empathy and Related Emotional Responses* (pp. 9–24). San francisco: Jossey-Bass Inc.

Fogel, A., & Bramco, A. U. (1997). Metacommunication as a source of indeterminism in relationship development. In A. Fogel, M. Lyra, & J. Valsinger (eds.), *Dynamics and Indeterminism in Developmental and Social Processes* (pp. 65–92). Mahweh, N.J.: Erlbaum.

Fox, N. A. (1991). If it's not left, it's right. Electroencephalograph asymmetry and the development of emotion. *American Psychologist*, **46**, 863–872.

Fox, N. A., Calkins, S. D., & Bell, M. A. (1994). Neural plasticity and development in the first two years of life: evidence from cognitive and socioemotional domains of research. *Development and Psychopathology*, **6**, 677–696.

Fox, N. A., Schmidt, L. A., & Henderson, H. A. (2000). Developmental psychophysiology: conceptual and methodological perspectives. In J. T. Cacioppo, L. G. Tassinary, & G. G. Berntson (eds.), *Handbook of Psychophysiology*, 2nd edn. Cambridge: Cambridge University Press.

Freud, S., & Breuer, J. (1895). *Studies on Hysteria (The Pelican Freud Library)* (Vol. 3), J. Strachey, A. Strachey, & J. Richards (eds.). Harmondsworth: Penguin.

Gainotti, G. (1989). Disorders of emotions and affect in patients with unilateral brain damage. In R. Boller, & J. Grafman (eds.), *Handbook of Neuropsychology* (Vol. 3) (pp. 345–361). Amsterdam: Elsevier.

Gallese, V. (2003). The roots of empathy: the shared manifold hypothesis and the neural basis of intersubjectivity. *Psychopathology*, **36**, 171–180.

Glaser, D. (2000). Child abuse and neglect and the brain – a review. *Journal of Child Psychology and Psychiatry*, **41(1)**, 97–116.

Grattan, L. M., & Eslinger, P. J. (1989). Higher cognition and social behavior: changes in cognitive flexibility and empathy after cerebral lesions. *Neuropsychology*, **3**, 175–185.

Greenough, W., & Black, J. (1992). Induction of brain structure by experience: substrate for cognitive development. In M. Gunnar, & C. Nelson (eds.), *Minnesota Symposia of Child Psychology 24: Developmental Behavioral Neurosciences* (pp. 155–200). Hillsdale, N.J.: Lawrence Erlbaum.

Gunnar, M. (1998). Quality of early care and buffering of neuroendocrine stress reactions: potential effects on the developing brain. *Preventative Medicine*, **27**, 208–211.

Harlow, J. M. (1868). Recovery after severe injury to the head. *Publication of the Massachusetts Medical Society*, **2**, 327–346.

Hofer, M. (1994). Hidden regulators in attachment, separation, and loss. *Monographs for the Society for Research in Child Development*, **59**, 192–207.

Hoffman, M. L. (2000). *Empathy and Moral Development: Implications for Caring and Justice.* New York: Cambridge University Press.

Hornak, J., Bramham, J., Rolls, E. T., *et al.* (2003). Changes in emotion after circumscribed surgical lesions of the orbitofrontal and cingulated cortices. *Brain*, **126**, 1691–1712.

Iacoboni, M., & Lenzi, G. L. (2002). Mirror neurons, the insula and empathy. *Behavioral and Brain Sciences*, **25**, 39–40.

Ito, Y., Teicher, M., Glod, C., & Ackerman, E. (1998). Preliminary evidence for aberrant cortical development in abused children: a quantitative EEG study. *Journal of Neuropsychiatry and Clinical Neurosciences*, **10**, 298–307.

Jaffe, J., Beebe, B., Feldstein, S., Crown, C. L., & Jasnow, M. D. (2001). Rhythms of dialogue in infancy. *Monographs of the Society for Research in Child Development*, **66**(2, 265).

James, W. (1884). What is emotion? *Mind*, **9**, 188–205.

Jones, N. A., Field, T., & Davalos, M. (2000). Right frontal EEG asymmetry and lack of empathy in preschool children of depressed mothers. *Child Psychiatry Human Development*, **30**, 189–204.

Jones, N. A., Field, T., Davalos, M., & Pickens, J. (1997). EEG stability in infants/children of depressed mothers. *Child Psychiatry Human Development*, **28**, 59–70.

Jones, N. A., Field, T., Fox, N. A., *et al.* (1998). Newborns of mothers with depressive symptoms are physiologically less developed. *Infant Behavior and Development*, **21**, 537–541.

Jones, N. A., Field, T., Fox, N. A., Lundy, B., & Davalos, M. (1997). EEG activation in 1-month-old infants of depressed mothers. *Development and Psychopathology*, **9**, 491–505.

Kandel, E. R., Schwartz, J. H., & Jessel, T. M. (2000). *Principles of Neural Science*, 4th edn. Columbus, Ohio: McGraw Hill.

LeDoux, J. E. (1996). *The Emotional Brain: The Mysterious Underpinning of Emotional Life.* New York: Simon and Schuster.

Levenson, R. W., & Ruef, A. M. (1992). Empathy: a physiological substrate. *Journal of Personality and Social Psychology*, **63(2)**, 234–246.

Lundy, B. L., Jones, N. A., Field, T., *et al.* (1999). Prenatal depression effects on neonates. *Infant Behavior and Development*, **22**, 121–137.

Lyoo, I., Han, M., & Cho, D. (1998). A brain MRI study in subjects with borderline personality disorder. *Journal of Affective Disorders*, **50(2–3)**, 235–243.

Nunez, P. L., Wingeier, B. M., & Silberstein, R. B. (2001). Spatial–temporal structures of human alpha rhythms: theory, microcurrent sources, multiscale measurements, and global binding neural networks. *Human Brain Mapping*, **13**, 125–164.

Panksepp, J. (2000). Affective consciousness and the instinctual motor system. The neural sources of sadness and joy. In R. Ellis, & N. Newton (eds.), *The Caldron of Consciousness: Motivation, Affect and Self-Organization: Advances in Consciousness Research Series* (Vol. 16). Amsterdam: John Benjamins.

Pivik, R. T., Broughton, R. J., Coppola, R., *et al.* (1993). Guidelines for the recording and quantitative analysis of electroencephalographic activity in research contexts. *Psychophysiology*, **30**, 547–558.

Plotsky, P., & Meaney, M. (1993). Early, postnatal experience alters hypothalamic corticotropin-releasing factor (CRF) mRNA, median eminence CRF content and stress-induced release in adult rats. *Molecular Brain Research*, **18**, 195–200.

Porges, S. W. (2003). The polyvagal theory: phylogenetic contributions to social behavior. *Physiology and Behavior*, **79**, 503–513.

Raine, A., Lenez, T., Bihrle, S., LaCasse, L., & Colletti, P. (2000). Reduced prefrontal gray matter volume and reduced autonomic activity in antisocial personality disorder. *Archives of General Psychiatry*, **57**, 119–127.

Robinson, R. G., Kubos, K. L., Starr, L. B., Rao, K., & Price, T. R. (1984). Mood disorders in stroke patients: importance of location of lesion. *Brain*, **107**, 81–91.

Schore, A. N. (1996). The experience-dependent maturation of a regulatory system in the orbital prefrontal cortex and the original of developmental psychopathology. *Development and Psychopathology*, **8**, 59–87.

Shamay-Tsoory, S. G., Tomer, R., Berger, B. D., & Aharon-Peretz, J. (2003). Characterization of empathy deficits following prefrontal brain damage: the role of the right ventromedial prefrontal cortex. *Journal of Cognitive Neuroscience*, **15**(3), 324–337.

Teicher, M., Glod, C., Surrey, J., & Swett, C. (1993). Early childhood abuse and limbic system ratings in adult psychiatric outpatients. *Journal of Neuropsychiatry and Clinical Neurosciences*, **5**, 301–306.

Thatcher, R. W., & John, E. R. (1977). *Functional Neuroscience: I. Foundations of Cognitive Processes*. Oxford: Lawrence Erlbaum.

Tomarken, A. J., Davidson, R. J., & Henriques, J. B. (1990). Resting frontal brain asymmetry predicts affective responses to films. *Journal of Personality and Social Psychology*, **59**, 791–801.

Tranel, D., Bechara, A., & Denburg, N. I. (2002). Asymmetric functional roles of right and left ventromedial prefrontal cortices in social conduct, decision-making, and emotional processing. *Cortex*, **38**, 589–612.

Trevarthen, C., & Aitken, K. J. (1994). Brain development, infant communication, and empathy disorders: intrinsic factors in child mental health. *Development and Psychopathology*, **6**, 597–633.

Urry, H. L., Nitschke, J. B., Dolski, I., *et al.* (2004). Making a life worth living: neural correlates of well-being. *Psychological Science*, **15**, 367–372.

Völlm, B., Richardson, P., Stirling, J., *et al.* (2004). Neurobiological substrates of antisocial and borderline personality disorder: preliminary results of a functional fMRI study. *Criminal Behavior and Mental Health*, **14**, 39–54.

Young, S. K., Fox, N. A., & Zahn-Waxler, C. (1999). The relation between temperament and empathy in 2-year-olds. *Developmental Psychology*, **35**, 1189–1197.

Zahn-Waxler, C., Cole, P. M., Welsh, J. D., & Fox, N. A. (1995). Psychophysiological correlates of empathy and prosocial behaviors in preschool children with behavior problems. *Development and Psychopathology*, **7**, 27–48.

Zahn-Waxler, C., Robinson, J. L., & Emde, R. E. (1992). The development of empathy in twins. *Developmental Psychology*, **28**, 1038–1047.

Zahn-Waxler, C., Schmitz, S., Fulker, D., Robinson, J., & Emde, R. (1996). Behavioral problems in 5-year-old monozygotic and dizygotic twins: genetic and environmental influences, patterns of regulation, and internalization of control. *Development and Psychopathology*, **8**, 103–122.

The cognitive neuropsychology of empathy

Jean Decety[1], Philip L. Jackson[2] and Eric Brunet[3]

[1]Department of Psychology, University of Chicago
[2]Department of Psychology, University of Laval, Canada
[3]Institute for Learning and Brain Sciences, University of Washington

14.1 Introduction

Despite the plethora of definitions of empathy, most authors generally agree that it implies at least three different aspects: feeling what another person is feeling; knowing what another person is feeling; and having the intention to respond compassionately to another person's distress. Note that these aspects may be experienced independently from one another and constitute different levels of complexity ranging from empathic mimicry to sympathy. Moreover, regardless of the particular terminology used by different scholars, there is broad agreement that empathy involves three primary elements: (1) an affective response to another person, which often, but not always, entails sharing that person's emotional state; (2) a cognitive capacity to adopt the perspective of the other person; and (3) some monitoring and self-regulatory mechanisms that keep track of the origins of self and other feelings (e.g. Batson, 1991; Decety & Jackson, 2004; Ickes, 1997). The multidimensionality of the empathy construct makes it less amenable to traditional methods of study and investigation.

We propose in light of the current knowledge in neuropsychology and cognitive neuroscience a model of empathy that relies on four intertwined major functional components that dynamically interact to produce this intersubjective experience. The first component, affective sharing, is based on a perception-action coupling mechanism and resulting shared representations between self and other (Preston & de Waal, 2002). Self-other awareness constitutes the second component. Empathy requires that there is no confusion between self and other even though some temporary identification between the observer and its target may occur. The third component, mental flexibility, is essential if one is to adopt the subjective perspective of the other and set aside one's own current perspective. Finally, the last component, emotion regulation including emotion reappraisal, is necessary to

Empathy in Mental Illness, eds. Tom F. D. Farrow and Peter W. R. Woodruff. Published by Cambridge University Press. © Cambridge University Press 2007.

produce an appropriate response to the other, which necessitates some control over one's own affective state.

In our view, none of these components can solely account for the expression of human empathy. Rather, the four are intertwined and interact with one another to produce the subjective experience of empathy. For instance, sharing emotion without self-awareness and any form of regulation leads to emotional contagion, which takes the form of total identification without discrimination between one's feelings and those of the other. Furthermore, experiencing another person's pain or distress state in the same way as one's own experience would lead to 'empathic over-arousal', in which the focus then becomes one's own feelings of stress rather than the other's need.

Like many emotion-related processes, some components of empathy occur automatically, and sometimes without awareness. This is the case for instance of the affective sharing aspect. Other components require intentional processing, such as perspective-taking and some aspects of emotion regulation.

14.2 Affective sharing between self and other

Emotional expression and perception are an integral part of human interactions. At one level, emotional expressions are governed by rules and can be elicited by simple stimuli, as in the example of disgust in the presence of bitter taste. However, humans and other animals also use bodily expressions to communicate various types of information to members of their own species. Understanding other people's emotional signals has clear adaptive advantage and is especially important in the formation and maintenance of social relationships.

The mechanism that accounts for the automatic mapping between self and other is primarily based on perception-action cycles, which has been comprehensively described as the common coding theory (Prinz, 1997). This theory states that perception of an action activates one's own action representations to the degree that the perceived and the represented action are similar (Knoblich & Flach, 2003). Furthermore, when two individuals socially interact with one another, this overlap creates shared representations, i.e. neural networks that are temporarily and simultaneously activated in the brain of the two agents for the same action (Decety & Sommerville, 2003; Jeannerod, 1999). This sharing explains how we come to understand each other, that is the isomorphism between action representations allows the individual to implicitly know the goals of others with the use of her/his own action representation system.

In neuroscience, evidence for this perception-action coupling ranges from electrophysiological recordings in monkeys showing that mirror neurones in the ventral premotor cortex fire during both goal-directed actions and the observation of the same actions performed by another individual (Rizzolatti *et al.*, 2001), to functional neuroimaging experiments in humans which demonstrate that the neural circuit involved in action execution overlaps with that activated when actions are observed or even imagined (Blakemore & Decety, 2001). This neural network includes the premotor cortex, the posterior parietal cortex, the supplementary motor area and the cerebellum.

The shared representations mechanism accounts (at least partly) for emotion processing and empathy as suggested by Preston and de Waal (2002). In this context, perception of emotion activates the neural mechanisms that are responsible for the generation of emotions. Such a system prompts the observer to resonate with the emotional state of another individual, with the observer activating the motor representations and associated autonomic and somatic responses that stem from the observed target, i.e. a sort of inverse mapping.

At the behavioural level, there is ample evidence for this shared mechanism in the recognition of emotion from facial expression in healthy volunteers. For instance, viewing facial expressions triggers subtle expressions on one's own face, even in the absence of conscious recognition of the stimulus (e.g. Wallbott, 1991). Likewise, making a facial expression is associated with feeling the corresponding emotion and generates specific changes in the autonomic nervous system (Levenson *et al.*, 1990).

The finding of paired deficits between emotion production and emotion recognition also provides neurophysiological arguments in favour of the perception-action coupling mechanism. Notably, a lesion study carried out with a large number of neurological patients by Adolphs and colleagues (2000) found that damage within the right somatosensory-related cortexes, including primary and secondary somatosensory cortexes, insula and anterior supramarginal gyrus, impaired the judgement of other people's emotional states from viewing their face. The same authors also reported an association between the impaired somatic sensation of one's own body and the impaired ability to judge other people's emotions. A subsequent study of brain-damaged individuals found that recognizing emotions from prosody is dependent on integrity of the right fronto-parietal cortex (Adolphs *et al.*, 2002). This last result is consistent with the hypothesis that the recognition of emotion in others requires the perceiver to reconstruct images of somatic and motor components that would normally be associated with producing and experiencing the emotion depicted in the stimulus.

Several dramatic case reports support the idea that similar neural systems are involved in both the recognition and the expression of specific emotion. For instance, patient S.M., whose amygdala was bilaterally destroyed by a metabolic disorder, was found to be impaired at both the recognition of fear from facial expressions as well as in the phenomenological experience of fear (Adolphs *et al.*,

1995). Another case, N.M, who suffered from bilateral amygdala damage and a left thalamic lesion, was found to be impaired at recognizing fear from facial expressions and exhibited an equivalent deficit affecting fear recognition from body postures and emotional sounds (Sprengelmeyer *et al.*, 1999). The patient also reported reduced anger and fear in his everyday experience of emotion. There is also evidence for paired deficits for the emotion of disgust. Another interesting case, patient N.K., who suffered left insula and putamen damage, was selectively impaired at recognizing social signals of disgust from multiple modalities (facial expressions, non-verbal sounds and emotional prosody), and was less disgusted than controls by disgust-provoking scenarios (Calder *et al.*, 2000). However, N.K.'s general knowledge of the concept of disgust was not impaired, nor did his scores on anger and fear questionnaires significantly differ from those of the control subjects.

Neuroimaging investigations have provided evidence for the perception-action coupling mechanism involved in emotion processing. Ekman and Davidson (1993) were able to demonstrate similar patterns of electroencephalographic activity for spontaneous and voluntary forms of smiling. Recently, a functional magnetic resonance imaging (fMRI) experiment confirmed and extended these findings by showing that when participants are required to observe or to imitate facial expressions of various emotions, increased haemodynamic activity is detected in the superior temporal sulcus, the anterior insula and the amygdala, as well as in areas of the premotor cortex corresponding to the facial representation (Carr *et al.*, 2003). Phillips *et al.* (1997) have shown that normal volunteers presented with both strong and mild expressions of disgust activated anterior insular cortex but not the amygdala, and that strong disgust also activated structures linked to a limbic cortico–striatal–thalamic circuit. Another fMRI study has extended these findings by showing that similar brain networks were involved in both the recognition (watching videoclips of facial expression) and the experience (inhaling odorants) of disgust (Wicker *et al.*, 2003). The authors found that observing facial expressions and feeling disgust activated the same sites in the anterior insula and to a lesser degree the anterior cingulate cortex (ACC).

14.3 Beyond the perception-action coupling

Although expressing emotions and perceiving emotions in others produce some overlap in neurohaemodynamic patterns, a number of studies have also pointed out important differences. For example, a study investigated the neural response to externally versus internally generated emotions, by comparing the cerebral blood flow responses to watching emotional-laden film clips versus autobiographical scripts (Reiman *et al.*, 1997). Both film-generated emotion and recall-generated emotion were associated with symmetrical increases in the medial prefrontal cortex and thalamus. The former condition also resulted in activation of the hypothalamus, the amygdala, the anterior temporal cortex and the occipito-tempo-parietal junction, while the latter condition was specifically associated with activation in the anterior insula and orbitofrontal cortex. There is thus an overlap between externally and internally produced emotions, but this overlap is partial.

Congruence between the different cues provided by other individuals also seems to be of importance when considering the extent of the shared neural network for emotion processing. A neuroimaging study has demonstrated the involvement of shared neural representations (in both emotion-processing areas and the fronto-parietal network) when subjects feel sympathy (i.e. the affinity, association, or relationship between persons or things wherein whatever affects one similarly affects the other) for another individual (Decety & Chaminade, 2003). In this study, participants were presented with a series of video-clips showing individuals telling sad and neutral stories, as if they had personally experienced them. These stories were told with either congruent or incongruent motor expression of emotion. At the end of each movie, subjects were asked to rate the mood of the actor and also rate how likeable they found that person. Watching sad stories versus neutral stories was associated with increased activity in emotion-processing related structures (including the amygdala and parieto-frontal areas) predominantly in the right hemisphere. This network was not activated when subjects watched incongruent social behaviour.

The expression of pain provides a crucial social signal, which can induce affective states as well as motivate helping behaviours in others. Pain thus offers a unique affective state to investigate the neural underpinning of empathy. Interestingly, a single-neurone recording study of pain processing in neurological patients has shown that there are pain-related neurones in the ACC that respond to both actual stimulation and the observation of the same stimuli delivered to another individual (Hutchison *et al.*, 1999). This study provided one of the first pieces of evidence for a shared mechanism between the perception of pain in self and in others and inspired subsequent studies. One fMRI experiment demonstrated that part of the ACC, the anterior insula, cerebellum and brainstem were activated when subjects experienced a painful stimulus, as well as when they observed a signal indicating that their partner was receiving a similar stimulus (Singer *et al.*, 2004). Consistent results were found in an fMRI study with healthy volunteers showing that both feeling a moderately painful pinprick and witnessing another person undergoing a similar stimulation were associated with activity in a common region of the right dorsal ACC (Morrison *et al.*, 2004). Jackson *et al.* (2005a) also conducted an fMRI study to identify the extent of the neural network engaged in the perception of pain in other individuals, and the possible somatotopy of the representation of pain. The participants were shown still photographs depicting right hands and feet in painful or neutral everyday-life situations, and asked to imagine the level of pain that these situations would produce to another person. Significant activation in regions involved in the affective aspects of the pain-processing network, notably the ACC and the anterior insula, was detected, but no activity in the somatosensory cortex. Moreover, the level of activity within the ACC was strongly correlated with subjects' mean ratings of pain attributed to the different situations. In a follow-up fMRI study, Jackson and colleagues (2006), again using pictures of hands and feet in painful scenarios, instructed the participants to imagine and rate the level of pain perceived from two different perspectives (self versus other). The results indicated that both the self and the other perspectives are associated with activation in the neural network involved in the affective aspect of pain processing, including the ACC and the insula. However, the self-perspective yielded higher pain ratings and involved the pain matrix more extensively, including the secondary somatosensory cortex and the posterior part of the subcalosal cingulate cortex. Adopting the perspective of the other was associated with increased activity in the right temporo-parietal junction. In addition, distinct subregions were activated within the insular cortex for the two perspectives. These findings highlight both the similarities and self–other distinctiveness as important aspects of human empathy, and they are also coherent with the view that empathy does not require a complete self–other merging (see also Lawrence *et al.*, 2006).

However, in the studies of pain and empathy mentioned above, the lack of activation in the somatosensory cortex during conditions of perception of pain for others points to a limitation of the sharing mechanism for pain, with the exception of imagining oneself in painful situations (see Jackson *et al.*, 2006, but see Avenanti *et al.*, 2005). Moreover, it should be noted that the ACC activations are located within the cognitive-motor subdivision of the ACC rather than within the more ventral-anterior affective one (Bush *et al.*, 2000). Therefore, one cannot exclude an alternate interpretation for the findings in these studies, namely that the perception and assessment of pain in others lead to an unspecific state of arousal and anxiety (Critchley, 2004), which puts the subjects in an avoidance stance. Hence, the relationship between pain and other negative emotions remains to be elucidated.

Altogether, shared representations between self and other at the cortical level have been found for action understanding, emotion recognition and for the perception of pain in others. The perception-action coupling mechanism offers an interesting foundation for intersubjectivity because it provides a functional bridge between first-person (self) information and third-person (other) information, an implicit connection between the self and the other (Decety & Sommerville, 2003). Moreover, there is a primacy of the self in the sense that the other is understood on the basis of the self. There is not one specific cortical site for shared representations: their neural underpinnings are widely distributed and the pattern of activation (and also presumably deactivation) varies according to the processing domain, the particular emotion and the stored information. However, as already pointed out, such a mechanism is necessary but not sufficient for empathic understanding. Moreover, it should be noted that the overlap between cortical areas involved in self-related actions/emotions and other-related actions/emotion is not complete. There are specific sub-circuits within the premotor, prefrontal and parietal cortexes that account for either the self or the other (e.g. Ruby & Decety, 2004; Seger *et al.*, 2004). In addition, very little is known regarding the temporal dynamics of the neural activation of the similar networks engaged in self and other. It seems, nevertheless, that in normal circumstances (except for certain pathological conditions such as patients with schizophrenia who experience passivity phenomenon) there is no confusion between self and other. We propose that self-awareness constitutes a prerequisite component of empathy.

14.4 Agency and self-awareness

Agency is a major aspect in our sense of ourselves as subjects. The ability to recognize oneself as the cause of an action, thought, or desire is crucial for attributing a behaviour to its proper agent. Indeed, to be an agent presupposes that one is simultaneously in the world and has the ability to separate himself or herself from it. Thus, the distinction between self-generated signals and signals produced by others is a key function for self-recognition (Jeannerod, 2003). Such a tracking or monitoring mechanism is necessary for an empathic response to take place, and is responsible for the lack of confusion regarding the source of the emotional state. Furthermore, self-aware individuals, as evidenced by being able to become the object of their own attention, experience a sense of psychological continuity over time and space (Gallup, 1998). It has been speculated that any organisms capable of self-recognition would have an introspective awareness of their own mental states and the ability to ascribe mental states to others (Humphrey, 1990). Having a clear sense of self may have evolved to solve at least two kinds of adaptive issues: (1) the self is the repository of the social feedback one receives from others, and (2) it allows one to model and understand the internal, subjective worlds of others, making it easier to infer the intentions and causes that lie behind observed behaviours, thus improving interaction efficacy. Interestingly, the development of self and other mental state understanding is functionally linked to that of executive functions, which in turn is related to the maturation of the prefrontal cortex. This means that the direct perception-action link and its resulting shared representation cannot solely account for intersubjective transactions between self and other. Executive function and particularly executive inhibition are needed to monitor intentions and their consequences.

Self-awareness does not rely upon a specific brain region, nor is it mediated by a unitary system. Rather, this subjective entity arises from complex interactions among networks distributed in the brain, especially within the prefrontal cortex and the inferior parietal lobule, and for which the right hemisphere seems to play a prominent role. Neuropsychological observations support a pre-eminent role of the right frontal lobe in self-related processing. For instance, Keenan and his group (Keenan *et al.*, 2003) demonstrated that patients undergoing a Wada test were temporarily desensitized with regards to the recognition of their own faces when the right hemisphere was anaesthetized. This was not the case when the left hemisphere was anaesthetized. Right hemisphere damage has also been found to be linked with impairments in autobiographical memory and self-evaluation (Stuss & Levine, 2002).

Based on these studies (and many others not reviewed here), Keenan *et al.* (2003) argued that the right hemisphere is a key player in self-awareness and mental state attribution. Note that their original definition of consciousness includes awareness of one's own thoughts as well as awareness of others' thoughts. Similar (but not identical) neural processing for self and other raises the question of how we distinguish between representations activated by the self and those activated by other.

Neuropsychological research indicates that the right inferior parietal cortex in conjunction with the prefrontal cortex is critical in distinguishing the self from the other, and therefore navigating shared representations (Decety & Sommerville, 2003). The inferior parietal cortex is a multimodal association area, which receives input from the lateral and posterior thalamus, as well as visual, auditory, som-esthetic and limbic areas. It has reciprocal connections to the prefrontal cortex, and to the temporal lobes (Eidelberg & Galaburda, 1984). These multiple connections confer on this region a role in the elaboration of an image of the body in space and in time on which the sense of agency depends. The insular cortex is also involved in body awareness, particularly in relation to the emotional aspect of it. Accumulating functional neuroimaging evidence indicates that an area in the right hemisphere at the junction between the posterior temporal and inferior parietal cortex (TPJ) plays a major role in the sense of agency, in distinguishing between self-produced actions and actions generated by others – comparing visuomotor and proprioceptive signals. For instance, the right parietal lobule is significantly more activated when subjects control a moving dot on a computer screen in comparison with the condition in which the dot is controlled by someone else and moved along a different trajectory from the subject's movements (see Jackson & Decety, 2004, for a review). Importantly, this region is directly connected with the medial prefrontal cortex. Frith and Frith (2003) have proposed that this area is involved in detecting the behaviour of agents, and analysing the goals and outcomes of this behaviour. It is worth noting that this region is activated not only during mentalizing tasks but also during the perception of actions made by others. A number of studies have shown that the right TPJ is recruited when distinguishing the perspectives of the self from those of others (see Decety & Grezes, 2006), an ability that is relevant to knowing that the contents of other people's minds can be different from our own.

All the aforementioned evidence strongly indicates that the inferior parietal cortex, in conjunction with the prefrontal cortex and the insula, plays a pivotal role in the implicit sense of self by monitoring the source of sensory signals, whether they originate from the self or from the environment, including information induced by the mirror system. We suggest that this circuit plays a crucial role in empathy by monitoring emotional signals originating from the self and maintaining a distinction between the self and other.

14.5 Adopting the perspective of the other

One may intentionally adopt another individual's psychological point of view, without compromising the distinction between self and other. This perspective-taking ability is a complex process that is necessary to overcome our egocentric tendency and understand the other as someone similar, yet different from oneself. Batson and his colleagues (1997) have demonstrated that imagining how a person feels has been found to evoke altruistic motivation; whereas imagining how one would feel in that person's situation evokes a more complex mix of other-oriented empathy and self-oriented personal distress, which has been found to evoke egoistic motivation (see also Jackson et al., 2006). This conception is compatible with accumulative empirical evidence showing that people are fundamentally egocentric and have difficulty getting beyond their own perspective and that our default mode of reasoning about others is biased (e.g., Keysar, 1994; Royzman et al., 2003). This default mode of reasoning about others, biased towards the self-perspective, constitutes a general feature of human cognition by which one experiences one's own point of view more directly. It also suggests that people have difficulty getting beyond their own perspective when anticipating what others are thinking or feeling. Usually, people are unaware of this projective tendency. Indeed, it operates at an unconscious level. Furthermore, such bias is coherent with the primacy of the self in the shared representations mechanism. One sees others through one's own embodied cognition and uses one's own knowledge (including beliefs, opinions, attitudes and feelings) as the primary basis for understanding others (Decety & Jackson, 2004).

For successful social interaction, and empathic understanding in particular, an adjustment must operate on these shared representations. While the projection of self-traits onto the other does not necessitate any significant store of knowledge about the other, empathic understanding requires the inclusion of other characteristics within the self. However, a complete merging or confusion of one's own and other's feelings is not the goal of empathy. Hence, mental flexibility is an important aspect of empathy. One needs to calibrate one's own perspective that has been activated by the interaction with the other, or even by its mere imagination. Such calibration requires executive functions that are mediated by the prefrontal cortex, as demonstrated by neuroimaging studies in healthy participants as well as neuropsychological observations.

A number of neuroimaging studies have investigated the neural underpinning of perspective taking in different modalities of self–other representations. In one study, participants were scanned while they were asked to imagine themselves performing a variety of everyday actions, or when imagining the experimenter doing similar actions (Ruby & Decety, 2001). Both conditions were associated with common activation in the supplementary motor area (SMA), premotor cortex and the occipito-temporal region, corresponding to the shared motor representations between the self and the other. Taking the perspective of the other to simulate his/her behaviour resulted in selective activation of the frontopolar cortex and right inferior parietal lobule. In another study, medical students were shown a series of affirmative health-related sentences and were asked to judge their truthfulness according to either their own perspective (i.e. as experts in medical knowledge), or that of a layperson (Ruby & Decety, 2003). The set of regions recruited when the participants put themselves in the shoes of a lay-person included the medial prefrontal cortex, the frontopolar and the right inferior parietal lobule. In a third study, the participants were presented with short written sentences that depicted real-life situations that are likely to induce social emotions, or other situations that were emotionally neutral (Ruby & Decety, 2004). In one condition they were asked to imagine how they would feel, while in another condition they were asked to imagine how their mother would feel in those situations. Activation was detected in the frontopolar cortex, the ventromedial prefrontal cortex, the medial prefrontal cortex and the right inferior parietal lobule when the participants adopted the perspective of their mother, regardless of the affective content of the situations depicted. Cortical regions that are involved in emotional processing were found to be activated in the conditions that integrated emotional-laden situations, including the amygdala and the temporal poles.

In an fMRI study, Seger *et al.* (2004) asked participants to make food preference judgements about themselves or about someone else (a person they knew fairly well). Self-judgements were associated with increased activity in the medial

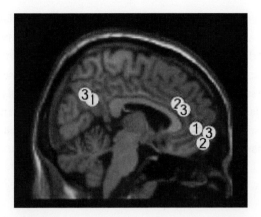

Figure 14.1. Brain areas (frontopolar, medial prefrontal/anterior paracingulate and posterior cingulate
cortexes) found activated when participants overtly adopt the perspective of another
individual versus self-perspective. The activated clusters, represented by white circles,
are superimposed onto an MRI sagittal section. Numbers correspond to experimental
condition in which participants imagined actions (1: Ruby & Decety, 2001), knowledge
(2: Ruby & Decety, 2003) or feelings (3: Ruby & Decety, 2004). Haemodynamic changes
in these regions are more pronounced in the right hemisphere. The systematic
activation of the right temporoparietal junction during third-person perspective taking is
not shown

prefrontal cortex, the anterior insula and secondary somatosensory areas. Other-
judgements resulted in activation of the medial prefrontal cortex, the frontopolar
cortex and the posterior cingulate.

One of the most striking findings of these studies that investigated self versus
others' perspectives is the systematic involvement of the frontopolar cortex,
medial prefrontal cortex, posterior cingulate and right temporoparietal junction
when the participants adopt the perspective of another person (see Figure 14.1).

Converging evidence from clinical neuropsychology and neuroscience suggests
that the frontopolar cortex is chiefly involved in inhibitory or regulating processing. Frontal damage may result in impaired perspective-taking ability and a lack of
cognitive flexibility (Eslinger, 1998). Interestingly, Anderson et al. (1999) reported
the cases of two patients with early damage to the anterior prefrontal cortex
(encompassing the frontopolar cortex) who, when tested on moral dilemmas,
exhibited an excessively egocentric perspective. A major study with neurological
patients with limited focal lesions reported dissociation of performance within the
frontal lobes when tested for visual perspective taking and detecting deception
(Stuss et al., 2001). Right frontal lobe lesions were associated with impaired visual
perspective taking, and medial frontal lesions, particularly right ventral, with
impaired detection of deception.

Another interesting fact is that perspective-taking tasks elicit similar haemo-dynamic changes in the medial paracingulate cortex to those of Theory of Mind tasks. It has been proposed that such activation reflects a 'decoupling' mechanism, which allows us to hold representations detached from the apparent reality (Frith & Frith, 2003). We suggest that the extent of the medial prefrontal activation during empathy is correlated with the cognitive load measured in terms of dis-engagement of the representation of others' feelings from the explicit social cues that are perceived and mapped to the self-representation.

14.6 Emotion regulation

Empathy requires some level of emotion regulation to manage and optimize intersubjective transactions between self and other. Emotion regulation refers to the processes by which individuals influence which emotions they have, when they have them and how they experience and express these emotions (Gross, 1998). This terminology also applies to the modulation of the behavioural and the physiological dimension of emotion. It is likely that the emotional state and affective consequences generated by the perception of the other's situation need regulation and control for the experience of empathy. Indeed, without such control, the mere activation of the perception-action coupling, including the associated autonomic and somatic responses, could lead to emotional contagion, anxiety and emotional distress. Such a regulation is also crucial when modulating one's own vicarious emotion so that it is not always experienced as aversive. It is worth noting that previous research has shown that emotion regulation is pos-itively related to feelings of concern for the other person (e.g. Derryberry & Rothbart, 1988). In contrast, people who experience their emotions intensely, especially negative emotions, are prone to personal distress, i.e. an aversive emo-tional reaction, such as anxiety or discomfort based on the recognition of another's emotional state or condition (Eisenberg *et al.*, 1991). Chronic incapacity to suppress negative emotion may be a key factor in anxiety, aggressive and violent behaviour (Jackson *et al.*, 2000).

A circuit that includes several regions of the prefrontal cortex, the amygdala, hippocampus, anterior cingulate cortex, insular cortex and ventral striatum has been implicated in various aspects of emotion regulation (Davidson, 2002). In neurology, a 'self-regulatory disorder' has been coined by Levine and colleagues (1999) for the syndrome exhibited by patients with ventromedial prefrontal cortex damage. This syndrome is defined as the inability to regulate behaviour according to internal goals and constraints. It arises from the inability to hold a mental representation of the self on-line and to use this self-related information to inhibit inappropriate responses. Both the orbitofrontal-ventromedial and dorsolateral cortexes have been reported in the neurological literature to be involved in empathy. Damage of the orbitofrontal cortex is associated with a wide range of social emotional deficits including impaired social judgement and disinhibited behaviour. For instance, Stone *et al.* (1998) reported that patients with bilateral lesions of the orbitofrontal cortex are impaired in the 'faux pas' task. Such a task requires both an understanding of false or mistaken belief, and an appreciation of the emotional impact of a statement on the listener.

Recent neuroimaging studies have begun to investigate the neural mechanisms involved in affective reappraisal, a cognitive strategy used to regulate emotion. For instance, an fMRI experiment has shown neural correlates of emotion reappraisal in the lateral prefrontal and medial prefrontal cortices, and decreased activity in the medial orbitofrontal cortex and the amygdala (Ochsner *et al.*, 2002). Another study identified a circuit composed of the right orbitofrontal, right dorsolateral prefrontal cortex and anterior cingulate for voluntary suppression of sadness (Lévesque *et al.*, 2003).

Although the specification of the cognitive and neural processes that support emotion regulation during empathic experience has not yet been the target of specific investigations (e.g. which strategy is at play), this top-down control likely plays a key role in empathy.

14.7 Multiple facets of empathy disorders

Although the loss of empathy has mainly been described after lesion of the frontal lobe, more specifically the prefrontal cortex, our model suggests that there may be distinct disorders related to empathy rather than a unique deficit. Furthermore, since our model assumes that empathy relies on dissociable components, it predicts a variety of structural or functional dysfunctions depending on which aspect is disturbed. We believe that this view is quite coherent with the broad range of disorders that are related to empathy, and with its multidimensional basis. Indeed, we do not think it is reasonable to assume a single source of empathy deficit in very different conditions such as sociopathy, conduct disorders, narcissistic personality disorder, Asperger's syndrome, stroke or traumatic brain injury. This section focuses on the various acquired empathy disorders stemming from neuropsychological disorders.

It is well accepted that empathic processing may be impaired after focal lesions of the prefrontal cortex. A study conducted by Stuss and colleagues (2001) demonstrated that lesions throughout the frontal lobe, with a more important role of the right hemisphere, are associated with impaired perspective taking. They have also shown that medial lesions, particularly in the right side, impaired mentalizing abilities. In addition, several other patient studies reported a relationship between the deficit in empathy and the performance of cognitive flexibility tasks among patients with lesions in the dorsolateral cortex, while those with orbitofrontal cortex lesions were more impaired in empathy but not in cognitive flexibility (Grattan *et al.*, 1994). Furthermore, a study by Shamay-Tsoory *et al.* (2003) reported that among patients with posterior lesions, only those with damage to the right hemisphere (parietal cortex) were impaired in empathy. Another recent study by the same authors tested patients with lesions of the ventromedial prefrontal cortex or dorsolateral prefrontal cortex with three Theory of Mind (second-order beliefs and faux pas) differing in the level of emotional processing involved (Shamay-Tsoory *et al.*, 2005). They found that patients with ventromedial lesions were most impaired in the faux pas task but presented normal performance in the second-order belief tasks. They further argued that, in order to detect faux pas, one is required not only to understand the knowledge of the other but also to have empathic understanding of their feelings.

These aforementioned studies point out that different parts of the right prefrontal cortex are involved in the capacity to reason about the feelings of others, including the ability to adopt the perspective of others. Yet, although these two aspects seem dissociable, future research is needed to elucidate what specific subprocess (in terms of computation) each subregion subserves. In that context single case studies can provide valuable information. For instance, one study showed an intermediate position between patients with profound neurobehavioural deficits and patients with impaired real-life social cognition despite intact neuropsychological performance, following orbitofrontal damage (Cicerone & Tanebaum, 1997). The patient had traumatic orbitomedial frontal lobe damage and demonstrated good neurocognitive recovery but a lasting profound disturbance of emotional regulation and social cognition. While classical measures associated with frontal lobe functions were found to be normal, the patient remained impaired on tasks requiring the interpretation of social situations, which mirrored her impairment in real life functioning. This disturbance in social cognition appeared to be related to difficulty appreciating and integrating the relatively subtle social and emotional cues required for an appropriate interpretation of events.

This interpretation is further supported by an experiment involving five cases with similar orbito-frontal lesions (Beer *et al.*, 2003). These authors compared healthy individuals and the five patients on a number of social/emotional measures, and suggested that deficient behavioural regulation is associated with inappropriate self-conscious emotions, or faulty appraisal, that reinforce maladaptive behaviour. Moreover, the authors provided evidence that deficient behavioural regulation is associated with impairments in interpreting the self-conscious emotions of others. They interpreted their results based on the idea that self-conscious emotions are important for regulating social behaviour.

The study of degenerative neurological diseases has also supplied evidence for relatively distinct routes to social cognition and empathy deficits. For instance, Snowden *et al.* (2003) have shown that patients with a frontotemporal dementia (FTD), a predominantly neocortical disorder associated with deficits in frontal executive functions, as well as patients with Huntington's disease (HD), a predominantly subcortical disorder characterized by involuntary movements, present difficulties in tasks of social cognition. However, the two patient groups display qualitatively different patterns of results. This suggests that the deficits of patients with a FTD may be attributed to a breakdown in Theory of Mind, while those of patients with HD appear to be associated with faulty inferences drawn from social situations. Interestingly, patients with HD and those with FTD lack sympathy and empathy, but for different reasons. In the former group, the loss of empathy arises at more an emotional than a cognitive level, while FTD patients live in an egocentric world in which they do not ascribe independent mental states to others. A compatible finding from a voxel-based morphometry analysis (i.e. a technique used for comparison of brain volume and detection of regional brain atrophy) on FTD patients revealed that atrophy in bilateral temporal lobe and medial orbito-frontal structures correlated with loss of cognitive empathy and that atrophy to the temporal pole correlated significantly with loss of emotional empathy (Rankin *et al.*, 2003). These findings are consistent with the idea of distinct neural underpinnings for the cognitive and affective aspects of empathy.

Lesions of the amygdala can produce deficits in mental state reasoning as demonstrated by Stone and colleagues (2003), who found right-sided lesions associated with affective state attributions. The role of the amygdala in detecting emotional states of others was further investigated in a large group of neurological patients by Shaw *et al.* (2004). They found that such deficit was observed in individuals who had amygdala damage during childhood but not when the lesion occurred later.

Overall, the neuropsychological evidence reviewed here strongly suggests that lesions to different cortical and subcortical structures or circuits can lead to an alteration of empathy or even a lack of empathic ability. However, qualitative differences exist in the nature of underlying deficits, and this supports our assertion that empathy entails a number of distinct components mediated by isolable neural systems. It is possible that psychopathological disorders such as depression, schizophrenia or autism, in which social breakdown are predominant for various reasons, will benefit from this neuropsychological model.

14.8 From covert to overt representation of others' mental states

The way our nervous system is organized and tailored by evolution provides the basic mechanism for resonating with others. This shared representations

mechanism (i.e. distributed neural patterns temporarily activated by actual perception or evoked from memory) driven by the common coding between perception and action provides the default mode (or tendency) of self-processing to
implicitly relate to others (Decety & Sommerville, 2003). This tendency needs to be
calibrated and regulated when sharing emotions or when adopting the perspective
of others in order to understand their feelings. This requires additional processing
mechanisms including the monitoring and manipulation of internal information
generated by activation of the shared representations (see Figure 14.2).

One of the main components of empathy is based on an unconscious mental
simulation of the emotional state of others. This idea is far from new. For instance,
Ax (1964) suggested that empathy might be thought of 'as an autonomic nervous
system state which tends to simulate that of another person'. Note that this
simulation may operate on-line or off-line. However, this simulation is not
exclusively under automatic management and may fall under conscious control.
This makes empathy as described here (as opposed to emotional contagion or
mimicry) an intentional capacity. Without self-awareness and emotion-regulation
processing, there is no true empathy. The constant and un-modulated activation
of shared representations would instead lead to anxiety, discomfort or emotional
distress. Such emotional states are generally associated with egoistic helping (i.e.
helping oriented to increasing the helper's own welfare by reducing her/his felt
distress). In contrast, empathic concern may be associated with altruistic helping
(i.e. helping directed at increasing the other's welfare). Such a formulation is
consistent with the observation that prosocial behaviours, which stem from
empathy, emerge in parallel with self-conscious emotions and the maturation of
self-regulation (Eisenberg *et al.*, 1991). Interestingly, these emotions require self-
evaluation and comparison with other selves, as well as some form of regulation.
Forming an explicit representation of another person's feeling, such as an intentional agent, necessitates additional mechanisms beyond the shared representation
level, such as memory and knowledge (e.g. Ickes, 1997). It also requires that
second-order representations of the other are available to consciousness (a decoupling mechanism between first-person information and second-person information), in which the anterior paracingulate cortex plays a unique function (Frith &
Frith, 2003). Thus, empathy cannot be described as a simple resonance of affect
between the self and other. It involves an explicit representation of the subjectivity
of the other, and presupposes a prosocial stance (Batson, 1991). Recent neuroimaging investigations of the perception of pain in others discussed above support
such a view. These studies have shown that only part of the network (i.e. affective-
motivational in nature; including the anterior cingulate cortex and the insula)
mediating pain experiences is shared when empathizing or evaluating the pain in
others, as opposed to a more global mirror representation which would involve

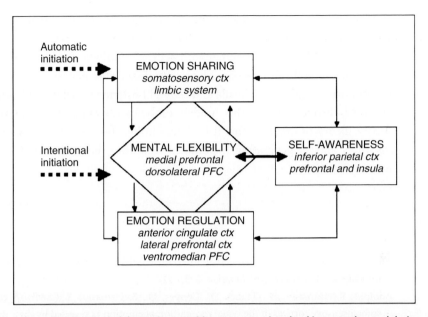

Figure 14.2. Schematic overview of the major cognitive processes involved in empathy, and their putative neural underpinnings. This model combines both the representational aspects (i.e. memories that are localized in distributed neural networks, e.g. shared affective representations), and processes (i.e. computational procedures that are neurally localized and are independent of the nature or modality of the stimulus that is being processed, e.g. decoupling mechanism between self and other). The medial prefrontal cortex/paracingulate sulcus plays a key role in decoupling between first-person and third-person information. The ventromedial prefrontal cortex has been described as a convergence zone in which information from amygdala, hippocampus and sensory regions interacts to influence social behaviour. The lateral prefrontal cortex and the anterior cingulate are part of a circuit that regulates emotion. Note the bidirectional links between the areas in which representation of emotions are temporarily activated (including autonomic and somatic responses) during empathic experience and the areas involved in emotion regulation. Each area has unique patterns of cortico-cortical connections, which determine its function, and differences in neural activity during the experience of empathy are produced by distributed subsystems of brain regions. Even though there is massive parallel processing, the dynamics of activation in these regions is also an important aspect to be investigated further

sensory components. Most importantly and often neglected in previous models of empathy, this process necessitates emotion regulation in which the ventral prefrontal cortex, with its strong connections with the limbic system, dorsolateral and medial prefrontal areas, plays an important role. Finally, empathy, like most complex social skills, is modulated by top-down processing involving cultural values, concepts, personal experience and the like.

To sum up, empathy is described as a complex process that involves four major aspects: affective sharing, mental flexibility, emotion regulation and self-awareness. Functional imaging data, together with neuropsychological evidence indicate that this cognitive ability is mediated by partly dissociable neural circuits, including the anterior cingulate, the insula and the right inferior parietal lobule, that can be selectively broken down. This model combines the simulation theory and the theory-theory of other minds. It has clear implication for the study of empathy disorders and in generating hypotheses regarding the neural underpinning of intersubjectivity.

REFERENCES

Adolphs, R., Damasio, H., & Tranel, D. (2002). Neural systems for recognition of emotional prosody: a 3-D lesion study. *Emotion*, **2**, 23–51.

Adolphs, R., Damasio, H., Tranel, D., Cooper, G., & Damasio, A. (2000). A role for the somatosensory cortices in the visual recognition of emotion as revealed by three dimensional lesion mapping. *Journal of Neuroscience*, **20**, 2683–2690.

Adolphs, R., Tranel, D., Damasio, H., & Damasio, A. (1995). Fear and the human amygdala. *Journal of Neuroscience*, **15**, 5879–5891.

Anderson, S. W., Bechara, A., Damasio, H., Tranel, D., & Damasio, A. R. (1999). Impairment of social and moral behavior related to early damage in human prefrontal cortex. *Nature Neuroscience*, **2**, 1032–1037.

Avenanti, A., Bueti, D., Galati, G., & Aglioti, S. M. (2005). Transcranial magnetic stimulation highlights the sensorimotor side of empathy for pain. *Nature Neuroscience*, **8**, 955–960.

Ax, A. A. (1964). Goals and methods of psychophysiology. *Psychophysiology*, **1**, 8–25.

Batson, C. D. (1991). Empathic joy and the empathy-altruism hypothesis. *Journal of Personality and Social Psychology*, **61**, 413–426.

Batson, C. D., Early, S., & Salvari, G. (1997). Perspective taking: imagining how another feels versus imagining how you would feel. *Personality and Social Psychology Bulletin*, **25**, 751–758.

Beer, J. S., Heerey, E. A., Keltner, D., Scabini, D., & Knight, R. T. (2003). The regulatory function of self-conscious emotion: insights from patients with orbitofrontal damage. *Journal of Personality and Social Psychology*, **85**, 594–604.

Blakemore, S.-J., & Decety, J. (2001). From the perception of action to the understanding of intention. *Nature Reviews Neuroscience*, **2**, 561–567.

Bush, G., Luu, P., & Posner, M. I. (2000). Cognitive and emotional influences in anterior cingulate cortex. *Trends in Cognitive Science*, **4**, 215–222.

Calder, A. J., Keane, J., Manes, F., Antoun, N., & Young, A. W. (2000). Impaired recognition an experience of disgust following brain injury. *Nature Neuroscience*, **3**, 1077–1078.

Carr, L., Iacoboni, M., Dubeau, M. C., Mazziotta, J. C., & Lenzi, G. L. (2003). Neural mechanisms of empathy in humans: a relay from neural systems for imitation to limbic areas. *Proceedings of National Academy of Science USA*, **100**, 5497–5502.

Cicerone, K. D., & Tanebaum, L. N. (1997). Disturbance of social cognition after traumatic orbitofrontal brain injury. *Archives of Clinical Neuropsychology*, **12**, 173–188.

Critchley, H. D. (2004). The human cortex responds to an interoceptive challenge. *Proceedings of the National Academy of Science USA*, **101**, 6333–6334.

Davidson, R. J. (2002). Anxiety and affective style: role of prefrontal cortex and amygdala. *Biological Psychiatry*, **51**, 68–80.

Decety, J., & Chaminade, T. (2003). Neural correlates of feeling sympathy. *Neuropsychologia*, **41**, 127–138.

Decety, J., & Grezes, J. (2006). The power of simulation: imagining one's own and other's behavior. *Brain Research*, **1079**, 4–14.

Decety, J., & Jackson, P. L. (2004). The functional architecture of human empathy. *Behavioral and Cognitive Neuroscience Reviews*, **3**, 71–100.

Decety, J., & Sommerville, J. A. (2003). Shared representations between self and others: a social cognitive neuroscience view. *Trends in Cognitive Science*, **7**, 527–533.

Derryberry, D., & Rothbart, M. K. (1988). Arousal, affect, and attention as components of temperament. *Journal of Personality and Social Psychology*, **55**, 958–966.

Eidelberg, D., & Galaburda, A. M. (1984). Inferior parietal lobule. *Archives of Neurology*, **41**, 843–852.

Eisenberg, N., Shea, C. L., Carlo, G., & Knight, G. (1991). Empathy related responding and cognition: A 'chicken and the egg' dilemma. In W. Kurtines, & J. Gewirtz (eds.), *Handbook of Moral Behavior and Development* (Vol. 2). *Research* (pp. 63–68). Hillsdale, N. J.: Erlbaum.

Ekman, P., & Davidson, R. J. (1993). Voluntary smiling changes regional brain activity. *Psychological Science*, **4**, 342–345.

Eslinger, P. J. (1998). Neurological and neuropsychological bases of empathy. *European Neurology*, **39**, 193–199.

Frith, U., & Frith, C. D. (2003). Development and neurophysiology of mentalizing. *Philosophical Transactions of the Royal Society, London B*, **358**, 459–473.

Gallup, G. G. (1998). Self-awareness and the evolution of social intelligence. *Behavioural Processes*, **42**, 239–247.

Grattan, L. M., Bloomer, R. H., Archambault, F. X., & Eslinger, P. J. (1994). Cognitive flexibility and empathy after frontal lobe lesion. *Neuropsychiatry, Neuropsychology, and Behavioral Neurology*, **7**, 251–257.

Gross, J. J. (1998). The emerging field of emotion regulation: an integrative review. *Review of General Psychology*, **2**, 271–289.

Humphrey, N. (1990). The uses of consciousness. In J. Brockman (ed.), *Speculations: The Reality Club* (pp. 67–84). New York: Prentice Hall.

Hutchison, W. D., Davis, K. D., Lozano, A. M., *et al.* (1999). Pain-related neurons in the human cingulate cortex. *Nature Neuroscience*, **2**, 403–405.

Ickes, W. (1997). *Empathic Accuracy.* New York: The Guilford Press.

Jackson, D. C., Malmstadt, J. R., Larson, C. L., & Davidson, R. J. (2000). Suppression and enhancement of emotional responses to unpleasant pictures. *Psychophysiology*, **37**, 512–522.

Jackson, P. L., Brunet, E., Meltzoff, A. N., & Decety, J. (2006). Empathy examined through the neural mechanisms involved in imagining how I feel versus how you feel: an event-related fMRI study. *Neuropsychologia*, **44**, 752–761.

Jackson, P. L., & Decety, J. (2004). Motor cognition: a new paradigm to study self other interactions. *Current Opinion in Neurobiology*, **14/2**, 259–263.

Jackson, P. L., Meltzoff, A. N., & Decety, J. (2005). How do we perceive the pain of others: a window into the neural processes involved in empathy. *NeuroImage*, **24**, 771–779.

Jeannerod, M. (1999). To act or not to act: perspective on the representation of actions. *Quarterly Journal of Experimental Psychology*, **52A**, 1–29.

Jeannerod, M. (2003). The mechanisms of self-recognition. *Behavioural Brain Research*, **142**, 1–15.

Keenan, J. P., Gallup, G. G., & Falk, D. (2003). *The Face in the Mirror: The Search for the Origins of Consciousness.* New York: HarperCollins Publishers.

Keysar, B. (1994). The illusory transparency of intention: linguistic perspective taking in text. *Cognitive Psychology*, **26**, 165–208.

Knoblich, G., & Flach, R. (2003). Action identity: evidence from self-recognition, prediction, and coordination. *Consciousness and Cognition*, **12**, 620–632.

Lawrence, E. J., Shaw, P., Giampietro, V. P., *et al.* (2006). The role of 'shared representations' in social perception and empathy: an fMRI study. *Neuroimage*, **29**, 1173–1184.

Levenson, R. W., Ekman, P., & Friesen, W. V. (1990). Voluntary facial action generates emotion-specific autonomic nervous system activity. *Psychophysiology*, **27**, 363–384.

Lévesque, J., Eugène, F., Joanette, Y., *et al.* (2003). Neural circuitry underlying voluntary suppression of sadness. *Biological Psychiatry*, **53**, 502–510.

Levine, B., Freedman, M., Dawson, D., Black, S. E., & Stuss, D. T. (1999). Ventral frontal contribution to self-regulation: convergence of episodic memory and inhibition. *Neurocase*, **5**, 263–275.

Morrison, I., Lloyd, D., di Pellegrino, G., & Roberts, N. (2004). Vicarious responses to pain in anterior cingulate cortex: is empathy a multisensory issue. *Cognitive, Affective, and Behavioral Neuroscience*, **4**, 270–278.

Ochsner, K. N., Bunge, S. A., Gross, J. J., & Gabrieli, J. D. E. (2002). Rethinking feelings: an fMRI study of the cognitive regulation of emotion. *Journal of Cognitive Neuroscience*, **14**, 1215–1229.

Phillips, M. L., Young, A. W., Senior, C., *et al.* (1997). A specific neural substrate for perceiving facial expressions of disgust. *Nature*, **389**, 495–498.

Preston, S. D., & de Waal, F. B. M. (2002). Empathy: its ultimate and proximate bases. *Behavioral and Brain Sciences*, **25**, 1–72.

Prinz, W. (1997). Perception and action planning. *European Journal of Cognitive Psychology*, **9**, 129–154.

Rankin, K. P., Gorno-Tempini, M. L., Weiner, M. W., & Miller, B. L. (2003). Neuroanatomy of impaired empathy in frontotemporal dementia. 55th Annual Meeting of the American Academy of Neurologists, Honolulu.

Reiman, E. M., Lane, R. D., Ahern, G. L., *et al.* (1997). Neuroanatomical correlates of externally and internally generated emotion. *American Journal of Psychiatry*, **154**, 918–925.

Rizzolatti, G., Fogassi, L., & Gallese, V. (2001). Neurophysiological mechanisms underlying the understanding and the imitation of action. *Nature Review Neuroscience*, **2**, 661–670.

Royzman, E. B., Cassidy, K. W., & Baron, J. (2003). I know you know: epistemic egocentrism in children and adults. *Review of General Psychology*, **7**, 38–65.

Ruby, P., & Decety, J. (2001). Effect of subjective perspective taking during simulation of action: a PET investigation of agency. *Nature Neuroscience*, **4**, 546–550.

Ruby, P., & Decety, J. (2003). What you believe versus what you think they believe: a neuroimaging study of conceptual perspective taking. *European Journal of Neuroscience*, **17**, 2475–2480.

Ruby, P., & Decety, J. (2004). How would you feel versus how do you think she would feel? A neuroimaging study of perspective taking with social emotions. *Journal of Cognitive Neuroscience*, **16**, 988–999.

Seger, C. A., Stone, M., & Keenan, J. P. (2004). Cortical activations during judgments about the self and an other person. *Neuropsychologia*, **42(9)**, 1168–1177.

Shamay-Tsoory, S. G., Tomer, R., Berger, B. D., & Aharon-Peretz, J. (2003). Characterization of empathy deficits following prefrontal brain damage: the role of right ventromedial prefrontal cortex. *Journal of Cognitive Neuroscience*, **15**, 1–14.

Shamay-Tsoory, S. G., Tomer, R., Berger, B. D., Goldsher, D., & Aharon-Peretz, J. (2005). Impaired affective theory of mind is associated with ventromedial prefrontal damage. *Cognitive and Behavioral Neurology*, **18**, 55–67.

Shaw, P., Lawrence, E. J., Radbourne, C., *et al.* (2004). The impact of early and late damage to the human amygdala on 'theory of mind' reasoning. *Brain*, **127**, 1535–1548.

Singer, T., Seymour, B., O'Doherty, J., *et al.* (2004). Empathy for pain involves the affective but not sensory components of pain. *Science*, **303**, 1157–1161.

Snowden, J. S., Gibbons, Z. C., Blackshaw, A., *et al.* (2003). Social cognition in frontotemporal dementia and Huntington's disease. *Neuropsychologia*, **41**, 688–701.

Sprengelmeyer, R., Young, A. W., Schroeder, U., *et al.* (1999). Knowing no fear. *Proceedings of the Royal Society (Series B: Biology)*, **266**, 2451–2456.

Stone, V. E., Baron-Cohen, S., Calder, A., Keane, J., & Young, A. (2003). Acquired theory of mind impairments in individuals with bilateral amygdala lesions. *Neuropsychologia*, **41**, 209–220.

Stone, V. E., Baron-Cohen, S., & Knight, R. T. (1998). Frontal lobe contributions to theory of mind. *Journal of Cognitive Neuroscience*, **10**, 640–646.

Stuss, D. T., Gallup, G., & Alexander, M. P. (2001). The frontal lobes are necessary for theory of mind. *Brain*, **124**, 279–286.

Stuss, D. T., & Levine, B. (2002). Adult clinical neuropsychology: lessons from studies of the frontal lobes. *Annual Review of Psychology*, **53**, 401–433.

Wallbott, H. G. (1991). Recognition of emotion from facial expression via imitation? Some indirect evidence for an old theory. *British Journal Social Psychology*, **30**, 207–219.

Wicker, B., Keysers, C., Plailly, J., *et al.* (2003). Both of us disgusted in my insula: the common neural basis of seeing and feeling disgust. *Neuron*, **40**, 655–664.

The genetics of empathy and its disorders

Henrik Anckarsäter[1] and C. Robert Cloninger[2]

[1]The Forensic Psychiatric Clinic, Malmö University Hospital
[2]Washington University School of Medicine

15.1 Introduction

Substantial evidence now shows that the differences between individuals in their empathy for one another are influenced by multiple genetic and environmental factors. In this chapter, we will first describe the way empathy can be decomposed into multiple traits that can be reliably measured for genetic investigation. The results of genetic studies will then be reviewed, showing that empathy is a multi-faceted phenomenon with complex dynamics influenced by non-linear interactions among biological, psychological and social processes. Available data suggest important clues to possible genetic mechanisms that underlie individual differences in the development of empathy, but as a wide variety of measures have been used, it is essential to begin with a critical discussion of their limitations and interpretation.

15.2 Deconstructing empathy

Empathy is an active process, or set of processes, in the relationship of one human being with another. Empathy may be spontaneous or calculated. It may be processed emotionally or by discursive reasoning, and it may be facilitated or impeded by volition (i.e. intentions involving particular goals and values). As it involves two or more humans (even if one of them is for example described in a book), empathy is dependent on social context. Our ability to empathize with others is, among innumerable other factors, influenced by our general well-being, prejudices, attitudes and position in the encounter.

As a result of the importance of social context for empathy, a major pitfall in research on empathy is the error of reification, where empathy is studied as an independent object, separate and measurable in isolation. In this review, we will report findings about a variety of measures of different aspects of empathy,

Empathy in Mental Illness, eds. Tom F. D. Farrow and Peter W. R. Woodruff. Published by Cambridge University Press. © Cambridge University Press 2007.

but we will try to avoid any suggestion that empathy can be reduced to a single entity or trait. Instead, empathy will be considered as a multi-faceted phenomenon with a complex biopsychosocial nature that leads to substantial differences between individuals in several traits related to the different aspects of empathy, including intentions, emotions, social relations and intellectual perspective.

In addition to there being individual differences in several traits related to empathy, it is often assumed that the differences between individuals are larger than the differences within an individual across situations and across time during lifetime development. Otherwise genetic differences are likely to have only a minor role in the development of empathy, and non-genetic influences would have greater importance. In fact, a substantial body of data shows moderate to strong heritability for traits related to empathy. However, these traits involve a wide variety of divergent measurement approaches, most of which will reduce intra-individual variations in actual empathy. Accordingly, we will consider a broad range of clinical indicators of empathy, including measures that make the questionable assumption that empathy is a simple and stable phenomenon. It is important, therefore, for the reader to keep in mind that there are many interdependent dynamic factors that influence the capacity of a person for empathy. Taken together, available data suggest that empathy is the expression of a non-linear dynamic system, not a fixed and stable property of a small number of variables. We will attempt to provide a sketch of the psychobiology of the interacting processes that influence empathy, so that future research can clarify these mechanisms in ways that are clinically and biologically meaningful.

15.3 The component processes leading to empathy

Several distinct psychological abilities have been proposed to play central roles in empathic processes. The most prominent ability is called the capacity for 'Theory of Mind' (ToM), originally defined as the ability to predict what's going on in other people's minds and to understand that their actions are guided by their understanding of reality, rather than by reality itself (Premack & Woodruff, 1978). Individual differences in ToM are commonly measured using 'False Belief Tasks', which are generally solved by children before the age of 4 (Hogrefe et al., 1986). Children who have problems understanding that other people may act upon misrepresentations also have difficulties understanding that they may do so themselves (Gopnik & Astington, 1988). ToM may be a necessary cognitive ability for some forms of affective and emotional processing important in empathy, but it does not exhaust the range of emotional processing involved in empathy-related processes.

The more intuitive and complex ability to recognize emotional states in others through observation and mimicry of gazes and voice may be tested by interpreting unknown emotions expressed by actors through a limited array of social cues, such as gaze or intonation only. Linguistic emotional processing is tested through changes in psychophysiological reactions and processing speed when confronted with emotionally charged or neutral words, as in 'Lexical Decision Tests'. The test conditions in lexical decision tasks are usually neutral in intention, and do not differ between understanding others for benevolent or callous purposes. Nevertheless, emotional understanding without any emotional identification appears to be unlikely, as suggested by one of the two most influential hypotheses about ToM (the 'simulation theory' as compared to the 'theory-theory'). Empirical data support the existence of mirror systems where identification and imitation are used for understanding mental states (Buccino *et al.*, 2001), although they may not fully account for the creation of a theoretical understanding. For example, substantial discrepancies have been observed between the development of awareness of desires versus perceptions that precede the development of awareness of cognitive phenomena (Gopnik & Wellman, 1992). The notion of ToM as a specific 'theoretical' process going beyond emotional identification as a higher level of meta-cognition (i.e. thinking about thinking) seems plausible, and defines one component of the processes that can lead to the development of empathy.

Benevolence is often assumed to be a hallmark of empathy in common language and in personality research. However, the intention of empathy is often not included in phenotype definitions, leaving the understanding of empathy on a personality level incomplete as the role of volition and the motivational forces behind it are not taken into account. Any understanding of empathy must include the processing of intentions, emotions and intellectual perspective in a social context.

15.4 Autism and empathy

A strong interest for research into the psychological and neurological basis for empathy has been attracted by the progress made in the understanding of autism, which is increasingly considered to be the 'prototypical' disorder of empathy. Autism is defined through severe, early-onset and persistent behavioural aberrations in three areas: social interaction, communication through language and flexibility in behavioural routines (Wing, 1981). Other problem constellations in the same areas are referred to as 'autism spectrum disorders' (mainly Asperger's syndrome, 'high-functioning' autism and atypical autism) or 'broader phenotypes', such as autistic traits in combination with other mental problems or expressed as personality traits rather than as a disorder (Wing, 1996). It has long been asked if the three criterion areas in autism (i.e. social aloofness, language deficits and repetitive non-social behaviour) represent separate problems that may vary independently, or if they are broadly associated with each other. Studies from patient groups (Constantino *et al.*, 2004; Spiker *et al.*, 2002; Szatmari *et al.*, 2002) suggest that the three areas are indeed associated, forming a single dimension of social interaction problems, completed in patients only by another separate dimension of general cognitive functioning, roughly corresponding to intelligence quotient (IQ). This conclusion, however, may depend on sampling with enrichment of autistic cases and phrasing questions to depend on the social context of the observer. For example, Constantino's Social Responsiveness Scale asks about all three areas diagnostic of autism, but does so from the social perspective of an external observer in order to simplify the rating task for non-clinicians. In contrast, when a questionnaire about the internal motivation of children is used by parents and teachers of 7-year-old twins with no enrichment with severe cases of autism, different genetic influences for social interactional and non-social (repetitive and stereotypic behaviours) symptoms of autism spectrum disorders were identified (Ronald *et al.*, 2006), with substantial heritability for both scales (54%–71%), largely influenced by *independent* genetic factors, suggesting genetic heterogeneity for autism spectrum disorders. Replication of this study is necessary before any firm conclusions can be drawn, particularly because the number of subjects with clear-cut dysfunctions was small.

Problems with mentalizing or ToM have been placed at the centre of autism since the 1980s, when it was first proposed by Uta Frith and her colleagues (Baron-Cohen *et al.*, 1985) as a possible explanation for the 'enigma' of autism, using various false belief tests in which the ability to understand that other people's actions are guided by their (sometimes mistaken) assumptions of the world is experimentally challenged. In a PET study of regional brain metabolism during work with ToM tasks, adult subjects with Asperger's syndrome did not activate a specific region on the border between Brodmann areas 8 and 9 in the left medial prefrontal cortex that had previously been found to be activated by this and similar tests in controls; instead, Asperger subjects activated a less specific brain area that was more ventrally located between Brodmann areas 9 and 10 (Happé *et al.*, 1996).

Christopher Gillberg proposed in the 1991 Emmanuel Miller memorial lecture that autism is a subclass among 'disorders of empathy' (Gillberg, 1992). He pointed to the important hiatus between emotions and empathy/ToM in autism, where unreflective social 'feelings' are more available than the ability to make sense of feelings. Defining empathy as 'the ability to conceptualize other people's inner worlds and to reflect on their thoughts and feelings' (Gillberg, 1992, p. 835), he proposed that empathy deficits are also important in tics/Tourette syndrome, attention-deficit hyperactivity disorder (ADHD) with motor/perceptual problems, anorexia nervosa and obsessive compulsive disorder (OCD). He suggested that the autism spectrum disorders may represent an extreme tail in a normal distribution of empathic ability. Subsequently, autistic traits have indeed been confirmed to be over-represented in anorexia nervosa (Wentz Nilsson *et al.*, 1999), OCD (Bejerot *et al.*, 2001), adolescent and criminal offenders (Siponmaa *et al.*, 2001; Soderstrom *et al.*, 2004), and in subjects with special abilities, such as absolute pitch (Brown *et al.*, 2003). Likewise, the notion of broader autistic phenotypes and 'shadow syndromes' characterized by social interaction difficulties, flexibility problems and aberrant communication has gained popular notice (Rathey & Johnson, 1997). Taken in Gillberg's cognitively oriented sense, empathy may stand out as a hallmark dysfunction in psychiatric disorders characterized by repetitive and stereotypical behaviours, problems with social reciprocity, allocentric thinking, or perception. Deficient empathy may also be one face of a coin where problems with self-regulation and control is the other face, synergistic and interacting through development.

Cognitive ToM deficits are thus not specific for autism, nor do they constitute a sufficient explanation for the 'enigma' of autism. Symptoms and signs of autism are generally present before the development of ToM proper at 2½ to 4 years of age (Perner & Lang, 1999), and the deficient ToM may be the end result of primary perceptual problems, e.g. in interpreting the face and the gaze of the mother and other caregivers as meaningful wholes rather than piecemeal. Specific problems with understanding other people's emotions from gazes, mimicry and voice have been demonstrated in autism (Baron-Cohen *et al.*, 1997; Rutherford *et al.*, 2002), and a weak 'central coherence' and a lack of drive towards creating coherent structures (more or less equivalent with 'Gestalts') have been proposed as core deficits, demonstrated through superior performances on the 'Embedded Figures Test' (Jolliffe & Baron-Cohen, 1997), and the Block Design subtest (compared to the object assembly subtest) in the Wechsler tests (Ehlers *et al.*, 1997). Because the ability to interpret social percepts and unite them to meaningful Gestalts may lie at the basis of the development of cognitive ToM skills, alternative theories of 'basic' psychological aberrations in autism may not be contradictory but rather complementary descriptions of processes that interact with one another as components of a non-linear dynamical system in the development of personality. 'High functioning' adults with autism spectrum disorders or autistic traits may also succeed all these tests, but perhaps they use unusual styles of information processing. The poor intuitive recognition of relations within a whole that is characteristic of individuals with autism spectrum disorders is similar to the deficit symptoms observed in some patients with schizophrenia, including asexuality (or perversions such as fetishism), avolition, asociality, alogia and autistic deficits in recognizing that the visual perspective of others may differ from one's own, corresponding to low temperament and character inventory (TCI) self-transcendence with a low intuitive insight into holistic relationships.

15.5 Autism and personality

Recently, empirical data on a 'broader phenotype' of autistic traits, over-represented among relatives of autistic probands and encompassing up to 10 % of the normal population, have supported the notion of autism representing a lowermost tail of a normally distributed variable measuring individual differences in social ease and responsiveness (Briskman *et al.*, 2001; Constantino & Todd, 2003). However, it is questionable whether a single variable measuring social responsiveness can fully capture individual differences in susceptibility to autism or to deficits in empathy. Except for cases of autism that are symptomatic of specific medical disorders, there are no data to show that the 'autism spectrum' disorders are discrete entities or taxons. The notion of a broader phenotype blending into the autism spectrum and autism proper may be regarded as a very promising hypothesis with a good deal of data supporting it and little evidence speaking against it. However, a single personality variable cannot account for variation in the multiple dimensions of human personality that are related to individual differences in the development of empathy. Substantial work on the autism spectrum condition has already shown that deficits in empathy are asso-ciated with multiple aspects of temperament and character. For example, subjects with autism spectrum disorders in studies using the TCI, detailed later, are high in Harm Avoidance (i.e. anxious and pessimistic), low in Novelty Seeking (i.e. rigid and preferring structured routines), low in Reward Dependence (i.e. aloof and detached), low in Self-directedness (i.e. immature and inept) and low in Cooperativeness (i.e. egocentrical and uncompassionate). These different aspects of personality interact to influence the degree of a person's empathy and quality of social relationships.

Hans Asperger initially defined the constellation of social interaction problems, monomanic fixations and communication abnormalities that has come to bear his name as a personality disorder ('Psychopathie' in German terminology). From the adult personality horizon, similar deficits in social bonding, communication and understanding have been proposed to form one core deficit in personality disor-ders, albeit described in a different terminology. Such overlap between definitions does not imply a perfect match, as exemplified by the fact that, although low on the group level, a number of adults with Asperger's syndrome have described them-selves as high in Reward Dependence (i.e. sociable and wanting approval), espe-cially in their emotional need for social stimulation (Soderstrom *et al.*, 2002), corresponding to the 'outgoing but odd' subtype of autism (Wing, 1983). These individuals may experience a significant need for social rewards and stimuli, even if they have difficulties in creating social relationships that may satisfy this longing, and are perceived by external observers as aloof. Such heterogeneity in personality among subjects with autism spectrum disorders shows the importance of the assessment of multiple personality dimensions from comprehensive inventories of the internal motivation of subjects, rather than overemphasis on a single dimension or externally observed social responsiveness.

In a classical description of a 'prototypical' personality disorder, psychopathy, Harvey Cleckley postulated that the core nucleus of the disorder lay in a deficient emotional processing of language (Cleckley, 1941), even if the disorder is generally described in much less functional, more social terms. Theories of personality often start from descriptions of how normal humans differ from each other to approach dysfunctional variants, whereas neuropsychiatry usually begins with clinical descriptions of clearly deficient abilities before later expanding consideration to broader phenotypes. A theoretical attempt to bridge the gap between these perspectives is offered by Cloninger's biopsychosocial model of personality.

Cloninger's seven-factor model contains both temperamental reaction patterns and dimensions of character maturation. For example, 'Cooperativeness' consists of the subscales 'Social Acceptance', 'Empathy', 'Helpfulness', 'Compassion' and 'Integrated Conscience', and is one of two major determinants of personality maturity versus disorder as defined traditionally in psychiatry. The other major determinant of personality maturity versus disorder is called 'Self-directedness' (Svrakic et al., 1993). In descriptions of adult personality disorders, problems in relation to others are often seen as another facet to problems in self-regulation (American Psychiatric Association, 1994; Cloninger et al., 1993). Self-monitoring and executive control may not only be developed in parallel with, but also play an important role in the development of, mentalizing about others, and both a cognitive Theory of Mind (ToM) and an awareness of self and others may be prerequisites for self-directedness (Cloninger, 2004; Perner & Lang, 1999). Autistic traits may be reflected in terms such as low 'Sociability' or low 'Reward Dependence', which is a temperamental pattern of impaired sensitivity to social cues. However, it is still necessary to ask to what extent individual differences in sensitivity to social cues brings us closer to the concept of 'empathy'. In fact, the temperamental dimension of Reward Dependence is empirically lower in subjects with autism spectrum disorders (Anckarsäter et al., 2006; Soderstrom et al., 2002). This dimension is also correlated with individual differences in the development of the empathy subscale of the character dimension cooperativeness (Cloninger et al., 1994). Consequently, individual differences in Reward Dependence do contribute to explaining individual differences in the development of empathy, in concert with other neurobiological and psychosocial processes

(Cloninger, 2004). For example, girls are higher on average in Reward Dependence than are boys, and also are higher in Cooperativeness (Cloninger *et al.*, 1994) and lower in their risk of autism spectrum conditions (Gillberg, 1995).

Adult subjects with Asperger's syndrome and other autism spectrum disorders describe themselves as severely deficient in both TCI Self-directedness and TCI Cooperativeness (Soderstrom *et al.*, 2002; Anckarsäter *et al.*, 2006). Self-transcendence has also consistently shown an abnormal structure in that subjects on the autistic spectrum are high in their capacity to be absorbed in details but are not well aware of the whole context (Frith, 1989), as indicated by higher scores on the self-forgetful subscale than on other subscales of TCI Self-transcendence (Anckarsäter *et al.*, 2006). In these groups, both Self-directedness and Cooperativeness have also been consistently negatively correlated with Harm Avoidance, indicating that anxiety, stress intolerance and pessimism are associated with an increased risk of personality immaturity and social interaction problems. Other temperamental foundations for character development may be illustrated by specific, positive associations between Reward Dependence and Cooperativeness, and negative associations between Novelty Seeking and Self-directedness, especially in subjects with ADHD (Anckarsäter *et al.*, 2006).

15.6 Empathy and personality

These findings with the TCI indicate that individual differences in each of the three branches of mental self-government, the executive functions measured by Self-directedness, legislative functions measured by Cooperativeness, and judicial functions measured by Self-transcendence, contribute to the development of empathy (Cloninger, 2004; Cloninger *et al.*, 1993). These three branches of mental self-government have also been described as skills in mentalizing, social inter-action and Gestalt formation. Each of these higher cognitive functions plays complementary roles in awareness of oneself, relationships to others and partici-pation in the world as a whole. They also have unique genetic determinants that contribute to different styles of information processing (Gillespie *et al.*, 2003), forming components of mental structure that influence vulnerability to a wide range of mental disorders (Cloninger, 2004).

Early-onset problems with mentalizing, social interaction and Gestalt formation may be dependent on deficient development of the right hemisphere, which is thought to be especially important for the infant's reactions to, and interactions with, the mother. The development of the 'social brain' is also thought to depend on adequate stimulation of the brain neonatally by oxytocin and vasopressin, which are themselves trophically guided by and influenced by the early develop-ing monoaminergic systems originating in the brainstem. Early-onset autism is associated with more prominent perceptual abnormalities than are seen even in patients with later-onset deficits in higher cognitive functioning. This suggests that the abnormal sensory functioning in autism may be the result of early neurodevelopmental deficits in the right hemisphere or in inter-hemispheric connectivity (Nydén *et al.*, 2004). Psycho-functional mechanisms hampering this maturation may involve problems in guiding and sustaining attention (which are required for a person to become aware of the complexity in social interactions and self-monitoring) and differences in impulse control (which requires the ability to be aware of consequences and context).

In Cloninger's more recent theory of self-awareness, the awareness of self and that of others are integrated as interactive components in the development of empathy. Empathy can be considered as a level of self-aware consciousness involving at least accurate social reciprocity or perhaps allocentric awareness, which is defined as being aware and accepting of others without judging and blaming. This development is influenced by other emotional drives, such as those toward repetitive and stereotyped behaviour (low Novelty Seeking), low sociability (aloof, low Reward Dependence), and problems with character maturation leading to deficient development of Self-directedness, Cooperativeness and Self-transcendence. From Cloninger's perspective, the development of empathy can be blocked by poor self-awareness, poor cognitive flexibility and/or deficits in contemplative thinking. In other words, the development of empathy is a complex adaptive process in which there are many psychobiological processes with distinct neurobiological and psychosocial influences (Cloninger, 2004). This can be described by considering the importance of aspects of Novelty Seeking, Reward Dependence, Self-directedness, Cooperativeness and Self-transcendence, being distinct psychobiological traits that interact through non-linear dynamic processes in the development of empathy, having distinct genetic determinants and distinct brain circuitry.

In a broad, non-psychiatric sense, empathy must be interpreted as the resulting overall behavioural and psychological manifestations of abilities involved in social perception, understanding, communication and interaction, as well as volitional processes and the effects of situational opportunity or restriction. Emotional capacity, affective states and psychosocial well-being exert important modulatory influences over a person's empathy. The non-static nature of empathy is demonstrated through the interplay of within-person and interpersonal dynamics. In Cloninger's biopsychosocial personal theory, empathy is partly, but not wholly, determined by the temperament dimension of Reward Dependence, which includes basic social reactive patterns using emotional processing. For example, sentimentality is a social component of Reward Dependence, which measures individual differences in emotional sensitivity and responsiveness to social cues.

This basic reactive, perceptual pattern of Reward Dependence is completed by a cognitive, conceptual set in the form of the character dimension Cooperativeness, which contains the subscale 'empathy'. As a subscale of TCI Cooperativeness, 'empathy' is the ability to look at things from the perspective of another, and it is moderately correlated with other subscales of Cooperativeness, which include the ability to be forgiving and compassionate (rather than being revengeful), to be helpful (rather than hostile), tolerant (rather than prejudicial) and principled (rather than opportunistic). Well-developed empathy requires the elevation of thought in self-aware consciousness to an allocentric perspective through the development of the higher cognitive functions measured by the three TCI character traits (Cloninger, 2004).

15.7 Empathy and psychiatric taxonomy

Deficient ability to reason about self and others may indeed be the core nucleus of the problems with self-regulation and social interaction that characterize mental disorders at large. ToM problems have been demonstrated in schizophrenia (Frith & Corcoran, 1996), uni- and bipolar mood disorders (Inoue *et al.*, 2004), 'social immaturity' (Muris *et al.*, 1998) and conduct disorder (Happé & Frith, 1996). Individual differences in the activation of the medial prefrontal cortex are important in self-referential thinking, such as the evaluation of internal cues of what is pleasant and unpleasant, which is an executive function that contributes to many mental disorders. These differences in activation of medial prefrontal cortex are strongly correlated with individual differences in the personality trait of Self-directedness measured in the TCI (Cloninger, 2004). Self-directedness is poorly developed in patients with Asperger's disorder, so poor Self-directedness is another contributor, besides Reward Dependence, to individual differences in the development of empathy.

Psychiatric research into the psychological mechanisms, aetiology and pathophysiology of deficient self-awareness and mentalizing has hitherto been hampered by the terminological and theoretical frame shift between child and adolescent psychiatry on the one hand and adult psychiatry and personality theory on the other. We now know that developmental disorders in childhood, involving neurological, behavioural and psychosocial functioning, are not rare. They affect at least 5% of children in severe forms and many more as broader phenotypes (Constantino & Todd, 2003; Kadesjo & Gillberg, 1998; Kadesjo *et al.*, 1999). Childhood-onset developmental disorders do not remit spontaneously in the majority of cases and are associated with a vast comorbid spectrum of mental health problems when followed up into adolescence or adulthood (Billstedt *et al.*, 2005; Rasmussen & Gillberg, 2000; Wolff, 1991). The child and adolescent psychiatric literature is usually based on studies of disorders that are described categorically (such as autism, ADHD, Tourette syndrome and OCD), whereas adult research on personality mainly uses quantitative descriptions. The difference in diagnostic practice and perspective between research traditions has created an artificial gap in information across the lifespan at about 18 years of age, which is unlikely to reflect any natural genetic mechanisms. It is clear that the dominant child psychiatric perspective that disorders are categories or taxons is not supported by evidence. Comorbidity is the rule rather than the exception (van Praag, 1996). Prevalence studies have always used categorical diagnostic criteria, assuming that discontinuities delineating natural classes of pathology really do exist. It is far more probable that the core features thought to be associated with such disorders (e.g. social interaction problems, attention or learning problems) affect more persons in 'shadow' forms than those meeting strict diagnostic criteria for caseness.

In adult personality research, the perspective has differed markedly from that in child psychiatric research. Even though the DSM system uses categorical definitions, it is generally assumed among professionals and lay persons alike that variation in personality is quantitative and multidimensional. Genetic variants associated with differences in such traits have been extensively studied by assessing differences in ratings of certain traits between carriers of polymorphisms in genes coding for proteins that influence neurotransmission and information processing in the brain. A growing body of literature has also used both categorical and quantitative assessments across the lifespan.

15.8 The genetics of empathy

We will now summarize available information on possible genetic mechanisms involved in interpersonal functioning and empathy from all these traditions, thus broadening the available information that may guide us in an area which has hitherto attracted far too few comprehensive programmes of research to understand the genetics of empathy. To do this with available data we will synthesize available information from several methodological approaches so that individual pieces of the epigenetic puzzle can be assembled like building blocks for a more complete picture of the reality of empathy. The study of genetic mechanisms involved in the development of social abilities and, on a higher level, of empathy is complicated by a number of obstacles. That hereditary factors play a role in creating differences in socially related traits or disorders is strongly supported by a wide range of studies, using adoptive children reared together or apart or comparisons of corresponding traits in dizygotic (DZ) and monozygotic (MZ) twin pairs. However, the genetics of empathy is far from established and understood in a contextual framework. Studies have hitherto largely neglected that hereditary and environmental factors may have different roles across social situations. Other familial, interpersonal and environmental mechanisms involved are not sufficiently known to chisel out the role of hereditary factors in the undoubtedly complex interplay of biological and psychosocial factors underlying the development of empathic and social abilities, which are among the most complex and unique in the human psychological apparatus.

Another challenge is the heterogeneity of assessment methods. Assessments of social, interpersonal and empathetic abilities in clinical practice and research are based either on psychological ratings of 'traits' associated with these abilities or of disordered 'states'. In contrast, the psychometric tests supposed to measure empathic abilities focus either on the identification of severely disordered states ('caseness') or on specific mechanisms involved which have an unclear bearing on a holistic understanding of empathy. For example, consider scales that identify symptoms of Asperger's syndrome, as well as laboratory tests measuring the ability to identify the emotional states of others in procedures, such as viewing faces of actors. We have a paucity of literature using quantitative measures of social abilities that may be perceived and assessed across situational and environmental modulatory influences. Most genetic work has been directed towards complex disordered states such as autism or personality disorder, taken as taxons assumed to be characterized by specific genetic aberrations, even though the evidence for a taxonomic structure of such states is doubtful. The literature review of this paper is based on comprehensive literature searches in PubMed using the search terms 'empathy' combined with either 'gene' (10 hits, January 2005) and 'genetics' (84 hits, January 2005), plus specific searches of genetic literature on childhood disorders and problems related to autism, and adult personality traits related to social interaction.

Genetic research into hereditary mechanisms involved in the development of a complex trait such as empathy/social interaction follow four main lines.

15.8.1 Adoption, twin and extended family research

There is clear and consistent evidence for genetic contributions to normal and abnormal personality traits, whether they are measured as quantitative traits or as clusters of personality disorders. Most data are about quantitative personality traits in adults. Abnormal traits defining adult personality disorders have been measured in twins using the Differential Assessment of Personality Pathology (DAPP). Monozygotic twins are consistently more concordant than dizygotic twins for abnormal personality traits, including traits related to empathy (see Table 15.1), such as callousness (56%), intimacy problems (48%), restricted expression of affect (41%), and social avoidance (53%) (Jang *et al.*, 1996). Aloof

Table 15.1: Heritability and concordances in 236 monozygotic (*MZ*) twin pairs and 247 dizygotic (*DZ*) twin pairs for the 18 basic scales of the Differential Assessment of Personality Pathology in Canada (Jang *et al.*, 1996)

Scale label	MZ correlation	DZ correlation	Heritability
Affective lability	0.49	0.12	0.45
Anxiousness	0.42	0.25	0.44
Callousness	0.56	0.32	0.56
Cognitive distortion	0.48	0.31	0.49
Compulsivity	0.40	0.19	0.37
Conduct problems	0.53	0.36	0.56
Identity problems	0.51	0.28	0.53
Insecure attachment	0.45	0.27	0.48
Intimacy problems	0.47	0.24	0.48
Narcissism	0.51	0.22	0.53
Oppositionality	0.41	0.29	0.46
Rejection	0.33	0.19	0.35
Restricted expression	0.48	0.26	0.41
Self-harm	0.39	0.26	0.41
Social avoidance	0.52	0.27	0.53
Stimulus-seeking	0.38	0.21	0.40
Submissiveness	0.41	0.29	0.45
Suspiciousness	0.42	0.29	0.45

Table 15.2: A study of categorical personality disorders (PDs), assessed by SCID-II interviews, in 92 MZ twin pairs and 129 DZ twin pairs in Norway (Torgersen *et al.*, 2000)

Diagnoses	MZ correlation	DZ correlation	Heritability
Any PD	0.58 ± 0.10	0.36 ± 0.10	0.44 ± 0.20
Any cluster A	0.37 ± 0.14	0.09 ± 0.11	0.37 ± 0.25
Any cluster B	0.60 ± 0.11	0.31 ± 0.12	0.59 ± 0.23
Any cluster C	0.61 ± 0.09	0.23 ± 0.11	0.59 ± 0.20

personality disorders, categorically defined, are also heritable according to a small study done in Norway (Torgersen *et al.*, 2000) (Table 15.2). Large-scale twin studies of comprehensive inventories that specify both normal and abnormal traits have shown that there are unique genetic determinants for every aspect of temperament and character, including those aspects of personality that are important in the development of empathy such as executive (i.e. TCI Self-directedness 34%), legislative (TCI Cooperativeness 27%), and judicial

Table 15.3: The total genetic effects (that is, heritability) of each of the 7 TCI personality dimensions estimated in 2517 twins in Australia (Gillespie *et al.*, 2003). Unique effects exclude genetic contributions shared with other personality dimensions

Personality dimension	Genetic effects	
	Total %	Unique %
Harm Avoidance	42	29
Novelty Seeking	39	32
Reward Dependence	35	20
Persistence	30	23
Self-directedness	34	25
Cooperativeness	27	16
Self-transcendence	45	26

functions (TCI Self-transcendence 45%), as well as relevant temperament traits such as Novelty Seeking (39%) and Reward Dependence (35%) (Gillespie *et al.*, 2003) (Table 15.3). With correction for the reliability of the short forms of the TCI used in these studies, the heritability of each of the seven TCI dimensions of personality is approximately 50%.

Studies of problems in social interaction among children provide additional evidence for genes contributing to individual differences in the development of empathy. In particular, when studied as categorical syndromes, the autism spectrum disorders are among the most heritable disorders that have been studied in psychiatry (Rutter, 1997). Several studies have shown an increase in risk for siblings of cases compared to controls, and higher concordances among MZ than DZ twins (Folstein & Rutter, 1977; Steffenburg *et al.*, 1989), yielding heritability estimates of nearly 90% for liability to autism that is not explained by specific medical conditions (Rutter *et al.*, 1999).

However, the heritability of liability to caseness for the most disabling forms of autism may be considerably higher than for the broader variants. Recent twin studies of quantitative autistic traits in the general population, such as social responsiveness, have shown considerably lower heritability (Constantino & Todd, 2003; Constantino *et al.*, 2003). An older study of the heritability of self-rated altruistic traits in twins from London, however, also showed strong heritability estimates: 56% for altruism, 68% for empathy and 72% for nurturance (Rushton *et al.*, 1984).

ADHD is another common child psychiatric disorder that is often associated with deficits in empathy (Kadesjo & Gillberg, 2001) and personality disorder

(Soderstrom *et al.*, 2005). Family (Biederman *et al.*, 1986), adoption (Cadoret & Stewart, 1991) and twin (Levy *et al.*, 1997; Sherman *et al.*, 1997) studies have shown a strong hereditary influence in ADHD and its components, both when studied as a categorical diagnosis and as continuous, dimensional measures (Larsson *et al.*, 2004; Thapar *et al.*, 2000). Hereditary factors for oppositional defiant disorder and conduct disorder have also been demonstrated through twin and adoption studies (Rhee & Waldman, 2002). Genetic influences seem to be more important for temperamental, aggressive antisocial behaviour that is persistent into adulthood as compared to non-aggressive, adolescent-limited behaviour (Eley *et al.*, 2003). Strong genetic effects have also been suggested for tic disorders, Tourette syndrome and OCD, although the early suggestions for Mendelian single-gene inheritance has not been supported by linkage trials, which remain inconclusive (Pauls *et al.*, 1991; Rutter *et al.*, 1999). Anorexia nervosa and bulimia nervosa are both strongly influenced by hereditary risk factors (Hudson *et al.*, 2003; Mangweth *et al.*, 2003; Strober *et al.*, 2000), and have been associated with empathy problems and alexithymia (Wentz Nilsson *et al.*, 1999).

A wide array of child and adolescent disorders associated with empathy problems are thus strongly genetic in their origins, and related to personality disorders and other mental disorders in adulthood. The child and adolescent precursors to the adult disorders provide intermediate developmental phenotypes that help to unravel the contributions of multiple genes and environmental factors to the development of empathy in adulthood.

15.8.2 Association with specific genetic disorders

Another possible line of study is to search for medical disorders caused by known genetic abnormalities and that influence the capacity for empathy. For example, autism is clearly over-represented in several genetic syndromes, Fragile X and tuberous sclerosis being the most common (Gillberg, 1995). Such associations also point to possible genetic mechanisms for very specific aspects of social interaction problems. Fragile X autism is characterized by specific gaze aversion, expressing an extreme sensitivity to meet other people's gaze (Gillberg, 1995). William's syndrome has often been used as a contrast to autism as it is characterized by mental retardation and hypersociability, with a relative ease in creating contact and maintaining 'cocktail' conversations. This disorder is due to a hemizygous deletion in chromosome band 7q11.23, in which the severity is possibly related to the size of the deletion (Donnai & Karmiloff-Smith, 2000; Doyle *et al.*, 2004).

15.8.3 Linkage studies

Susceptibility regions for autism have been identified in several large-scale projects assembling families, parent-child trios, or affected sib-pairs with autism. Many susceptibility sites have been found in one of these studies but have not been replicated, as is expected when gene–gene and gene–environment interactions are important. The regions that provide the most consistent evidence in meta-analyses include candidate regions on chromosomes 2q32 (IMGSAC, 2001), 3q25–27 (Auranen *et al.*, 2002) [both significant in a recent meta-analysis (Veenstra-Vanderweele *et al.*, 2004)], 7q21–36 (IMGSAC, 2001) especially 21–22 and 32–36 (the latter also related to language impairments, reviewed in Veenstra-VanderWeele & Cook, 2004), 16p13 (IMGSAC, 2001) and 17q (IMGSAC, 2001) (all these regions have shown linkage in more than one study according to the cited meta-analysis). For several, linkage has increased when only subjects with delayed speech development have been included in the analyses (Muhle *et al.*, 2004). These regions all contain many genetic polymorphisms, so it is not possible at present to identify specific genes with a known pathophysiology leading to autism based on linkage analyses alone.

15.8.4 Candidate gene research

When the pattern of inheritance is complex, as it appears to be for empathy and its disorders, association studies can be more powerful than linkage studies to demonstrate the effects of a specific gene. For example, some candidate genes for autism were suggested by their location on chromosome 15q11–13 because of frequent findings of cytogenetic aberrations in this area in subjects with autism (Gillberg, 1998) and of the occurrence of autism in Angelmann and Prader–Willi syndromes, which are caused by deletions in this area. Specifically, a gamma-aminobutyric acid (GABA) receptor A β3 subunit (GABRB3) polymorphism has been associated with autism in several studies (Cook *et al.*, 1998; Martin *et al.*, 2000).

A variable number tandem repeat (VNTR) polymorphism in the promoter gene for the serotonin transporter (5-HTTLPR) (17q12) is identified as functional and associated with personality, particularly social anxiety and Cooperativeness (Hamer *et al.*, 1999; Sabol *et al.*, 1999). This polymorphism has also been found to be associated with autism in some, but not all, studies (Cook *et al.*, 1997; Klauck *et al.*, 1997; Persico *et al.*, 2000). In contrast, the gene for the serotonin transporter (5-HTT) on chromosome 17p11.2 contains several VNTR, none of which has been associated with autism (Betancur *et al.*, 2002).

Several candidate genes have been studied because of evidence for abnormal prenatal development of the central nervous system in autism, including genes involved in neural development and neural tube closure during the first trimester of gestation, which is similar to the increased risk of autism following early exposure to valproic acid or thalidomide (Arndt *et al.*, 2005). In particular, the HOXA1 gene, a member of the gene family of homeobox transcription factors, is critical for the development of hindbrain neural structures and cranial features that are often abnormal in autism. The HOXA1 A218G polymorphism has been associated with autism, particularly cases with enlarged head circumference and dysmorphic features (Conciatori *et al.*, 2004).

Similarly, the reelin gene (RELN, potentially involved in neural migration during early development) located in the putative susceptibility region on chromosome 7q22 is associated with a rare disorder called autosomal recessive lissencephalopathy and may contain a long trinucleotide repeat polymorphism in the 5′ region which was overrepresented in autism in one study (Persico *et al.*, 2001), but not in others (Krebs *et al.*, 2002; Zhang *et al.*, 2002).

Likewise, mutations in the neuroligin genes (NLGN3, NLGN4, involved in synaptogenesis) on chromosome X (Xq13.1 and Xp22.3) were associated with autism in two families (Jamain *et al.*, 2003), and have later been found in mental retardation (Laumonnier *et al.*, 2004).

The glutamate receptor subunit GluR6 (GRIK2) (6q21) has three known polymorphisms for which a pattern of maternal transmission has been identified and linked to autism (Jamain *et al.*, 2002).

The vasopressin receptor 1 A (AVPR1A) has been associated with autism in a transmission disequilibrium test involving 115 trios with autism (Kim *et al.*, 2002). This association is particularly interesting because AVPRlA is also associated with individual differences in TCI Reward Dependence among anorexic subjects (Bachner-Melman *et al.*, 2005). The most common allele of the microsatellite RS1 of the vasopressin receptor gene is strongly associated with low Reward Dependence.

Oxytocin has been putatively implied in autism and social impairments, and two studies have found linkage for autism to the oxytocin receptor gene (OTR) on 3p25–26 (Auranen *et al.*, 2002; Shao *et al.*, 2002).

Several animal knock-out studies where behavioural effects of gene deletions are studied have reported genetic effects on stereotyped behaviours, especially mice with no functional dopamine transporter gene (DAT) (Rodriguiz *et al.*, 2004). In humans, highly stereotyped behaviours including self-injurious behaviours are frequently encountered in Rett syndrome, Prader–Willi, Lesch–Nyhan and other genetic syndromes (Gillberg & Soderstrom, 2003).

Studies have yielded a number of positive associations between dopamine-related genes and ADHD (Bobb *et al.*, 2004), some of which have been possible to replicate. Studies on genes influencing noradrenaline, which is another catecholamine of putative importance for cognition and focused attention, have also shown promising candidates for ADHD (Park *et al.*, 2004). A recent study suggested an association between a glutamate receptor and ADHD (Turic *et al.*, 2004). Genetic studies have also implicated various serotonin-related genes are associated with aggression in subjects with ADHD (Beitchman *et al.*, 2003; Retz, *et al.*, 2004).

15.9 Importance of gene–gene and gene–environment interactions for empathy

Findings about specific individual candidate genes have often proven to be inconsistently replicable when they are studied by independent groups, as has been the case with the association of the DRD4 dopamine receptor and Novelty Seeking (Kluger *et al.*, 2002; Schinka *et al.*, 2002). Such inconsistent results need to be evaluated within the general context of the role of personality dimensions as moderator variables in non-linear adaptive systems that are important for understanding complex processes such as the development of empathy and its disorders. As a result of their non-linear function as moderators, the inheritance of personality is expected to involve gene–gene and gene–environment interactions (Keltikangas-Jarvinen *et al.*, 2004; Kluger *et al.*, 2002). For most quantitative traits, individuals with intermediate values are better adapted than individuals with extremely high or low values, and individuals at each extreme are more prone to disorders. Unless the relevant interacting biopsychosocial variables are simultaneously measured, results with individual variables in different samples are expected to be inconsistent despite their validity in some contexts.

Molecular genetic studies on Novelty Seeking confirm the importance of non-linear gene–gene and gene–environment interactions in Novelty Seeking, which is usually low in autism spectrum disorders. A polymorphism of DAT is associated with individual differences in initiating and continuing to smoke cigarettes, an effect that is mediated by the joint association of cigarette smoking and the dopamine transporter with Novelty Seeking (Sabol *et al.*, 1999). In addition, the dopamine receptor DRD4 exon II seven-repeat allele has been associated with high Novelty Seeking and increased risk of opiate dependence (Kotler *et al.*, 1997). Other work has shown that Novelty Seeking is associated with the ten-repeat allele of the dopamine transporter DAT1 when the DRD4 seven-repeat allele is absent (Van Gestel *et al.*, 2002).

Novelty Seeking also depends on the three-way interaction of DRD4 with COMT and the serotonin transporter promoter's regulatory region (5-HTTLPR). In the absence of the short 5-HTTLPR allele (5HTTLPR L/L genotype) and in the presence of the high-activity COMT Val/Val genotype, Novelty Seeking scores are higher in the presence of the DRD4 seven-repeat allele (Benjamin *et al.*, 2000). Furthermore, within families, siblings who shared identical genotype groups for all three polymorphisms (COMT, DRD4 and 5-HTTLPR) had significantly correlated Novelty Seeking scores (intraclass correlation = 0.39 in 49 subjects, $p < 0.008$), while sibs with dissimilar genotypes in at least one polymorphism showed no significant correlation (intraclass coefficient $= 0.18$ in 110 subjects, $p = 0.09$). Similar interactions were also observed between these three polymorphisms and Novelty Seeking in an independent sample of unrelated subjects (Benjamin *et al.*, 2000) which has been replicated by independent investigators (Strobel *et al.*, 2003). A similar three-way interaction has been described for the temperament dimension Persistence with dopamine receptor genes type 4 (D4DR) and type 3 (D3DR), and the serotonin receptor gene type 2c (5-HT2c) (Ebstein *et al.*, 1997).

Gene–environment interaction has also been demonstrated for TCI Novelty Seeking in prospective population-based studies (Ekelund *et al.*, 1999; Keltikangas-Jarvinen *et al.*, 2003; Keltikangas-Jarvinen & Heinonen, 2003). The TCI was administered to two large birth cohorts of Finnish men and women, and the individuals who scored in the top 10% and bottom 10% of TCI Novelty Seeking were genotyped for the exon-3 repeat polymorphism of DRD4. The two-repeat and five-repeat alleles, which are rare in the Americas and Africa, were more than three times as frequent (16% versus 5%) in Finns who were very high in Novelty Seeking than in those who were very low in Novelty Seeking (Ekelund *et al.*, 1999; Keltikangas-Jarvinen *et al.*, 2003), and this difference was replicated in an independent sample (Keltikangas-Jarvinen *et al.*, 2003). The association with the two-repeat and five-repeat alleles was strongest for the two most adaptive aspects of Novelty Seeking, exploratory excitability and impulsive decision-making (Keltikangas-Jarvinen *et al.*, 2003). Finnish men and women with the two-repeat and five-repeat alleles of the exon three DRD4 polymorphism were higher in Novelty Seeking as adults if they experienced a hostile childhood environment, as measured by maternal reports of emotional distance and a strict authoritarian disciplinary style with physical punishment (Keltikangas-Jarvinen & Heinonen, 2003). The mother's reports of childhood environment were obtained when the children were aged 18–21 years, and genotyping and personality assessment of Novelty Seeking was done independently 15 years later. If children had the two-repeat or five-repeat alleles of the DRD4 polymorphism, their TCI Novelty Seeking scores were high if they were reared in a hostile childhood environment and their Novelty Seeking was low if they were reared in a kind and cooperative environment. Children with certain genotypes are likely to evoke a characteristic pattern of responses from their parents and others, and to select for themselves certain aspects from the available environments (Scarr & McCartney, 1983). However, therapeutic environments such as kind and cooperative parenting can evoke positive adaptation by modifying gene expression, which depends on the orchestrated interaction of many genes and environmental influences (Keltikangas-Jarvinen & Heinonen, 2003). Such complex gene–gene and gene–environmental interactions are well documented for other common diseases, such as coronary artery disease and hypertension (Sing *et al.*, 1996; Zerba *et al.*, 2000).

These studies provide a model of what needs to be done in future work to understand the epigenesis of empathy and autism spectrum disorders. Genetic research in child psychiatry has often been limited to categorical diagnoses and has not considered possible gene–environment or gene–gene interactions. The relative paucity of linkage findings in comparison to the number of families studied suggests that complex interactional patterns and heterogeneity are important in the development of empathy and its disorders. New approaches are called for as knowledge grows that the 'pure' syndromes of 'classical' autism or ADHD without any important comorbidity are not characteristic of the problem constellations encountered in clinical practice or epidemiological studies in the general population. Genetic heterogeneity is to be expected, and autistic problems may be a common developmental endpoint of a number of disturbances (Gillberg & Coleman, 2000). High-functioning cases, expressed rather as personality types than as severe disorders, may prove to be crucial phenotypes for genetic research, especially in efforts to characterize the interactions among genetic and environmental variables in the development of empathy.

These findings show that the regulation of gene expression related to the development of empathy is mediated by complex adaptive systems made up of multiple genetic and environmental factors. Personality is comprised of multiple heritable dimensions made up of unique but partially overlapping sets of epistatic genes (i.e. genes that interact non-additively with other genes). These developmental systems modulate brain states by modifying the transitory connections between changing distributed networks of neurones. The prominence of gene–gene and gene–environmental interactions is characteristic of most common diseases and quantitative phenotypes such as the personality traits related to the development of empathy (Cloninger, 2004).

15.10 Implications for further research

Further research on the genetics of empathy and its disorders is needed for specific reasons including:

1. Further understanding of, and acceptance for, individual differences in the basic mechanisms involved in social functioning may form the basis of treatments or other efforts aiming to promote cooperativeness and maturation even in persons with basic problems in these areas.

2. Further elucidation of these individual differences may help us understand the reactions of other persons, including perceived enemies or alien people on a societal macro-level, in a more truly empathic way, giving more success to social interaction strategies in handling conflict.
3. The identification of genes important for social functioning may point to specific brain circuits that may be targeted through pharmacological and psychological treatments in the future to alleviate the suffering inferred by deficient empathy in a range of mental disorders.

REFERENCES

American Psychiatric Association. (1994). *Diagnostic and Statistical Manual of Mental Disorders* (4th edn.). Washington, DC: American Psychiatric Association Press.

Anckarsäter, H., Stahlberg, O., Larson, T., *et al.* (2006). The impact of ADHD and autism spectrum disorders on temperament, character and personality development. *American Journal of Psychiatry*, **163(7)**, 1239–1244.

Arndt, T. L., Stodgell, C. J., & Rodier, P. M. (2005). The teratology of autism. *International Journal of Developmental Neuroscience*, **23(2–3)**, 189–199.

Auranen, M., Vanhala, R., Varilo, T., *et al.* (2002). A genomewide screen for autism-spectrum disorders: evidence for a major susceptibility locus on chromosome 3q25–27. *American Journal of Human Genetics*, **71(4)**, 777–790.

Bachner-Melman, R., Zohar, A. H., & Ebstein, R. P. (2005). The TPQ profile of anorexic women and its relationship to recovery. Paper presented at the World Congress of Psychiatry, Vienna.

Baron-Cohen, S., Leslie, A. M., & Frith, U. (1985). Does the autistic child have a 'theory of mind'? *Cognition*, **21(1)**, 37–46.

Baron-Cohen, S., Wheelwright, S., & Jolliffe, T. (1997). Is there a 'language of the eyes'? Evidence from normal adults and adults with autism or Asperger syndrome. *Visual Cognition*, **4(3)**, 311–331.

Beitchman, J. H., Davidge, K. M., Kennedy, J. L., *et al.* (2003). The serotonin transporter gene in aggressive children with and without ADHD and nonaggressive matched controls. *Annals of the New York Academy of Science*, **1008**, 248–251.

Bejerot, S., Nylander, L., & Lindstrom, E. (2001). Autistic traits in obsessive-compulsive disorder. *Nordic Journal of Psychiatry*, **55(3)**, 169–176.

Benjamin, J., Osher, Y., Kotler, M., *et al.* (2000). Association between tridimensional personality questionnaire (TPQ) traits and three functional polymorphisms: dopamine receptor D4 (DRD4), serotonin transporter promoter region (5-HTTLPR) and catechol O-methyltransferase (COMT). *Molecular Psychiatry*, **5(1)**, 96–100.

Betancur, C., Corbex, M., Spielewoy, C., *et al.* (2002). Serotonin transporter gene polymorphisms and hyperserotonemia in autistic disorder. *Molecular Psychiatry*, **7(1)**, 67–71.

Biederman, J., Munir, K., Knee, D., *et al.* (1986). A family study of patients with attention deficit disorder and normal controls. *Journal of Psychiatric Research*, **20(4)**, 263–274.

Billstedt, E., Gillberg, I. C., & Gillberg, C. (2005). Autism after adolescense: a population-based 13- to 22- year follow-up study of 120 individuals with autism diagnosed in childhood. *Journal of Autism and Developmental Disorders*, **35(3)**, 351–360.

Bobb, A. J., Castellanos, F. X., Addington, A. M., & Rapoport, J. L. (2004). Molecular genetic studies of ADHD: 1991 to 2004. *American Journal of Medical Genetics B Neuropsychiatric Genetics*, **132(1)**, 109–125.

Briskman, J., Happé, F., & Frith, U. (2001). Exploring the cognitive phenotype of autism: weak 'central coherence' in parents and siblings of children with autism: II. Real-life skills and preferences. *Journal of Child Psychology and Psychiatry*, **42(3)**, 309–316.

Brown, W. A., Cammuso, K., Sachs, H., *et al.* (2003). Autism-related language, personality and cognition in people with absolute pitch: results of a preliminary study. *Journal of Autism and Developmental Disorders*, **33(2)**, 163–167.

Buccino, G., Binkofski, F., Fink, G. R., *et al.* (2001). Action observation activates premotor and parietal areas in a somatotopic manner: an fMRI study. *European Journal of Neuroscience*, **13(2)**, 400–404.

Cadoret, R. J., & Stewart, M. A. (1991). An adoption study of attention deficit/hyperactivity/ aggression and their relationship to adult antisocial personality. *Comprehensive Psychiatry*, **32(1)**, 73–82.

Cleckley, H. (1941). *The Mask of Sanity*. St. Louis, Mo.: Mosby.

Cloninger, C. R. (2004). *Feeling Good: The Science of Well-Being*. New York: Oxford University Press.

Cloninger, C. R., Przybeck, T. R., Svrakic, D. M., & Wetzel, R. D. (1994). *The Temperament and Character Inventory: A Guide to Its Development and Use*. St. Louis, Mo.: Washington University Center for Psychobiology of Personality.

Cloninger, C. R., Svrakic, D. M., & Przybeck, T. R. (1993). A psychobiological model of temperament and character. *Archives of General Psychiatry*, **50(12)**, 975–990.

Conciatori, M., Stodgell, C. J., Hyman, S. L., *et al.* (2004). Association between HOXA1 A218G polymorphism and increased head circumference in patients with autism. *Biological Psychiatry*, **55**, 413–419.

Constantino, J. N., Gruber, C. P., Davis, S., *et al.* (2004). The factor structure of autistic traits. *Journal of Child Psychology and Psychiatry*, **45(4)**, 719–726.

Constantino, J. N., Hudziak, J. J., & Todd, R. D. (2003). Deficits in reciprocal social behavior in male twins: evidence for a genetically independent domain of psychopathology. *Journal of the American Academy of Child and Adolescent Psychiatry*, **42(4)**, 458–467.

Constantino, J. N., & Todd, R. D. (2003). Autistic traits in the general population: a twin study. *Archives of General Psychiatry*, **60(5)**, 524–530.

Cook, E. H., Jr., Courchesne, R. Y., Cox, N. J., *et al.* (1998). Linkage-disequilibrium mapping of autistic disorder, with 15q11–13 markers. *American Journal of Human Genetics*, **62(5)**, 1077–1083.

Cook, E. H., Jr., Courchesne, R., Lord, C., *et al.* (1997). Evidence of linkage between the serotonin transporter and autistic disorder. *Molecular Psychiatry*, **2(3)**, 247–250.

Donnai, D., & Karmiloff-Smith, A. (2000). Williams syndrome: from genotype through to the cognitive phenotype. *American Journal of Medical Genetics*, **97(2)**, 164–171.

Doyle, T. F., Bellugi, U., Korenberg, J. R., & Graham, J. (2004). 'Everybody in the world is my friend' hypersociability in young children with Williams syndrome. *American Journal of Medical Genetics A*, **124(3)**, 263–273.

Ebstein, R. P., Segman, R., Benjamin, J., *et al.* (1997). 5-HT2C (HTR2C) serotonin receptor gene polymorphism associated with the human personality trait of reward dependence: interaction with dopamine D4 receptor (D4DR) and dopamine D3 receptor (D3DR) polymorphisms. *American Journal of Medical Genetics*, **74(1)**, 65–72.

Ehlers, S., Nydén, A., Gillberg, C., *et al.* (1997). Asperger syndrome, autism and attention disorders: a comparative study of the cognitive profiles of 120 children. *Journal of Child Psychology and Psychiatry*, **38(2)**, 207–217.

Ekelund, J., Lichtermann, D., Jarvelin, M. R., & Peltonen, L. (1999). Association between novelty seeking and the type 4 dopamine receptor gene in a large Finnish cohort sample. *American Journal of Psychiatry*, **156(9)**, 1453–1455.

Eley, T. C., Lichtenstein, P., & Moffitt, T. E. (2003). A longitudinal behavioral genetic analysis of the etiology of aggressive and nonaggressive antisocial behavior. *Developmental Psychopathology*, **15(2)**, 383–402.

Folstein, S., & Rutter, M. (1977). Infantile autism: a genetic study of 21 twin pairs. *Journal of Child Psychology and Psychiatry*, **18(4)**, 297–321.

Frith, C. D., & Corcoran, R. (1996). Exploring 'theory of mind' in people with schizophrenia. *Psychological Medicine*, **26(3)**, 521–530.

Frith, U. (1989). *Autism: Explaining the Enigma*. Oxford: Basil Blackwell.

Gillberg, C. (1992). The Emanuel Miller Memorial Lecture 1991. Autism and autistic-like conditions: subclasses among disorders of empathy. *Journal of Child Psychology and Psychiatry*, **33(5)**, 813–842.

Gillberg, C. (1995). *Clinical Child Neuropsychiatry*. Cambridge: Cambridge University Press.

Gillberg, C. (1998). Chromosomal disorders and autism. *Journal of Autism and Developmental Disorders*, **28(5)**, 415–425.

Gillberg, C., & Coleman, M. (2000). *The Biology of the Autistic Syndromes*, 3rd edn. London: Mac Keith.

Gillberg, C., & Soderstrom, H. (2003). Learning disability. *Lancet*, **362(9386)**, 811–821.

Gillespie, N. A., Cloninger, C. R., Heath, A. C., & Martin, N. G. (2003). The genetic and environmental relationship between Cloninger's dimensions of temperament and character. *Personal and Individual Differences*, **35(8)**, 1931–1946.

Gopnik, A., & Astington, J. W. (1988). Children's understanding of representational change and its relation to the understanding of false belief and the appearance-reality distinction. *Child Development*, **59(1)**, 26–37.

Gopnik, A., & Wellman, H. M. (1992). Why the child's theory of mind really is a theory. *Mind Language*, **7(1–2)**, 145–171.

Hamer, D. H., Greenberg, B. D., Sabol, S. Z., & Murphy, D. L. (1999). Role of the serotonin transporter gene in temperament and character. *Journal of Personality Disorders*, **13**(4), 312–327.

Happé, F., Ehlers, S., Fletcher, P., *et al.* (1996). 'Theory of mind' in the brain. Evidence from a PET scan study of Asperger syndrome. *Neuroreport*, **8**(1), 197–201.

Happé, F., & Frith, U. (1996). Theory of mind and social impairment in children with conduct disorder. *British Journal of Developmental Psychology*, **14**, 385–398.

Hogrefe, J. G., Wimmer, H., & Perner, J. (1986). Ignorance versus false belief: a developmental lag in attribution of epistemic states. *Child Development*, **57**(3), 567–582.

Hudson, J. I., Mangweth, B., Pope, H. G., Jr., *et al.* (2003). Family study of affective spectrum disorder. *Archives of General Psychiatry*, **60**(2), 170–177.

IMGSAC. (2001). A genomewide screen for autism: strong evidence for linkage to chromosomes 2q, 7q, and 16p. *American Journal of Human Genetics*, **69**(3), 570–581.

Inoue, Y., Tonooka, Y., Yamada, K., & Kanba, S. (2004). Deficiency of theory of mind in patients with remitted mood disorder. *Journal of Affective Disorders*, **82**(3), 403–409.

Jamain, S., Betancur, C., Quach, H., *et al.* (2002). Linkage and association of the glutamate receptor 6 gene with autism. *Molecular Psychiatry*, **7**(3), 302–310.

Jamain, S., Quach, H., Betancur, C., *et al.* (2003). Mutations of the X-linked genes encoding neuroligins NLGN3 and NLGN4 are associated with autism. *Nature Genetics*, **34**(1), 27–29.

Jang, K. L., Livesley, W. J., Vernon, P. A., & Jackson, D. N. (1996). Heritability of personality disorder traits: a twin study. *Acta Psychiatrica Scandinavica*, **94**(6), 438–444.

Jolliffe, T., & Baron-Cohen, S. (1997). Are people with autism and Asperger syndrome faster than normal on the Embedded Figures Test? *Journal of Child Psychology and Psychiatry*, **38**(5), 527–534.

Kadesjo, B., & Gillberg, C. (1998). Attention deficits and clumsiness in Swedish 7-year-old children. *Developmental Medicine and Child Neurology*, **40**(12), 796–804.

Kadesjo, B., & Gillberg, C. (2001). The comorbidity of ADHD in the general population of Swedish school-age children. *Journal of Child Psychology and Psychiatry*, **42**(4), 487–492.

Kadesjo, B., Gillberg, C., & Hagberg, B. (1999). Brief report: autism and Asperger syndrome in seven-year-old children: a total population study. *Journal of Autism and Developmental Disorders*, **29**(4), 327–331.

Keltikangas-Jarvinen, L., Elovainio, M., Kivimaki, M., *et al.* (2003). Association between the type 4 dopamine receptor gene polymorphism and novelty seeking. *Psychosomatic Medicine*, **65**(3), 471–476.

Keltikangas-Jarvinen, L., & Heinonen, K. (2003). Childhood roots of adulthood hostility: family factors as predictors of cognitive and affective hostility. *Child Development*, **74**(6), 1751–1768.

Keltikangas-Jarvinen, L., Raikkonen, K., Ekelund, J., & Peltonen, L. (2004). Nature and nurture in novelty seeking. *Molecular Psychiatry*, **9**(3), 308–311.

Kim, S. J., Young, L. J., Gonen, D., *et al.* (2002). Transmission disequilibrium testing of arginine vasopressin receptor 1 A (AVPR1A) polymorphisms in autism. *Molecular Psychiatry*, **7**(5), 503–507.

Klauck, S. M., Poustka, F., Benner, A., Lesch, K. P., & Poustka, A. (1997). Serotonin transporter (5-HTT) gene variants associated with autism? *Human Molecular Genetics*, **6(13)**, 2233–2238.

Kluger, A. N., Siegfried, Z., & Ebstein, R. P. (2002). A meta-analysis of the association between DRD4 polymorphism and novelty seeking. *Molecular Psychiatry*, **7(7)**, 712–717.

Kotler, M., Cohen, H., Segman, R., *et al.* (1997). Excess dopamine D4 receptor (D4DR) exon III seven repeat allele in opioid-dependent subjects. *Molecular Psychiatry*, **2(3)**, 251–254.

Krebs, M. O., Betancur, C., Leroy, S., Bourdel, M. C., Gillberg, C., & Leboyer, M. (2002). Absence of association between a polymorphic GGC repeat in the 5′ untranslated region of the reelin gene and autism. *Molecular Psychiatry*, **7(7)**, 801–804.

Larsson, J. O., Larsson, H., & Lichtenstein, P. (2004). Genetic and environmental contributions to stability and change of ADHD symptoms between 8 and 13 years of age: a longitudinal twin study. *Journal of the American Academy of Child and Adolescent Psychiatry*, **43(10)**, 1267–1275.

Laumonnier, F., Bonnet-Brilhault, F., Gomot, M., *et al.* (2004). X-linked mental retardation and autism are associated with a mutation in the NLGN4 gene, a member of the neuroligin family. *American Journal of Human Genetics*, **74(3)**, 552–557.

Levy, F., Hay, D. A., McStephen, M., Wood, C., & Waldman, I. (1997). Attention-deficit hyperactivity disorder: a category or a continuum? Genetic analysis of a large-scale twin study. *Journal of the American Academy of Child and Adolescent Psychiatry*, **36(6)**, 737–744.

Mangweth, B., Hudson, J. I., Pope, H. G., *et al.* (2003). Family study of the aggregation of eating disorders and mood disorders. *Psychological Medicine*, **33(7)**, 1319–1323.

Martin, E. R., Menold, M. M., Wolpert, C. M., *et al.* (2000). Analysis of linkage disequilibrium in gamma-aminobutyric acid receptor subunit genes in autistic disorder. *American Journal of Medical Genetics*, **96(1)**, 43–48.

Muhle, R., Trentacoste, S. V., & Rapin, I. (2004). The genetics of autism. *Pediatrics*, **113(5)**, e472–486.

Muris, P., Steerneman, P., & Merckelbach, H. (1998). Difficulties in the understanding of false belief: specific to autism and other pervasive developmental disorders? *Psychological RepoA*, **82(1)**, 51–57.

Nydén, A., Carlsson, M., Carlsson, A., & Gillberg, C. (2004). Interhemispheric transfer in high-functioning children and adolescents with autism spectrum disorders: a controlled pilot study. *Developmental Medicine and Child Neurology*, **46(7)**, 448–454.

Park, L., Nigg, J. T., Waldman, I. D., *et al.* (2004). Association and linkage of alpha-2 A adrenergic receptor gene polymorphisms with childhood ADHD. *Molecular Psychiatry*, **10(6)**, 572–580.

Pauls, D. L., Raymond, C. L., Stevenson, J. M., & Leckman, J. F. (1991). A family study of Gilles de la Tourette syndrome. *American Journal of Human Genetics*, **48(1)**, 154–163.

Perner, J., & Lang, B. (1999). Development of theory of mind and executive control. *Trends in Cognitive Science*, **3(9)**, 337–344.

Persico, A. M., Militerni, R., Bravaccio, C., *et al.* (2000). Lack of association between serotonin transporter gene promoter variants and autistic disorder in two ethnically distinct samples. *American Journal of Medical Genetics*, **96(1)**, 123–127.

Persico, A. M., D'Agruma, L., Maiorano, N., *et al.* (2001). Reelin gene alleles and haplotypes as a factor predisposing to autistic disorder. *Molecular Psychiatry*, **6(2)**, 150–159.

Premack, D., & Woodruff, G. (1978). Does the chimpanzee have a theory of mind? *Behavioral and Brain Science*, **1**, 515–526.

Rasmussen, P., & Gillberg, C. (2000). Natural outcome of ADHD with developmental coordination disorder at age 22 years: a controlled, longitudinal, community-based study. *Journal of the American Academy of Child and Adolescent Psychiatry*, **39(11)**, 1424–1431.

Rathey, J. J., & Johnson, C. (1997). *Shadow Syndromes*. New York: Pantheon Books.

Retz, W., Retz-Junginger, P., Supprian, T., Thome, J., & Rosler, M. (2004). Association of serotonin transporter promoter gene polymorphism with violence: relation with personality disorders, impulsivity, and childhood ADHD psychopathology. *Behavioral Sciences and the Law*, **22(3)**, 415–425.

Rhee, S. H., & Waldman, I. D. (2002). Genetic and environmental influences on antisocial behavior: a meta-analysis of twin and adoption studies. *Psychological Bulletin*, **128(3)**, 490–529.

Rodriguiz, R. M., Chu, R., Caron, M. G., & Wetsel, W. C. (2004). Aberrant responses in social interaction of dopamine transporter knockout mice. *Behavioral Brain Research*, **148(1–2)**, 185–198.

Ronald, A., Happé, F., & Plomin, R. (2006). Autistic-like features in a community sample of 7-year-olds: genetic evidence for separate social and non-social components. In press.

Rushton, J. P., Fulker, D. W., Neale, M. C., Blizard, R. A., & Eysenck, H. J. (1984). Altruism and genetics. *Acta Geneticae Medicae et Gemellologiae (Roma)*, **33(2)**, 265–271.

Rutherford, M. D., Baron-Cohen, S., & Wheelwright, S. (2002). Reading the mind in the voice: a study with normal adults and adults with Asperger syndrome and high functioning autism. *Journal of Autism and Developmental Disorders*, **32(3)**, 189–194.

Rutter, M. (1997). Implications of genetic research for child psychiatry. *Canadian Journal of Psychiatry*, **42(6)**, 569–576.

Rutter, M., Silberg, J., O'Connor, T., & Simonoff, E. (1999). Genetics and child psychiatry: II Empirical research findings. *Journal of Child Psychology and Psychiatry*, **40(1)**, 19–55.

Sabol, S. Z., Nelson, M. L., Fisher, C., *et al.* (1999). A genetic association for cigarette smoking behavior. *Health Psychology*, **18(1)**, 7–13.

Scarr, S., & McCartney, K. (1983). How people make their own environments: a theory of genotype greater than environment effects. *Child Development*, **54(2)**, 424–435.

Schinka, J. A., Letsch, E. A., & Crawford, F. C. (2002). DRD4 and novelty seeking: results of meta-analyses. *American Journal of Medical Genetics*, **114(6)**, 643–648.

Shao, Y., Wolpert, C. M., Raiford, K. L., *et al.* (2002). Genomic screen and follow-up analysis for autistic disorder. *American Journal of Medical Genetics*, **114(1)**, 99–105.

Sherman, D. K., Iacono, W. G., & McGue, M. K. (1997). Attention-deficit hyperactivity disorder dimensions: a twin study of inattention and impulsivity-hyperactivity. *Journal of the American Academy of Child and Adolescent Psychiatry*, **36**(6), 745–753.

Sing, C. F., Haviland, M. B., & Reilly, S. L. (1996). Genetic architecture of common multi-factorial diseases. *Ciba Foundation Symposium*, **197**, 211–229; discussion 229–232.

Siponmaa, L., Kristiansson, M., Jonson, C., Nydén, A., & Gillberg, C. (2001). Juvenile and young adult mentally disordered offenders: the role of child neuropsychiatric disorders. *Journal of the American Academy of Psychiatry and the Law*, **29**(4), 420–426.

Soderstrom, H., Nilsson, T., Sjodin, A. K., Carlstedt, A., & Forsman, A. (2005). The childhood-onset neuropsychiatric background to adulthood psychopathic traits and personality disorders. *Comprehensive Psychiatry*, **46**(2), 111–116.

Soderstrom, H., Rastam, M., & Gillberg, C. (2002). Temperament and character in adults with Asperger syndrome. *Autism*, **6**(3), 287–297.

Soderstrom, H., Sjodin, A. K., Carlstedt, A., & Forsman, A. (2004). Adult psychopathic personality with childhood-onset hyperactivity and conduct disorder: a central problem constellation in forensic psychiatry. *Psychiatry Research*, **121**(3), 271–280.

Spiker, D., Lotspeich, L. J., Dimiceli, S., Myers, R. M., & Risch, N. (2002). Behavioral phenotypic variation in autism multiplex families: evidence for a continuous severity gradient. *American Journal of Medical Genetics*, **114**(2), 129–136.

Steffenburg, S., Gillberg, C., Hellgren, L., *et al.* (1989). A twin study of autism in Denmark, Finland, Iceland, Norway and Sweden. *Journal of Child Psychology and Psychiatry*, **30**(3), 405–416.

Strobel, A., Lesch, K. P., Jatzke, S., Paetzold, F., & Brocke, B. (2003). Further evidence for a modulation of Novelty Seeking by DRD4 exon III, 5-HTTLPR, and COMT val/met variants. *Molecular Psychiatry*, **8**(3), 371–372.

Strober, M., Freeman, R., Lampert, C., Diamond, J., & Kaye, W. (2000). Controlled family study of anorexia nervosa and bulimia nervosa: evidence of shared liability and transmission of partial syndromes. *American Journal of Psychiatry*, **157**(3), 393–401.

Svrakic, D. M., Whitehead, C., Przybeck, T. R., & Cloninger, C. R. (1993). Differential diagnosis of personality disorders by the seven-factor model of temperament and character. *Archives of General Psychiatry*, **50**(12), 991–999.

Szatmari, P., Merette, C., Bryson, S. E., *et al.* (2002). Quantifying dimensions in autism: a factor-analytic study. *Journal of the American Academy of Child and Adolescent Psychiatry*, **41**(4), 467–474.

Thapar, A., Harrington, R., Ross, K., & McGuffin, P. (2000). Does the definition of ADHD affect heritability? *Journal of the American Academy of Child and Adolescent Psychiatry*, **39**(12), 1528–1536.

Torgersen, S., Lygren, S., Orien, P. A., *et al.* (2000). A twin study of personality disorders. *Comprehensive Psychiatry*, **41**(6), 416–425.

Turic, D., Langley, K., Mills, S., *et al.* (2004). Follow-up of genetic linkage findings on chromosome 16p13: evidence of association of *N*-methyl-D aspartate glutamate receptor 2 A gene polymorphism with ADHD. *Molecular Psychiatry*, **9**(2), 169–173.

Van Gestel, S., Forsgren, T., Claes, S., *et al.* (2002). Epistatic effects of genes from the dopamine and serotonin systems on the temperament traits of novelty seeking and harm avoidance. *Molecular Psychiatry*, **7(5)**, 448–450.

van Praag, H. M. (1996). Comorbidity (psycho) analysed. *British Journal of Psychiatry Supplement*, **30**, 129–134.

Veenstra-Vanderweele, J., Christian, S. L., & Cook, E. H., Jr. (2004). Autism as a paradigmatic complex genetic disorder. *Annual Review of Genomics and Human Genetics*, **5**, 379–405.

Veenstra-Vanderweele, J., & Cook, E. H., Jr. (2004). Molecular genetics of autism spectrum disorder. *Molecular Psychiatry*, **9(9)**, 819–832.

Wentz Nilsson, E. W., Gillberg, C., Gillberg, I. C., & Rastam, M. (1999). Ten-year follow-up of adolescent-onset anorexia nervosa: personality disorders. *Journal of the American Academy of Child and Adolescent Psychiatry*, **38(11)**, 1389–1395.

Wing, L. (1981). Language, social, and cognitive impairments in autism and severe mental retardation. *Journal of Autism and Developmental Disorders*, **11(1)**, 31–44.

Wing, L. (1983). Social and interpersonal needs. In E. Schopler, & G. B. Mesibov (eds.), *Autism in Adolescents and Adults* (pp. 337–354). New York: Plenum Press.

Wing, L. (1996). Autistic spectrum disorders. *British Medical Journal*, **312(7027)**, 327–328.

Wolff, S. (1991). 'Schizoid' personality in childhood and adult life: I. The vagaries of diagnostic labelling. *British Journal of Psychiatry*, **159**, 615–620, 634–635.

Zerba, K. E., Ferrell, R. E., & Sing, C. F. (2000). Complex adaptive systems and human health: the influence of common genotypes of the apolipoprotein E (ApoE) gene polymorphism and age on the relational order within a field of lipid metabolism traits. *Human Genetics*, **107(5)**, 466–475.

Zhang, H., Liu, X., Zhang, C., *et al.* (2002). Reelin gene alleles and susceptibility to autism spectrum disorders. *Molecular Psychiatry*, **7(9)**, 1012–1017.

16

Empathogenic agents: their use, abuse, mechanism of action and addiction potential

Dan Velea and Michel Hautefeuille

Addictions Unit, Marmottan Hospital

Many substances promote empathy, but the most common are ecstasy (MDMA) like and some newer chemical molecules like ketamine, phencyclidine and LSD. We suggest however that substances that are not inherently empathetic (e.g. smart drugs) can also fulfil this function.

Research underlines the possible role of serotonergic neurotransmitters and the involvement of mirror neurons in this type of empathy seeking behaviour. From a clinical point of view, it is important to highlight the difference between these two situations, as it will impact on the type of care proposed and on the global understanding we have of drug consumption phenomena, especially among young people, most of whom are recreational users.

16.1 Introduction

In a society driven by 'performance worship' (Ehrenberg, 1991), and where the notion of individuality is breaking up, relationships between individuals are more and more based on power and competition. Solitude, feelings of incompleteness, withdrawal into oneself and difficulties being noticed by peers are signs of being a misfit and of poor psychosocial integration (Alexander, 1990; Erickson, 1963). The recourse to self-medication and psychoactive substances that can modify one's state of consciousness, mood and thought processes (sometimes using prescription medicines, but mainly illegal drugs) is continuously growing. This recourse to self-medication can be seen as a behavioural adaptation and a way of dealing with problems in life (addiction, marginality, criminality, self-consciousness, anxiety, depression and suicidality).

The problems therefore to be considered are that of a society using chemicals for enjoyment, to promote empathy and happiness and to enhance

Empathy in Mental Illness, eds. Tom F. D. Farrow and Peter W. R. Woodruff. Published by Cambridge University Press. © Cambridge University Press 2007.

performance – problems that are encountered in all social classes: stressed managers looking to increase their intellectual performance, athletes doping to increase their physical abilities and students and ordinary employees abusing psychoactive medicines. The various substances used can be seen as 'chemical crutches' (Velea, 2002a, 2005) as they facilitate the creation of new social relationships induced by drug use and abuse. In this context, social constraints become bearable and the individual feels independent while remaining within society. Ultimately, the problem of the individual's autonomy and independence is solved by the use of stimulant products. In a way, drugs are becoming a means for 'social and relational integration' (Ehrenberg, 1991). The image of marginality, alienation and social deviance that has previously been associated with drug use has been replaced with an image of socialization and social integration. Psychotropic medicines are becoming the means for the chemical control of social unrest.

Psychoactive substances are also often used to promote empathy within the rave and club scene. The image of young people looking for social interaction and recognition, and using/abusing drugs known for their empathogenic quality (MDMA – ecstasy, MDA, MBDM, MDEA) has mainly negative connotations. Very few studies have looked into these users' real motivations, their uneasiness about life and integration, the pain resulting from a lack of social and individual recognition and of real personal relationships. This chapter will also look into aspects of solitary drug use seen as a pursuit of 'self-empathy' – a concept that includes self-acceptance and management of alexithymia (the inability to express one's feelings).

16.2 The empathy concept

The simplest definition of 'empathy' concerns the ability of a person to imagine being in another's place and to understand their feelings, desires, representations and actions. This concept was first used in 1759 (Smith, 1759) under the term 'sympathy', which implied identification with another person and the sharing of feelings and emotions in the context of inter-individual relationships. Vischer (1873) and Lotze (1923) analysed the human ability to understand inanimate objects and various animal species by taking their perspective (Gallese, 2003). Empathy is a translation of the German word Einfülhung, introduced by Lipps (1903a) in the field of intersubjectivity and the observation and imitation of other people's movements and actions (*ich fühle mich so in him = I feel myself so much in him*) (Lipps, 1903b). Other authors (Sheets-Johnstone, 1999) introduced the idea of the 'living body' as a tool with which to share both emotional and sensorial experiences. According to Stein (1964), *empathy* not only covers the understanding of another's feelings and emotions, but also implies an element of experimentation, imitation and even identifying with another through the sharing of experiences.

For empathy to exist requires self-awareness or insight. Without self-awareness and without being able to express one's emotions, a situation arises where the pursuit of empathy can only be achieved by drug use. This is often the case in people suffering from alexithymia who cannot express their feelings and emotions (Sifneos, 1973). Alexithymia includes a difficulty in communicating feelings to others, the inability to identify one's own emotions and poverty of imagination (Taylor *et al.*, 1997). All these inabilities are perceived by users as capable of being overcome by drug use.

One of the aetiological hypotheses for alexithymia puts forward the idea of an inadequate connection between the limbic system (the part of the brain related to emotion that connects to the amygdala) and the language areas of the neocortex due to a regulation disturbance by the basal ganglia (Sifneos, 1996). Another hypothesis is based around the asymmetry between the brain hemispheres and the functional balance between them (Farges & Farges, 2002).

Several studies (Havilland, *et al.*, 1994; Keller *et al.*, 1995; Krystal, 1979; Wurmser, 1974) report links between alexithymic characteristics and addictive behaviours – particularly those involving empathogenic and/or psychoactive drugs (Farges & Farges, 2002). This has led to the idea that the use of psychoactive substances may modulate emotions and impulses and allow their expression.

Regarding the clinical assessment of patients using drugs to promote empathy, we hypothesize that, for patients with characteristics of alexithymia, empathogenic drug use could have a self-medicating role in their search for self-empathy (both self-acceptance and help in expressing one's own emotions). Unlike narcissism, self-empathy involves self-acceptance.

16.3 Raves and the pursuit of empathy

The rave scene provides good examples of individuals seeking an empathic experience. At raves, the psychological state of individuals looking for a state of modified consciousness is influenced by several factors: the context, the collective trance phenomenon, the musical atmosphere, especially the rhythm of the music, projected images (often fractals) and, most important, the other participants. For many, participating in a rave allows an escape from their daily cultural and social conditioning.

An aspect that is often emphasized by ravers is the absence, or rather the simplicity, of the language used. Communication occurs at a non-verbal level through gestures and imitation. The communication process becomes a sharing of emotions and sensations.

We will analyse the use of, and dependency caused by, current psychoactive and empathogenic substances as well as other drugs used at raves to achieve an empathic experience, individuality and integration into a group. Our analysis will review the substrates and neurological mechanisms involved in empathy, based on the psychological effects of each substance, taking the effects of MDMA (ecstasy) as a comparator.

16.4 The concept of recreational use and addiction

It should be emphasized here that most users of psychoactive/empathogenic substances participate in recreational use without any dependency occurring. Recreational use is characterized by the fact that drug use happens in particular circumstances (e.g. enjoyable use in the context of a party, often in a group). The most frequently used recreational drugs are cannabis and ecstasy. The user seeks a feeling of pleasure, of well-being, appeasement or disinhibition, communication and self-knowledge or self-insight. The search for sensation and novelty, for social interaction, adherence to a group, transgression of conventions, and for initiatory rituals are also part of users' motivations. Some users can show signs of problematic behaviours (Jessor, 1998), but the common aim remains the enhancement of empathy. This type of use generally has no negative socioprofessional consequences.

Definitions of dependence and addiction are given in international classifications such as the *Diagnostic and Statistical Manual of Mental Disorders* (DSM-IV; American Psychiatric Association, 2004) or the Goodman criteria (Goodman, 1990).

A very important dimension, which we have already mentioned, is the search for sensation and novelty. This is expressed by the need for new, complex and varied experiences, and the willingness to take physical and social risks to obtain and maintain a high level of brain stimulation. This sensation-seeking behaviour implies a disinhibition that is often encountered among individuals who are looking for ways to enhance empathy. The unpredictable nature of these experiences and the high level of risk-taking facilitate increased levels of excitation. The level of an individual's sensation-seeking behaviour can be objectively measured with tools such as the Zuckermann sensation-seeking scale (Zuckermann, 1994); Figure 16.1.

The highest incidence of sensation seeking is often encountered among people who are highly dependent on pharmaceutics, such as alcohol and drug users, and among those exhibiting risky behaviour. These people are extrovert in nature, on a permanent search for stimulation and often have equally non-conforming and risk-taking partners. Their antisocial way of life is the result of activities required to continuously satisfy their impulses. Social conventions and laws are often transgressed in order to obtain excitement at any price. It is also true that users who suffer from a lack of social and emotional interactions (psychopathic or dissocial

Marvin Zuckermann developed the SSS, a 40-item self-report scale, which has been widely used and influential in the study of sensation seeking. The SSS has four clusters of items (each of them containing ten questions) which reflect the primary expressions of sensation seeking:
- *Thrill and Adventure Seeking (SAS)*: these questions indicate a desire to do things that involve physical risk (sports and behaviours implying speed and danger) and the search for excitement in socially acceptable ways.
- *Experience Seeking (ES)*: these questions reflect a search for new experiences through living in a non-conforming way, a search for artistic, musical and intellectual expression, and for travel with like-minded people.
- *Disinhibition (DIS)*: these items correspond to the need for social release, possibly through drinking, gambling and sex.
- *Boredom Susceptibility (BS)*: these questions indicate low tolerance for activities or people that are routine or repetitive. Those who endorse these items tend to get jumpy and restless when little external stimulation is available.

Figure 16.1. The Zuckermann sensation-seeking scale (SSS-V) (from Zuckermann, 1994)

personalities) seldom have the opportunity to have empathic experiences (Decety & Jackson, 2004).

16.5 Ordeal and near-death experience

In 1976, two French authors (Valleur & Charles-Nicolas, 1982) showed the similarities that exist between the risks taken by drug users and the way that God's judgement was applied to suspects in the Middle Ages. In the Middle Ages, to ascertain whether a suspect was guilty, they were exposed to a violent and dangerous ordeal. If they survived, it was interpreted that God had protected them and consequently that they were innocent.

'Ordeal behaviours' are those that engage an individual in recurrent episodes that can endanger life, but whose ending cannot be predicted. Underlying these behaviours, the 'ordealic fantasy' could consist of putting one's life in the hands of God's or another, leaving the outcome to chance and subsequently, through survival, prove one's right to life and even immortality. The repetition of risk taking is interpretable as an attempt to have access to a better world. Choosing someone else to decide one's own right to life ultimately questions the legitimacy of the law.

Drug use (especially of stimulant drugs) appears to be an attempt at seeking new sensations, including ones that play with death, and consists of exploring or challenging limits, e.g. in the quest for near-death experiences.

The ordeal dimension is very prominent in modern-day near-death experiences that consist of using toxic substances to reach a point very close to clinical death before coming back (Hautefeuille & Velea, 2002). This quest involves trying to discern what might exist after death. We will come back to this subject within the later examination of 'flatliner' substances.

16.6 The dopaminergic rewarding mechanism

All addictive substances activate the brain systems involved in the dopaminergic reward mechanism. Electric self-stimulation of specific parts of the brain has elucidated which cerebral structures are involved in dependence. The anatomical reward circuit corresponds to the mesocorticolimbic system, which is essentially a dopaminergic mediator. The dopaminergic neurones are situated in the brainstem (A_{10} neurones) at the level of the ventral tegmental area (VTA) and project towards the limbic system nuclei (nucleus accumbens, amygdala, septal nucleus) and the prefrontal cortex.

The reward system works through neuromediators (essentially dopamine, but also opioids, serotonin and gamma-aminobutyric acid or GABA). The implicated dopaminergic receptors are types D_1, D_2 and D_3. All psychoactive substances achieve their neurobiochemical effects via the dopaminergic receptors of the nucleus accumbens, and in the case of psychostimulants additionally the serotonergic pathways.

16.7 Empathogenic substances

The use of plants to induce altered states of consciousness has existed since the origin of human beings. From the Stone Age, we have records of shamanic experiences and of tribal initiation rituals based on the ingestion of plant concoctions. Most of the plants were hallucinogenic and included opium, cannabis, coca mixtures and others that we have lost, such as the Indian soma. The common point of all these experiences was the achievement of an altered state of consciousness which has been described as '... *experiences in which the individual gets the feeling that the current functioning of his self-consciousness is out of order and that he is experiencing another connection with the world, with himself, his body, and his identity*' (Lapassade, 1987).

The use of empathogenic substances additionally facilitates communication, self-worth and, above all, acceptance in a group. Using these substances is seen as proof of active participation in a group. It may also provide well-being resulting from feelings of control and power.

16.8 Designer drugs

The term 'designer drugs' started to be used in the 1960s to cover a group of psychoactive drugs derived from phenylethylamines, which had new properties compared to the more classical ones. The concept of drugs 'à la carte' is very interesting for initiates on the social scene (Hautefeuille, 2002). In the beginning, their use was the result of work by small groups such as those led by Alexander Shulgin (Shulgin & Shulgin, 1991) a pharmacist who, for over 30 years, carried out research on the effects of about 200 phenylethylamines by synthesizing and experimenting with them. Psychostimulants which had exciting and euphoric properties were then classed as a group called 'empathogens' (Metzner, 1985) among which the best known is ecstasy (MDMA).

It is noteworthy the types of designs and logos that are engraved on ecstasy tablets. These logos are very suggestive of users' emotional participation, are messages for initiates and, in some cases, have special packaging for a particular event. Sometimes the logo represents 'love' in relation to ecstasy's reputation for its promotion, hence ecstasy is often referred to as 'the love pill'.

Currently, several classes of designer drugs are used on the party scene, or privately, for their empathogenic effects:

- Amphetamine-type stimulants (ATS) whose leading representative is ecstasy (MDMA). Most of them are phenylethylamines: MDA (3,4-methylenedioxy-amphetamine), MBDB [2-methylamino-1-(3,4-methylenedioxyphenyl) butane], MDEA (3,4-methylenedioxy-*N*-ethylamphetamine), as well as less popular ones: 2C-B (4-bromo-2,5-dimethoxy-phenylethylamine), DOB (2,5-dimethoxy-4-bromoamphetamine), DOM or STP (2,5-dimethoxy-4-methylamphetamine)
- Tryptamines: DMT (Dimethyltryptamine), DPT (*N, N*-dipropyltryptamine)
- Arylcyclohexylamines: PCP (phencyclidine) and ketamine

According to the National Institute of Drug Abuse (NIDA), 'club drugs' include phenylethylamines, but also: lysergic acid diethylamide (LSD), gamma-hydroxy-butyrate (GHB; and its precursor gamma-butyrolactone, GBL), 2C-B, ketamine, flunitrazepam (Rohypnol®) and amphetamines.

According to a World Health Organization (WHO) report (2004) '. . . *the use of amphetamine-type stimulants (ATS) is a global and growing phenomenon and in recent years, there has been a pronounced increase in the production and use of ATS worldwide. Over the past decade, use of ATS has infiltrated its way into the main-stream culture in certain countries. Younger people in particular seem to possess a skewed sense of safety about these substances, believing rather erroneously that they are safe and benign. Meanwhile, ATS are posing a serious threat to the health, social and economic fabric of families, communities and countries. For many countries, the problem of ATS is relatively new, growing quickly and unlikely to go away'.*

16.9 Smart drugs

This class of substances covers medications whose secondary use is founded on their real medicinal properties. Their use in groups, or individually, is in seeking well-being, self-worth, happiness, increased intellectual performance and increased communication abilities. Their use can be considered as a quest for 'self-empathy', seeking self-acceptance through better psychosocial adaptation and integration. Named 'nootropics', this class includes mixed medications such as piracetam (to improve intellectual performance), dehydroepiandrosterone (DHEA; to improve the sense of well-being, alertness and stamina, and to enhance sexual interest and libido), procaine hydrochloride (anti-aging), GHB (anaesthetic, aphrodisiac, hallucinogenic), herbal ecstasy (ephedrine), melatonin (anti-insomniac, anti-aging, improves sexual performance) and modafinil (stimulates and maintains wakefulness).

Paradoxically, substances used in the search for general well-being, self-knowledge and empathy also include psychodysleptics such as cannabis and alcohol, which have a sedative effect in contrast to the alerting effects of empathogenic psychostimulants. Psychodysleptics are sometimes used to reduce the 'speed' effects of ATS, but also to facilitate a connection with others. In this case, the desired effect is social disinhibition.

Many users say that LSD use is increasing: it is sought for its hallucinogenic and 'trip' properties. Cocaine is used at parties, or individually, for its psychostimulant properties and its ability to increase performance (e.g. in the socioprofessional environment with its associated high levels of stress).

16.10 Ecstasy, an empathogenic and entactogenic molecule

16.10.1 History

After LSD, ecstasy is the most well known synthetic drug. A derivative of phenylethylamine, its structure is close to that of catecholamines (adrenaline, vegetal alkaloids such as the ephedrine or the cathinone isolated from khat). Because of the increasing number of products mixed with the basic molecule (including atropine, benzodiazepines, ketamine and amphetamines), though it is still sold under the generic name of 'ecstasy', we will use the term MDMA. It was first synthesized in 1891 by a German chemist, Fritz Haber. It was patented in 1914 as an anorexigenic drug by Merck laboratories.

In 1965, Alexander Shulgin re-synthesized MDMA in his laboratory, and published the results of his experimentations (Nichols & Shulgin, 1976). MDMA was included in the list of banned substances in 1985 in the USA, and in 1986 in France. In the last two decades, MDMA has been used clinically to complement individual and group psychotherapies (Grob, 1998; Metzner, 1998).

16.10.2 Presentation

Ecstasy is found in the form of coloured tablets or pills, each one with a suggestive logo (love pound, love drug, money), and sometimes as a white powder. It is generally swallowed or, more rarely, snorted. There is considerable danger in the wide range of mixtures marketed as ecstasy, which often contain very little MDMA. Diluting products are very varied and include: caffeine, ephedrine, amphetamines, LSD, hallucinogenic mushrooms, MDA, MDE, DOB, ketamine and benzodiazepines. There are several hundred 'street names' in use for the ecstasy pills (Hautefeuille & Velea, 2002).

16.10.3 Effects

Ecstasy is mainly used at raves and in nightclubs, but is increasingly being used among groups of friends at home. There are also increasing numbers of lone consumers. Effects can be particularly strong on the social scene: rhythmic music, the need to overcome fatigue, intense and continuous physical activity (sometimes for 24 h without a break), polyconsumption (MDMA, alcohol, cannabis) and water loss without rehydration. Effects start 30–60 min after oral ingestion and increase very quickly. They generally last 3–4 h, before a latency period (of 2–6 h) and eventual return to a normal state, during which time falling asleep is impossible. The pharmacokinetic properties of MDMA are non-linear, with high doses producing disproportionate rises in plasma levels (Cami *et al.*, 1997).

MDMA is widely distributed in the body and crosses the blood–brain barrier. Between 3% and 7% is converted by the liver to the active substance 3,4-methylenedioxyamphetamine (MDA), 28% is biotransformed to other metabolites, and around 65% is eliminated, unchanged, via the kidneys. The half-life of MDMA in plasma is 7.6 h. This information is relevant when treating intoxication: 6–8 half-lives are necessary for complete elimination of MDMA, giving a total time of around 48 h for the drug to be completely eliminated. At a plasma level of 8 mg/l – considered to be the level of severe intoxication – more than 24 h is necessary for a decrease to a plasma level lower than 1 mg/l, which produces less clinical effects. Therefore, 24 h would be the estimated time of intensive care needed by intoxicated patients who had taken a few ecstasy tablets (WHO, 2004).

MDMA's primary characteristic is linked to its properties and, unlike LSD, it modifies and amplifies sensations without impairing intellectual processes, at least when the dose is normal and the substance is not mixed with others. A high-level dose may however generate hallucinogenic effects. This sensorial amplification property is why, whilst Metzner classified it as 'empathogenic', Shulgin and Nichols classified it as 'entactogenic' (allowing contact with one's own body).

A major effect expected by users on the rave scene is that it has aphrodisiac properties, which are actually rarely obtained with ecstasy. This prompted Saunders to say, 'Ecstasy is a sensual drug and not a sexual drug' (Sueur *et al.*, 2000).

Psychological effects consist of an increase in empathy towards others and oneself, increased self-confidence and a state of euphoria. These effects can be analysed through impulsivity, venturesomeness, empathy (IVE) questionnaires (Morgan, 1998; Parrot *et al.*, 2000). The hallucinogenic potency of MDMA is very low compared with that of LSD, 2C-B or ketamine. MDMA is anorexigenic, with an amphetamine-like effect on weight.

The risk of an amphetamine-like pharmacopsychosis, which appears to concern few users, is dependent on dose, duration of use, the age of the user, and any pre-existing psychological problems. Panic attacks with a quick onset and remission can sometimes be observed among users. Chronic use at high doses can generate chronic psychotic episodes and/or characteristic depressive states (loss of momentum and self-confidence and development of a guilt complex). These states are related to the serotonergic effects of MDMA.

Somatic effects cover muscular pain, spasms and dehydration due to physical effort and ambient heat. Other symptoms often include tachycardia, tremor, nausea, bruxism, perspiration, vomiting, an increased sensitivity to cold, light and colours, ataxia and nystagmus. There are descriptions of an 'MDMA acute intoxication syndrome' (including hyperthermia and rhabdomyolysis) which appears quickly after ingestion (Sueur *et al.*, 2000). Other reported symptoms include acute liver intoxication appearing about 15 days after ingestion and possible neurological problems including cerebrovascular accidents, Parkinsonism and cognitive decline.

Research concerning the therapeutic effects of psychoactive substances was central to Timothy Leary's empirical experiments in the 1960s. At the time, research concerned LSD, ketamine, ayahuasca and marijuana. Presently, the disinhibition, well-being and empathogenic effects of MDMA are being studied in the USA with patients in the terminal phases of cancer (Halpern, McLean Hospital and Mithoefer, South Carolina MDMA project).

The authors of these studies emphasize that the main researched effect of MDMA is not its anxiolytic properties, but rather its empathogenic capacity. Halpern comments on how MDMA facilitates conversational dialogue with anxious patients and decreases panic attacks in these patients. Halpern suggests that the medical use of ecstasy could provide a therapeutic alternative to benzodiazepines at strong doses. American specialists such as Rick Doblin (founder and head of Multidisciplinary Association for Psychedelic Studies – MAPS) further emphasizes the importance of these studies, having investigated the use of ecstasy in the treatment of post-traumatic stress disorder (PTSD).

16.10.4 Testing

The large number of products and mixtures available that are sold as ecstasy in France led to the development of testing practices. These practices, which take place within a risk-reduction policy on the rave scene, aim to analyse the pills' contents and warn users about the possible negative effects of particular mixtures, and even to discover other analogues of yet unknown substances. Testing also allows constructive contact with users. The Marquis test can be used to find out which molecules are present in a so-called ecstasy pill: including MDMA, MDA, MBDB, amphetamine and 2C-B. However, ultimately only a qualitative analysis done in a laboratory is completely reliable (Velea & Hautefeuille, 1999), though chromatography allows a relatively complete, reliable and precise identification of the constituent products.

16.10.5 Neurobiochemical aspects

The psychological effects of psychoactive drugs are characterized by an alternate state of consciousness, euphoria or dysphoria, elation and empathy, and are the result of interactions between the substance and various neurotransmitters. The affinity of MDMA to bind to neurotransmitters varies from very strong to low (Battaglia & De Souza, 1989).

Two optical isomers of the MDMA molecule exist: the $S(+)$ and the $R(-)$ forms. The $S(+)$ form is more active then the $R(-)$ form at eliciting psychotropic effects in humans (Steele *et al.*, 1994) and also the most active at serotonin re-uptake sites. The $R(-)$ form, very active on serotonin receptors, is implicated in the genesis of hallucinations (hallucinogenic drugs such as LSD intensively stimulate the 5-HT$_2$ receptors) (Nash *et al.*, 1994).

Because MDMA has a low binding affinity for noradrenaline and dopamine re-uptake sites, it also has less psychostimulant potency than amphetamine (Wall *et al.*, 1995). There is also a lower binding affinity with adrenergic receptors (particularly alpha-2) (Battaglia *et al.*, 1988). MDMA's interaction with muscarinic receptors is very low.

16.10.6 Ecstasy and the serotonergic system

Serotonergic neurones are present in all parts of the human brain, but in relatively low numbers (of the order of several tens of thousands) (Jacobs & Fornal, 1995). Serotonin (5-HT) is synthesized from tryptophan. Three types of receptors are present in the synapse: 5HT$_1$, 5HT$_2$ and 5HT$_3$. Most of the serotonergic neurones are situated in the raphe nuclei (situated in the midline of the medulla oblongata). Neurones project from here to the whole brain, but especially to the hippocampus, amygdala, thalamus and hypothalamus (Cottereau *et al.*, 1990).

Studies performed on rats (Spanos & Yamamoto, 1989) showed that the presence of MDMA and serotonergic neurones promotes repetitive motor behaviours (this partly explains why, during raves, MDMA users have repetitive movements – dance and trance-like – apparently without effort and appear disconnected from their environment). Other studies underline that this hyperactivity is mainly due to increased serotonin release in the brain, with dopamine's role being minor (Callaway *et al.*, 1991). A recent report suggests a biphasic action of the phenyl-ethylamines, namely serotonergic and dopaminergic interaction. In its first phase, MDMA's action on synapses stimulates increased serotonin release (Gudelsky & Nash, 1996). This serotonin release (to 20 times normal levels) is maximal at 30–60 min after MDMA ingestion. The release is facilitated via an exchange mechanism of serotonin and MDMA in the synapse (MDMA tending to replace serotonin in the synaptic vesicle; Wall *et al.*, 1995). The effect is also reported for other MDMA analogues: MDA, MDEA and MBDB.

One important effect of MDMA consumption, even acutely, is a decrease in cerebral serotonin and its metabolite 5-hydroxyindole acetic acid (5-HIAA). The serotonin levels return to normal 24 h after consumption. With long-term chronic consumption, cerebral serotonin depletion is due to re-uptake inhibition. It has been suggested that this depletion could be due to serotonergic receptor destruction (Wilson & Molliver, 1994). This suggestion has been strengthened by positron emission tomography (PET) scanning studies demonstrating a significant decrease of serotonin transportation which is directly correlated with MDMA use (McCann *et al.*, 1998).

The mechanism of MDMA neurotoxicity on serotonergic receptors is not well understood, but it has been hypothesized that it may be an indirect mechanism. As direct injections of MDMA into the brain have no neurotoxic effects (Paris & Cunningham, 1992), it has been hypothesized that an MDMA metabolite may be acting (Lim & Foltz, 1991), suggesting that the neurotoxicity could be the result of neurotransmitters released by the MDMA ingestion. This second hypothesis is backed up by the role that dopamine appears to play as an intermediate agent in MDMA neurotoxicity. Dopamine release (especially in the nucleus accumbens) during the second phase of phenylethylamine action destroys serotonergic neurons (Nash & Nichols, 1991; Sprague *et al.*, 1998).

16.10.7 The serotonergic deficiency syndrome

The concept of such a syndrome comes from research on depression with its well-known association with a serotonin deficiency (Pöldinger *et al.*, 1991). Two questions can be asked. First, is there a primary serotonergic deficiency in individuals who suffer from a lack of confidence and problems with interpersonal skills and who seek increased empathy, insight and emotional expression? As a matter of fact, clinical analysis proves that the use of empathogenic substances represents a kind of self-medication.

The second question involves the issue of the effects of serotonergic depletion caused by phenylethylamine use such as MDMA, and the subsequent attempts to restore serotonergic homeostasis through the repetitive use of MDMA. This hypothesis is confirmed by the choice of the empathogenic substances as part of this self-medication.

16.10.8 Neuroendocrine modifications

Grob (1998) observed that the secretion of a variety of hormones [cortisol, adrenocorticotropic hormone (ACTH), prolactin] is significantly increased 1 h after MDMA ingestion. These secretions return to normal within about 5 h. This mechanism, which involves the hypothalamo-pituitary-adrenal (HPA) axis, may be pertinent in relation to the emergence of stress reactions among MDMA users. The first phase of stress appears as an immediate response (after about 10 s) to physical and psychological aggression and represents a preparation for fighting. The rapid response of the sympathetic nervous system generates catecholamine release (adrenaline through the adrenal gland, and noradrenaline through post-ganglionic fibres). During the adaptation phase that follows, there is a stimulation of the HPA axis. In response to the previous adrenergic stimulation, the paraventricular nucleus (PVN) of the hypothalamus synthesizes corticotrophic releasing factor (CRF). These CRF neurones are regulated by the amygdala and hippocampus. At the pituitary level, the release of CRF induces the release of ACTH starting from its precursor, pro-opiomelanocortin (POMC). All these reactions end with the release of glucocorticoids (cortisol) through the adrenal glands (Velea, 2002b). The ACTH and cortisol increase is partially induced by serotonin, which stimulates the HPA axis. Another study suggests that MDMA use induces a decrease of striatal and hippocampal corticosteroid receptors (Yau *et al.*, 1994).

16.10.9 Empathy and imitation behaviours

Regarding MDMA users, the link between their imitative and repetitive movements and their pursuit of empathy leads to an interesting reflection on the role of the mirror neurones. The ventral premotor cortex (Broca's area F5) hosts the 'canonical neurones' which are activated during an individual's actions. Another category of neurones exists, the 'mirror neurones' (Rizollatti *et al.*, 1996), which, as well as being activated during an individual's actions, are also activated by observing others' actions. Neuroimaging studies suggest that the ability to predict another's intentions and psychological (affective) states is mediated by the prefrontal cortex (Farrow *et al.*, 2001).

During the imitation and observation of emotions (the relevant neurones being located in the upper temporal lobe, linked to the ventral premotor cortex via the lower parietal lobe – Rizollatti *et al.*, 1996), a strong activation of the amygdala (Carr *et al.*, 2003) and limbic system also occurs.

A recent model (Meltzoff & Decety, 2003) proposes a three-phase developmental process, from imitation to empathy. In the first phase, babies express their innate ability to create links between their actions and those of others. In the second phase, children are able to express emotions via facial mimicry. The final phase occurs when children realize that other people share the same facial expressions and thereby realize that others must feel the same emotions as them when they have these facial expressions.

It is interesting to note here the involvement of both the limbic system and the amygdala, which are also involved in alexithymia. Their important role in the expression of emotion may suggest a link between empathy, alexithymia and the stress adaptation reaction.

16.11 Other empathogenic substances of the phenylethylamine type

MDMA – ecstasy – is the reference substance in empathogenic effect. We now present some other substances that possess empathogenic effects, of different degrees. As is well known to addiction specialists, these empathogenic effects are partially dependant on subjective circumstances (personality, environment, cultural and sociological determinants).

To date, no studies have compared scientifically the empathogenic properties of these different substances. Therefore, each quoted study involves analysis of each molecule in an independent way.

16.11.1 MDA

MDA is a hallucinogenic psychostimulant. Its molecular structure is very close to that of MDMA (it is produced by the metabolism of MDMA). In its pure state, MDA is a white powder, but the version found on the streets is often yellow or brown. Oral ingestion of 100–200 mg leads to intense effects. Psychological effects begin with feelings of calm, peace, joy, intense feelings of empathy (they are called 'love drugs'), and increased vigilance and perception. With a higher dosage (more than 300 mg), the hallucinogenic effects (delirious flush) are similar to those found with MDMA. The somatic effects include tachycardia, disseminated intravascular coagulation [a haemorrhagic disorder, characterized by multiple ecchymoses (bleeding under the skin), mucosal bleeding and depletion of platelets and clotting factors in the blood] and respiratory depression, effects that can occasionally lead to death among MDA users.

16.11.2 MDEA

This substance's action is slower and less intensive than that of MDMA (lasting 3–5 h). Its empathetic action is very low and is essentially due to the ingestion of mixtures which also contain MDMA.

16.11.3 MBDB

MBDB's molecular structure and effects are very similar to those of MDMA, but the duration and intensity of its action are lower. It is sold under the name 'Eden, methyl-J'. Current doses are around 120–150 mg, and the effects last about 4–6 h. The empathogenic, euphoric and psychedelic effects are also less than those of MDMA. According to its designer (DE Nichols), MBDB does not induce any hallucinogenic effects.

16.11.4 2C-B

2C-B is sold under names such as 'Nexus', 'Eve', and even 'XTC' (sometimes producing confusion with ecstasy). Its recreational use is rapidly increasing on the rave scene. 2C-B is a hallucinogenic substance, synthesized by the American chemist Alexandre Shulgin (in 1974). Its chemical formula shows some similarities with mescaline, a drug used in initiatory rituals by American Indians. 2C-B produces coloured visual hallucinations, psychedelic sensations, distortions of forms and surfaces, and feelings of increased extrasensorial perception. Its aphrodisiac properties are very strong: the substance is well known for increasing sexual desire and performance, unlike ecstasy which also had this (false) reputation. The effects of 2C-B last 3–8 h and are stronger than those of MDMA. A small dose, of around 5–10 mg, rapidly produces hallucinogenic and psychedelic effects. The security margin between desired effects and negative ones (i.e. bad trips) is very narrow. A good binding affinity with brain serotonergic receptors has been reported.

16.11.5 DOM or STP

STP and DOM are two names for the same hallucinogenic and psychostimulant molecule. It is currently found in the form of a powder of white or off-white colour. At a low dosage (1–2 mg), DOM is slightly euphoric and generates psychological stimulation. At a higher dose (more than 5 mg), it induces mescaline-like or LSD-like effects: visual hallucinations, distortions, visual and auditory illusions. The residual hallucinogenic effect can last 8–24 h after ingestion of more than 5 mg.

16.12 Tryptamine-type empathogenic substances

16.12.1 DMT

DMT's molecular structure is similar to that of psilocin (a hallucinogenic alkaloid present in hallucinogenic mushrooms). It is seen in the form of a white, crystalline powder and is often sold under the street name of 'Dimitri'. Injected or inhaled at a dosage of around 50–60 mg, it produces psychological effects similar to those of other hallucinogenic substances such as LSD or mescaline. The similarities in these effects can be explained by molecular similarities and by a quasi-identical binding affinity for the 5-HT2 receptor. Its intravenous use produces behavioural changes, hypersensitivity, visual and auditory hallucinations, and euphoria. Unlike other hallucinogens, the hallucinogenic effects of DMT (which have a remarkable intensity) appear quickly and do not last for long (30–60 min). This explains one of its street names: 'businessman's lunch'.

16.13 Arylhexylamine-type empathogenic substances

16.13.1 PCP or phencyclidine

Initially used as an anaesthetic product in humans, PCP is currently mostly used in the veterinary field. Its use in humans was stopped in 1965 due to problems on wakening, particularly agitation and confusional states. PCP can be found in the form of a white crystalline power, quickly soluble in water or alcohol, or in the form of tablets or pills. Among its effects at low or average doses (under 20 mg) are relaxation, impaired motor function, changes in the perception of space and body, audiovisual distortions, feeling of depersonalization, isolation and mutism. A high incidence of violent actions (against oneself or others) has been reported.

16.13.2 Ketamine: [2-(2-chlorophenyl)-2-methylamino-cyclohexan-1-one]

Ketamine is an anaesthetic of dissociative-type: patients can feel detached from reality (Hautefeuille & Velea, 2002). For several years, its diverse use has been observed, especially within the rave scene where it can be found under various names: ket, special K, kit kat, keller, super acid. It belongs to what are known as 'chill-out drugs' ('drogues couches' in French), as it has no stimulant effect and does not promote a desire to dance. It is mainly snorted. It is used either for its own hallucinogenic effects or as an inducer of the effects of other products such as ecstasy and LSD. Users experience hallucinogenic effects, extrasensorial perceptions, or mystical revelations. Frequently, users describe experiences of clinical death ('near-death experiences'); the reason why it is also called 'flatliner', a reference to the film of the same title (Flatliners, USA, 1990).

16.14 Other psychoactive substances

16.14.1 GHB: gamma-hydroxybutyric acid, Gamma-OH™

GHB was first synthesized in the 1960s, by Henri Laborit, a French doctor who also discovered neuroleptics. GHB was used as a general anaesthetic, particularly in gynaecology and obstetrics. GHB was found to be an endogenous compound, naturally occurring in the brain of mammals where it is synthesized from GABA. GHB increases the level of dopamine in the brain and acts on endorphins (endogenous precursors of opioids). In the 1980s, GHB was heavily used by bodybuilders who used it for its ability to stimulate the release of growth hormones, thus favouring a decrease in fat levels and an increase in bodily muscle mass (Velea & Hautefeuille, 1999).

GHB is available in the form of a colourless, odourless and flavourless liquid. It is well known under names such as 'liquecstasy' or 'liquid X', because its socializing effects are similar to ecstasy's empathetic effect. The most commonly reported effects, for moderate doses, are: calmness, sensuality, mild euphoria and a tendency to talk a lot. These types of effects characterize GHB as a 'chill-out' drug as it does not promote a desire to dance.

Its aphrodisiac effects have been the subject of several studies within the medico-legal services, following rapes committed under its influence. Its ability to increase sexual performance makes GHB a valuable drug for some adults. Since the dangers of GHB use have been made clear, and since its prohibition, chemists have produced GHB precursor substances, which, once ingested, are changed into gamma-hydroxybutyrate known as 'natural cleaners': gamma-butyrolactone (GBL), 2(3H), furanone di-hydro, and 1, 4-butanediol (BD).

16.14.2 LSD

LSD was discovered by the Swiss chemist Albert Hofmann in 1938. When pure, LSD takes the form of an odourless white, crystalline powder. It is frequently sold in the form of small pieces of blotting paper or in small pills of various forms and colours.

LSD generally acts in 20–60 min with effects lasting 6–8 h, followed by an end phase (with sleeping difficulties) of 1–2 h. Psychological effects are central and start with a feeling of euphoria and dizziness. The 'psychedelic' experience includes visual and pseudo-hallucinogenic perceptions (the user remains aware that the experience is not real), time distortion (a minute seems to be as long as an hour), distortions of space, of the body (lack of corporal limits, a feeling of floating). Another classical effect is synaesthesia (a merging of the senses leading to the perception of experiences in another modality such as 'seeing' music, or 'listening' to colours). These phenomena are called 'simultaneous perceptions'. There is also an increased intensity of sensorial perceptions and emotions.

Some users can experience unpleasant feelings (fear, anguish, panic attacks). A 'bad trip' is a negative experience that can happen at the start of the high, but may also begin several hours after the first effects. Users also sometimes describe a loss of identity, feelings of disintegration and terrifying hallucinations.

Long-term effects are characterized by 'flash-backs': chronic hallucinations persisting through periods of abstinence invoking memories of experiences when under the drug's influence. Hallucinations are generally visual (varying from colours without form to frightening visions). Acute psychotic episodes (of paranoid schizophrenia type) can occasionally appear after a single LSD experience (pharmacopsychosis).

16.15 CONCLUSIONS

In general, the use of psychoactive substances always has an underlying function that gives the addictive behaviours a self-therapy dimension. In the case of the abovementioned substances, the ultimate goal of their use is often to facilitate empathy. We suggest however that substances that are not inherently empathetic can also fulfil this function.

Therefore, the use of these products plays an important role for people having difficulties managing their emotions within a group and creating interpersonal relationships. This is especially the case for people suffering from alexithymia, and for people who want to create an 'artificial empathy', one that can be very powerful.

In raves, and on the party scene the use of such substances facilitates imitative behaviours, induces gestural mimicry, and increases feelings such as acceptance, social integration and individual recognition. Through analysis of the possible role of serotonergic neurotransmitters and the involvement of mirror neurones in this type of behaviour, research should focus on what may be called 'mirror empathy'. In other cases, research should focus on the emotional experience at a more personal level, on self-acceptance: on what we have called 'self-empathy'.

From a clinical point of view, it seems important to highlight the difference between these two types of situation, as it will impact on the type of care proposed and on the global understanding we have of drug consumption phenomena, especially among young people, most of whom are recreational users.

REFERENCES

Alexander, B. K. (1990). The empirical and theoretical bases for an adaptive model of addiction. *Journal of Drug Issues*, **20**(**1**), 37–65.

American Psychiatric Association. (2004). *Diagnostic and Statistical Manual of Mental Disorders*, 4th edn. Arlington, Va.: APA.

Battaglia, G., & De Souza, E. B. (1989). Pharmacologic profile of amphetamine derivatives at various brain recognition sites: selective effects of serotonergic systems. *NIDA Research Monograph*, **94**, 240–258.

Battaglia, G., Yeh, S. H., & De Souza, E. B. (1988). MDMA-induced neurotoxicity: parameters of degeneration and recovery of brain serotonin neurons. *Pharmacology, Biochemistry, and Behavior*, **94**, 269–274.

Callaway, C. W., Johnson, M. P., Gold, L. H., Nichols, D. E., & Geyer, M. A. (1991). Amphetamine derivates induce locomotor hyperactivity by acting as indirect serotonin agonists. *Psychopharmacology*, **104**, 293–310.

Cami, J., de la Torre, R., Ortuno, J., *et al.* (1997). Pharmacokinetics of ecstasy (MDMA) in healthy subjects. *European Journal of Clinical Pharmacology*, **52**, 168.

Carr, L., Iacoboni, M., Dubeau, M. C., Maziotta, J. C., & Lenzi, G. L. (2003). Neural mechanism of empathy in humans: a relay from neural systems for imitation to limbic area. *Proceedings of the National Academy of Sciences of the USA*, **100(9)**, 5497–5502.

Cottereau, M. J., Manus, A., & Martin A. (1990). *Manuel de Thérapeutique Psychiatrique*. Paris: Masson.

Decety, J., & Jackson P. L. (2004). The functional architecture of human empathy. *Behavioural and Cognitive Neuroscience Reviews*, **10(10)**, 1–30.

Ehrenberg, A. (1991). *Le Culte de la Performance*. Paris: Calman-Lévy.

Erickson, E. H. (1963). *Childhood and Society*. New York: Norton.

Farges, F., & Farges, S. (2002). Alexithymie et substances psychoactives: revue critique de la littérature. *Psychotropes*, **8(2)**, 47–74.

Farrow, T. F. D., Zheng, Y., Wilkinson, I. D., *et al.* (2001). Investigating the functional anatomy of empathy and forgiveness. *Neuroreport*, **12(11)**, 2433–2438.

Gallese, V. (2003). The roots of empathy: the shared manifold hypothesis and the neural basis of intersubjectivity. *Psychopathology*, **36**, 171–180.

Goodman, A. (1990). Addiction: definition and implication. *British Journal of Addiction*, **85**, 1403–1408.

Grob, C. S. (1998). MDMA research: preliminary investigations with human subjects. *International Journal of Drug Policy*, **9(1)**, 102.

Gudelsky, G. A., & Nash, J. F. (1996). Carrier-mediated release of serotonin by 3,4-methylen-dioxymethamphetamine: implications for serotonin-dopamine interactions. *Journal of Neurochemistry*, **66**, 243–249.

Hautefeuille, M. (2002). *Les Drogues à la Carte*. Paris: Payot.

Hautefeuille, M., & Velea, D. (2002). *Les Drogues de Synthèse*. Paris: PUF.

Havilland, M. G., Hendrix, M. S., Shaw, D. G., & Henry, J. P. (1994). Alexithymia in women and men hospitalized for psychoactive substance dependence. *Comprehensive Psychiatry*, **35**, 124–128.

Jacobs, B. L., & Fornal, C. A. (1995). Serotonin and behaviour: a general hypothesis. In F. E. Bloom, D. J. Kupper (eds.), *Psychopharmacology: The Fourth Generation of Progress* (pp. 461–469). New York: Raven Press.

Jessor, R. (1998). New perspectives on adolescent risk behavior. In *Adolescent Risk Behavior*. New York: Cambridge University Press.

Keller, D. S., Caroll, K. M., Nich, C., & Rounsaville B. J. (1995). Alexithymia in cocaine abusers. *American Journal of Addiction*, **4**, 234–244.

Krystal, H. (1979). Alexithymia and psychotherapy. *American Journal of Psychotherapy*, **33**, 17–31.

Lapassade, G. (1987). *Les États Modifiés de Conscience*. Paris: PUF.

Lim, H. K., & Foltz, R. L. (1991). In vivo formation of aromatic hydroxylated metabolites of 3,4-(methylenedioxy)methamphetamine in the rat: identification by ion trap (MS/MS and MS/MS/MS) techniques. *Biological Mass Spectrometry*, **20**, 677–686.

Lipps, T. (1903a). *Grundlegung der Aesthetik*. Hamburg: Engelmann.

Lipps, T. (1903b). Einfühlung, innere Nachahmung und Organempfindung. *Archives of General Psychiatry*, **1**. Leipzig: Engelmann.

Lotze, H. (1923). Mikrokosmos. Ideen zur Naturgeschichte und Geschichte der Menschheit. Versuch einer Anthropologie (6th edn.) (Vol 2). Leipzig: Meiner.

McCann, U. D., Szabo, Z., Scheffel, U., Dannals, R. F., & Ricaurte, G. A. (1998). Positron emission tomographic evidence of toxic effects of MDMA (ecstasy) on brain serotonin neurones in human beings. *Lancet*, **352**, 1433–1437.

Meltzoff, A. N., & Decety, J. (2003). What imitation tells us about social cognition: a rapprochement between developmental psychology and cognitive neuroscience. *Philosophical Transactions of the Royal Society, London B*, **358**, 491–500.

Metzner, R. (1985). *Through the Gateway of the Heart*. San Francisco: Four Trees Press.

Metzner, R. (1998). Hallucinogenic drugs and plants in psychotherapy and shamanism. *Journal of Psychoactive Drugs*, **30(4)**, 333–341.

Morgan, M. J. (1998). Recreational use of 'Ecstasy' (MDMA) is associated with elevated impulsivity. *Neuropsychopharmacology*, **19(4)**, 252–264.

Nash, J. F., & Nichols, D. E. (1991). Microdialysis studies on 3,4-(methylendioxy)-methamphetamine and structurally related analogues. *European Journal of Pharmacology*, **4**, 79–84.

Nash, J. F., Roth, B. L., Brodkin, J. D., Nichols, D. E., & Gudelsky, G. A. (1994). Effects of the $R(-)$ and $S(+)$ isomers of MDA and MDMA on phosphatidyl inositol turnover in cultured cells expression 5-HT(2A) or 5-HT(2C) receptors. *Neuroscience Letters*, **177**, 111–115.

Nichols D. E., & Shulgin A. T. (1976). Sulfur analogs of psychotomimetic amines. *Journal of Pharmacological Science*, **65(10)**, 1554–1556.

Paris, J. M., & Cunningham, K. A. (1992). Lack of serotonin neurotoxicity after intraraphe microinjections of $(+)$ 3,4-(methylendioxy)-methamphetamine (MDMA). *Brain Research Bulletin*, **28**, 115–119.

Parrot, A. C., Sisk, E., & Turner, J. J. D. (2000). Psychobiological problems in heavy ecstasy (MDMA) polydrug users. *Drug and Alcohol Dependence*, **60**, 105–110.

Pöldinger, W., Calanchini, B., & Schwarz, W. (1991). A functional-dimensional approach to depression: serotonin deficiency as a target syndrome in a comparison of 5-hydroxytryptophan and fluvoxamine. *Psychopathology*, **24**, 53–81.

Rizollatti, G., Fadiga, L., Gallese, V., & Fogassi, L. (1996). Premotor cortex and the recognition of motor actions. *Cognitive Brain Research*, **3**, 131–141.

Sheets-Johnstone, M. (1999). *The Primacy of Movement* (pp. 1–44). Amsterdam: Benjamins Publishing.

Shulgin, A., & Shulgin, A. (1991). *PIHKAL. A Chemical Love Story*. Berkeley: Transform Press.

Sifneos, P. E. (1973). The prevalence of 'alexithymic' characteristics in psychosomatic patients. *Pyschotherapy Psychosomatics*, **22**, 255–262.

Sifneos, P. E. (1996). Alexithymia: past and present, *American Journal of Psychiatry*, **153**(7), 137–142.

Smith, A. (1759). In D. D. Raphael, A. L. Macfie (eds.), *The Theory of Moral Sentiments*. Oxford: Oxford University Press, 1976.

Spanos, L. J., & Yamamoto, B. K. (1989). Acute and subacute effects of methylendioxymethamphetamines [(+ / −) MDMA] on locomotion and serotonin syndrome behavior in the rat. *Pharmacology, Biochemistry, and Behavior*, **34**, 697.

Sprague, J. E., Everman, S. L., & Nichols, D. E. (1998). An integrated hypothesis for the serotonergic axonal loss induced by 3, 4-methylenedioxymethamphetamine. *Neurotoxicology*, **19**(3), 427–441.

Steele, T. D., McCann, U. D., & Ricaurte, G. A. (1994). 3,4-Methylendioxy-amphetamine (MDMA, 'Ecstasy'): pharmacology and toxicology in animals and humans. *Addiction*, **89**, 539–551.

Stein, E. (1964). *On the Problem of Empathy*. The Hague: Martinus Nijhoff.

Sueur, C., Cammas, R., & Lebeau, B. (2000). L'Ecstasy au sein de la famille des substances psychédéliques: effets et dangerosité. *Psychotropes*, **6**(2), 9–73.

Taylor, G. J., Bagby, M., & Parker, J. D. A. (1997). *Disorders of Affect Regulation: Alexithymia in Medical and Psychiatric Illness*. Cambridge: Cambridge University Press.

Valleur, M., & Charles-Nicolas, A. (1982). Les conduites ordaliques. In C. Olivenstein (ed.), *La Vie du Toxicomane*. Paris: PUF.

Velea, D. (2002a). Une société de médiation chimique. *Dépendance*. Lausanne, **2**, 17, 22–25.

Velea, D. (2002b). Neurobiologie des addictions. In J. M. Thurin, N. Baumann (eds.), *Stress, Pathologie et Immunité* (pp. 110–109). Paris: Flammarion.

Velea, D. (2005). *Toxicomanie et Conduites Addictives*. Paris: Heures de France.

Velea, D., & Hautefeuille, M. (1999). Les nouvelles drogues de synthèse empathogènes. *L'Encéphale*, **XXV**, 508–514.

Vischer, R. (1873). *Über das Optische Formgefühl: Ein Beitrag zur Ästhetik. In drei Schriften zum ästhetischen Formproblem*. Halle: Niemeyer.

Wall, S. G., Gu H., & Rudnick, G. (1995). Biogenic amine flux mediated by cloned transporters stably expressed in cultured cells lines: amphetamine specificity for inhibition and efflux. *Molecular Pharmacology*, **47**, 544–550.

WHO (2004). *Neuroscience of Psychoactive Substance Use and Dependence*. Geneva: WHO.

Wilson, M. A., & Molliver, M. E. (1994). Microglial response to degeneration of serotonergic axon terminals. *Glia*, **11**, 18–34.

Wurmser, S. L. (1974). Psychoanalytic considerations of the etiology of compulsive drug use. *Journal of the American Psychoanalytic Association*, **22**, 820–843.

Yau, J. L. W., Kelly, P. A. T., Sharkey, J., & Seckl, J. R. (1994). Chronic 3,4-(methylendioxy)-methamphetamine administration decreases glucocorticoid and mineralocorticoid receptor, but increases 5-hydroxytryptamine (IC) receptor gene expression in the rat hippocampus. *Neuroscience*, **61**, 31–40.

Zuckermann, M. (1994). *Behavioural Expressions and Biosocial Bases of Sensation Seeking*. New York: Cambridge University Press.

Existential empathy: the intimacy of self and other

Marco Iacoboni

Brain Research Institute, David Geffen School of Medicine at UCLA

17.1 Imitation and empathy between self and other

Empathy is the ability to imagine oneself in another's place, and understand the other's feelings. The aspect of *understanding* the feelings of others critically defines empathy, as opposed to sympathy, in which one has a feeling corresponding to that which another feels. How does this understanding occur? Understanding is the ability to make sense of things. As such, it is often assumed that understanding is a mental ability. However, one of the background assumptions of the research I am going to discuss here is that understanding is not exclusively mental but is essentially corporeal as well. The other central aspect of the definition of empathy is that it requires a sense of self and a sense of the other. Without self-awareness and awareness of the other, one cannot 'imagine oneself in another's place'. Thus, the foundational aspects of empathy are a sense of self, a sense of the other, and an embodied relational process between self and other. Such an embodied relational process between self and other can be easily identified in imitative behaviour. Imitation is a central component of non-verbal communication in pre-verbal toddlers. In fact, when dyads and triads of children of different ages interact in settings with two or three identical sets of attractive objects, imitation is the predominant form of interaction between 18 and 30 months of age (Nadel, 2002). The effect of setting is reduced in older children with verbal abilities. This suggests that imitation serves as the main form of communication in pre-verbal children, whereas in older children with verbal abilities imitation becomes one of the possible forms of communication (Nadel, 2002). The role of imitation as a form of non-verbal communication actually continues in adulthood, albeit in an automatic, largely non-conscious form. The phenomenon of the Chameleon effect has been described repeatedly and studied in several laboratories (Barsalou *et al.*, 2003; Hatfield *et al.*, 1994; Niedenthal *et al.*, 2005). It refers to non-conscious

Empathy in Mental Illness, eds. Tom F. D. Farrow and Peter W. R. Woodruff. Published by Cambridge University Press. © Cambridge University Press 2007.

mimicry of the postures, mannerisms and facial expressions of people while they interact in a social situation (Chartrand & Bargh, 1999; Hatfield *et al.*, 1994). A series of experiments has shown not only that people tend to imitate automatically and unintentionally the motor behaviour of strangers, but also that being imitated facilitates interactions and increases liking, and that individual variability in the tendency to imitate others correlate with scores on empathy (Chartrand & Bargh, 1999). What are the neural bases of these phenomena?

17.2 Neural precursors of imitation and empathy

In our laboratory, we have investigated in the last few years the neural mechanisms of imitation and empathy. Our research has been inspired by findings in single-cell recording studies in macaques. These studies revealed functional properties in ventral premotor and inferior parietal neurones that seemed quite relevant to imitation. In fact, these neurones, collectively called mirror neurones, fire when the monkey performs object-oriented actions such as grasping, holding, manipulating and tearing, and when the monkey sees somebody else performing the same actions (diPellegrino *et al.*, 1992; Gallese *et al.*, 1996). Interestingly, mirror neurones will not fire at the sight of a pantomimed action (Gallese *et al.*, 1996). However, mirror neurones fire even when the actual grasp of the object is occluded from vision, as long as the animal has witnessed the initial reach of the hand going to grasp the object (Umilta *et al.*, 2001). Moreover, mirror neurones also fire, in complete darkness, at the sound associated with an action (Kohler *et al.*, 2002). The motor properties of these neurones are also interesting. In fact, some of these neurones fire when the monkey grasps an object with the left hand, or with the right hand, or with the mouth (Gallese *et al.*, 1996). Taken together, these data suggest that the firing of these neurones is associated with achieving or witnessing the achievement of the goal of an action. Some mirror neurones in the parietal lobe have complex properties that seem relevant to some higher order aspects of motor behaviour, for instance sequencing. It has been shown that some parietal mirror neurones fire at the sight of a hand grasping an object and fire also while the monkey bites the objects with the mouth (Gallese *et al.*, 2002). This suggests a hand-to-mouth sequence.

Mirror neurones in the ventral premotor cortex are located in a cortical area called F5 (Matelli *et al.*, 1985), whereas parietal mirror neurones are located in a rostral inferior parietal area, area PF (Gallese *et al.*, 2002). Area F5 and area PF are reciprocally connected (Rizzolatti & Luppino, 2001). Area PF in the inferior parietal lobule is in turn connected with the superior temporal cortex (Seltzer & Pandya, 1994). In the superior temporal cortex, and precisely in the superior temporal sulcus (STS), there are higher order visual neurones that fire at the sight of object-oriented actions (Perrett *et al.*, 1989). Similarly to the visual properties of mirror neurones, these STS neurones do not fire at the sight of a hand approaching a graspable object but not grasping it. The STS–PF–F5 circuit has the anatomical connectivity pattern and the functional properties of a whole cortical circuit dedicated to the understanding of actions of self and other. Thus, this circuit of the macaque brain seems a good candidate for being a precursor of a similar system in the human brain relevant to imitation, a process that requires the mapping of actions of others onto actions of self.

17.3 Human homologues of macaque mirror neurone areas

We tested the hypothesis that macaque mirror neurones are precursors of human neural systems for imitation in a series of brain imaging experiments largely based on functional magnetic resonance imaging (fMRI). The rationale behind the studies was the following: if one looks at the activity in mirror neurones during the execution and observation of action, the firing rate during observation is approximately half the firing rate recorded during the execution of the action (Gallese *et al.*, 1996). Thus, we predicted that areas with mirror neurone properties in the human brain should have an increased signal during motor execution – compared to a resting baseline – twice as large as the one obtained during observation of an action. Moreover, given that imitation yields both observation and execution of an action, we posited that in human mirror neurone areas the increased signal during imitation should amount to approximately the sum of the increased signal during execution only and observation only. This profile of activity was observed in the pars opercularis of the inferior frontal gyrus and in the rostral part of the posterior parietal cortex during imitation of finger movements (Iacoboni *et al.*, 1999). These two regions are anatomically compatible with the macaque regions containing mirror neurones, area F5 in the inferior frontal cortex and area PF in the rostral part of the posterior parietal cortex.

With regard to the human homologue of macaque STS, several laboratories have independently reported that the posterior STS in the human brain responds to biological motion (Allison *et al.*, 2000; Puce *et al.*, 1998; Puce & Perrett, 2003). In our imitation studies we also observed an area in posterior STS that responded more to biological motion than to static pictures of hands. Importantly, this region seems functionally connected to fronto-parietal mirror neurone areas in that it seems to be the recipient of efferent copies of motor commands originating from fronto-parietal mirror neurone areas (Iacoboni *et al.*, 2001). Efferent copies of motor commands are useful for predicting the sensory consequences of planned actions. Given that STS seems to provide a higher order description of the action to be imitated, we proposed that when STS receives efferent copies of motor commands during imitation, it performs a matching process between the visual description of the action and the predicted sensory consequences of the planned imitative action (Iacoboni *et al.*, 2001).

We have also proposed that the activity in the inferior frontal region with mirror neurone properties, most likely Brodmann area 44, is associated with the goal of the imitative action (Iacoboni *et al.*, 1999). In fact, the activity in Brodmann area 44 is reliably higher during imitation of actions with visible goals compared to actions with no visible goal, even though the motor aspect of the action is identical in both cases (Koski *et al.*, 2002). Interestingly, Brodmann area 44 also shows higher activity during imitation of an action as in a mirror (for instance, when model and imitator are face to face, the model is using the left hand while the imitator is imitating with the right hand) compared to imitation of the same action with the anatomically corresponding hand (for instance, when model and imitator are face to face, the model is using the right hand while the imitator is imitating with the right hand). Imitating as in a mirror is the predominant form of imitation early in development (Wapner & Cirillo, 1968). In this form of imitation, the model and the imitator share the same sector of space; they get physically closer. Taken together, this evidence suggests that one of the goals of the imitative process is to create some form of intimacy between the model and the imitator. This concept of intimacy fits well with the links between imitation and empathy and it has been largely neglected in the behavioural studies of imitation of the last decades that have been dominated by a cold, cognitive approach to the investigation of imitative behaviour.

17.4 Imitation and empathy: the links between mirror neurones and the limbic system

So far we have described cortical areas that are relevant to imitation and do not seem to belong to the classical neural systems associated with emotions. So, the question we decided to address was the following: how does the cortical architecture for imitation composed of STS, the rostral part of the posterior parietal cortex and inferior frontal cortex connect anatomically and functionally with areas classically linked to emotional behaviour?

To address this question we first looked at the available anatomical evidence. In the primate brain there seems to be at least one area connecting the limbic system with the three cortical systems – superior temporal cortex, posterior parietal cortex and inferior frontal cortex – that are critical to imitation. This area is the dysgranular sector of the insular lobe (Augustine, 1996). We posited that the dysgranular sector of the insula might play a key role in a large-scale neural network for empathy comprising areas relevant to emotion and to imitation. This hypothesis fulfilled the original proposal of Lipps (as cited by Gallese, 2001), according to which a form of inner imitation of the action of others was critical to generating empathy. This hypothesis was also supported by evidence suggesting that the insula receives slow-conducting unmyelinated fibres that respond to caress/light touch and may be relevant to emotional and affiliative behaviour between individuals (Olausson *et al.*, 2002). To test empirically this model, we used fMRI while subjects were either observing or imitating facial emotional expressions. We reasoned that if the way to empathy goes through some forms of inner imitation of actions of others, then even the simple observation of emotional facial expression should activate the same brain regions used to perform and imitate those emotional facial expressions. However, overt imitation of those emotional facial expressions should yield greater activity in this large-scale network, which comprises the human fronto-parietal mirror neurone system, STS, the insula and the limbic system, due to the simultaneous encoding of the sensory input and planning of the motor output (Carr *et al.*, 2003). We did observe such a pattern of activity in this neural circuit (Carr *et al.*, 2003). Of particular interest is that the limbic area that demonstrated the predicted pattern of activity was the right amygdala. A study on conscious and unconscious processing of emotional facial expression had suggested that the right amygdala is associated with unconscious processing of emotional facial expressions (Morris *et al.*, 1998). This is in line with the kind of unconscious imitation observed in empathic individuals (Chartrand & Bargh, 1999) and suggests that the kind of empathic mechanism we are tapping into here does not require an explicit representational content of the emotional states of others.

In this first study on imitating emotional facial expressions we treated different emotions as a single entity, but different emotions are obviously not a single entity and often are associated with different neural systems. In the large-scale study on emotions in adolescence that we are currently performing we are now comparing the observation and imitation of different kinds of emotions. An interesting preliminary finding of some interim analyses shows that when subjects – in this case 21 10-year-old children with no neurological or psychiatric disorder – imitate a happy face, there is increased activity in medial prefrontal cortex, encompassing also the orbitofrontal sector, compared to imitating a face with a neutral emotional expression (Figure 17.1). The medial part of the orbitofrontal cortex has been associated with monitoring the reward value of different kinds of reinforcers (Kringelbach & Rolls, 2004). Indeed, also the ventral striatum, strongly associated with reward value, was activated by this contrast. Imitating a happy face of others seems for the self a rewarding experience. The self enjoys participating with a resonant bodily expression in the happiness of others. Again, the intimacy of self and other seems transparent during empathic resonance.

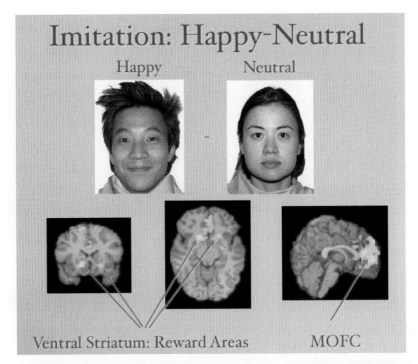

Figure 17.1. In a study on 21 adolescents imitating facial emotional expressions, in which gender and race were equally balanced across emotions, medial orbitofrontal (MOFC) and ventral striatum were more active when imitating a happy face compared to when imitating a face with a neutral expression

17.5 The mirror neurone system and self-recognition

Interestingly, several studies on the sense of self have used a technique called the morphing technique, according to which the face of self and the face of various kinds of others are morphed in a single face to varying degrees. This technique has been prevalently used in tasks requiring self-recognition, rather than any form of empathic resonance. Surprisingly, in a recent study on self-recognition from our group using fMRI and the morphing technique we observed a clear-cut involvement of the mirror neurone system in recognizing morphs prevalently made of self. In this experiment, we used morphs composed only of self and highly familiar others (people that spent several hours a day with the subjects or were long-time close friends of the subjects). Previous studies of this kind had mostly adopted the approach of using famous people as others. With this approach, one controls nicely for familiarity of the stimulus, because presumably the face of a famous person is a face that the subjects had seen several times. However, this approach does not control for the significance of the other to the self. If there is no personal

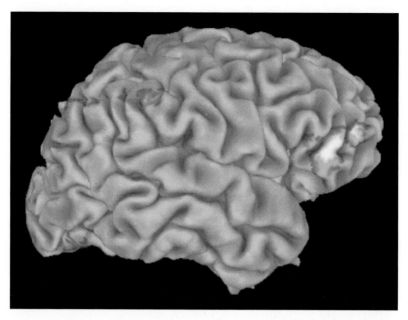

Figure 17.2. Increased activity in right inferior frontal and rostral inferior parietal areas during a self-recognition task while watching morphs of self and other faces composed prevalently of self

relationship with the other, the other is probably perceived in a detached way. In contrast, when the other is a highly familiar person, the perception of the other is presumably linked to a sense of engagement, commitment, closeness and intimacy. In our study, where the other was always represented by a highly familiar personal friend, self-recognition of morphs was associated with increased activity in frontal and parietal mirror neurone areas in the right hemisphere (Figure 17.2) for increasing percentage of self in the morph (Uddin *et al.*, 2005). That is, the greater the contribution of self in the morph, the greater the increase of signal in fronto-parietal mirror neurone areas. How do we explain this signal increase in mirror neurone areas during self-recognition of morphs of self and a highly personally familiar other? After all, mirror neurone areas map actions of others onto actions of self, and at prima facie they seem to support a mechanism for assimilating self and other, rather than a mechanism for distinguishing between them. However, it has been shown that even passive viewing of a static face activates premotor activity (Leslie *et al.*, 2004). Thus, watching a face seems to induce some form of motor imagery. Here, when subjects watch morphs composed of self and highly familiar and personally close others, mirror neurone areas are activated due to the highly relevant social relation of self and other and more so for morphs composed prevalently of self because of the ease with which one can map oneself onto one's own motor system. What emerges from this study is a sense that notions such as self and other cannot be assimilated to static representations, but are actually highly dynamic and interdependent. Mirror neurone areas seem to monitor this interdependence, this intimacy, this sense of collective agency that comes out of social interactions and that is tightly linked to the ability to form empathic resonance (Chartrand & Bargh, 1999).

17.6 Existential empathy and existential neuroscience

Rather than the product of a Cartesian self that contemplates others and infers their emotional states, or the other kind of Cartesian self that simulates the emotional states of others by activating the same neural system that would be activated when personally feeling those emotions, mirror neurone activity linking self and other emotionally and empathically seems to support the view of an existential self that understands the emotional states of other people by committing authentically to other people's involvement in the world into which the self is thrown. Thus, empathy, and especially empathy via imitation, as we have seen above, is not a simulation made by an agent of some mental states of other agents. Rather, it is the accomplishment of collective agents.

This is reminiscent of recurrent themes in the continental philosophy known as existential phenomenology (Dreyfus, 1991; Heidegger, 1927; Merleau-Ponty, 1945). This is why I call this approach existential neuroscience. The existence of mirror neurones only makes sense for agents fully interacting with other people and their environment, in which the basic dichotomies inherited by classical cognitivism melt down completely. These basic dichotomies are the subject/world and the inner/outer dichotomies; these assume that the cognitive agent or subject understands the objects of the world and by doing so produces knowledge, and that these internal mental states represent outer objects of the world – independently – in an inner mental world. The observation of your smiling face triggers a cascade of neural activity in my brain, from inferior frontal (mirror) neurones controlling my facial musculature down to anterior insula neurones and to limbic neurones such that I suddenly and deeply feel your happiness. Your happiness is in my body.

This sharing of mental states across individuals enabled by mirror neurones seems not just restricted to emotions. We have recently reported how mirror neurones enable the understanding of the intentions of other people (Iacoboni *et al.*, 2005). We performed an fMRI experiment in which subjects were observing three different types of stimuli. The first type we call CONTEXT. There are two different kinds of scenes with the same objects: a teapot, a cup, cookies (Figure 17.3). In one case, the objects are neatly organized, suggesting that somebody is going to have tea. In the other case, there are cookie crumbles, a dirty

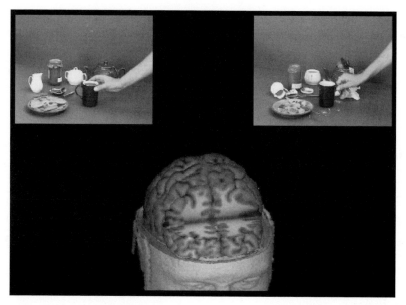

Figure 17.3. Right inferior frontal area that shows increased activity for observation of grasping actions embedded in contexts that suggest the intention behind the action

napkin, etc., suggesting that somebody has already had tea. We call the second type of stimulus ACTION. Here subjects watch only a grasping action of a hand directed at a cup in an objectless background. We call the third type of stimulus INTENTION. Here subjects watch the grasping action directed at the cup while the action is embedded in one of the two scenes presented in the CONTEXT stimulus. The idea behind the experiment is that the same action can be associated with different intentions. In this case, grasping a cup may be associated with drinking or cleaning. The context in which the action occurs may provide an important clue to the observer with regard to the intention of the agent. How do we understand this? Through an inferential process? Apparently not. The crucial comparison, the one between INTENTION and ACTION, revealed that additional neural activity for INTENTION was observed only in the dorsal part of the pars opercularis of the inferior frontal gyrus, a human area with strong mirror neurone properties. Thus, it seemed that mirror neurones also provide a mechanism for understanding the intentions of others. But how does it work? After all, classically described mirror neurones should fire to both ACTION and INTENTION, a grasping action being present in both cases. There are different classes of mirror neurones and among them there are neurones called 'logically related' because they do not fire at the execution and observation of the same action, but rather of a logically related action, say observing a grasping action and performing a hand-to-mouth action. Thus, what likely occurred in our study was that the INTENTION condition would activate not only classical mirror neurones for grasping but also 'logically related' mirror neurones that would be associated with the action that would logically follow the observed one according to the context in which the action occurred. Thus, intention understanding is implemented in human mirror areas by activating a chain of mirror neurones. Indeed, we also found that the drinking INTENTION was associated with greater activity than the cleaning INTENTION. This makes sense if one considers that drinking is a much more primary intention than cleaning and that neuronal chains for drinking are likely more represented than neuronal chains for cleaning in the grasping circuit. Understanding intentions corresponds to predicting a forthcoming goal, and that is something that the motor system is able to perform automatically. As Merleau-Ponty wrote in his '*Phenomenology of Perception*' several decades before mirror neurones were discovered, 'It is as if the other person's intentions inhabited my body and mine his'.

17.7 Conclusion

In this chapter, I have addressed the theoretical implications of recent neuroscience work on the neurobiology of imitation and empathy. The central role of the human mirror neurone system in human interactions suggests an alternative framework to classical cognitivism, dominant in cognitive neuroscience. This alternative framework is reminiscent of themes recurrent in existential phenomenology. Thus, I suggest calling this framework existential neuroscience.

REFERENCES

Allison, T., Puce, A., & McCarthy, G. (2000). Social perception from visual cues: role of the STS region. *Trends in Cognitive Science*, **4**, 267–278.

Augustine, J. R. (1996). Circuitry and functional aspects of the insular lobes in primates including humans. *Brain Research Reviews*, **2**, 229–294.

Barsalou, L. W., Niedenthal, P. M., Barbey, A. K., & Ruppert, J. A. (2003). Social embodiment. In B. H. Ross (ed.), *The Psychology of Learning and Motivation* (Vol. 43) (pp. 43–92). San Diego: Academic Press.

Carr, L., Iacoboni, M., Dubeau, M. C., Mazziotta, J. C., & Lenzi, G. L. (2003). Neural mechanisms of empathy in humans: a relay from neural systems for imitation to limbic areas. *Proceedings of the National Academy of Sciences of the USA*, **100(9)**, 5497–5502.

Chartrand, T. L., & Bargh, J. A. (1999). The chameleon effect: the perception-behavior link and social interaction. *Journal of Personality & Social Psychology*, **76(6)**, 893–910.

diPellegrino, G., Fadiga, L., Fogassi, L., Gallese, V., & Rizzolatti, G. (1992). Understanding motor events: a neurophysiological study. *Experimental Brain Research*, **91**, 176–180.

Dreyfus, H. L. (1991). *Being-in-the-World: A Commentary on Heidegger's Being and Time, Division I.* Cambridge, Mass.: MIT Press.

Gallese, V. (2001). The 'shared manifold' hypothesis. *Journal of Consciousness Studies*, **8(5–7)**, 33–50.

Gallese, V., Fadiga, L., Fogassi, L., & Rizzolatti, G. (1996). Action recognition in the premotor cortex. *Brain*, **119**, 593–609.

Gallese, V., Fogassi, L., Fadiga, L., & Rizzolatti, G. (2002). Action representation and the inferior parietal lobule. In W. Prinz, & B. Hommel (eds.), *Attention and Performance XIX. Common Mechanisms in Perception and Action* (pp. 247–266). Oxford: Oxford University Press.

Hatfield, E., Cacioppo, J. T., & Rapson, R. L. (1994). *Emotional Contagion.* Paris: Cambridge University Press.

Heidegger, M. (1927). *Being and Time.* New York: Harper & Row.

Iacoboni, M., Koski, L. M., Brass, M., *et al.* (2001). Reafferent copies of imitated actions in the right superior temporal cortex. *Proceedings of the National Academy of Sciences of the USA*, **98(24)**, 13995–13999.

Iacoboni, M., Molnar-Szakacs, I., Gallese, V., *et al.* (2005). Grasping the intentions of others with one's own mirror neuron system. *Public Library of Science Biology*, **3(3)**, e79.

Iacoboni, M., Woods, R. P., Brass, M., *et al.* (1999). Cortical mechanisms of human imitation. *Science*, **286(5449)**, 2526–2528.

Kohler, E., Keysers, C., Umilta, M. A., *et al.* (2002). Hearing sounds, understanding actions: action representation in mirror neurons. *Science*, **297(5582)**, 846–848.

Koski, L., Wohlschlager, A., Bekkering, H., *et al.* (2002). Modulation of motor and premotor activity during imitation of target-directed actions. *Cerebral Cortex*, **12(8)**, 847–855.

Kringelbach, M. L., & Rolls, E. T. (2004). The functional neuroanatomy of the human orbito-frontal cortex: evidence from neuroimaging and neuropsychology. *Progress in Neurobiology*, **72(5)**, 341–372.

Leslie, K. R., Johnson-Frey, S. H., & Grafton, S. T. (2004). Functional imaging of face and hand imitation: towards a motor theory of empathy. *Neuroimage*, **21(2)**, 601–607.

Matelli, M., Luppino, G., & Rizzolatti, G. (1985). Patterns of cytochrome oxidase activity in the frontal agranular cortex of the macaque monkey. *Behavioural Brain Research*, **18**, 125–136.

Merleau-Ponty, M. (1945). *Phenomenology of Perception.* London: Routledge.

Morris, J. S., Ohman, A., & Dolan, R. J. (1998). Conscious and unconscious emotional learning in the human amygdala. *Nature*, **393(6684)**, 467–470.

Nadel, J. (2002). Imitation and imitation recognition: functional use in preverbal infants and nonverbal children with autism. In A. N. Meltzoff, & W. Prinz (eds.), *The Imitative Mind: Development, Evolution, and Brain Bases* (pp. 42–62). Cambridge: Cambridge University Press.

Niedenthal, P. M., Barsalou, L. W., Winkielman, P., Krauth-Gruber, S., & Ric, F. (2005). Embodiment in attitudes, social perception, and emotion. *Personality & Social Psychology Review*, **9(3)**, 184–211.

Olausson, H., Lamarre, Y., Backlund, H., *et al.* (2002). Unmyelinated tactile afferents signal touch and project to insular cortex. *Nature Neuroscience*, **5(9)**, 900–904.

Perrett, D. I., Harries, M. H., Bevan, R., *et al.* (1989). Frameworks of analysis for the neural representation of animate objects and actions. *Journal of Experimental Biology*, **146**, 87–113.

Puce, A., Allison, T., Bentin, S., Gore, J. C., & McCarthy, G. (1998). Temporal cortex activation in humans viewing eye and mouth movements. *Journal of Neuroscience*, **18**, 2188–2199.

Puce, A., & Perrett, D. (2003). Electrophysiology and brain imaging of biological motion. *Philosophical Transactions of the Royal Society of London, Series B, Biological Sciences*, **358(1431)**, 435–445.

Rizzolatti, G., & Luppino, G. (2001). The cortical motor system. *Neuron*, **31**, 889–901.

Seltzer, B., & Pandya, D. N. (1994). Parietal, temporal, and occipital projections to cortex of the superior temporal sulcus in the rhesus monkey: a retrograde tracer study. *Journal of Comparative Neurology*, **343**, 445–463.

Uddin, L., Kaplan, J., Molnar-Szakacs, I., Zaidel, E., & Iacoboni, M. (2005). Self-face recognition activates a frontoparietal 'mirror' network in the right hemisphere: an event-related fMRI study. *NeuroImage*, **25(3)**, 926–935.

Umilta, M. A., Kohler, E., Gallese, V., *et al.* (2001). I know what you are doing. A neuro-physiological study. *Neuron*, **31**, 155–165.

Wapner, S., & Cirillo, L. (1968). Imitation of a model's hand movement: age changes in transposition of left-right relations. *Child Development*, **39**, 887–894.

18

Empathizing and systemizing in males, females and autism: a test of the neural competition theory

Nigel Goldenfeld[1], Simon Baron-Cohen[2], Sally Wheelwright[2], Chris Ashwin[2] and Bhismadev Chakrabarti

[1]Centre for Mathematical Sciences, University of Cambridge and Department of Physics, University of Illinois at Urbana – Champaign
[2]Autism Research Centre, Department of Psychiatry, University of Cambridge

18.1 Empathizing and systemizing: sex differences

Two key modes of thought are systemizing and empathizing (Baron-Cohen, 2002). Systemizing is the drive to understand the rules governing the behaviour of a system and the drive to construct systems that are lawful. Systemizing allows one to predict and control such systems. Empathizing is the drive to identify another person's thoughts or emotions, and to respond to their mental states with an appropriate emotion. Empathizing allows one to predict another person's behaviour at a level that is accurate enough to facilitate social interaction. A growing body of data suggests that, on average, females are better than males at empathizing, and males are better than females at systemizing (Geary, 1998; Maccoby, 1999). In this chapter, we review evidence that these abilities strongly differentiate the male and female brain types, and re-analyse some published data to show that these abilities compete, so that despite sex differences in cognitive style, there is no overall sex difference in cognitive ability.

18.2 Autism

Individuals with autism spectrum conditions have severe social difficulties and an 'obsessional' pattern of thought and behaviour (American Psychiatric Association, 1994). Such diagnostic features may arise as a result of their significant disabilities in empathizing (Baron-Cohen et al., 1999, 2001a;

Empathy in Mental Illness, eds. Tom F. D. Farrow and Peter W. R. Woodruff. Published by Cambridge University Press. © Cambridge University Press 2007.

Baron-Cohen and Wheelwright, 2003) as well as their stronger drive to systemize (Baron-Cohen *et al.*, 2001b; Jolliffe & Baron-Cohen, 1997). Such a cognitive profile, together with significant sex bias in incidence rate, is compatible with the theory that autism is an extreme of the male brain (Baron-Cohen, 2002, 2003).

18.3 The empathy quotient (EQ) and the systemizing quotient (SQ)

In order to quantify systemizing and empathizing, two self-report questionnaires have been developed (Baron-Cohen *et al.*, 2003): the systemizing quotient (SQ) and the empathy quotient (EQ). In that study, these two questionnaires were tested in two groups: Group 1 comprised 114 males and 163 females randomly selected from the general population. Group 2 comprised 33 males and 14 females diagnosed with Asperger's syndrome (AS) or high-functioning autism (HFA). The mean scores of this study confirmed both the sex difference in the general population (i.e. a male superiority in systemizing and a female superiority in empathizing), and the extreme male brain theory of autism.

Full details about the construction of the SQ and EQ questionnaires are available elsewhere (Baron-Cohen *et al.*, 2003; Baron-Cohen & Wheelwright, 2004). The EQ and SQ were designed to be short, easy to complete and easy to score. They have a forced-choice format, and are self-administered. Both the SQ and EQ comprise 60 questions, 40 assessing systemizing or empathizing (respectively), and 20 filler (control) items. Approximately half the items are worded to produce a 'disagree' response, and half an 'agree' response, for the systemizing/empathizing response. This is to avoid a response bias either way. Items are randomized. An individual scores 2 points if they strongly display a systemizing/empathizing response, and 1 point if they slightly display a systemizing/empathizing response.

In this chapter, we have re-analysed the data reported in the earlier study (Baron-Cohen *et al.*, 2003) to test for a correlation between the scores for each individual on these tests. The maximum score on both questionnaires was 80. We plotted the raw scores from all individuals (from both groups) on a single chart, whose axes were labelled by the SQ and EQ scores, as shown in Figure 18.1a. The means of each test were taken from Group 1 in the earlier data set, and in this way represent a sex-blind mean of the general population. As can be seen, the results cluster in the SQ-EQ space and do not randomly fill the chart. This suggests that it may not be possible to score anywhere in SQ-EQ space, and that there may be constraints operating, such that SQ and EQ are not independent.

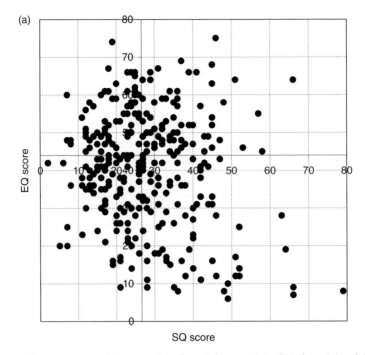

Figure 18.1a. SQ scores versus EQ scores for all participants. Note that the origin of the graph is at the controls' mean SQ and EQ scores. Visual inspection of the data shows that scores are not randomly scattered in all four quadrants of EQ and SQ space, but cluster significantly. Shown in black, it is unclear if these clusters are linked to sex, or diagnosis, but such associations are revealed in Figure 18.1b (in colour)

18.4 Do the EQ and SQ 'sex' the brain? A re-analysis of the 2003 dataset

We separated out the scores from the three groups: males from the general population (henceforth, male controls), females from the general population (female controls), and individuals with AS/HFA, as shown in colour in Figure 18.1b. Inspection of this plot strongly suggests three distinct populations. To explore the variations around the mean, we transformed the raw SQ and EQ scores into the two new variables: $S \equiv (SQ - <SQ>)/80$ and $E \equiv (EQ - <EQ>)/80$, i.e. we first subtracted the control population mean (denoted by $<\ldots>$) from the scores, then divided by the maximum possible score, 80. The means were: 26.66 (SQ) and 44.01 (EQ). To reveal the differences between the populations we essentially factor analysed the results by performing a rotation of the original SQ and EQ axes by 45°. We normalized by the factors of ½, as is appropriate for an axis rotation. These new variables are defined as follows:

$D = (S - E)/2$ (i.e. the difference between the normalized SQ and EQ scores) and $C = (S + E)/2$ (i.e. the sum of the normalized SQ and EQ scores).

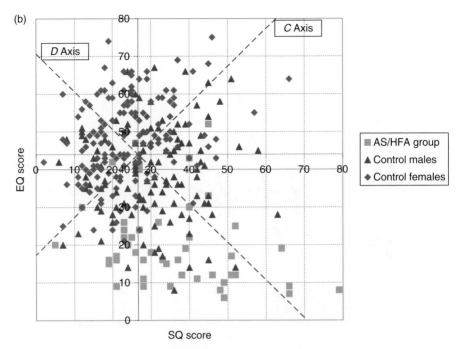

Figure 18.1b. SQ scores versus EQ scores for all participants, separated into the three groups. Note that the origin of the graph is at the controls' mean SQ and EQ scores. Also shown are the C axis (the combined EQ and SQ scores) and the D axis (the difference between the SQ and EQ scores). Whilst Figure 18.1a was blind to sex and diagnosis (all participants are shown in a single colour), here it becomes immediately apparent that more females are clustering towards the upper left quadrant, that more males are clustering towards the lower left quadrant, and that more people with Asperger's syndrome/high-functioning autism (AS/HFA) are clustering deep in the lower left quadrant

D scores represent the difference in ability at systemizing and empathizing for each individual. A high D score can be attained either by being good at systemizing or poor at empathizing, or both. C scores test if systemizing and empathizing stand in a reciprocal, competitive relationship with each other, such that as one scores higher on one of these dimensions, one scores lower on the other. Competition might arise at the neural level [since space is limited in the cortex (Kimura, 1999)] or might arise because both depend on some other biological resource [e.g. the hormone fetal testosterone (Knickmeyer et al., 2005)]. If systemizing and empathizing are reciprocal, one would expect no difference in C scores between the sexes. These new D and C axes are shown in dotted lines on Figure 18.1b.

Figure 18.1b shows that the data have approximate boundaries that lie parallel to the C axis; in other words, the data vary significantly along the D dimension, but much less so along the C dimension. Our rotation was chosen to exhibit precisely

(a)

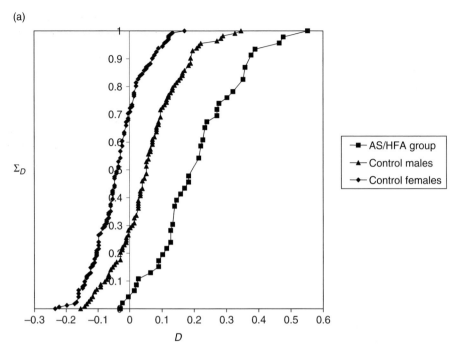

Figure 18.2a. Cumulative distribution function (Σ_D) of *D*. This graph dramatically reveals that the *difference* scores (*D*) between EQ and SQ significantly differentiate between the three populations (males, females and individuals with a diagnosis of AS/HFA)

this feature, but what was unexpected was that the rotation of 45° had such a natural interpretation, as explained below. Figure 18.1b suggests that the male control data have greater weight than the female data on the positive *D* axis, and the AS/HFA group has weight even further to the right along that axis than the male controls. By contrast, there is no significant trend along the *C* axis.

To explore this further, we have plotted the cumulative distributions of our data along the *D* and *C* directions, making separate plots for control male, control female and AS/HFA groups. We define the cumulative distribution $\Sigma_D(D)$ along the *D* direction as the fraction of data points whose *D* value is less than D' irrespective of the *C* value (see Figure 18.2a). Similarly, we define the cumulative distribution $\Sigma_C(C)$ along the *C* direction as the fraction of data points whose *C* value is less than C', irrespective of the *D* value (see Figure 18.2b).

The means and standard deviations of the *C* and *D* scores for the different populations are as follows. *D* scores: control females $= -0.039$ (0.006); control males $= 0.055$ (0.011); AS/HFA $= 0.21$ (0.018). *C* scores: control females $= 0.007$ (0.011); control males $= -0.0$ (0.012); AS/HFA $= -0.092$ (0.010).

Figure 18.2a shows the cumulative distribution along the *D* direction, Σ_D, plotted for the three different groups: control female, control male and AS/HFA.

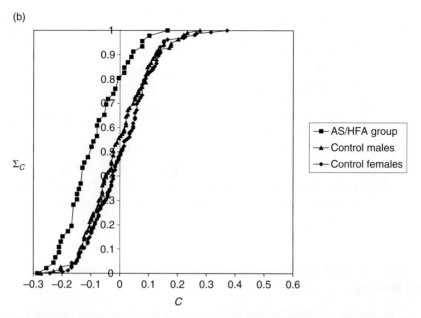

Figure 18.2b. Cumulative distribution function (Σ_C) of C. This graph reveals that when EQ and SQ scores are *summed*, the resulting C scores do not differ between males and females. This means that, overall, neither sex is superior, and that there is neural compensation: the more EQ one has, the less SQ, and vice versa. Such a relationship does not hold for individuals with AS/HFA, who remain with a lower overall C score, evidence of their empathy deficit

The cumulative distributions are widely spaced apart, much further than the fluctuations in the raw data, indicating that these groups really do represent three distinct populations and are not sampled from the same underlying distribution. We quantified this observation by performing a between-subjects single-factor analysis of variance (ANOVA). There was a significant effect of group [$F(2, 321) = 121, p < 0.0001$]. Post-hoc Tukey tests confirmed that all three groups differed significantly from one another.

Figure 18.2b shows the cumulative distribution along the C direction, Σ_C, plotted for the three different groups: control female, control male and AS/HFA. It is apparent that the control male and control female plots are indistinguishable up to the sample fluctuations, but both are well separated from the plots for the AS/HFA group. We have quantified this observation by performing a between-subjects single-factor ANOVA. As expected, there was a significant effect of group [$F(2, 321) = 16.2, p < 0.0001$]. Post-hoc Tukey tests confirmed that there was no significant difference between control males and females, but both of these groups were significantly different from the AS/HFA group.

18.5 Interpretation

These results indicate that the control male and female groups show distinct and significant differences in their cognitive style. The male group scores higher than the female group along the D dimension (relatively higher systemizing and lower empathizing), but there is no difference between the sexes in the measure of C (combined scores). Apparently, females' relatively high empathizing ability compensates for their less developed systemizing ability, and conversely males' high systemizing ability compensates for their less well-developed empathizing skills. The AS/HFA group has a lower C score. This is because, although they outperform both male and female controls on the systemizing measure, this does not compensate for their much lower scores on the empathizing measure.

18.6 A taxonomy of brain types, based on the difference between empathy and systemizing

Previously, a classification of brain types was proposed (Baron-Cohen, 2002), based in part on the empirical evidence suggesting that, as a group, males score higher on the SQ, but lower on the EQ, relative to females (Baron-Cohen *et al.*, 2003). These data also suggested the possibility of a weak inverse relation between SQ and EQ scores. This inverse relationship is fully exposed by the analysis presented here. In particular, because the sex-differences are only discernible along the D dimension, regions of similar brain type are bounded by lines that are parallel to the C axis, or in terms of the original raw data, lines that lie parallel to the lower-left to upper-right diagonal of the SQ–EQ plot. Since there is no unique way to break up the results of our data analysis into identifiable groups along the D dimension, we propose a classification based upon the cumulant plot of Figure 18.2a. This generates five brain types, as follows:

1. A significant proportion of individuals in the general population is likely to have a 'balanced' brain (or be of Type B), that is, their E and the S are not significantly different from each other. This can be expressed as $E \approx S$. In practice, we defined this as individuals whose D score lay between the median of the control male and female populations.
2. A proportion of the general population is likely to have an 'extreme S' Type brain, that is, having a D score larger than the median of the AS/HFA group. This can be expressed as $S \gg E$.
3. A proportion of the general population is likely to have an 'extreme E' Type brain, symmetrically opposite to the extreme S Type brain. This can be expressed as $E \gg S$. (We are not aware of any known clinical group which corresponds to this.)

4. The S Type brain can then be defined as those individuals who lie between the Type B and the extreme Type S brains. This can be expressed as $S > E$.

5. The E Type brain can then be defined as those individuals who lie between the Type B and the extreme Type E brains. This can be expressed as $E > S$.

These five brain type definitions are based upon median scores, rather than a priori criteria based upon the mean and standard deviation. This obviates the need to make special assumptions about the form of the distributions. Table 18.1 shows the percentage of each of the three groups of individuals falling into each of the five Types of brain, using the median definitions above.

Table 18.1 also shows that similar results were obtained by using a classification based upon the control males and females and simply taking a range of percentiles that separated out the tails of the distribution and the centre.

These natural groupings can be defined in terms of the deviations of the SQ and EQ scores from the means over the control populations. Thus, the balanced (B) brain type refers to individuals whose scores are close to the respective means, while S and E are brain types where the deviation from the mean is much greater in S (E) than for E (S). Similarly, extreme S and extreme E are extreme forms of brain types S and E respectively.

With the median definitions as given in Table 18.1, we note that there are significant sex differences in the populations of the different brain types. In the balanced brain type, males and females are present in virtually equal proportions. However, in S-type brains, males outnumber females by a factor of nearly 3:1. In E-type brains, females outnumber males by about the same factor. Finally, among the extreme S-type brains, individuals diagnosed with AS/HFA outnumber males by a factor of nearly 10. Unfortunately, there are not enough data to make any determination of sex-related trends within the AS/HFA group. We hope that future studies will be able to address this interesting question. These trends, rather than the precise boundaries we have chosen between the brain types, are the key differences that our SQ and EQ studies expose, and are not very sensitive to whether the median or percentile classification is used.

In order to present these results in a practical form, we show in Figure 18.3 our results for the different brain types (using the median definitions), translated back into raw scores on the SQ and EQ tests. Figure 18.3 can be directly used to classify an individual's brain type as represented by their responses to the SQ and EQ tests.

18.7 The brain basis of empathy: further distinctions?

Philosophical (Stein, 1989) and evolutionary (Brothers, 1990; Levenson, 1996; Preston & de Waal, 2002) accounts have suggested that empathizing is not a unitary construct. Possible constituent fractions include cognitive empathy (CE)

Table 18.1: Classifications of brain type based upon median positions of the subpopulation control males, females and those with Asperger's syndrome/high-functioning autism (AS/HFA) (data from Figure 18.2a), and upon percentiles of the entire sample (data from Figure 18.1a). Both classifications give similar results. Noteworthy are that more females have a brain of Type E, more males have a brain of Type S, and more individuals with AS/HFA have brain of Extreme Type S

Parameter	Brain type				
	Extreme E	E	B	S	Extreme S
Brain sex	Extreme female	Female	Balanced	Male	Extreme male
Defining characteristic	$S \ll E$	$S < E$	$S \approx E$	$S > E$	$S \gg E$
Brain types based on median positions of the three subpopulations male, females, AS/HFA					
Brain boundary (median)	$D < -0.16$	$-0.16 < D < 0.035$	$-0.035 < D < 0.052$	$0.052 < D < 0.21$	$D > 0.21$
Female %	7	47	32	14	0
Male %	0	17	31	46	6
AS/HFA %	0	0	13	40	47
Brain types based on percentiles of male and female controls					
Brain boundary (percentile)	$D < -0.16$	$-0.16 < D < -0.048$	$-0.048 < D < 0.027$	$0.027 < D < 0.21$	$D > 0.21$
Percentile (per)	Per < 2.5	$2.5 \leq$ per < 35	$35 \leq$ per < 65	$65 \leq$ per < 97.5	per ≥ 97.5
Female %	4.3	44.2	35.0	16.5	0
Male %	0	16.7	23.7	53.5	6.1
AS/HFA %	0	0	12.8	40.4	46.8

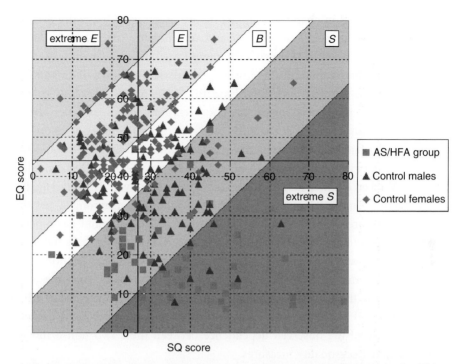

Figure 18.3. SQ scores versus EQ scores for all participants with the proposed boundaries for the different brain types. Five clear bands or brain types are justified: (1) more males fall in zone S (type S, where $S > E$); (2) more females fall in zone E (type E, where $E > S$); (3) many individuals show a type B (balanced profile, where $E = S$), in the white zone; (4) more individuals with AS/HFA fall in the extreme S zone (extreme type S, where $S \gg E$); and (5) some females (but no males) fall in the extreme E dark yellow zone (extreme type E, where $E \gg S$)

(attributions about other's mental states); emotional contagion (EC) ('the tendency to automatically mimic and synchronize facial expressions, vocalizations, postures and movements with those of another person, and, consequently, to converge emotionally' (Hatfield *et al.*, 1992); and sympathy (SY), which involves a 'concern mechanism' (Nichols, 2001) that is often associated with a prosocial/altruistic behavioural component. Our current self-report measure (EQ) provides a composite score of all these three components of empathy (Baron-Cohen & Wheelwright, 2004; Lawrence *et al.*, 2004). Example questions tapping into these individual components are as follows:

1. CE: I often find it difficult to judge if something is rude or polite
2. EC: I get upset if I see people suffering on news programmes
3. SY: I really enjoy caring for other people

Current experiments are underway in our laboratory to test the neurophysiological validity of such conceptual dissociations of empathy. Such a dissociation could help in characterizing the nature of observed 'empathy deficits' in clinical conditions such as autism and psychopathy (Russell & Sharma, 2003). Neuroimaging experiments have implicated different brain areas for performing tasks that tapped into one or more of these 'fraction's of empathy'. Traditional 'Theory of Mind' (cognitive empathy) tasks have consistently shown activity in medial prefrontal cortex, superior temporal gyrus and the temporo-parietal junctions (Frith & Frith, 2003; Saxe *et al.*, 2004). Studies of emotional contagion have demonstrated involuntary facial mimicry (Dimberg *et al.*, 2000) as well as activity in the mirror-neurone-rich regions of the brain (Decety & Jackson, 2004; Wicker *et al.*, 2003). Sympathy has been relatively less investigated, with one study implicating the left inferior frontal gyrus, among a network of other structures (Decety & Chaminade, 2003). While it would be somewhat phreno-logical to expect classical double-dissociations among these individual fractions of empathy, the clinical significance of such a finding cannot be underplayed. There may also be further fractionation of empathy into the comprehension versus the response elements. Our current fMRI studies of the brain basis of EQ and SQ scores may shed light on the neural nature and conceptual signifi-cance of the observed dependence between these two non-orthogonal psycho-metric personality measures.

18.8 Conclusions

We have shown that a re-analysis of the data from an earlier study using the EQ and SQ (Baron-Cohen *et al.*, 2003) reliably sexes the brain when analysed blind. In addition, although females show stronger empathizing and males show stronger systemizing, their *combined* scores do not differ, suggesting that empa-thizing and systemizing compete neurally in the brain. This also leads to the gratifying conclusion that, overall, neither sex is superior. We also confirm earlier reports that people with AS or HFA have stronger systemizing scores than normal, but our new analysis shows that this does not compensate for their weaker empathy: thus their combined scores do not equal those of the normal groups. This result lends support to the extreme male brain theory of autism, and confirms that autism spectrum conditions arise from a cognitive deficit in empathizing.

Acknowledgments

S.B.C. and S.W. were supported by the Medical Research Council of the United Kingdom. N.G. was supported by the US National Science Foundation during the period of this work. C.A. was supported by NAAR, and B.C. was supported by Trinity College. We thank Johnny Lawson and Akio Wakabayashi for valuable discussions around the model being tested here.

REFERENCES

American Psychiatric Association (1994). *DSM-IV Diagnostic and Statistical Manual of Mental Disorders* (4th edn.). Washington DC: American Psychiatric Association Press.

Baron-Cohen, S. (2002). The extreme male brain theory of autism. *Trends in Cognitive Sciences*, **6**, 248–254.

Baron-Cohen, S. (2003). *The Essential Difference: Men, Women and the Extreme Male Brain.* London: Penguin.

Baron-Cohen, S., O'Riordan, M., Jones, R., Stone, V., & Plaisted, K. (1999). A new test of social sensitivity: detection of faux pas in normal children and children with Asperger syndrome. *Journal of Autism and Developmental Disorders*, **29**, 407–418.

Baron-Cohen, S., Richler, J., Bisarya, D., Gurunathan, N., & Wheelwright, S. (2003). The Systemising Quotient (SQ): an investigation of adults with Asperger syndrome or high functioning autism and normal sex differences. *Philosophical Transactions of the Royal Society, Series B, Special issue on 'Autism Mind and Brain'*, **358**, 361–374.

Baron-Cohen, S., & Wheelwright, S. (2003). The Friendship Questionnaire (FQ): an investigation of adults with Asperger syndrome or high functioning autism, and normal sex differences. *Journal of Autism and Developmental Disorders*, **33**, 509–517.

Baron-Cohen, S., & Wheelwright, S. (2004). The Empathy Quotient (EQ). An investigation of adults with Asperger syndrome or high functioning autism, and normal sex differences. *Journal of Autism and Developmental Disorders*, **34**, 163–175.

Baron-Cohen, S., Wheelwright, S., Hill, J., Raste, Y., & Plumb, I. (2001a). The 'Reading the Mind in the eyes' test revised version: a study with normal adults, and adults with Asperger syndrome or high-functioning autism. *Journal of Child Psychiatry and Psychiatry*, **42**, 241–252.

Baron-Cohen, S., Wheelwright, S., Scahill, V., Lawson, J., & Spong, A. (2001b). Are intuitive physics and intuitive psychology independent? *Journal of Developmental and Learning Disorders*, **5**, 47–78.

Brothers, L. (1990). The neural basis of primate social communication. *Motivation and Emotion*, **14**, 81–91.

Decety, J., & Chaminade, T. (2003). Neural correlates of feeling sympathy. *Neuropsychologia*, **41**, 127–138.

Decety, J., & Jackson, P. (2004). The functional architecture of human empathy. *Behavioural and Cognitive Neuroscience Reviews*, **3**, 71–100.

Dimberg, U., Thunberg, M., & Elmehed, K. (2000). Unconscious facial reactions to emotional facial expressions. *Psychological Science*, **11**, 86–89.

Frith, U., & Frith, C. (2003). Development and neurophysiology of mentalizing. *Philosophical Transactions of the Royal Society*, **358**, 459–473.

Geary, D. C. (1998). *Male, Female: The Evolution of Human Sex Differences*. Washington DC: American Psychological Association.

Hatfield, E., Cacioppo, J. T., & Rapson, R. L. (1992). Emotional contagion. In M. S. Clark (ed.), *Review of Personality and Social Psychology: Emotion and Behaviour*. Newbury Park, Calif.: Sage Publications.

Jolliffe, T., & Baron-Cohen, S. (1997). Are people with autism or Asperger's syndrome faster than normal on the embedded figures task? *Journal of Child Psychology and Psychiatry*, **38**, 527–534.

Kimura, D. (1999). *Sex and Cognition*. Cambridge, Mass.: MIT Press.

Knickmeyer, R., Baron-Cohen, S., Raggatt, P., & Taylor, K. (2005). Foetal testosterone, social cognition, and restricted interests in children. *Journal of Child Psychology and Psychiatry*, **45**, 1–13.

Lawrence, E. J., Shaw, P., Baker, D., Baron-Cohen, S., & David, A. S. (2004). Measuring empathy – reliability and validity of the empathy quotient. *Psychological Medicine*, **34**, 911–919.

Levenson, R. W. (1996). Biological substrates of empathy and facial modulation of emotion: two facets of the scientific legacy of John Lazetta. *Motivation and Emotion*, **20**, 185–204.

Maccoby, E. (1999). *The Two Sexes: Growing Up Apart, Coming Together*: Princeton, N.J.: Harvard University Press.

Nichols, S. (2001). Mindreading and the cognitive architecture underlying altruistic motivation. *Mind and Language*, **16**, 425–455.

Preston, S. D., & de Waal, F. B. M. (2002). Empathy: its ultimate and proximate bases. *Behavioural and Brain Sciences*, **25**, 1–72.

Russell, T., & Sharma, T. (2003). Social cognition at the neural level: investigations in autism, psychopathy and schizophrenia. In M. Brune, H. Ribbert & W. Schiefenhovel (eds.), *The Social Brain: Evolution and Pathology*. New York: John Wiley & Sons Limited.

Saxe, R., Carey, S., & Kanwisher, N. (2004). Understanding other minds: linking developmental psychology and functional neuroimaging. *Annual Review in Psychology*, **55**, 87–124.

Stein, E. (1989). *On the Problem of Empathy*. Washington, DC: ICS Publications.

Wicker, B., Keysers, C., Plailly, J., *et al.* (2003). Both of us disgusted in *My* insula: the common neural basis of seeing and feeling disgust. *Neuron*, **40**, 655–664.

19

Motivational-affective processing and the neural foundations of empathy

India Morrison

Centre for Cognitive Neuroscience, University of Wales Bangor

... Candace, howling oh-my-God-oh-my-God, holds up her hand, which is gushing blood from a deep gash that extends from her thumbnail almost to her palm. The blood is everywhere – down her arm, in the elaborate grooves she's been carving in the back of her chair ... Looking at all the blood, Tick feels her own left arm begin to throb the way it always does in anticipation of hypodermic needles at the doctor's office, and at horror movies when somebody gets slashed.

Richard Russo, *Empire Falls*

19.1 Introduction

Pleasure and pain, comfort and discomfort, hot and cold – we are creatures for whom states of affairs are imbued with goodness or badness. When they are bad, we experience the need to avoid or terminate the experience. Sometimes, like the character Tick in the quote above, we feel comparable subjective sensations when we see someone else in aversive circumstances, even though we ourselves might be quite safe from them.

Recent research hints that we, as body owners, perceive even the actions and sensations of other people through a 'filter' of our own bodily representations. Visual information about the goal-directed actions of others can engage action-preparation pathways in the brains of passive observers (di Pellegrino *et al.*, 1992; Gallese *et al.*, 1996; Rizzolatti *et al.*, 1996). This visual sensitivity might even reflect a general functional principle, not limited to motor areas, but extending to other cortical systems such as those subserving disgust (Phillips, *et al.*, 1997; Wicker *et al.*, 2003) and pain (Jackson *et al.*, 2005; Morrison *et al.*, 2004; Singer *et al.*, 2004). These results suggest a basic *type* of mechanism for the social brain to take third-person visual information about others and transform it into first-person, bodily terms. Many researchers have come to regard this as a crucial predicate for empathy (e.g. Decety & Jackson 2004; Gallese 2001, 2003; Keysers *et al.*, 2004).

Empathy in Mental Illness, eds. Tom F. D. Farrow and Peter W. R. Woodruff. Published by Cambridge University Press. © Cambridge University Press 2007.

My approach to this research is a relatively bottom-up one. Though it may seem odd in a book devoted to the subject, I shall temporarily suspend the broad, vernacular word 'empathy', except for its occasional use as a covering term. Instead, I refer to the visual modulation of body-related brain areas by *others'* situations or expressions as 'vicarious responding'. Vicarious responding is a descriptive term pitched at the level of neural coding. It is important to note that although vicarious responding may facilitate subjective feeling states, it is *not* taken as sufficient to instigate full-blown emotions or overt actions. Vicarious responding can occur in regions associated with particular domains, such as motor action, body sensation and affect.

In the search for basic building blocks of empathy, then, I turn to specific systems – pain in particular – to investigate the ways in which the motivational-affective nature of processing in these systems may contribute to aversive reactions to others' distress. The strategy of this chapter is to ask first what these systems do for the organism itself, and then to explore what it may mean for the nature of empathy when visual modulation of these systems gives rise to vicarious responses in the observer. Of particular interest are those networks involved in the learning and preparation of motivated, affectively valenced, skeletomotor movements of aversion.

When placed in the wider motivational-affective framework presented here, vicarious responses may be examined with respect to a variety of affective response components, including facial expressions. Intriguingly, formal properties of vicarious responding in the motivational-affective domain point to a deep analogy with those in the action representation domain. This analogy has implications for the way we conceptualize the organization of the social brain and the nature of intersubjective processing, and is probed further in the final section.

19.2 Vicarious responding in a motivational-affective (M-A) framework

One of empathy's quintessential features is that it has a certain 'from-the-inside' feel that ranks it with other varieties of emotional experience. Vicarious responding in emotional networks may represent a basic condition for the characteristic affective buzz so often associated with the visual perception of *others'* emotional states (Carr *et al.*, 2003; Gallese, 2001, 2003). To pursue this line of thinking requires a clarification of what it would entail in functional terms. Towards this end, the following sections will concentrate on aspects of functional processing in two domains that have shown evidence of vicarious responding: pain and disgust.

19.2.1 Studying vicarious responding

Human neuroanatomical studies that have bearing on vicarious responding in the emotional domain can be roughly divided into two types: one that hinges on the perception or recognition of emotions generally, and one that relates perception or recognition to the experience of emotion, usually targetting a specific emotion. Both types of study frequently present static facial expressions as emotion stimuli. Dynamic facial displays, point-light body displays, scripts, actors and emotion imitation have also been used (Atkinson *et al.*, 2004; Carr *et al.*, 2003; Decety & Chaminade, 2003; Farrow *et al.*, 2001; Heberlein *et al.*, 2004; Leslie *et al.*, 2004). The facial expression stimuli typically presented to subjects are photographs depicting Ekman's six basic emotion categories: anger, fear, sadness, happiness, disgust and surprise (Ekman & Friesen, 1971). Because these categories of emotion expression are panculturally recognized, they are accepted as robustly validated means for tapping into immediate, automatic emotion-related processing.

Most studies of the first type seek to investigate emotion processing in a general sense, cutting across categories of emotion. For example, Adolphs *et al.* (2000) found that patients with damage to right somatosensory cortexes were selectively impaired in the recognition of emotional expressions. Because the right somatosensory cortexes are also implicated in the generation of emotional expressions in healthy adults (Adolphs, 2002; Adolphs *et al.*, 2000), Adolphs reasoned that both the generation and the recognition of emotional expressions draw upon some of the same perceptual and somatosensory resources. This supports the view that areas associated with body representation are not committed to processing only those signals from one's own body, but are susceptible to 'infiltration' by affective information related to other people.

Studies of the second type tend to focus on particular emotions, such as fear or disgust, or sensory domains that are not usually classed alongside the basic emotions, such as pain or touch (e.g. Keysers *et al.*, 2004). The emphasis here is not on perception or recognition alone, but on the experience of that particular emotion or state. The kinds of stimuli used include basic facial expressions, but can also involve attempts to produce that particular state in the subject. For disgust, this can take the form of administering a bad odour or taste, for example; for pain, submitting volunteers to painful stimuli such as localized electric shocks. When neuroimaging techniques are employed, the processing of certain emotions or states in the subject's brain can then be directly compared to the processing related to the subject's perception of those states in others. In what follows I shall focus on this type of study, mostly with respect to pain, but making the occasional incursion into the realm of disgust as well.

19.2.2 Domain-specific vicarious responses: pain and disgust

Preliminary evidence for vicarious responding in pain networks came from a neurophysiological study recording from cortical cells of human patients awaiting brain surgery (Hutchison *et al.*, 1999). Using microelectrodes, Hutchison *et al.*

recorded from the anterior cingulate cortex (ACC) of 11 patients as several types of painful stimuli were applied to their hands: painful heat, painful cold and mechanical 'pinpricks' from a sharp probe. They found stimulus-specific pain responses in area 24b of dorsal ACC (24b' of Vogt *et al.*, 1995a), including cells that discharged preferentially to the pinprick stimulus. When an experimenter quite serendipitously pricked himself with this sharp probe, one of these cells discharged (Hutchison *et al.*, 1999; W. D. Hutchison, pers. comm.). Thus this particular cell appears to have been sensitive not only to pain-related input originating from the hand, but also to visual input carrying information about another person's hand.

This effect was corroborated in healthy subjects in a functional magnetic resonance imaging (fMRI) experiment by Morrison *et al.* (2004). Volunteers underwent aversive stimulation of one hand with a needle-like sharp probe while in the scanner. In another condition, they watched videos of someone else's hand being pricked by a hypodermic needle. The same region – ACC 24b – was the only region that showed overlapping haemodynamic activity while both seeing and feeling pain. The locus of overlapping activity fell squarely within the recording site reported by Hutchison *et al.* (1999).

A similar result was obtained by Singer *et al.* (2004). Here, female subjects viewed their own hand alongside that of their romantic partner as electrode shocks were delivered to one or the other at either high or low levels of stimulation. Visual cues projected on a screen behind the hands indicated to the subject whether the shock would occur to herself or to her partner, as well as whether the stimulation would be low (not painful) or high (painful). Activity in both the ACC and another region, the anterior insula, was shared between the self and other conditions when the shock was painful.

This part of the ACC (above the corpus callosum) is variously termed dorsal ACC (Bush *et al.*, 2002) and midcingulate cortex (Vogt *et al.*, 2003). Although the latter designation is more systematically grounded in anatomical, functional and cytoarchetectonic distinctions, I shall use the term dorsal ACC here for the sake of consistency with the empathy neuroimaging literature (see Figure 19.1). Both the dorsal ACC and the anterior insula are among those cortical areas most reliably activated in neuroimaging studies of pain (Peyron *et al.*, 2000). The Morrison *et al.* (2004) study showed that a specific region in the pain network shows selectivity to ecological pain cues in relation both to oneself and to strangers. Singer *et al.* (2004) demonstrate that pain-related regions are likewise engaged by symbolic cues in situations in which there is an imminent and ongoing threat of pain both to oneself and to a loved one. In another fMRI experiment, subjects viewed a demonstrator's hand and foot encountering a variety of everyday mishaps, such as being slammed in a car door or cut with a knife while slicing cucumbers (Jackson *et al.*, 2005). Observing others' painful situations activated

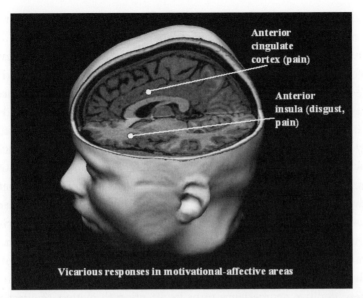

Figure 19.1. A cutaway view of the brain showing areas in which vicarious responses have been observed in caudal regions of the medial dorsal anterior cingulate cortex (for pain) and the anterior insula (for olfactory disgust and pain). These two areas are important in relating bodily information to potential behavioural responses. (Rendered MRI image shows $x = -1$ and $z = 4$ in Talairach space)

the same region of the dorsal ACC and anterior insula implicated in the other imaging studies (Figure 19.1).

The anterior insula, at the head of a length of infolded cortical tissue buried in the sylvian fissure, has also been implicated in nausea and disgust (Calder *et al.*, 2001). Patients with lesions to the insula show a selective deficit in recognizing facial expressions of disgust (Phillips *et al.*, 1997). One patient with bilateral insular lesions presented a 'disgust blindness' that pertained not only to the recognition of disgusted facial expressions, which in one case he spontaneously ventured to label 'hungry and thirsty', but extended even to displays of retching and regurgitating food – it was 'delicious', he hazarded (Adolphs *et al.*, 2003). These findings have also been supported in healthy subjects using fMRI (Phillips *et al.*, 1998). Consistent with this, Wicker *et al.*' s (2003) fMRI investigation of disgust showed vicarious responding in the anterior insula, with overlapping activation when subjects smelled offensive odours while in the scanner and observed demonstrators' apparently disgusted reactions to the smells.

These studies are instructive in that they explore the specificity of vicarious responses with respect to networks associated with given domains such as pain and disgust. They also raise questions about the function of these systems. What are such representations *for*? How might they benefit the organism, and in what wider terms might they be more generally understood?

Increasingly, the neuroscience of emotion has begun to adopt a biology-inspired perspective that views emotions as dispositions to act (Brothers, 1990; Panksepp, 1998). In this view, the function of emotion is ultimately to produce specific responses which prepare the organism to approach or avoid certain objects or contexts. These responses can occur at various levels, whether physiological or overtly behavioural, so a given affective response usually comes as a 'package' that can include autonomic and endocrine as well as muscular responses. One of the most salient features of this perspective is its functionalist spirit: such responses are adaptive, and are shaped by evolution, learning, or both. Emotions are no longer seen as pathological disruptions of rational thought, but as doing very sophisticated, useful things. Organisms come equipped with the wherewithal to orient to, remember and even anticipate the complexities of the world through complicated (if now and then imperfect) suites of dispositional mechanisms.

When cognitive neuroscience turns its attention to matters of affect, considerations regarding the functions and adaptiveness of emotions become framed in information-processing terms. To say that a neural structure is involved in a given process is to say that it has a systematic effect that plays a role in performing a certain job designated in the experimenter's hypothesis – such as 'feeling pain' or 'recognizing facial expressions of disgust'. Given that emotions function to influence action dispositions, what terms would most usefully describe the kind of information processing in neural pathways in which vicarious responses have been observed?

19.2.3 A motivational-affective framework

Information processing in neural pathways that include ACC and anterior insula have been characterized as 'motivational-affective' (Melzack, 1999; Price, 2000; Rainville *et al.*, 1999). Mammals have evolved learning mechanisms that go beyond reactive affective responses – mechanisms which play essential roles in evaluating and learning complex contingencies as well as in selecting, changing and controlling relevant response elements. 'Motivation' is a general concept used by behavioural neuroscientists in hypotheses about the many ways in which organisms change their behaviour. (It should be noted that the concept of motivation has a rich history in social psychology too. The concept of motivation used here is the neuroscientist's.) Essentially in the service of bioregulation, motivation in the behaving organism often manifests in learning processes that contribute to the ways in which behaviour becomes modified with respect to rewarding or aversive objects or situations (Berridge, 2004).

The ACC comes to the fore in motivation (Bush *et al.*, 2002; Devinsky *et al.*, 1995; Hadland *et al.*, 2003; Walton *et al.*, 2003) as well as response selection

(Hadland *et al.*, 2003; Paus, 2001; Rushworth *et al.*, 2003). The role of primate dorsal ACC in particular is tightly linked to the relating of reward information with response preparation and selection, as when changing reward contingencies demand modifications in motor response (Bush *et al.*, 2002; O'Doherty *et al.*, 2003; Shima & Tanji, 1998). This sort of learning in the dorsal ACC occurs under conditions in which stimuli are novel, salient (Devinsky *et al.*, 1995; Downar *et al.*, 2003; Huettel *et al.*, 2004), and infrequent, uncertain, or unpredictable (Hsieh *et al.*, 1999; Huettel *et al.*, 2004). Moreover, ACC activation in fMRI studies decreases with learning and error reduction (Gusnard *et al.*, 2001; Raichle, 1998), indicating a role for this area in early stages of learning when greater control is required.

The learning, preparation and production of flexible behaviour are deeply bound up with the valenced evaluation of objects and their contexts. These evaluations can be accompanied by positively or negatively hedonic subjective experiences. Some objects come with built-in hedonic value, such as food and water. But hedonic value can also be learned and modified, influencing the kinds of behaviour we make towards a hedonic object, as well as the effort we are willing to put into obtaining a pleasant stimulus or avoiding an unpleasant one. Hedonic value can also attach to objects that appear in the same context as hedonic objects, independently of a cognitive appreciation of the relevant cause-and-effect relationships or the instrumental means to obtain or avoid them (Berridge, 2004). In humans, socially relevant and semantic cues have also been shown to modify motivated behaviour. Happy face primes increase the quantity of food and drink consumed, whereas angry faces curb it (Winkielman *et al.*, 2005); and positively valenced words potentiate approach movements, whereas negative ones potentiate withdrawal movements (Chen & Bargh, 1999).

The ACC has been consistently linked to subjective qualities such as pleasantness or unpleasantness, feelings of effort accompanying concentration of attention or performance of a difficult task, and consciousness (Posner & Rothbart, 1998; Rainville *et al.*, 1997, 1999; Walton *et al.*, 2003). Indeed, in his model of consciousness Damasio (1994, 1999) identifies the ACC as one of the key areas involved in the subjective awareness of bodily changes that occur with respect to an object. He proposes that a first-order representation of the body – the viscera, the skin, hormone levels and so forth – is supported by certain brainstem structures alongside somatosensory cortexes and insula. When the bodily situation changes in response to objects in the world (for example, your thudding heartbeat when a bear noses around your tent), second-order 'images' of the corresponding activity in these first-order maps are coded in areas such as ACC and orbitofrontal cortexes. This dynamic re-mapping is thought to be accompanied by subjective awareness of emotional states and to contribute to flexible, goal-directed behaviour via an influence on response dispositions and motivated decision-making.

Along similar lines, Craig (2003a) proposes an interoceptive network concerning afferent information about the physiological condition of internal tissues. In humans, phylogenetically unique projections from (1) the thalamus to anterior insula, and (2) dorsal ACC to anterior insula are postulated to form the basis of a higher-order subjective awareness of self. In Craig's model, the anterior insula's role goes beyond first-order mapping and into the realms of conscious emotional experience. An fMRI study of heartbeat detection implicating the right anterior insula and dorsal ACC prompted Critchley *et al.* (2004) to conclude that these two areas work in concert, with the right anterior insula possibly more directly involved in body mapping and the ACC in mobilizing a behavioural response (Bechara & Naqvi, 2004; Craig, 2004).

Drawing together these aspects of affective response disposition, motivational learning and subjective experience yields a potentially fruitful theoretical framework for vicarious responding. A motivational-affective (M-A) framework identifies relevant information-processing aspects of neural systems and provides explanatory resources within which to situate hypotheses about empathy. Not least, it is capable of producing constrained, testable hypotheses.

19.3 M-A systems in pain and disgust

The concerted workings of affective and motivational processes drench our perceptual world with value and run deep in our heritage as organic creatures. At the heart of M-A systems lie bioregulatory processes whose job it is to avoid damage to precious tissues both without and within. Section 19.2 introduced the notion that affective responses and motivational processes are functionally intertwined on several levels. This section concentrates on the skeletomotor element in particular, with a view to elucidating its role in M-A pain and disgust processing.

19.3.1 Parsing pain

The pioneering neuroscientist Charles Scott Sherrington characterized pain as a heuristic category of perception, referring to its rough-and-ready role in learning about tissue damage through specialized channels of perception (Sherrington, 1948). Modern pain researchers invoke the International Association for the Study of Pain's definition, which also emphasizes the detection of tissue damage or the threat of tissue damage (Price, 1999). At least part of what pain *is*, then, has to do with learning contingencies that involve harm or the looming prospect of harm. But pain is not just a sort of sensory push to which the organism replies with a behavioural pull. Learning about pain also means learning about objects and contexts – and just as there are plentiful sources of harm in the environment, there are many ways in which the organism can prepare and deploy an appropriate reaction.

A straightforward way of avoiding pain or removing oneself from a painful situation is simply to move. Leaping up from your chair if you have sat on a wasp is perhaps not very graceful, but is an elegant solution to the immediate problem. In information-processing terms, a reaction like this is made possible by several computations, which may occur at least partly in parallel (Price *et al.*, 2002). The wasp sting must be detected and its location (your posterior), intensity (high), and nature (stinging) discriminated, its significance must be evaluated (bad), and efferent motor signals sent to orchestrate the aversive movement (leaping from your chair).

Current models of pain processing reflect just such a division of labour in the way the brain codes various aspects of the same painful experience. The coding of pain is divisible into two major dimensions that are empirically dissociable: the sensory-discriminative (S-D) and the motivational-affective (M-A). The S-D dimension supports the spatial localization and intensity encoding of painful stimuli. In a complementary manner, the M-A dimension is involved in coding the affective unpleasantness and motivational relevance of nociceptive (noxious) information. These two dimensions also follow relatively distinct pathways from the spinal cord to subcortical and cortical regions in the brain. On the whole, sensory-discriminative processing has been associated with nerve fibres ascending through lateral nuclei of the thalamus to somatosensory cortexes. M-A processing is associated primarily with medial thalamic pathways, with terminations in cortical areas including the ACC and insula (Sewards & Sewards, 2002, 2003; Vogt & Sikes, 2000).

With the exception of a few key neuroimaging studies (Price, 2000; Rainville *et al.*, 1997, 1999), evidence for the functional distinction between M-A and S-D dimensions of pain processing has come from mammals such as rats and monkeys. Observations from humans are rare, but instructive. Ploner *et al.* (1999) reports a patient with selective damage to the right postcentral gyrus and parietal operculum, which include somatosensory areas for the skin of the hands. When stimulated with a laser, the patient was unable to localize a painful stimulus on the left (contralateral) hand. However, he appeared to have intact motivational processing, identifying the painful sensation as 'something he wanted to avoid' despite not being able to discriminate its sensory characteristics (Ploner *et al.*, 1999). In keeping with this, stimulation of anterior cingulate cortex in humans produces reports of unspecific motivation or urges, and feelings of 'wanting or planning to do something' (Bancaud & Talairach, 1992). It is perhaps telling that damage to the ACC, a cortical target for medial fibre projections, can alter pain perception without impairing localization, yet microstimulation does not produce feelings of pain (Davis *et al.*, 1994; Hutchison *et al.*, 1999).

Intriguingly, neuroimaging studies of vicarious pain have consistently failed to show significant vicarious effects in S-D pathways such as somatosensory cortexes

(Jackson *et al.*, 2005; Morrison *et al.*, 2004; Singer *et al.*, 2004), even when body-part-specific effects are hypothesized (e.g. hand versus foot; Jackson *et al.*, 2005). However, a potential role for somatosensory cortices should not be ruled out on the basis of its silence in the analyses reported in these fMRI studies (see e.g. Avenanti *et al.*, 2004). For instance, it is possible that any such role may escape the logic of conjunction (overlap or common activation) used in Morrison *et al.* (2004) and Singer *et al.* (2004). It may also depend on various aspects of the experimental design and stimulus parameters, such as perceived intensity (Jackson *et al.*, 2005; S. Aglioti, pers. comm.), and even the measures used, which remain to be systematically explored.

19.3.2 From motivation to movement

The motivated feeling of wanting to move corresponds subjectively to what we would label an urge. Motivational urges in themselves may not intrinsically specify a particular effector. Cortical M-A-related regions such as the dorsal ACC do not contain a meticulously delineated sensorimotor topography of the body as S-D regions do (Barch *et al.*, 2001; Vogt *et al.*, 1995a, 2003). Outside of the caudal cingulate motor areas (CMAs), any 'mapping' here may be conceived more in terms of motivational salience, and in any case is not especially spatially acute (Mesulam, 1999). This squares well with the uncomfortable but ill-localized subjective experience of vicarious pain, which is of a variety vividly termed 'all-overishness' by William James: "If our friend goes near to the edge of a precipice, we get the well-known feeling of 'all-overishness', and we shrink back, although we positively *know* him to be safe, and have no distinct imagination of his fall" (James, 1892).

As discussed in section 19.2, the dorsal ACC is well-placed to relate fluctuating reward outcomes to motor responses. The dorsal ACC sits above the corpus callosum, distinct from the eye, forelimb, hand and voice motor representation of adjacent cingulate motor areas with which it interacts (Isomura & Takada, 2004; Vogt *et al.*, 1995a). It receives indirect projections from superior temporal areas associated with higher-level, semantic visual processing (Vogt & Pandya, 1987). Within the dorsal regions that include those implicated in vicarious pain, pain-related neurones have been found among the same populations as reward-related neurones (Koyama *et al.*, 2001) and those that anticipate painful stimuli (Koyama *et al.*, 1998; Porro *et al.*, 2003). Projections from dorsal ACC reach supplementary motor, premotor, cingulate motor and primary motor cortexes, influencing the selection of skeletomotor responses to painful stimuli (Devinsky *et al.*, 1995; Matelli *et al.*, 1991; Vogt *et al.*, 1995a).

Pain, then, is more than an unpleasant subjective state. On the functional level, many computations interact in different ways, and among different effector systems, to produce particular responses. The same is true of disgust. Disgust, of course, is closely associated with mechanisms that expel distasteful or noxious substances from the body. When an offensive item is swallowed, brainstem areas coordinate complicated emetic reflexes such as retching and vomiting. Before matters reach such a pass, however, orofacial movements of aversion or expulsion can preempt the need for vomiting. These movements are of a skeletomotor nature and are more susceptible to voluntary control than retching and vomiting. The anterior insula and basal ganglia are involved in disgust and nausea (Calder, *et al.*, 2000, 2001), and may play a role in learning about distasteful items for the purposes of altering behaviour in future circumstances.

Just as pain can be considered a heuristic category of perception, nausea – which precedes and accompanies emetic reflexes – can also be thought of as a subjective warning bell based on past experience. From the inside, nausea has an 'urgish' feel too. Direct stimulation of the anterior insula in human epilepsy patients has produced nausea (Penfield & Rasmussen, 1955), as well as unpleasant, urgent M-A feelings in the throat and nose (Krolak-Salmon *et al.*, 2003). It is possible that the insula, via its olfactory and gustatory involvement and connections with the motor-related basal ganglia (Augustine, 1996), contributes to the potentiation of orofacial aversive or expulsive movements.

19.3.3 From learning to communication

Facial expressions have evolved as part of the affect 'package' in emotions such as disgust. An evolutionary approach treats facial expressions as traits that can be investigated phylogenetically (that is, by finding instances of it on the family tree of mammals). For example, the bitter taste of quinine produces gaping and aversive head movements that are shared among rodents and primates, including us (Berridge 2000, 2004; Erikson & Schulkin, 2003). Grimacing and 'squinching' the eyes is shared among great apes, but is not seen in rodents or Old and New World monkeys (Steiner *et al.*, 2001). Grimacing (pulling the corners of the mouth back and down with lips tightly over the teeth) is also a feature of the face shared by macaques and humans when tense or anticipating something unpleasant, and in this capacity it is unrelated to disgust (Redican, 1982). Exploring what we share, or do not share, with other species allows us to extrapolate into evolutionary history to make inferences about the history and function of disgust expressions.

For humans, to see someone with a disgusted look on their face is *not* to see the horizontal wrinkles on the nose or that the eyebrows are lowered without being drawn together. It is simply to perceive that they are disgusted. Influential current theories treat disgust as a multicomponent appraisal mechanism, at the core of which is assessing the risk of contamination (Curtis *et al.*, 2004; Marzillier & Davey, 2004; Rozin *et al.*, 2000). The disgusted facial expression gives clues to conspecifics about the outcome of such evaluations. Expressions are one way of making that heuristic warning bell ring out a bit more publicly. If we, as social animals, use others' efferent facial signals as heuristic in themselves – especially if their perception comes along with congruent subjective evaluations – we are saved the perils of discovering first-hand that something is dangerous or noxious.

Communicative facial expressions also exist for pain, though they appear to be less reliably perceived (Prkachin et al., 1994; Williams, 2002). Contracting the orbital muscles and drawing the eyebrows together becomes more pronounced the more intense the pain (Prkachin et al., 1994). The inaccuracy or conservatism of judgement for pain facial displays increases with longer exposure times (Prkachin et al., 2004). In fact, faked pain displays take longer to play out and are less coordinated than real ones (Hill & Craig, 2002). This is consistent with a model of vicarious responding at the psychological level, in which information-laden cognitive factors interact with quick – perhaps automatic – vicarious responses in empathic judgements (Eisenberg, 1991). The ability to detect pain from faces becomes more refined as the child gets older (Deyo et al., 2004). There is fMRI evidence that the dorsal ACC is also engaged when individuals view video clips featuring the painful facial expressions of chronic pain patients (Botvinick et al., 2005).

The potentially advantageous circumvention of trial-and-error learning by observational learning is not limited to facial expression information. The pain empathy research discussed earlier suggests that situational cues can also give hints to the observer about the aversive nature of objects. The sight of a needle coming into contact with skin (Morrison et al., 2004), flinching, blood, or even an arbitrary cue associated with pain (Singer et al., 2004), may all be examples of information-laden situational cues. Controlled studies dealing specifically with observational learning and pain empathy in other animals are rare, but there is some evidence intimating that chimpanzees react aversively to others' pain (Itakura, 1994; Parr, 2001). Parr (2001) showed that when chimps watched videos of the vet visiting conspecifics to give them hypodermic injections, their finger temperature decreased, indicative of parasympathetic ('dampening down') nervous activation.

So far there is no cohesive research programme on M-A observational learning in primates as there is for imitation. Preston and de Waal (2002) cover some germane research in primates and rodents in light of empathy. There is also evidence that observation of conspecific behaviour influences positive reward learning in capuchin monkeys, a New World primate much more distantly related to humans than chimpanzees (Brosnan & de Waal, 2004).

19.3.4 Beyond vicarious responding

Where empathy is concerned, considering vicarious responding in a M-A framework may go some way towards explaining our ability to identify another's circumstances as aversive based on situational or expressive cues. It may also partially account for the 'oomph' in empathy – why we are actually *motivated* to remove the source of discomfort, even though the body in question is not our own. When discomfort cannot be helped, or after a distressing event, primates often comfort each other with grooming gestures. In primates, grooming is not just about hygiene. It has taken on a new significance as a form of bonding, reinforcing alliances, and sometimes even as a palliative measure after a fracas (de Waal & van Roosmalen, 1979; Dunbar 1996).

Part of the calming effect of being groomed may have to do with the concomitant production of endogenous opiates (Dunbar, 1996; Keverne *et al.*, 1989). With respect to pain, it is interesting to note that opioids have analgesic properties and that the ACC contains a wealth of opioid receptors postulated to play a role in the modulation of the M-A dimension of pain (Vogt *et al.*, 1995b). The benefits of comforting a hurt person by touching and stroking them may even apply at the level of the spinal cord. Gentle stimulation of large-diameter afferent fibres in the skin can inhibit nociceptive interneurones in the dorsal horn, which may explain why rubbing a wound alleviates pain (Craig, 2003b; Melzack, 1999) – regardless of who is doing the rubbing!

If it is ultimately advantageous for systems sensitive to potential harm to react to false-positives to avoid the risk of false-negatives, then pain observation may be a 'runaway' form of anticipation that is not always truth-preserving (Griffiths, 1997). But if an overt response has even the slightest use as an information-bearing signal, it can take on new propensities in new contexts over the course of social and cultural evolution (Guilford & Dawkins, 1993). Competition among members of the same social group can also result in the exploitation of others' responses to communicative signals (Byrne & Whiten, 1997). This can take the form of outright deception, but can also manifest in the strategic deployment or exaggeration of a display. Or now and then, in human interactions, it can take the form of social lubrication, as when we put on a pitying expression to communicate that we understand the other person's distress even though we actually remain relatively unmoved by it (Bavelas *et al.*, 1987; Poole & Craig, 1992). Disjunctions between the experiential and communicative roles of pain and disgust displays should be borne in mind in developing a cognitive neuroscience of empathy.

19.4 The analogy with mirror neurones

Vicarious responding effects in M-A networks would not have been so eagerly sought, nor their significance quite so readily grasped, if it had not been for the prior discovery of mirror neurones in action representation networks. Mirror neurones provide the paradigmatic example of how a common coding mechanism can collapse perceptual with motor information (Prinz, 1990; Rizzolatti *et al.*, 1996). But how deep does the analogy go? Have we now discovered *affective* mirror neurones? In this section I argue that M-A and action representation networks handle different kinds of information, but that there are numerous formal points of similarity which nudge us closer to a functional understanding of organizational principles in the social brain.

19.4.1 Comparison between M-A and action representation networks

The premotor and parietal action representation circuits discussed elsewhere in this book provide the model case for vicarious responding. They contain mirror neurones, a type of visuomotor cell that fires both during the generation of a goal-directed action and also during the observation of a similar action made by someone else. Their postulated role in empathy has been interpreted as being relatively direct (e.g. Carr *et al.*, 2003; Leslie *et al.*, 2004). I am not inclined to assign a direct or necessary role to action representation in the recognition and interpretation of others' affective states. But I do believe that mirror neurones are a rich source for analogy when it comes to understanding general principles of perception-response transformations in the social domain.

19.4.2 Similarities

In making the following comparisons, I consider only those areas in which microelectrode recordings in macaques or humans have demonstrated vicarious responding – that is, visual modulation of response-related neural populations. These are monkey premotor area F5, monkey parietal area PF (7b), and human ACC area 24b. Perhaps this criterion is a bit stringent, but it will also be interesting to see whether future studies reveal any new vicarious-responding areas sharing the properties discussed here. These formal properties may even serve as a guide for where in the brain vicarious responses are more likely to be discovered.

At least five major similarities between these M-A and premotor-parietal action representation (A-R) regions can be drawn. They are: *(1) transformational coding; (2) goal-level coding; (3) movement preparation; (4) relationship to sensory integration processes* and *(5) cytological heterogeneity* (Table 19.1). Premotor F5, parietal PF and dorsal ACC each subserve a translation of sensory information into early response codes. The clearest illustrations of this are provided by neural populations in macaque premotor F5, which transform visual shape- and space-related object information into a motor-specific vocabulary of potential actions (Kakei *et al.*, 2003; Rizzolatti & Luppino, 2001; Rizzolatti *et al.*, 2002). These transformations are based on object features or other relevant cues, as in the case of 'canonical' neurones (Grèzes *et al.*, 2003; Rizzolatti & Craighero 2004). In the case of mirror neurones, the relevant transformations are based upon the observation

Table 19.1: Similarities between action-representation and motivational-affective areas observed to respond vicariously

Property	Monkey premotor F5	Monkey parietal PF	Human dorsal ACC
Transformational coding (perception/response)	Visual and auditory object features in space/egocentric motor code	Proprioceptive and visual/motor code	Nociceptive, visual/motor code
Goal-level coding	Grasping, tearing, etc; intentions	Grasping embedded in action chains	Aversive motivational urges
Movement preparation	Actions of hand and mouth	Distal, proximal limb and face movements	Aversive, nocifensive skeletomotor responses
Relationship to sensory integration	Inputs from parietal multisensory areas	Inputs from multiple sensory modalities	Inputs from temporal and parietal multisensory areas
Cytological heterogeneity (functional or morphological)	Hand-, face-, and arm-visual- and motor-selective cells	Proprioceptive face and arm, visual-, touch-, motor-selective cells	Pain, reward; pyramidal, spindle cells

of others' actions (di Pellegrino *et al.*, 1992; Rizzolatti *et al.*, 1996). Mirror neurones have been observed to discharge when the object of the action is out of sight (Umiltá *et al.*, 2001), as well as in response to sounds associated with certain actions, such as tearing a paper or cracking open a peanut (Keysers *et al.*, 2003). There is also compelling early evidence that a proportion of mirror neurones are sensitive to intransitive ingestive and communicative facial gestures (Buccino *et al.*, 2004; Ferrari *et al.*, 2003).

However, the 'motor vocabularies' in which F5 and ACC trade are relatively flexible with regard to specific effectors. The potential actions coded by F5 neurones pertain to the hand, foot and mouth (Godschalk *et al.*, 1995), but representation here exists at the level of the *goal* of action, not the particular effector. There are neurones that fire when the monkey makes a tearing action, regardless of whether it is the hands or the mouth that is actually carrying out the tearing (Rizzolatti & Luppino, 2001). In a comparable manner, ACC neurones may operate at the level of 'urge representation', a notion supported by the human microstimulation reports referred to in Section 19.3.1 (Bancaud & Talairach, 1992; Matsumoto *et al.*, 2004). (For a discussion of goal states, values, and intentionality, see Metzinger & Gallese, 2003). Emerging research also shows that goal-level representation exists in inferior parietal cortex, which includes PF, when monkeys perform the same actions with different goals (Fogassi *et al.*, 2005).

Parietal area PF (7b) is associated with face and arm representation. In the monkey, the inferior and superior posterior parietal areas chiefly receive visual inputs from striate cortex, but are also the first regions along the dorsal visual stream to integrate these retinally derived signals with other sensory signals (such as somatosensory and proprioceptive afferents) to form a higher-order representation of visual space (Driver & Mattingley, 1998). Like F5 and dorsal ACC, the cell types in PF are not functionally segregated (Rizzolatti & Craighero, 2004). More importantly, however, PF contains neurones that discharge when the monkey performs specific movements. Mirror neurones with both visual and motor properties have been discovered here too (Rizzolatti & Craighero, 2004; Rizzolatti *et al.*, 2002).

Found among these mixed populations are also *pain*-related sensory neurones with visual properties (Dong *et al.*, 1994). A proportion of these fired both when a part of the skin on the face was stimulated with noxious heat, and when the monkey viewed a threatening stimulus coming towards or hovering near that part of the skin. Moreover, the responses of these cells closely matched the behavioural response curves for the tolerance-escape task the monkeys performed. In nearby ventral intraparietal sulcus (VIP), part of the fronto-parietal action circuit, microstimulation has produced eye, lip and arm movements comparable to those elicited by an airpuff into the eyes (Cooke *et al.*, 2003). This indicates a role for the parietal cortex in the orchestration of aversive movements that require the integration of visuotactile information into an egocentric coordinate frame.

Each of these areas, then, plays a more or less direct role in relating integrated sensory information to potential motor responses. That they interact with each other too is evidenced by the numerous reciprocal projections from PF to some of the key regions in the preparation of actions and motivated movements. PF sends connections to premotor and supplementary motor cortexes, to the cingulate cortex, and to the anterior insula (Dong *et al.*, 1994). It is quite plausible that reciprocal communication between PF and these other quarters of M-A and A-R circuitry influences the preparation and initiation of motor responses. When the stimulus possesses noxious associations or a negative hedonic impact based on past interactions, M-A processing may mediate motor response via cingulate motor, supplementary motor and premotor projections. Other complex aversive muscular responses (such as the airpuff reaction) that do not necessarily involve flexible, motivated response learning, but do require visuotactile, spatiotemporal integration within peripersonal space, may be mediated primarily by sensorimotor circuits in the parietal cortex via projections to premotor and motor cortexes.

Premotor F5, parietal PF and dorsal ACC are also cytologically heterogeneous areas (Matelli *et al.*, 1991; Strick *et al.*, 1998; Rizzolatti & Luppino, 2001; Vogt *et al.*, 1995a, 2003). This means that they contain mixed cell populations, in which either the morphological or response properties (or both) of the cells differ, even though they are found in the same neighbourhood of tissue. In the case of ACC, nociceptive and reward-sensitive neurones have been found in area 24 (Koyama *et al.*, 2001), as well as large clusters of pyramidal cells in layer V which are postulated to operate in a motor capacity (Vogt *et al.*, 1995a).

Analogies always rest on comparisons. The more resemblances there are between two systems, the greater one's confidence that these reflect a more fundamental relationship of similarity. Functional similarities frequently indicate comparable organizational constraints (think of insect wings and bird wings). The hypothesis that vicariously responding neurones in M-A regions belong in the same category as mirror neurones depends on how deep these similarities go. This is especially true for examining the nature of visual modulation in vicarious responding.

For instance, the response of the ACC pinprick cell observed by Hutchison *et al.* might have disappeared if the patient had closed his or her eyes, meaning that its nociceptive properties would not have been independent of visual information in the same way that mirror neurones' motor properties are (this was not tested as it was not part of the experimenters' hypothesis). An alternative explanation for the overlap in the Morrison *et al.* study is that this region of the ACC integrates information from two perceptual channels, vision and nociception, in a manner unrelated to response preparation or even emotion. Similarly, the overlapping activity in the Singer *et al.* study might be attributable to attentional or other higher-level demands in the experimental paradigm. These possibilities make it necessary to be circumspect and to take a wider view, looking towards the more general properties of the systems in which vicarious responses are found. The analysis presented here is intended merely as an initial step towards this end.

19.4.3 Differences: 'hot' versus 'cold' motor processing

By definition, M-A and A-R networks selectively process information from different domains. M-A networks are more concerned with potentially rewarding or aversive states of affairs. A-R networks, on the other hand, deal with relating kinesthetic and proprioceptive information to features of objects in space. This distinction may not always seem so obvious. Considering that motor output is the end result of the examples discussed here, one might be tempted to consolidate the M-A and A-R into a single framework. Conversely, one might wish to keep feelings and actions entirely separate, especially since M-A processing is not limited to skeletomotor efference, but also influences behavioural disposition and visceral responses via autonomic and endocrine channels too.

Yet computationally, M-A and A-R pathways are distinct but related axes for the encoding of perceptual information. They are neither divergent nor wholly convergent. The two axes probably intersect, especially the closer they get to motor efference – but the important difference is that they are essentially concerned with pulling apart and putting together different *kinds* of information. M-A systems have to do with learning flexible responses regarding the properties of objects: will it bite?, can I eat it? The A-R system, in contrast, is concerned with kinesthetic body representation and the more metrical properties of objects: where is it?, can I grab it?

Considering these functional differences, the two systems are likely to differ in more specific ways too. Spatial information, such as an object's coordinates within the visual field or a sensation's location on the body, may not be as important for M-A networks as they are for A-R networks. Although aversive responses do require context-dependent flexibility, they are not likely to necessitate such highly coordinated distal, digital manipulation as actions do. When encountering a threat to tissue, less precise movements often suffice to remove oneself from the offending object.

Because they both result in skeletomotor output, M-A and A-R systems are continuous and certainly overlapping. However, they each tend to cluster toward one or the other end of a conceptual hot–cold spectrum. Actions and intentions directed towards manipulating objects are at the 'cold' end – unhurried, coordinated, dispassionate. In contrast, the anticipation and execution of movements in response to potentially harmful objects or events are 'hot' – quick, valenced, and with that elusive subjective 'oomph'. Like their cold counterparts in the A-R domain, processing in M-A networks supports a generative (Haggard, 2001) representation of the noxious stimulus, producing behavioural outcomes that are not predictable from the nature of the stimulus alone.

19.4.4 Conclusions

Placing vicarious responding in a M-A framework may make it easier to ground the multifarious variables we face in the scientific study of empathy. A salient advantage of a M-A framework is that it is methodologically equipped to accommodate the subjective element, as much as that is possible. Yet we are still not in a position to make the explanatory leap from vicarious responding to the rich scope of full-fledged affective experience evoked by the word 'empathy.' At the very least, this will require further empirical testing and a continual examination of the assumptions supporting our interpretations of the data.

Acknowledgements

I am grateful to Tony Atkinson, Giuseppe di Pellegrino, Paul Downing, Andrea Heberlein and John Parkinson for invaluable comments on a previous draft; and to Marius Peelen for assistance in producing Figure 19.1 using BrainVoyager 2000® software.

REFERENCES

Adolphs, R. (2002). Neural systems for recognizing emotion. *Current Opinion in Neurobiology* **12:2**, 169–177.

Adolphs, R., Damasio, H., Tranel, D., Cooper, G., & Damasio, A. R. (2000). A role for somatosensory cortices in the visual recognition of emotion as revealed by three-dimensional lesion mapping. *The Journal of Neuroscience*, **20**, 2683–2690.

Adolphs, R., Tranel, D., & Damasio A. R. (2003). Dissociable neural systems for recognizing emotions. *Brain and Cognition*, **52**, 61–69.

Atkinson, A. P., Dittrich, W. H., Gemmell, A. J., & Young, A. W. (2004). Emotion perception from dynamic and static body expressions in point-light and full-light displays. *Perception*, **33**, 717–746.

Augustine, J. R. (1996). Circuitry and functional aspects of the insular lobe in primates including humans. *Brain Research Reviews*, **22**, 229–244.

Avenanti, A., Bufalari I., & Aglioti S. M. (2004). Other's pain embodied in one's own motor system. *CNS Annual Meeting*, April.

Bancaud, J., & Talairach, J. (1992). Clinical semiology of frontal lobe seizures. *Advances in Neurology*, **57**, 3–58.

Barch, D. M., Braver, T. S., Akbudak, E., Conturo, T., Ollinger, J., & Snyder, A. (2001). Anterior cingulate cortex and response conflict: effects of response modality and processing domain. *Cerebral Cortex*, **11**, 837–848.

Bavelas, J. B., Black, A., Lemery, C. R., & Mullett, J. (1987). Motor mimicry as primitive empathy. In N. Eisenberg, & J. Strayer (eds.), *Empathy and its Development* (pp. 317–338). Cambridge: Cambridge University Press.

Bechara, A., & Naqvi, N. (2004). Listening to your heart: interoceptive awareness as a gateway to feeling. *Nature Neuroscience*, **7**, 102–103.

Berridge, K. C. (2000). Measuring hedonic impact in animals and infants: microstructure of affective taste reactivity patterns. *Neuroscience and Biobehavioral Reviews*, **24**, 173–198.

Berridge, K. C. (2004). Motivation concepts in behavioral neuroscience. *Physiology and Behavior*, **81**, 179–209.

Botvinick, M., Jha, A. P., Bylsma, L. M., *et al.* (2005). Viewing facial expression of pain engages cortical areas involved in the direct experience of pain. *Neuroimage*, **25**, 312–319.

Brosnan, S. F., & de Waal, F. B. (2004). Socially learned preferences for differentially rewarded tokens in the brown capuchin monkey (*Cebus apella*). *Journal of Comparative Psychology*, **118**, 33–39.

Brothers, L. (1990). The social brain: a project for integrating primate behavior and neurophysiology in a new domain. *Concepts in Neuroscience*, **1**, 27–61.

Buccino, G., Lui, F., Canessa, N., Patteri, I., & Lagravinese, G. (2004). Neural circuits involved in the recognition of actions performed by non-conspecifics: an fMRI study. *Journal of Cognitive Neuroscience*, **16**, 1–14.

Bush, G., Vogt, B. A., Holmes, J., *et al.* (2002). Dorsal anterior cingulate cortex: a role in reward-based decision making. *Proceedings of the National Academy of Sciences of the USA*, **99**, 523–528.

Byrne, R. W., & Whiten, A. (1997). Machiavellian intelligence. In A. Whiten, & R. W. Byrne (eds.), *Machiavellian Intelligence II* (pp. 1–23). Cambridge: Cambridge University Press.

Calder, A. J., Keane, J., Manes, F., Antoun, N., & Young, A. W. (2000). Impaired recognition and experience of disgust following brain injury. *Nature Neuroscience*, **3:11**, 1077–1078.

Calder, A. J., Lawrence, A. D., & Young, A. W. (2001). Neuropsychology of fear and loathing. *Nature Reviews Neuroscience*, **2**, 352–363.

Carr, L., Iacoboni, M., Dubeau, M. C., Mazziotta, J. C., & Lenzi, G. L. (2003). Neural mechanisms of empathy in humans: a relay from neural systems for imitation to limbic areas. *Proceedings of the National Academy of Sciences of the USA*, **100**, 5497–5502.

Chen, M., & Bargh, J. A. (1999). Consequences of automatic evaluation: immediate behavioral predispositions to approach or avoid the stimulus. *Personality and Social Psychology Bulletin*, **25**, 215–224.

Cooke, D. F., Taylor, C. S. R., Moore, T., & Graziano, M. S. A. (2003). Complex movements evoked by microstimulation of the ventral intraparietal area. *Proceedings of the National Academy of Sciences of the USA*, **100**, 6161–6168.

Craig, A. D. (2003a). Interoception: the sense of the physiological condition of the body. *Current Opinion in Neurobiology*, **13**, 500–505.

Craig, A. D. (2003b). Pain mechanisms: labeled lines versus convergence in central processing. *Annual Review of Neuroscience*, **26**, 1–30.

Craig, A. D. (2004). Human feelings: why are some more aware than others? *Trends in Cognitive Science*, **8**, 239–241.

Critchley, H. D., Wiens, S., Rotshtein, P., Ohman, A., & Dolan, R. J. (2004). Neural systems supporting interoceptive awareness. *Nature Neuroscience*, **7**, 189–195.

Curtis, V., Aunger, R., & Rabie, T. (2004). Evidence that disgust evolved to protect from risk of disease. *Proceedings of the Royal Society of London B* **271** (Suppl), S131–S133.

Damasio, A. R. (1994). *Descartes' Error*. New York: Picador.

Damasio, A. (1999). *The Feeling of What Happens: Body and Emotion in the Making of Consciousness*. London: Harcourt Brace.

Davis, K. D., Hutchison, W. D., Lozano, A. M., & Dostrovsky, J. O. (1994). Altered pain and temperature perception following cingulotomy and capsulotomy in a patient with schizoaffective disorder. *Pain*, **59**, 189–199.

de Waal, F. B. M., & van Roosmalen, A. (1979). Reconcilation and consolation among chimpanzees. *Behavioral Ecology and Sociobiology*, **5**, 55–56.

Decety, J., & Chaminade T. (2003). Neural correlates of feeling sympathy. *Neuropsychologia*, **1483**, 1–12.

Decety, J., & Jackson P. L. (2004). The functional architecture of human empathy. *Behavioral and Cognitive Neuroscience Reviews*, **3**, 71–100.

Devinsky, O., Morrell, M. J., & Vogt, B. A. (1995). Contributions of anterior cingulate cortex to behaviour. *Brain*, **118**, 279–306.

Deyo, K. S., Prkachin, K. M., & Mercer, S. R. (2004). Development of sensitivity to facial expression of pain. *Pain*, **107**, 16–21.

di Pellegrino, G., Fadiga, L., Fogassi, L., Gallese, V., & Rizzolatti, G. (1992). Understanding motor events: a neurophysiological study. *Experimental Brain Research*, **91**, 176–180.

Dong, W. K., Chudler, E. H., Sugiyama, K., Roberts, V. J., & Hayashi, T. (1994). Somatosensory, multisensory, and task-related neurons in cortical area 7b (PF) of unanesthetized monkeys. *Journal of Neurophysiology*, **72**, 542–564.

Downar, J., Mikulis, D. J., & Davis, K. D. (2003). Neural correlates of the prolonged salience of painful stimulation. *NeuroImage*, **20**, 1540–1551.

Driver, J., & Mattingley, J. B. (1998). Parietal neglect and visual awareness. *Nature Neuroscience*, **1**, 17–22.

Dunbar, R. (1996). *Grooming, Gossip, and the Evolution of Language*. Cambridge, Mass.: Harvard University Press.

Eisenberg, N. (1991). Empathy-related responding and cognition: A 'chicken and the egg' dilemma. In W. M. Kurtines, & J. L. Gewirtz (eds.), *Handbook of Moral Behavior and Development (Vol. 2)*. Hillsdale, N.J.: Lawrence Erlbaum Associates.

Ekman, P., & Friesen, W. V. (1971). Constants across culture in face and emotion. *Journal of Personality and Social Psychology*, **17**, 124–129.

Erikson, K., & Schulkin, J. (2003). Facial expressions of emotion: a cognitive neuroscience perspective. *Brain and Cognition*, **52**, 52–60.

Farrow, T. F., Zheng, Y., Wilkinson, I. D., *et al.* (2001). Investigating the functional anatomy of empathy and forgiveness. *NeuroReport*, **12**, 2433–2438.

Ferrari, P. F., Gallese, V., Rizzolatti, G., & Fogassi, L. (2003). Mirror neurons responding to the observation of ingestive and communicative mouth actions in the monkey ventral premotor cortex. *European Journal of Neuroscience*, **17**, 1703–1714.

Fogassi, L., Ferrari, P. F., Gesierich, B., *et al.* (2005). Parietal lobe: from action organization to intention understanding. *Science*, **308(5722)**, 662–667.

Gallese, V. (2001). The shared manifold hypothesis: from mirror neurons to empathy. *Journal of Consciousness Studies*, **8**, 51–68.

Gallese, V. (2003). The manifold nature of interpersonal relations: the quest for a common mechanism. *Philosophical Transactions of the Royal Society of London, Biology*, **358**, 517–528.

Gallese, V., Fadiga, L., Fogassi, L., & Rizzolatti, G. (1996). Action recognition in the premotor cortex. *Brain*, **119**, 593–609.

Godschalk, M., Mitz, A. R., van Duin, B., & van der Burg, H. (1995). Somatotopy of monkey premotor cortex examined with microstimulation. *Neuroscience Research*, **23**, 269–279.

Grèzes, J., Armony, J. L., Rowe, J., & Passingham, R. E. (2003). Activations related to 'mirror' and 'canonical' neurones in the human brain: an fMRI study. *NeuroImage*, **18**, 928–937.

Griffiths, P. E. (1997). *What Emotions Really Are*. Chicago, Iu.: University of Chicago Press.

Guilford, T., & Dawkins, M. S. (1993). Receiver psychology and the design of animal signals. *Trends in Neurosciences*, **16**, 430–436.

Gusnard, D. A., Akbudak, E., Shulman, G. L., & Raichle, M. E. (2001). Medial prefrontal cortex and self-referential mental activity: relation to a default mode of brain function. *Proceedings of the National Academy of Sciences of the USA*, **98**, 4259–4264.

Hadland, K. A., Rushworth, M. F., Gaffan, D., & Passingham, R. E. (2003). The anterior cingulate and reward-guided selection of actions. *Journal of Neurophysiology*, **89**, 1161–1164.

Haggard, P. (2001). The psychology of action. *British Journal of Psychology*, **92**, 113–128.

Heberlein, A. S., Adolphs, R., Tranel, D., & Damasio, H. (2004). Cortical regions for judgments of emotions and personality traits from point-light walkers. *Journal of Cognitive Neuroscience*, **17**, 1142–1158.

Hill, M. L., & Craig, K. D. (2002). Detecting deception in pain expressions: the structure of genuine and deceptive facial displays. *Pain*, **98**, 135–144.

Hsieh, J. C., Stone-Elander, S., & Ingvar, M. (1999). Anticipatory coping of pain expressed in the human anterior cingulate cortex: a positron emission tomography study. *Neuroscience Letters*, **262**, 61–64.

Huettel, S. A., Misiurek, J., Jurkowski, A. J., & McCarthy, G. (2004). Dynamic and strategic aspects of executive processing. *Brain Research*, **1000**, 78–84.

Hutchison, W. D., Davis, K. D., Lozano, A. M., Tasker, R. R., & Dostrovsky, J. O. (1999). Pain-related neurons in the human cingulate cortex. *Nature Neuroscience*, **2**, 403–405.

Isomura, Y., & Takada, M. (2004). Neural mechanisms of versatile functions in primate anterior cingulate cortex. *Reviews in Neuroscience*, **15**, 279–291.

Itakura, S. (1994). Differentiated responses to different human conditions by chimpanzees. *Perceptual and Motor Skills*, **79**, 1288–1290.

Jackson, P. L., Meltzoff, A. N., & Decety, J. (2005). How do we perceive the pain of others? *Neuroimage*, **24**, 771–779.

James, W. (1892). *Psychology: The Briefer Course*. Reprinted in 1985. University of Notre Dame Press.

Kakei, S., Hoffman, D. S., & Strick, P. L. (2003). Sensorimotor transformations in cortical motor areas. *Neuroscience Research*, **46**, 1–10.

Keverne, E. B., Martensz, N. D., & Tuite, B. (1989). Beta-endorphin concentrations in cerebrospinal fluid of monkeys are influenced by grooming relationships. *Psychoneuroendocrinology*, **14**, 155–161.

Keysers, C., Kohler, E., Umiltá, M. A., *et al.* (2003). Ausiovisual mirror neurons and action recognition. *Experimental Brain Research*, **153**, 628–636.

Keysers, C., Wicker, B., Gazzola, V., *et al.* (2004). A touching sight: SII/PV activation during the observation and experience of touch. *Neuron*, **42**, 335–346.

Koyama, T., Kato, K., Tanaka, Y. Z., & Mikami, A. (2001). Anterior cingulate activity during pain-avoidance and reward tasks in monkeys. *Neuroscience Research*, **39**, 421–430.

Koyama, T., Tanaka, Y. Z., & Mikami, A. (1998). Nociceptive neurons in the macaque anterior cingulate cortex activate during anticipation of pain. *Neuroreport*, **9**, 2663–2667.

Krolak-Salmon, P., Henaff, M. A., Isnard, J., *et al.* (2003). An attention modulated response to disgust in human ventral anterior insula. *Annals of Neurology*, **53**, 446–453.

Leslie, K. R., Johnson-Frey, S. H., & Grafton, S. T. (2004). Functional imaging of face and hand imitation: towards a motor theory of empathy. *NeuroImage*, **21**, 601–607.

Marzillier, S. L., & Davey, G. C. L. (2004). The emotional profiling of disgust-eliciting stimuli: evidence for primary and complex disgusts. *Cognition and Emotion*, **18**, 313–336.

Matelli, M., Luppino, G., & Rizzolatti, G. (1991). Architecture of superior and mesial area 6 and the adjacent cingulate cortex in the macaque monkey. *Journal of Comparative Neurology*, **311**, 445–462.

Matsumoto, K., Suzuki, W., & Tanaka, K. (2004). Neuronal correlates of goal-based motor selection in the prefrontal cortex. *Science*, **11**, 229–232.

Melzack, R. (1999). From the gate to the neuromatrix. *Pain Suppl 6*, S121–S126.

Mesulam, M. M. (1999). Spatial attention and neglect: parietal, frontal and cingulate contributions to the mental representation and attentional targeting of salient extrapersonal events. *Philosophical Transactions of the Royal Society of London. Biology*, **354**, 1325–1346.

Metzinger, T., & Gallese, V. (2003). The emergence of a shared action ontology: building blocks for a theory. *Consciousness and Cognition*, **12**, 549–571.

Morrison, I., Lloyd, D. M, di Pellegrino, G., & Roberts, N. (2004). Vicarious responses to pain in anterior cingulate cortex: is empathy a multisensory issue? *Cognitive, Affective, and Behavioral Neuroscience*, **4**, 270–278.

O'Doherty, J., Critchley, H., Deichmann, R., & Dolan, R. J. (2003). Dissociating valence of outcome from behavioral control in human orbital and ventral prefrontal cortices. *Neuroscience*, **23**, 7931–7939.

Panksepp, J. (1998). *Affective Neuroscience: The Foundations of Human and Animal Emotions.* New York: Oxford University Press.

Parr, L. A. (2001). Cognitive and physiological markers of emotional awareness in chimpanzees (*Pan troglodytes*). *Animal Cognition*, **4**, 223–229.

Paus, T. (2001). Primate anterior cingulate cortex: where motor control, drive, and cognition interface. *Nature Reviews Neuroscience*, **2**, 417–424.

Penfield, W., & Rasmussen, T. (1955). *The Cerebral Cortex of Man: A Clinical Study of Localization of Function.* New York: Macmillan Company.

Peyron, R., Laurent, B., & Garcia-Larrea, L. (2000). Functional imaging of brain responses to pain: a review and meta-analysis. *Clinical Neurophysiology*, **30**, 263–288.

Phillips, M. L., Young, A. W., Scott, S. K., *et al.* (1998). Neural responses to facial and vocal expressions of fear and disgust. *Proceedings in Biological Sciences*, **265**, 1809–1817.

Phillips, M. L., Young, A. W., Senior, C., *et al.* (1997). A specific neural substrate for perceiving facial expressions of disgust. *Nature*, **2(389)**, 495–498.

Ploner, M., Freund, H. J., & Schnitzler, A. (1999). Pain affect without pain sensation in a patient with a postcentral lesion. *Pain*, **81**, 211–214.

Poole, G. D., & Craig, K. D. (1992). Judgments of genuine, suppressed, and faked facial expressions of pain. *Journal of Personality and Social Psychology*, **63**, 797–805.

Porro, C. A., Cettolo, V., Francescato, M. P., & Baraldi, P. (2003). Functional activity mapping of the mesial hemispheric wall during anticipation of pain. *NeuroImage*, **19**, 1738–1747.

Posner, M. I., & Rothbart, M. K. (1998). Attention, self-regulation and consciousness. *Philosophical Transactions of the Royal Society of London, Biology*, **29**, 1915–1927.

Preston, S., & de Waal, F. (2002). Empathy: its ultimate and proximate bases. *Behavioral Brain Sciences*, **25**, 1.

Price, D. D. (1999). *Psychological Mechanisms of Pain and Analgesia*. Seattle: IASP Press.

Price, D. D. (2000). Psychological and neural mechanisms of the affective dimension of pain. *Science*, **288**, 1769–1772.

Price, D. D., Barrell, J. J., & Rainville, P. (2002). Integrating experiential-phenomenological methods and neuroscience to study neural mechanisms of pain and consciousness. *Consciousness and Cognition*, **11**, 593–608.

Prinz, W. (1990). A common coding approach to perception and action. In O. Neumann, & W. Prinz (eds.), *Relationships Between Perception and Action: Current Approaches* (pp. 167–201). New York: Springer-Verlag.

Prkachin, K. M., Berzins, S., & Mercer, S. R. (1994). Encoding and decoding of pain expressions: a judgement study. *Pain*, **58**, 253–259.

Prkachin, K. M., Mass, H., & Mercer, S. R. (2004). Effects of exposure on perception of pain expression. *Pain*, **111**, 8–12.

Raichle, M. E. (1998). The neural correlates of consciousness: an analysis of cognitive skill learning. *Philosophical Transactions of the Royal Society of London, Biology*, **353**, 1889–1901.

Rainville, P., Carrier, B., Hofbauer, R. K., Bushnell, M. C., & Duncan, G. H. (1999). Dissociation of sensory and affective dimensions of pain using hypnotic modulation. *Pain*, **82**, 159–171.

Rainville, P., Duncan, G. H., Price, D. D., Carrier, B., & Bushnell, M. C. (1997). Pain affect encoded in human anterior cingulate but not somatosensory cortex. *Science*, **277**, 968–971.

Redican, W. K. (1982). An evolutionary perspective on human facial displays. In P. Ekman (ed.), *Emotion in the Human Face*, 2nd edn. (pp. 213–280). Cambridge: Cambridge University Press.

Rizzolatti, G., & Craighero, L. (2004). The mirror neuron system. *Annual Review of Neuroscience*, **27**, 169–192.

Rizzolatti, G., Fadiga, L., Gallese, V., & Fogassi, L. (1996). Premotor cortex and the recognition of motor actions. *Cognitive Brain Research*, **3:2**, 131–141.

Rizzolatti, G., Fogassi, L., & Gallese, V. (2002). Motor and cognitive functions of the ventral premotor cortex. *Current Opinion in Neurobiology*, **12**, 149–154.

Rizzolatti, G., & Luppino, G. (2001). The cortical motor system. *Neuron*, **27**, 889–901.

Rozin, P., Haidt J., & McCauley, C. R. (2000). Disgust. In M. Lewis, & J. M. Haviland-Jones (eds.), *Handbook of Emotions*, 2nd edn. (pp. 637–653). New York: Guilford Press.

Rushworth, M. F., Hadland, K. A., Gaffan, D., & Passingham, R. E. (2003). The effect of cingulate cortex lesions on task switching and working memory. *Journal of Cognitive Neuroscience*, **15**, 338–353.

Sewards, T. V. & Sewards, M. A. (2002). The medial pain system: neural representations of the motivational aspect of pain. *Brain Research Bulletin*, **59**, 163–180.

Sewards, T. V., & Sewards, M. A. (2003). Representations of motivational drives in medial cortex, medial thalmus, hypothalamus, and midbrain. *Brain Research Bulletin*, **61**, 25–49.

Sherrington, C. S. (1948). *The Integrative Action of the Nervous System*. Cambridge: Cambridge University Press.

Shima, K., & Tanji, J. (1998). Role for cingulate motor area cells in voluntary movement selection based on reward. *Science*, **282**, 1335–1338.

Singer, T., Seymour, B., O'Doherty, J., *et al.* (2004). Empathy for pain involves the affective but not sensory components of pain. *Science*, **20**, 1157–1162.

Steiner, J. E., Glaser, D., Hawilo, M. E., & Berridge, K. C. (2001). Comparative expression of hedonic impact: affective reactions to taste by human infants and other primates. *Neuroscience and Biobehavioral Reviews*, **25**, 53–74.

Strick, P. L., Dum, R. P., & Picard, N. (1998). Motor areas on the medial wall of the hemisphere. *Novartis Foundation Symposium*, **218**, 64–75.

Umiltá, M. A., Kohler, E., Gallese, V., *et al.* (2001). I know what you are doing. a neuro-physiological study. *Neuron*, **19**, 155–165.

Vogt, B. A., Berger, G. R., & Derbyshire, W. G. (2003). Structural and functional dichotomy of human midcingulate cortex. *European Journal of Neuroscience*, **18**, 3134–3144.

Vogt, B. A., Nimchinsky, E. A., & Hof, P. R. (1995a). Human cingulate cortex: surface features, flat maps, and cytoarchitecture. *Journal of Comparative Neurology*, **359**, 490–506.

Vogt, B. A., & Pandya, D. N. (1987). Cingulate cortex of the rhesus monkey: II. Cortical afferents. *Journal of Comparative Neurology*, **262**, 271–289.

Vogt, B. A., & Sikes, R. W. (2000). The medial pain system, cingulate cortex, and parallel processing of nociceptive information. *Progress in Brain Research*, **122**, 223–235.

Vogt, B. A., Wiley, R. G., & Jensen, E. L. (1995b). Localization of Mu and delta opioid receptors to anterior cingulate afferents and projection neurons and input/output model of Mu regulation. *Experimental Neurology*, **135**, 83–92.

Walton, M. E., Bannerman, D. M., Alterescu, K., & Rushworth, M. F. (2003). Functional specialization within medial frontal cortex of the anterior cingulate for evaluating effort-related decisions. *Journal of Neuroscience*, **23**, 6475–6479.

Wicker, B., Keysers, C., Plailly, J., *et al.* (2003). Both of us disgusted in my insula: the common neural basis of seeing and feeling disgust. *Neuron*, **40**, 655–664.

Williams, A. C. (2002). Facial expression of pain: an evolutionary account. *Behavioral and Brain Sciences*, **25**, 439–455.

Winkielman, P., Berridge, K. C., & Wilbarger, J. L. (2005). Unconscious affective reactions to masked happy versus angry faces influence consumption behavior and judgments of value. *Personality and Social Psychology Bulletin*, **31**, 121–135.

Face processing and empathy

Anthony P. Atkinson

Department of Psychology, University of Durham

20.1 Introduction

The central issue to be explored in this chapter is the relation between perceiving an emotion in another and the triggering or re-creation of one or more aspects of that emotional state in oneself. This is what I shall sometimes refer to as 'perceptually mediated empathy', as distinct from 'cognitive empathy', where the subject represents someone else's state through top-down processes such as imaginative projection (e.g. Goldie, 1999; Preston & de Waal, 2002).

It has been suggested that a primary function of perceptually mediated empathy is to enable the recognition of emotional expressions, via processes of emotional contagion and simulation (Adolphs, 2002; Gallese *et al.*, 2004; Goldman & Sripada, 2005). There is currently a lot of excitement about this idea. Is all the fuss justified? I shall demonstrate that while there is indeed cause for excitement, the evidence to date is far from able to warrant claims that processes of emotional contagion and simulation provide the sole, primary, or even an important means by which we come to know what others are feeling. There are several other possible functions of perceptually mediated empathy, about which I have little to say, other than some general thoughts at the end of the chapter about the developmental role of perceptually mediated empathy in enabling a more general 'mindreading' or 'Theory of Mind' capacity.

I ought to note two points of conceptual clarification before continuing. First, consider the distinction between *perception* and *recognition*. This reflects a distinction in philosophy between the *perception of things*, or non-epistemic perception, and the *perception of facts* or epistemic perception (Dretske, 1969). Perceiving an object or event, such as a fearful facial expression, does not require that the object or event be recognized or interpreted in any particular way; it does not require that we associate what we perceive with any additional knowledge about what it means. Perceiving a fact, on the other hand, means grasping the fact, and entails coming to know that it *is* a fact.

Empathy in Mental Illness, eds. Tom F. D. Farrow and Peter W. R. Woodruff. Published by Cambridge University Press. © Cambridge University Press 2007.

Epistemically seeing an expression of fear, for example, involves recognizing or coming to know this fact via the visual modality. In psychology and cognitive neuroscience, 'perception' is sometimes used to cover both non-epistemic and epistemic perception. At other times, however, the use of 'perception' is restricted to non-epistemic perception, while 'recognition' refers to epistemic perception. On this latter usage, which I shall endeavour to respect in what follows, 'perception' typically refers to processes that make explicit the distinct features of stimuli and their geometric configurations to allow discrimination among different stimuli on the basis of their appearance. In contrast, 'recognition' refers to processes that require additional knowledge that could not be obtained solely from an inspection of the features of the stimulus. For instance, recognition of fear from a facial expression may occur by linking the perceptual properties of the facial stimulus to the concept of fear, the lexical label 'fear', and the perception of the emotional fear response (or a central representation thereof) that the stimulus triggers in oneself.

My second point of conceptual clarification concerns some ambiguity in the use of the term 'emotional experience' in the literature. Sometimes the term is used to refer to the subjective feelings associated with emotional and mood states. At other times, it is used in a more general sense to refer to the possession or occurrence of an emotional state (e.g. fear), with its attendant physiological and behavioural, as well as subjective experiential, components. I interpret 'emotional experience' in this more general sense to mean the possession or occurrence of an emotional state, and thus to consist not only in certain feelings (the awareness of one's emotional state and what it is like to be in that state) but also in overt behaviour (e.g. facial expression) and physiological (especially autonomic) response. But that is not all. On the particular interpretation advocated here, one can have an emotional experience that may or may not be accompanied by a characteristic feeling. This interpretation stems from the view that measurements of feelings (via subjective report), behaviour, or physiology can be taken as evidence for an emotional state, but are not constitutive of that state. That is, although we use evidence of what people say and do to infer their emotional states, those emotional states are not to be identified with any one particular piece of that evidence (behaviour, physiology, vouched feeling), nor, indeed, with that evidence in the round. Thus, when it is suggested that perceiving an emotion in another can trigger the experience of that or a closely related emotion in oneself, it is possible to consider the question of whether that empathic response to the other's expressed emotion does or does not include the associated emotional feeling.

20.2 How might perceptually mediated empathy enable emotion recognition?

How do we come to know what emotional states others are experiencing? In addition to or in the absence of their verbal reports, we can gauge other people's emotional states by reading their faces and bodies for characteristic postures and movements. But how do we come to associate particular postures and movements of another's face and body with specific emotional states? As a first pass, we can distinguish two views about how this might happen. One view proposes what we might think of as a purely computational or rule-based system: we somehow come to learn that faces that look thus and so are expressing fear, for example, and that faces that look this way rather than any other are expressing anger, say. In other words, according to this view, our perceptual systems are able to construct representations based on the physical features of the stimulus (e.g. the shape and configuration of facial features, and how faces move) and on other information acquired in our formative years that are of sufficient detail for us to discriminate between and identify at least a basic set of emotional expressions. [For a more detailed exposition of this sort of account, see Goldman & Sripada's (2005) discussion of a 'theory-theory' account of emotion perception.] This first view has a lot to recommend it: it is computationally tractable, and there appears to be sufficient geometric, configural and spatial frequency information in emotional facial expressions to distinguish between a variety of emotions (e.g. Calder *et al.*, 2001; Dailey *et al.*, 2002), to at least some of which neural mechanisms known to be involved in face and emotion processing are sensitive (e.g. Winston *et al.*, 2003b). Moreover, there is a good deal of other evidence from psychology and neuroscience that is consistent with this view; see Adolphs (2002), for a review.

Why, then, should we be giving serious consideration to an alternative view? Because there is now a large, varied and fast-growing set of findings that points to an intimate relationship between the perception and experience of emotion, yet the first view of emotion perception and recognition, outlined above, does not require any such relationship at all, and indeed, on that view, there is little if any good reason to suppose that such a relationship exists. The bulk of this chapter is devoted to a critical survey of this evidence of an intimate relationship between emotion perception and experience, in an attempt to provide a clearer picture of the processes and neural mechanisms involved and of how they might underpin emotion recognition. This alternative (though not necessarily mutually exclusive) account of emotion recognition is that a capacity to experience a particular emotion (or emotions in general) underpins the ability to recognize expressions of that emotion (or emotions in general) in others. There are two basic and not necessarily incompatible ways in which this idea might be realized, as depicted in Figure 20.1: (A) A primitive form of emotional contagion might operate, such that viewing another's emotional expression triggers that emotion in oneself, either directly or via unintentional mimicry of that expression, which allows us then to infer the other's emotional state (e.g. Hatfield *et al.*, 1994; Wild *et al.*, 2001; for a review, see Preston & de Waal, 2002). (B) Alternatively, viewing another's

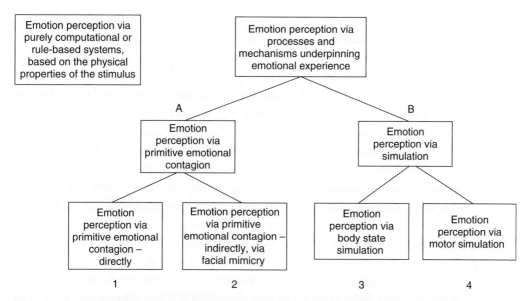

Figure 20.1. A tree diagram showing the four main theses, discussed in the text, as to the ways in which our perception of other's emotional expressions might be related to our capacity to experience emotions

emotional expression might involve simulating the viewed emotional state via the generation of representations of the associated body state (Adolphs, 2002), or simulating the motor programmes for producing the viewed expression (Carr *et al.*, 2003; Gallese *et al.*, 2004; Leslie *et al.*, 2004). Note that the simulation accounts, but not the emotional contagion accounts, allow for (even if they do not provide a direct account of) our capacity to respond to another's expressed emotion with some emotion other than that which we perceive: simulation can be taken offline, such that one does not actually experience the emotion one is simulating (that is, in such offline cases, one's feeling, behaviour and physiology do not correspond to the emotion one is simulating).

20.3 Relationships between emotional state and emotion recognition performance

Besides the evidence directly relevant to the emotional contagion and simulation proposals of emotion perception, which is discussed in Sections 20.4 and 20.5, respectively, there is some behavioural evidence consistent with both proposals, with which I shall begin. This evidence suggests a close relationship between the experience of emotions and the ability to recognize them. Numerous studies have shown that people with disorders of emotional experience, such as in schizophrenia and major depressive disorder, also process emotional information abnormally, including abnormal processing of emotional expressions. Research with healthy participants has also demonstrated influences of emotional or mood state on emotion recognition performance.

Core features of schizophrenia include abnormal emotional behaviour and experience, especially flattened affect and anhedonia, as shown by diminished facial expressivity, reduced expressive gestures, speaking in a monotone, and the like. Whether schizophrenics' subjective emotional feelings differ from normal is less clear, however, with some patients and measures showing abnormal (e.g. Dworkin et al., 1996) and others showing relatively normal feelings (e.g. Berenbaum & Oltmanns, 1992). That both the recognition and production of emotional expressions in schizophrenia are compromised, and that there may also be defective feeling deserve further investigation. Moreover, the particular inter-relationships between these capacities in schizophrenia are likely to shed light on these capacities more generally, and on the simulation and contagion theories of emotion processing in particular. Consider, for example, the finding that when schizophrenics' facial expressions were manipulated, their self-reported feelings of sadness, fear, and happiness, but not anger, were congruent with the adopted expressions, whereas only body postures of anger elicited greater emotion-congruent feelings (Flack et al., 1999). In contrast, higher ratings of emotional feeling congruent with the adopted facial or body posture were reported by healthy controls for all four emotions, whereas patients with depression showed this effect only for sadness, for both facial and body postures. Nevertheless, schizophrenics appear to produce normal facial electromyographic (EMG) responses to photographs of positive versus negative facial expressions. Kring et al. (1999) reported that, in both schizophrenic and non-schizophrenic participants, viewing positive facial expressions elicited an increase in the electrical activity of the zygomatic muscle, which elevates the lips in smiling, and viewing negative facial expressions elicited an increase in the electrical activity of the corrugator muscle, which is involved in frowning. While the corrugator muscle activity was greater in the schizophrenic group, the authors suggest good reasons for thinking that this increased activity reflects other processes not related to emotion. As I discuss in the Section 20.4, more emotion-specific patterns of facial EMG response to others' facial expressions have been recorded in healthy participants; whether individuals with schizophrenia also show these normal patterns of response has yet to be determined.

Numerous studies have demonstrated emotion recognition deficits accompanying major depressive disorder. For example, Rubinow and Post (1992) found that depressed patients were impaired in the recognition of sadness, happiness, and interest in facial expressions, but were not impaired in recognizing emotions in verbal expressions, suggesting the deficit is specific to vision. Asthana et al.

(1998) found that major depressives were impaired relative to non-depressed controls in judging whether two simultaneously presented faces expressed the same or different emotions (happy, sad, fear, anger, neutral). These patients were also impaired on visuospatial tasks involving both simple patterns and faces, suggesting a general visual perceptive deficit rather than a more specific emotion recognition deficit. Impairments in recognizing a range of emotions in facial expressions (fear, anger, surprise, disgust, happiness, sadness, indifference) were also reported by Persad and Polivy (1993), in both depressed university students and depressed psychiatric patients. However, a number of other studies have reported evidence of either valence-specific or emotion-specific impairments; indeed, several studies suggest that depression is associated with an emotion-congruent bias, that is for interpreting facial expressions as negative, and especially as sad (though see Surguladze *et al.*, 2004, as discussed below). Hale (1998), for example, had major depressives and healthy control participants rate how strongly schematic facial expressions displayed each of seven emotions (fear, anger, sadness, disgust, rejection, happiness, invitation). It was found that the more severe the depression upon admission, and the greater the persistence of the depression, the more likely the patients were to judge expressions as negative, whereas the judgement of positive emotions (happiness, invitation) was not related to the patients' depression. The patients were more likely than controls to classify expressions as sad, and this bias towards sadness judgements was the best predictor of the patients' depression persistence. Other studies have also found this tendency for depressed patients to recognize significantly more sadness in facial expressions than healthy control participants (e.g. Gur *et al.*, 1992). Bouhuys *et al.* (1995) even found a depression-related negative bias in the perception of facial displays in healthy participants, using music to induce a depressed mood. Compared to those induced into a positive mood with elating music, participants who felt depressed perceived more sadness and rejection in 'ambiguous' faces (i.e. faces expressing similar amounts of positive and negative emotions) and less invitation and happiness in 'clear' faces (i.e. faces showing a preponderance of positive or negative emotions).

The uncovering of depression-related deficits in emotion recognition may often require relatively subtle tests, typically involving measures of reaction time or very brief stimulus presentations. For example, Surguladze *et al.* (2004) showed that people with major depressive disorder were less accurate than healthy control participants in their ability to identify mild (50%) and more intense (100%) sad and, to a lesser extent, happy facial expressions presented for short (100 ms) durations in a three-alternative forced-choice task (sad, happy, neutral). The depressed patients did not significantly differ from controls in their ability to identify sad, happy and neutral expressions presented for longer (2000 ms) durations, however. Nor did the patients differ from controls on a recognition memory test of non-emotional face recognition, suggesting that their deficit was specific to facial emotion rather than a more general face perception deficit. Whereas healthy controls had a slight bias for identifying long-duration neutral and mildly happy (50% intensity) faces as happy, this bias was significantly weaker in the depressive patients. The patients' bias away from labelling facial expressions as happy was not associated with a bias towards labelling expressions as sad.

Before proceeding, it is important to note a caveat. Evidence that deficits or other abnormalities in emotional experience are accompanied by deficits or other abnormalities in emotion recognition does not necessarily imply that emotion recognition and experience have a direct causal link; there might instead be some causally prior set of processes whose disrupted functioning leads both to abnormal emotional experience and abnormal emotion recognition.

There is also a modicum of evidence from non-clinical populations that emotion recognition performance is influenced by the observer's mood. Socially anxious non-clinical subjects were found to be more sensitive than low-anxiety subjects in the detection of fear in morphed blends of photographic images of facial emotions, in a study by Richards et al. (2002). And compared to people with low levels of anxiety, moderately and highly anxious individuals are faster to respond to probes following briefly presented threatening (angry) than non-threatening faces (e.g. Bradley et al., 2000), indicating an initial vigilance for threat.

It is not just anxiety levels that can affect one's responses to another's emotion. By inducing certain moods in experimental participants, it is possible to enhance their sensitivity to emotion-congruent information, including other people's emotional expressions. For example, participants in Niedenthal et al.'s (2000) study were induced to feel happiness, sadness or neutral emotion, and were then presented with computer-animated photographic images of faces that began in an emotional expression and morphed to a neutral pose. The participants' task was to stop the animations at the point at which they believed the faces to be emotionally neutral. Emotion-congruent expressions were perceived to persist longer than those that were incongruent with the experienced mood. It is not even necessary for the participant's mood to be experimentally manipulated in order for their mood to influence their emotion perception performance. Durrani (2005) found that people with predominantly negative or positive mood traits were significantly worse in recognizing disgust (but not anger, fear, happiness or sadness) in dynamic body expressions than control subjects, who were in neither positive nor negative moods; similarly, people in a predominantly negative or positive mood state were significantly worse at recognizing disgust in emotional vocalizations compared to control subjects.

20.4 Emotion recognition via primitive emotional contagion

If the recognition of another's emotion can be achieved via a process of primitive emotional contagion, in a direct, unmediated fashion (branch A1 in Figure 20.1), then how might this occur? One idea, as depicted in Figure 20.2, is that after some initial visual processing, certain visual characteristics of a viewed face (the shape, configuration and movement of its features) would be sufficient to trigger a corresponding emotional state in the observer, or to alter the observer's current emotional state in the direction of the viewed emotion. Presumably induction of emotional states in this way would require that visual information pertaining to the expressed emotion is relayed directly to separate mechanisms underlying emotional experience, or that the perceptual mechanisms themselves also subserve emotional experience.

Some evidence that the perceptual mechanisms themselves might also subserve emotional experience comes from research with brain-damaged patients who have selective emotion-recognition deficits. There are indications that these patients may also have a corresponding circumscribed deficit in their experience of the same emotions they are unable to recognize. Patients with bilateral amygdala damage have particular difficulty recognizing fearful facial expressions, but have relatively little difficulty recognizing other emotions expressed in the face, such as disgust, happiness and sadness (e.g. Adolphs *et al.*, 1999; Calder *et al.*, 1996). In contrast, people with damage to the anterior insula have particular difficulty recognizing facial expressions of disgust, but are not so impaired at recognizing

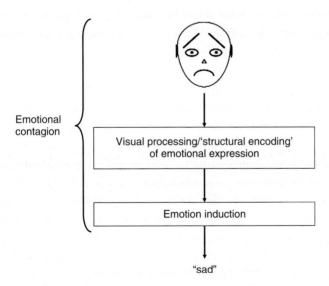

Figure 20.2. Emotion perception via emotional contagion – directly

other facial expressions, including fear, happiness and sadness (e.g. Calder *et al.*, 2000b). More recently, a selective impairment in the recognition of anger from facial expressions has been demonstrated in patients with damage to a region of the subcortical basal ganglia known as the ventral striatum (Calder *et al.*, 2004), as well as in healthy participants who are administered sulpride, an antipsychotic drug that reduces aggression and operates by blocking dopamine receptors (Lawrence *et al.*, 2002).

Sprengelmeyer *et al.* (1999) reported that a patient with bilateral amygdala damage, who was impaired at recognizing expressions of fear in faces, body postures and emotional sounds, also differed significantly from controls on questionnaires probing everyday experience of fear and anger but not on a questionnaire probing everyday experience of disgust. These questionnaires required the participants to rate a set of situations on the extent to which those situations would make them experience the emotion in question. The patient's lower scores indicated that situations that would normally evoke anger or fear would not do so for him. Moreover, this patient reported only one occasion in the 20 years prior to testing when he could remember having experienced fear, despite having engaged in numerous risky endeavours. Calder *et al.* (2000b) reported that a patient who was impaired at recognizing disgust in facial expressions and non-verbal sounds, due to a selective left hemisphere lesion primarily affecting insular cortex, also showed abnormal self-assessed experience of disgust, but not of fear or anger, using the same questionnaires as Sprengelmeyer *et al.* (1999). These findings are consistent with work implicating the amygdala and insula in the experience of various emotions, including fear and disgust (e.g. Damasio *et al.*, 2000). Finally, that the ventral striatum is involved in the experience of anger is consistent with animal studies identifying a role for this region in certain forms of aggression (for a review, see Calder *et al.*, 2004). Partial support for this thesis was provided by Calder *et al.* (2004): two of the four patients with ventral striatum lesions that they tested were found to have significantly abnormal experience of anger, as assessed by three self-report questionnaires: one manifest as heightened, the other as reduced, anger reactions. The responses of the other two patients to the questionnaires showed only minimal disruption in their experience of anger.

Not all patients with emotion perception deficits appear to have abnormal emotional experience, however. For example, amygdala lesions do not necessarily impair emotional experience, either as assessed by a questionnaire asking about the typicality of experienced positive and negative emotions, or by a daily diary record of experienced positive and negative emotions (Anderson & Phelps, 2002). Moreover, amygdala lesions do not always block generation of arousal skin conductance responses (SCRs; Tranel & Damasio, 1994), even though an arousal SCR consistently accompanies amygdala activity when, for example, neurologically intact participants view static fearful facial expressions (Williams *et al.*, 2001). Such findings raise the possibility that while emotion recognition may engage processes that are also involved in emotional experience, either the engagement of those processes is not necessary for emotion recognition, or, if those processes are necessarily engaged, then their operation may not necessarily produce the relevant emotional experience. Nonetheless, as very few patient studies have measured online emotional experience during emotion recognition tasks (whether behavioural or physiological measures, or measures of self-reported feelings or mood), the possibility is left open that any processes of contagion or simulation underpinning emotion recognition may involve, at least as a by-product, the subject experiencing the emotion they are viewing in another as and when they are viewing it.

Further evidence for common neural mechanisms underpinning emotion perception and experience comes from work in humans involving either neuroimaging or artificial neural stimulation. An fMRI study, conducted by Wicker *et al.* (2003), found that feeling disgusted and seeing someone else's expression of felt disgust have a common neural basis, specifically the anterior insula and perhaps also anterior cingulate cortex. Direct stimulation of insula neurones can generate reports of unpleasant disgust-related sensations in the throat spreading up to the mouth, lips and nose (Krolak-Salmon *et al.*, 2003). In contrast, direct electrical stimulation within medial temporal lobe, primarily of amygdala and hippocampus, can evoke unpleasant feelings that are predominantly reported as fear or anxiety (Halgren *et al.*, 1978). This finding tallies with more recent neuroimaging research suggesting a disproportionate role for human amygdala in the experience of negative emotions, especially fear; for example, the finding that procaine-induced feelings of intense fear are associated with significant left amygdala activity, compared to euphoric feelings (Ketter *et al.*, 1996).

If the recognition of another's emotion can occur via a process of primitive emotional contagion, this might happen in a more indirect fashion (branch A2 in Figure 20.1), perhaps mediated by mimicry of the viewed facial expression. According to this idea, viewing a face automatically initiates facial muscle activity in one's own face corresponding to the viewed facial expression, and feedback from that muscle activity induces the relevant emotional state (Figure 20.3). If such facial feedback does occur, then the mechanism likely involves proprioceptive sensation of the self-generated facial expression (e.g. Tomkins, 1981), an obvious neural substrate for which is the face region of primary somatosensory cortex (to be discussed in more detail in Section 20.5).

Certainly there is plenty of evidence that unintentional facial mimicry can and often does occur. Young infants are able to discriminate and respond to certain facial postures and movements of a live model, such as tongue or lip protrusions,

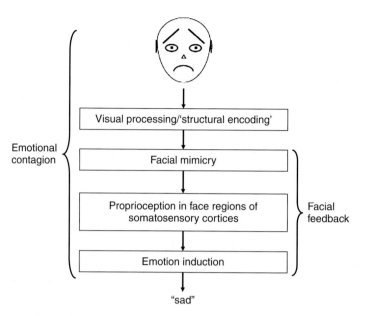

Figure 20.3. Emotion perception via emotional contagion – indirectly, via facial mimicry

mouth widening and expressions of joy, sadness and surprise, by imitating them (Field *et al.*, 1982; Meltzoff & Moore, 1983). In adults, unintentional facial mimicry tends to be a lot less obvious, but nevertheless detectable. Viewing static or dynamic facial expressions results in expressions on one's own face that may not be readily visible, but that can be measured with facial EMG (Dimberg, 1982). These spontaneous and rapid changes in the electrical activity of the facial muscles tend to mimic the expression shown in the stimulus (Hess & Blairy, 2001), and can occur even in the absence of conscious recognition of the face (Dimberg *et al.*, 2000). Moreover, they are often accompanied by changes in self-reported mood congruent with the viewed facial expressions. For example, as mentioned in the previous section, EMG responses to photographs of faces reliably distinguish positive and negative expressions. In particular, angry and fearful faces evoke increased activity in the corrugator muscle, compared to happy (and in some cases, neutral) faces, whereas happy faces evoke increased activity in the zygomatic muscle, compared to angry and fearful (and in some cases, neutral) faces (e.g. Dimberg, 1982; Dimberg *et al.*, 2000; Lundqvist & Dimberg, 1995). Happy faces also tend to evoke increased activity in *orbicularis oculi*, which is the muscle that narrows the eyes and closes the eyelids (Blairy *et al.*, 1999). Sad faces can evoke a moderate increase in corrugator activity, while disgust faces evoke increased activity in *levator labii*, which is the muscle that widens the nostrils and raises the upper lip (Blairy *et al.*, 1999; Lundqvist & Dimberg, 1995).

Viewed facial expressions are able to elicit changes in self-reported mood that tend to be congruent with the viewed facial expressions (Lundqvist & Dimberg, 1995), even when presented for as little as 500 ms (Wild *et al.*, 2001), with more intense expressions tending to produce more intense feelings (Blairy *et al.*, 1999; Wild *et al.*, 2001). For example, in Lundqvist and Dimberg's (1995) study, happy and sad expressions were found to evoke increased feelings of, respectively, happiness and sadness in the viewer, relative to neutral expressions, while angry faces evoked an increased experience of fear and disgust. In Wild *et al.*'s (2001) study, more intense static facial expressions of happiness and sadness evoked greater feelings of the congruent emotion than did less intense expressions, and in Blairy *et al.*'s (1999) study, both angry and fearful static faces evoked greater feelings of irritation or aggression than did happy faces, while greater feelings of repugnance were evoked by disgust than by happy faces.

Dynamic, as well as static, facial expressions of emotion elicit emotionally congruent facial EMG responses and modulate reported mood, at least in cases of happiness, sadness and anger (Hess & Blairy, 2001). Hess and Blairy (2001) did not find evidence that dynamic facial expressions of disgust modulate reported mood, which is surprising given their earlier finding with static expressions (Blairy *et al.*, 1999). Nevertheless, further investigations are warranted, given the rarity of studies using dynamic expressions to examine the relationship between facial mimicry and emotional contagion, and that Hess and Blairy did not examine responses to expressions of other emotions, such as fear.

Physiological responses reliably distinguish emotions in visual scenes and viewed faces. Yet it is unclear whether these responses index changes in emotional state initiated directly by the visual information (Figure 20.2), or indirectly, via mimicry and consequent facial feedback (Figure 20.3). For example, viewed emotional expression stimuli can elicit changes in the skin conductance response (SCR) and heart rate. Changes in SCR to static facial expressions of emotion have been recorded within the context of a conditioning paradigm (e.g. Öhman & Dimberg, 1978). Outside of such a conditioning paradigm, Dimberg (1982) found that viewed angry and happy static faces not only elicited increased facial EMG responses, relative to neutral faces, but also elicited decreased SCR and heart rate (though SCR and heart rate did not distinguish between these two emotions). A more recent study found increased SCR to fearful relative to neutral static faces during both conscious and unconscious stimulus presentations (Williams *et al.*, 2004).

What evidence is there of facial feedback, that is, of changes in one's facial expression altering one's emotional state? One line of evidence comes from studies demonstrating that the intentional production of visible facial postures and movements – which, unbeknownst to the experimental participant, correspond to particular emotional expressions – can lead to other, emotion-related somato-visceral responses in the person producing the expression, as well as to changes in feeling (e.g., Adelmann & Zajonc, 1989; but see Matsumoto, 1987, who argues that the evidence for facial feedback affecting subjective feeling is less than convincing). Moreover, there is evidence of emotion-specific patterns of response arising from this facial feedback. For instance, Levenson and colleagues (e.g. Levenson *et al.*, 1990) found that facial configurations corresponding to expressions of fear, anger, disgust, sadness, happiness and surprise were associated with distinctive patterns of SCR, heart rate and finger temperature. The patterns of autonomic activity distinguished between the negative and positive emotions and among all the negative emotions. SCR on its own clearly distinguished posed facial expressions of fear and disgust from happiness and surprise (though it did not distinguish between these individual emotions), and the SCR differences between anger, sadness, happiness and surprise were all very near the criterion significance level. Heart rate on its own clearly distinguished posed facial expressions of anger, fear and sadness from disgust and surprise (though did not distinguish between these individual emotions), while expressions of happiness produced a heart rate that was intermediate between these two groups and significantly different from that produced by expressions of anger, fear and surprise, but not from expressions of sadness or disgust. Finger temperature on its own distinguished only between posed expressions of fear and anger. Levenson and colleagues also found that these same voluntary facial expressions were associated with significant levels of subjective experience of the related emotion, and that the emotion-specific patterns of autonomic activity were stronger when experience of the associated emotion was reported. In a related study, Hess *et al.*'s (1992) participants were asked to (1) self-generate one of four emotional states (happiness, sadness, anger, peacefulness), (2) produce facial expressions of these emotions without trying to feel them, or (3) feel and express these emotions. Hess *et al.* found that measures of facial EMG, SCR and heart rate together differentiated these four emotions within each of the three tasks. Taken together, these findings add further weight to the idea that a primitive mode of emotional contagion can be mediated by facial mimicry.

No one measure of somatovisceral response is able to differentiate fully between discrete emotions such as anger, disgust, fear, happiness and sadness. Meta-analyses of numerous studies indicate that while combinations of such measures provide a clearer differentiation, it is clearest when positive and negative emotions are contrasted (stronger autonomic responses for negative than positive emotions) than when discrete emotions are contrasted (Cacioppo *et al.*, 2000). Moreover, there is individual variation in the extent to which people are emotionally responsive to the emotions they perceive in other people's faces. In the first of two experiments reported by Laird *et al.* (1994), participants who reported that

viewing various facial expressions had caused them to experience the corresponding emotion were, in a separate procedure, more likely than participants who
did not report such emotion-congruent changes in mood to mimic the behaviour
of an actor expressing startled fear in two brief film clips (jerking their heads
and bodies backwards in unison with the actor). In Laird *et al.*'s second experiment, participants watched three video clips depicting happy people. They did
so while: (1) inhibiting their facial movements; (2) not thinking about their faces
(natural movement); and (3) exaggerating any naturally occurring expressions.
Those participants who reported, in a separate procedure, that viewing various
facial expressions had caused them to experience the corresponding emotion
reported being less happy when they were asked to inhibit their facial movements,
compared to those who did not report such emotion-congruent changes in
mood upon exposure to the facial expressions. More recently, Sonnby-
Borgström *et al.* (2003) examined the relationship between facial mimicry (as
measured by facial EMG) and subsequent self-reported mood upon exposure to static facial expressions of anger and happiness, in participants who
were categorized as either high or low empathizers according to their scores on
a standard empathy questionnaire. The high-empathy participants produced
greater facial mimicry than the low-empathy participants, even at short exposure
times (up to 56 ms), suggesting that these mimicry responses are automatic.
Indeed, at these short exposure times, the low-empathy participants tended to
show inverse zygomaticus muscle reactions ('smiling') when exposed to an angry
face. There were no differences between high- and low-empathy participants in
self-reported feelings, either when looking at angry faces or when looking at happy
faces. Nevertheless, the high-empathy participants showed a higher correspondence between facial mimicry and self-reported feelings, with negative and positive
feelings being distinguished by the activity of both the zygomaticus and the
corrugator muscles of this group, but only by the activity of the zygomaticus
muscle for the low-empathy group, and in the opposite direction (a greater rather
than smaller 'smiling' response for negative than for positive feelings).

   Given all the evidence discussed so far, it is tempting to conclude that mimicry
mediates emotion recognition via a process of emotional contagion; that is, that
you can come to know what another is feeling by unintentionally mimicking their
facial expression, the feedback from which induces that same emotional state in
yourself, from which you are then easily able to infer that the other is feeling just as
you now do. Yet there is little if any direct evidence of this suggested causal
sequence, despite attempts to find some. For example, Hess and Blairy (2001)
did not find any relation between emotion recognition performance (on an
emotion rating task) and the tendency to mimic the dynamic facial displays of
happiness, sadness, anger and disgust (as measured by facial EMG). Nor did Hess

and Blairy find any relation between mimicry and emotional contagion (as measured by self-report), even though there was evidence of mimicry for all four emotions, and evidence of contagion from expressions of happiness and sadness. Moreover, a study of a rare patient suffering from a bilateral facial paralysis, who was unable to convey emotions through facial expressions, found that her reported emotional experience upon being presented with emotionally evocative slides did not differ from that of normal participants (Keillor *et al.*, 2002). This patient was also still able to detect, discriminate and image emotional expressions (Keillor *et al.*, 2002); similarly, people with Möbius syndrome, who also suffer from facial paralysis, are also not significantly impaired at recognizing facial expressions of emotions (Calder *et al.*, 2000a). Together, these findings are not consistent with the claim that facial feedback is necessary to experience emotion, or to the claim that facial mimicry mediates emotion recognition via a process of emotional contagion. Nevertheless, as relatively few studies have examined these issues, there may still yet be some truth to be found in the idea that at least sometimes unintentional facial mimicry mediates emotion recognition, either directly or by first triggering that same emotional state in the perceiver. Note, though, the difficulty of distinguishing between facial mimicry mediating emotion recognition directly, or by first triggering that same emotional state in the perceiver. Suppose that one had evidence that emotion recognition abilities are correlated with facial mimicry and other changes in emotional state, such as a change in reported mood, congruent with the viewed emotion. Such evidence would not necessarily indicate that facial mimicry instigates a change in emotional state, which in turn allows the inference that the other person is feeling what you are now feeling. For facial mimicry might mediate emotion recognition directly yet nonetheless produce a change in emotional state as a by-product (i.e. that any change in emotional state as a consequence of facial mimicry is epiphenomenal with respect to emotion recognition).

20.5 Emotion recognition via simulation

An alternative way in which one might catch another's emotion by virtue of viewing their expression is that the visual information directly modulates neural structures that represent changes related to body state and generate feelings (akin to Damasio's, 1994, 'as-if' loop), creating a simulation of the other's emotional state (Adolphs, 2002; Adolphs *et al.*, 2000). Whilst speculative, this idea (branch B3 in Figure 20.1; see also Figure 20.4) is motivated by some tantalizing evidence. Primary and secondary somatosensory cortexes (SI and SII) and insular cortex represent information related to body states – SI primarily somatosensory information and SII and insula primarily information about states of the viscera and

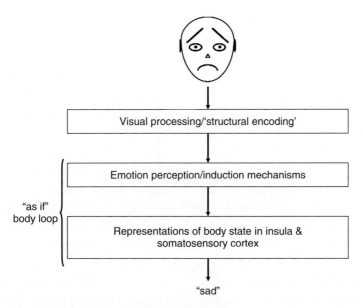

Figure 20.4. Emotion perception via body state simulation

autonomic nervous system (Craig, 2002) – and are thus proposed to have important roles in emotions, including emotional feelings (e.g. Craig, 2002; Damasio,
1994). As I discuss below, not only is there some evidence of somatosensory and
insular cortex involvement in emotional experience, but there is also evidence
implicating these regions in emotion recognition.

A different simulation proposal (branch B4 in Figure 20.1) is that what is
simulated is not the change in body states associated with the experience of the
emotion that one is viewing in another person, but rather the motor movements
comprising the relevant facial expression (Carr *et al.*, 2003; Gallese *et al.*, 2004;
Leslie *et al.*, 2004). This idea of motor simulation (Figure 20.5) raises the possibility of motor signals 'leaking out' to the periphery, in which case facial muscle
activity upon viewing another's expression would be a by-product of a process that
enables emotion recognition, not a stage in a causal sequence leading to emotion
recognition. Consider, also, that if either a motor or body-state simulation process
occurs, then it is possible that the simulation could be run 'offline', without
producing any measurable effect on the periphery (e.g. change in facial muscle
activity or SCR) or change in subjective feeling. In other words, if we have the
capacity to simulate the emotional states of others, then this might not always (or
even ever) result in one actually experiencing the viewed and simulated emotional
state (i.e. in emotional contagion).

If we do have the capacity to simulate either the body states or the motor
movements of people whose expressions we view, then one would expect some

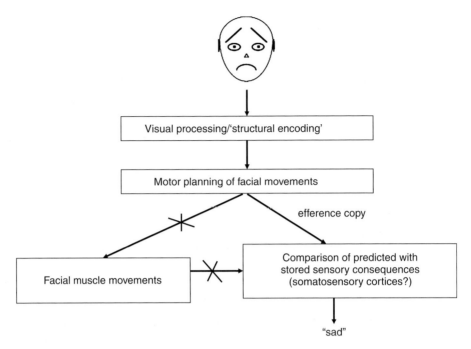

Figure 20.5. Emotion perception via motor simulation. As suggested in this diagram, motor simulation might enable emotion recognition by way of a process in which efference copies of facial motor commands are fed to a system that compares the predicted sensory consequences of that movement with previously experienced actual sensory consequences of such movements. (This schematic is based on forward models of motor planning and error correction, in which efference copies of motor commands are compared to the actual sensory consequences of the executed movements; see Wolpert *et al.*, 2003, for a review. The crossed arrows indicate that such a motor simulation process is run offline)

commonality amongst the neural systems that subserve emotion perception and those that generate somatosensory body images or those that generate motor movements involved in emotional expression. The evidence is consistent with, but not strongly supportive of, both forms of simulation.

Somatosensory cortex has been implicated in emotional experience. For example, somatosensory cortex was prominent amongst a set of regions engaged by the recall of personal episodes of happiness, sadness, anger and fear in a neuroimaging study (Damasio *et al.*, 2000). Interestingly, somatosensory cortex may even be involved in mediating emotional experience triggered by visual events that are not consciously perceived: in a recent study, it was reported that activation of left somatosensory cortex was correlated with negatively valenced feelings and the amplitude of the startle eyeblink in response to aversively conditioned faces with neutral expressions that were presented in the blind fields of blindsight patients, and thus not consciously perceived (Anders *et al.*, 2004). A possible neural pathway subserving this capacity is a subcortical route to the amygdala, which is thought to underpin residual visual abilities in blindsight (Cowey & Stoerig, 1991), and projections from the amygdala to primary and secondary somatosensory cortexes via insular cortex (Amaral & Price, 1984).

Somatosensory cortex has also been implicated in emotion recognition. Evidence comes from studies of people with somatosensory cortex damage, especially in the right hemisphere, and functional-imaging studies in healthy adults. In a study involving over 100 patients with focal brain damage, it was found that impaired recognition of facial emotion correlated best with lesions situated in the right somatosensory cortex (including SI, SII and insular cortex) (Adolphs *et al.*, 2000). A study using similar methods, but employing point-light displays of body movements instead of static facial expressions, found that impairments in judging emotions from these stimuli were also associated with damage to several components of a network of neural structures, with the most reliable region of lesion overlap associated with this impairment in right somatosensory cortex (Heberlein *et al.*, 2004). At the time of writing, only two functional imaging studies have been published that specifically examined the role of somatosensory cortex in emotion recognition, and the results of both are broadly consistent with these lesion studies. Winston *et al.* (2003a) found enhanced activation in somatosensory and ventromedial prefrontal cortices, as measured by fMRI, when participants made explicit as compared to implicit emotion judgements (which of two simultaneously presented faces is more emotional, versus which is more male). Similarly, Kilts *et al.* (2003) found that judging the emotional intensity of static angry and happy, compared to neutral, faces activated left (but not right) somatosensory cortex, amongst other regions. Activity in response to these emotional expressions, which was generally stronger than that in the somatosensory cortex, was also recorded in cortical motor-related regions, including primary motor and premotor cortexes, raising the possibility that the facial expressions were engaging processes of motor simulation, akin to 'mirror neurone' activity for facial emotional expressions.

Mirror neurones for facial expressions of emotion – i.e. neural mechanisms common to both the perception and production of facial expressions – are what we might expect to find if emotion recognition involves mimicking the viewed expression, or executing its motor programme offline. In the premotor cortex of monkeys, there are neurones that respond not only when the monkey prepares to perform an action itself, but also when the monkey observes the same visually presented action performed by someone else (e.g. Gallese *et al.*, 1996; Rizzolatti *et al.*, 1996). Various supportive findings have also been obtained in humans. Observing another's actions results in desynchronization in motor cortex as measured with magnetoencephalography (Hari *et al.*, 1998), and lowers the threshold for producing motor responses when transcranial magnetic stimulation is used to activate motor cortex (Strafella & Paus, 2000). Imitating another's actions via observation activates premotor cortex in functional imaging studies (Iacoboni *et al.*, 1999); moreover, such activation is somatotopic with respect to the body part that is observed to perform the action, even in the absence of any overt action on the part of the subject (Buccino *et al.*, 2001). It thus appears that primates construct motor representations suited to performing the same action that they visually perceive someone else perform, in line with both the contagion and simulation proposals. The existence of emotion-related mirror neurones is suggested by the activation of a largely similar neural network when subjects either passively view or deliberately imitate static facial expressions of basic emotions (Carr *et al.*, 2003) and dynamic smiling and frowning expressions (Leslie *et al.*, 2004). Premotor areas, especially the inferior prefrontal area responsible for face movement, were prominent in this network. Imitation elicited greater and more bilateral activation of these areas than passive viewing, corresponding to an additive effect of expression observation and execution. Other regions implicated in this network included superior temporal cortex (in both studies), insula and amygdala (in Carr *et al.*, 2003).

Interestingly, it was static but not dynamic angry and happy faces that elicited somatosensory and motor cortex activation in Kilts *et al.*'s (2003) study. This raises the possibility that the recognition of emotions in dynamic facial expressions relies less on motor simulation than on static facial expressions. Indeed, Kilts *et al.* claim that the results of their study 'suggest that the decoding of emotion messages in static, but not dynamic, expressions is solved by the activation of a network of brain regions that link by covert simulation the static percept to the mental representation of the emotion. Emotion perception in dynamic expressions apparently involves a lesser reliance on motor simulation'. (Kilts *et al.*, 2003, p. 165). But that is counterintuitive insofar as one might expect the dynamic production of an expression to be simulated more readily than a static expression. Moving moves, one might say. While Kilts *et al.* do not offer an explanation of why static facial expressions might generate greater activity than dynamic expressions in left somatosensory, primary motor and premotor cortexes, one plausible reason is that it is easier to decipher the emotion in dynamic than in static faces, and so the relevant neural systems have to 'try harder', as it were, when one is confronted with a static face. But that by itself does not necessitate Kilts *et al.*'s results without some further considerations. One such consideration would be that perhaps it takes the brain longer to process the static stimuli to figure out the emotion than it does to process the dynamic stimuli for the same purpose. Since the blood-oxygen-level-dependent (BOLD) response measured in fMRI will integrate signal over some seconds, the longer a particular region is engaged in processing, the more signal you get. Thus, the dynamic stimuli may have engaged a simulation process, as realized in a network involving somatosensory, primary motor and premotor cortexes, at least as much as the static stimuli, just more transiently. Functional MRI is limited in the extent to which one can use it to distinguish between a relatively large but short lived burst of activity in a particular neural region, and more prolonged activity of smaller magnitude. That requires a method with greater temporal resolution, such as the recording of event-related potentials using electroencephalography or magneto-encephalography. Clearly, then, more research is required to establish whether dynamic expressions engage neural structures presumed to underpin a simulation process more than do static expressions (or vice versa), and to establish whether this holds for body as well as facial expressions. Further research is also required to establish whether it is right or left somatosensory cortex (or both) that is crucial for emotion recognition, and whether its hemispheric involvement varies across emotions and means of expression.

We should note three caveats about somatosensory and motor cortex involvement in emotion recognition. First, functional imaging studies are correlational. No one has yet provided convincing demonstrations of a *causal* role for motor cortex in emotion recognition (there are no reports of lesions of these areas disrupting emotion recognition, for example), or for somatosensory cortex in emotional experience in humans, and, in particular, a causal role for just that region of somatosensory cortex shown to be important in emotion recognition (primarily right SII). So firm conclusions cannot yet be drawn. Second, note that even if somatosensory cortex is at least sometimes involved in both emotion recognition and experience, and thus possibly a major component in a neural network for simulating the emotional states of others, it may not be required for either the recognition or experience of at least some emotions. This is suggested by, for example, Wicker *et al.*'s (2003) finding that feeling disgusted and seeing someone else express disgust both activated the anterior insula and anterior cingulate, but that they appeared to do so directly, without the involvement of primary or secondary somatosensory cortices. Third, earlier I mentioned that if facial emotion recognition involves catching another's emotional state by unintentionally mimicking their facial expression, then an obvious candidate for a neural region that represents the proprioceptive information from this facial feedback is somatosensory cortex. Yet much of the evidence of somatosensory cortex involvement in emotion recognition is unable to distinguish between this idea and the proposal that this evidence is typically claimed to support; namely, that emotion recognition involves simulation of somatosensory states associated with the viewed emotion. If the latter proposal is to be supported over the former, then future studies will need to measure and preferably control for facial mimicry.

20.6 Concluding remarks

I have been depositing a little cold water on the idea that processes of emotional contagion and simulation underpin emotion recognition. While there is considerable evidence from a variety of sources that perceiving emotions in others and experiencing them for oneself are correlated, there is precious little evidence that these capacities are causally related in the way that many authors suggest, namely that we come to know what others are feeling by coming to know *how* they are feeling (i.e. by actually experiencing the same emotional state as they are experiencing, or by simulating one or more aspects of the viewed emotional state).

Despite my more cautious take on the idea that perceptually mediated empathy provides an important means by which we come to know the emotional states of others, I have no intention of being a killjoy; indeed, I think the idea deserves to be taken seriously. Not only is there suggestive (albeit not direct) evidence in favour of the idea, it also offers new and possibly promising prospects for understanding what people are *thinking* (believing, desiring, etc.), as well as what they are feeling (see Gallese *et al.*, 2004; Goldman & Sripada, 2005; Meltzoff & Decety, 2003). However, lest we get too excited about the prospects of such ideas providing the answers to all the important questions about how we mindread, we ought to heed Goldman and Sripada's (2005) warning that it cannot simply be assumed that processes underpinning facial emotion recognition can be extrapolated to other types of mindreading; for instance, coming to know what other people are thinking might require more complex processes than coming to know what they are feeling.

Finally, a few words on the distinction between self and other in relation to visually mediated empathy. Emotional contagion per se need not go along with a capacity to distinguish self from other. Indeed, there are functions that emotional contagion can conceivably serve without there being such a capacity in operation or even existing in an organism at all, such as the motivation of action in the face of danger that the creature does not itself perceive but which a conspecific does. But in order for emotional contagion to drive the recognition of emotion in others, and in the case of simulation-driven emotion recognition, presumably processes that distinguish self from others must be in place, for it would be not much good if a simulated or felt emotional state of another was misattributed to oneself. The sense of self and thus the ability to distinguish between self and others when attributing emotions, thoughts and actions develops as a consequence of interpersonal interactions and a capacity to imitate, and may well be implemented by a system involving the inferior parietal cortex in conjunction with the prefrontal cortex (Decety & Chaminade, 2003; Meltzoff & Decety, 2003).

Acknowledgements

The bulk of this chapter was written while the author was a Visiting Research Fellow in the Department of Neurology, University of Iowa Hospitals and Clinics, Iowa City, USA, a sojourn funded by a Short-term Fellowship from the Human Frontier Science Program. Thanks to Ralph Adolphs and India Morrison for their valuable input. The face shown in Figures 20.2–20.5 is from the FEEST database of facial expression stimuli (Young *et al.*, 2002).

REFERENCES

Adelmann, P. K., & Zajonc, R. B. (1989). Facial efference and the experience of emotion. *Annual Review of Psychology*, **40**, 249–280.

Adolphs, R. (2002). Neural systems for recognizing emotion. *Current Opinion in Neurobiology*, **12**, 169–177.

Adolphs, R., Damasio, H., Tranel, D., Cooper, G., & Damasio, A. R. (2000). A role for somatosensory cortices in the visual recognition of emotion as revealed by 3-D lesion mapping. *Journal of Neuroscience*, **20**, 2683–2690.

Adolphs, R., Tranel, D., Hamann, S., *et al.* (1999). Recognition of facial emotion in nine individuals with bilateral amygdala damage. *Neuropsychologia*, **37**, 1111–1117.

Amaral, D. G., & Price, J. L. (1984). Amygdalo-cortical projections in the monkey (*Macaca fascicularis*). *The Journal of Comparative Neurology*, **230**, 465–496.

Anders, S., Birbaumer, N., Sadowski, B., Erb, M., Mader, I., Grodd, W., & Lotze, M. (2004). Parietal somatosensory association cortex mediates affective blindsight. *Nature Neuroscience*, **7**, 339–340.

Anderson, A. K., & Phelps, E. A. (2002). Is the human amygdala critical for the subjective experience of emotion? Evidence of intact dispositional affect in patients with amygdala lesions. *Journal of Cognitive Neuroscience*, **14**, 709–720.

Asthana, H. S., Mandal, M. K., Khurana, H., & Haque-Nizamie, S. (1998). Visuospatial and affect recognition deficit in depression. *Journal of Affective Disorders*, **48**, 57–62.

Berenbaum, H., & Oltmanns, T. F. (1992). Emotional experience and expression in schizophrenia and depression. *Journal of Abnormal Psychology*, **101**, 37–44.

Blairy, S., Herrera, P., & Hess, U. (1999). Mimicry and the judgment of emotional facial expressions. *Journal of Nonverbal Behavior*, **23**, 5–41.

Bouhuys, A. L., Bloem, G. M., & Groothuis, T. G. (1995). Induction of depressed and elated mood by music influences the perception of facial emotional expressions in healthy subjects. *Journal of Affective Disorders*, **33**, 215–226.

Bradley, B. P., Mogg, K., & Millar, N. H. (2000). Covert and overt orienting of attention to emotional faces in anxiety. *Cognition & Emotion*, **14**, 789–808.

Buccino, G., Binkofski, F., Fink, G. R., *et al.* (2001). Action observation activates premotor and parietal areas in a somatotopic manner: an fMRI study. *European Journal of Neuroscience*, **13**, 400–404.

Cacioppo, J. T., Berntson, G. G., Larsen, J. T., Poehlmann, K. M., & Ito, T. A. (2000). The psychophysiology of emotion. In R. Lewis & J. M. Haviland-Jones (eds.), *The Handbook of Emotion*, 2nd edn. (pp. 173–191). New York: Guilford Press.

Calder, A. J., Burton, A. M., Miller, P., Young, A. W., & Akamatsu, S. (2001). A principal component analysis of facial expressions. *Vision Research*, **41**, 1179–1208.

Calder, A. J., Keane, J., Cole, J., Campbell, R., & Young, A. W. (2000a). Facial expression recognition by people with Möbius syndrome. *Cognitive Neuropsychology*, **17**, 73–87.

Calder, A. J., Keane, J., Lawrence, A. D., & Manes, F. (2004). Impaired recognition of anger following damage to the ventral striatum. *Brain*, **127**, 1958–1969.

Calder, A. J., Keane, J., Manes, F., Antoun, N., & Young, A. W. (2000b). Impaired recognition and experience of disgust following brain injury. *Nature Neuroscience*, **3**, 1077–1078.

Calder, A. J., Young, A. W., Rowland, D., *et al.* (1996). Facial emotion recognition after bilateral amygdala damage: differentially severe impairment of fear. *Cognitive Neuropsychology*, **13**, 699–745.

Carr, L., Iacoboni, M., Dubeau, M. C., Mazziotta, J. C., & Lenzi, G. L. (2003). Neural mechanisms of empathy in humans: a relay from neural systems for imitation to limbic areas. *Proceedings of the National Academy of Sciences of the USA*, **100**, 5497–5502.

Cowey, A., & Stoerig, P. (1991). The neurobiology of blindsight. *Trends in Neurosciences*, **14**, 140–145.

Craig, A. D. (2002). How do you feel? Interoception: the sense of the physiological condition of the body. *Nature Reviews Neuroscience*, **3**, 655–666.

Dailey, M. N., Cottrell, G. W., Padgett, C., & Adolphs, R. (2002). EMPATH: a neural network that categorizes facial expressions. *Journal of Cognitive Neuroscience*, **14**, 1158–1173.

Damasio, A. R. (1994). *Descartes' Error: Emotion, Reason, and the Human Brain*. New York: Grosset/Putnam.

Damasio, A. R., Grabowski, T. J., Bechara, A., *et al.* (2000). Subcortical and cortical brain activity during the feeling of self-generated emotions. *Nature Neuroscience*, **3**, 1049–1056.

Decety, J., & Chaminade, T. (2003). When the self represents the other: a new cognitive neuroscience view on psychological identification. *Consciousness and Cognition*, **12**, 577–596.

Dimberg, U. (1982). Facial reactions to facial expressions. *Psychophysiology*, **19**, 643–647.

Dimberg, U., Thunberg, M., & Elmehed, K. (2000). Unconscious facial reactions to emotional facial expressions. *Psychological Science*, **11**, 86–89.

Dretske, F. I. (1969). *Seeing and Knowing*. London: Routledge & Kegan Paul.

Durrani, S. J. (2005). Studies of emotion recognition from multiple communication channels. Unpublished PhD thesis, University of St. Andrews.

Dworkin, R. H., Clark, S. C., Amador, X. F., & Gorman, J. M. (1996). Does affective blunting in schizophrenia reflect affective deficit or neuromotor dysfunction? *Schizophrenia Research*, **20**, 301–306.

Field, T. M., Woodson, R., Greenberg, R., & Cohen, D. (1982). Discrimination and imitation of facial expression by neonates. *Science*, **218**, 179–181.

Flack, W. F., Jr., Laird, J. D., & Cavallaro, L. A. (1999). Emotional expression and feeling in schizophrenia: effects of specific expressive behaviors on emotional experiences. *Journal of Clinical Psychology*, **55**, 1–20.

Gallese, V., Fadiga, L., Fogassi, L., & Rizzolatti, G. (1996). Action recognition in the premotor cortex. *Brain*, **119**, 593–609.

Gallese, V., Keysers, C., & Rizzolatti, G. (2004). A unifying view of the basis of social cognition. *Trends in Cognitive Sciences*, **8**, 396–403.

Goldie, P. (1999). How we think of others' emotions. *Mind & Language*, **14**, 394–423.

Goldman, A. I., & Sripada, C. S. (2005). Simulationist models of face-based emotion recognition. *Cognition*, **94**, 193–213.

Gur, R. C., Erwin, R. J., Gur, R. E., *et al.* (1992). Facial emotion discrimination: II. Behavioral findings in depression. *Psychiatry Research*, **42**, 241–251.

Hale, W. W. (1998). Judgment of facial expressions and depression persistence. *Psychiatry Research*, **80**, 265–274.

Halgren, E., Walter, R. D., Cherlow, D. G., & Crandall, P. H. (1978). Mental phenomena evoked by electrical stimulation of the human hippocampal formation and amygdala. *Brain*, **101**, 83–117.

Hari, R., Forss, N., Avikainen, S., *et al.* (1998). Activation of human primary motor cortex during action observation: a neuromagnetic study. *Proceedings of the National Academy of Sciences of the USA*, **95**, 15061–15065.

Hatfield, E., Cacioppo, J. T., & Rapson, R. L. (1994). *Emotional Contagion*. New York: Cambridge University Press.

Heberlein, A. S., Adolphs, R., Tranel, D., & Damasio, H. (2004). Cortical regions for judgments of emotions and personality traits from point-light walkers. *Journal of Cognitive Neuroscience*, **16**, 1143–1158.

Hess, U., & Blairy, S. (2001). Facial mimicry and emotional contagion to dynamic emotional facial expressions and their influence on decoding accuracy. *International Journal of Psychophysiology*, **40**, 129–141.

Hess, U., Kappas, A., McHugo, G. J., Lanzetta, J. T., & Kleck, R. E. (1992). The facilitative effect of facial expression on the self-generation of emotion. *International Journal of Psychophysiology*, **12**, 251–265.

Iacoboni, M., Woods, R. P., Brass, M., *et al.* (1999). Cortical mechanisms of human imitation. *Science*, **286**, 2526–2528.

Keillor, J. M., Barrett, A. M., Crucian, G. P., Kortenkamp, S., & Heilman, K. M. (2002). Emotional experience and perception in the absence of facial feedback. *Journal of the International Neuropsychological Society*, **8**, 130–135.

Ketter, T. A., Andreason, P. J., George, M. S., *et al.* (1996). Anterior paralimbic mediation of procaine-induced emotional and psychosensory experiences. *Archives of General Psychiatry*, **53**, 59–69.

Kilts, C. D., Egan, G., Gideon, D. A., Ely, T. D., & Hoffman, J. M. (2003). Dissociable neural pathways are involved in the recognition of emotion in static and dynamic facial expressions. *NeuroImage*, **18**, 156–168.

Kring, A. M., Kerr, S. L., & Earnst, K. S. (1999). Schizophrenic patients show facial reactions to emotional facial expressions. *Psychophysiology*, **36**, 186–192.

Krolak-Salmon, P., Henaff, M. A., Isnard, J., *et al.* (2003). An attention modulated response to disgust in human ventral anterior insula. *Annals of Neurology*, **53**, 446–453.

Laird, J. D., Alibozak, T., Davainis, D., *et al.* (1994). Individual differences in the effects of spontaneous mimicry on emotional contagion. *Motivation and Emotion*, **18**, 231–247.

Lawrence, A. D., Calder, A. J., McGowan, S. W., & Grasby, P. M. (2002). Selective disruption of the recognition of facial expressions of anger. *NeuroReport*, **13**, 881–884.

Leslie, K. R., Johnson-Frey, S. H., & Grafton, S. T. (2004). Functional imaging of face and hand imitation: towards a motor theory of empathy. *NeuroImage*, **21**, 601–607.

Levenson, R. W., Ekman, P., & Friesen, W. V. (1990). Voluntary facial action generates emotion-specific autonomic nervous system activity. *Psychophysiology*, **27**, 363–384.

Lundqvist, L. O., & Dimberg, U. (1995). Facial expressions are contagious. *Journal of Psychophysiology*, **9**, 203–211.

Matsumoto, D. (1987). The role of facial response in the experience of emotion: more methodological problems and a metaanalysis. *Journal of Personality and Social Psychology*, **52**, 769–774.

Meltzoff, A. N., & Decety, J. (2003). What imitation tells us about social cognition: a rapprochement between developmental psychology and cognitive neuroscience. *Philosophical Transactions of the Royal Society of London, Series B: Biological Sciences*, **358**, 491–500.

Meltzoff, A. N., & Moore, M. K. (1983). Newborn infants imitate adult facial gestures. *Child Development*, **54**, 702–709.

Niedenthal, P. M., Halberstadt, J. B., Margolin, J., & Innes-Ker, A. H. (2000). Emotional state and the detection of change in facial expression of emotion. *European Journal of Social Psychology*, **30**, 211–222.

Öhman, A., & Dimberg, U. (1978). Facial expressions as conditioned stimuli for electrodermal responses: a case of 'preparedness'? *Journal of Personality and Social Psychology*, **36**, 1251–1258.

Persad, S. M., & Polivy, J. (1993). Differences between depressed and nondepressed individuals in the recognition of and response to facial emotional cues. *Journal of Abnormal Psychology*, **102**, 358–368.

Preston, D., & de Waal, F. B. M. (2002). Empathy: its ultimate and proximate bases. *Behavioral and Brain Sciences*, **25**, 1–72.

Richards, A., French, C. C., Calder, A. J., *et al.* (2002). Anxiety-related bias in the classification of emotionally ambiguous facial expressions. *Emotion*, **2**, 273–287.

Rizzolatti, G., Fadiga, L., Gallese, V., & Fogassi, L. (1996). Premotor cortex and the recognition of motor actions. *Cognitive Brain Research*, **3**, 131–141.

Rubinow, D. R., & Post, R. M. (1992). Impaired recognition of affect in facial expression in depressed patients. *Biological Psychiatry*, **31**, 947–953.

Sonnby-Borgström, M., Jönsson, P., & Svensson, O. (2003). Emotional empathy as related to mimicry reactions at different levels of information processing. *Journal of Nonverbal Behavior*, **27**, 3–23.

Sprengelmeyer, R., Young, A. W., Schroeder, U., *et al.* (1999). Knowing no fear. *Proceedings of the Royal Society of London. Series B: Biological Sciences*, **266**, 2451–2456.

Strafella, A. P., & Paus, T. (2000). Modulation of cortical excitability during action observation: a transcranial magnetic stimulation study. *Experimental Brain Research*, **11**, 2289–2292.

Surguladze, S. A., Young, A. W., Senior, C., Brebion, G., Travis, M. J., & Phillips, M. L. (2004). Recognition accuracy and response bias to happy and sad facial expressions in patients with major depression. *Neuropsychology*, **18**, 212–218.

Tomkins, S. S. (1981). The role of facial response in the experience of emotion: a reply. *Journal of Personality and Social Psychology*, **40**, 355–357.

Tranel, D., & Damasio, A. R. (1994). Intact electrodermal skin conductance responses after bilateral amygdala damage. *Neuropsychologia*, **27**, 381–390.

Wicker, B., Keysers, C., Plailly, J., *et al.* (2003). Both of us disgusted in My insula: the common neural basis of seeing and feeling disgust. *Neuron*, **40**, 655–664.

Wild, B., Erb, M., & Bartels, M. (2001). Are emotions contagious? Evoked emotions while viewing emotionally expressive faces: quality, quantity, time course and gender differences. *Psychiatry Research*, **102**, 109–124.

Williams, L. M., Liddell, B. J., Rathjen, J., *et al.* (2004). Mapping the time course of nonconscious and conscious perception of fear: an integration of central and peripheral measures. *Human Brain Mapping*, **21**, 64–74.

Williams, L. M., Phillips, M. L., Brammer, M. J., *et al.* (2001). Arousal dissociates amygdala and hippocampal fear responses: evidence from simultaneous fMRI and skin conductance recording. *NeuroImage*, **14**, 1070–1079.

Winston, J. S., O'Doherty, J., & Dolan, R. J. (2003a). Common and distinct neural responses during direct and incidental processing of multiple facial emotions. *NeuroImage*, **20**, 84–97.

Winston, J. S., Vuilleumier, P., & Dolan, R. J. (2003b). Effects of low-spatial frequency components of fearful faces on fusiform cortex activity. *Current Biology*, **13**, 1824–1829.

Wolpert, D. M., Doya, K., & Kawato, M. (2003). A unifying computational framework for motor control and social interaction. *Philosophical Transactions of the Royal Society of London, Series B: Biological Sciences*, **358**, 593–602.

Young, A. W., Perrett, D. I., Calder, A. J., Sprengelmeyer, R., & Ekman, P. (2002). Facial expressions of emotion: stimuli and tests (FEEST). Bury St. Edmunds: Thames Valley Test Company.

Part III

Empathy models, regulation and measurement of empathy

Balancing the empathy expense account: strategies for regulating empathic response

Sara D. Hodges and Robert Biswas-Diener

Department of Psychology, University of Oregon

21.1 Introduction

Is it *good* to be empathic? Even taking into account the wide spectrum of definitions associated with the term 'empathy', people are generally in favour of the concept. Psychological research and anecdotal evidence suggest that empathy is widely valued. Hogan's (1969) individual difference measure of empathy has items which suggest that high scorers are all-around good citizens in addition to being empathic (e.g. 'I usually take an active part in the entertainment at parties' and 'Most of the arguments or quarrels I get into are over matters of principle'). When Norman (1967) rank-ordered traits in terms of social desirability, empathy was rated on average at 6.7 on a 9-point scale, where 9 was the highest desirability. Many of the chapters in this book (e.g. chapters 2, 8) point to deficits in empathy or the absence of empathy as being prominent features of serious psychological disorders and mental disabilities. Indeed, respect for empathy is so great that many criminals, particularly sex offenders (e.g. Pithers, 1994), have been enrolled in 'empathy training' programmes (albeit some based on inconclusive research findings) as a part of rehabilitation. It appears that the ability to respond empathically is highly sought after.

However, there can be too much of a good thing, and although it has been said that one can never be too rich or too thin, there do appear to be costs to being too empathic, as well as costs associated with the more common other extreme (not being empathic enough). Thus, an individual's ideal level of empathy may not be that individual's maximal level of empathy, and having strategies for regulating empathy – both increasing and decreasing it – would be helpful. This chapter explores such strategies. First, we provide an overview of the major constructs associated with empathy that would be the target of these strategies. Next, we discuss the strategies themselves, including their effectiveness and costs. Finally, we

Empathy in Mental Illness, eds. Tom F. D. Farrow and Peter W. R. Woodruff. Published by Cambridge University Press. © Cambridge University Press 2007.

explore some cases of empathy regulation gone awry and the consequences of these regulatory misses, particularly those consequences related to mental health.

21.2 Defining empathy

It doesn't take much digging into the research on empathy to discover that there is quite a range of definitions and concepts associated with this concept (Chlopan *et al.*, 1985; Davis, 1983; Klein & Hodges, 2001). To make things more confusing, no consistent nomenclature is used to distinguish these strands of empathy, so that different researchers studying very different constructs may all claim to have found the cause, correlates or consequences of 'empathy'. This lack of precision may have emerged because everyday (i.e. lay) use of the term 'empathy' presupposes the presence of all the elements that make up this multi-dimensional construct (e.g. 'mindreading', concern for the other person, distress at another's plight and stepping outside of the self's egocentric frame), whereas many researchers have chosen to measure and/or manipulate only one element.

Despite the overabundance of operational definitions of empathy, consistent themes emerge. Empathic responses can be ordered along a continuum of simple to complex. The most rudimentary glimmers of empathy are found in emotional contagion (e.g. Hatfield *et al.*, 1993) and imitation – crying when another cries or opening one's mouth when another opens her mouth. These mirroring behaviours occur among the youngest of humans (e.g. Meltzoff & Moore, 1983), and the capacity to imitate is thought to be a fundamental and critical building block for other forms of empathy and perspective taking (Rizzolatti *et al.*, 2002). However, humans exhibit much more complex and impressive forms of empathy, and it is at these more advanced levels that another distinction in characterizing empathy becomes apparent, splitting the concept roughly into emotional and cognitive components.

Emotional empathy – an emotional response to another person – is what comes to mind for many people when they think of empathy. Emotional empathy itself has traditionally been further split into two additional constructs. The first, and the one that corresponds most closely to the concept referred to simply as 'empathy' in everyday conversations, is what we label 'empathic concern' in this chapter. Empathic concern entails feelings of compassion and warmth felt *for* the target of empathy. The second piece of emotional empathy, known as 'personal distress' can be every bit as emotionally charged as empathic concern, but in this case, the emotions are self-centred feelings of distress prompted *by* the target of empathy. Thus, watching a preteen engage in an awkward interaction with a romantic crush could prompt both – feelings of empathic concern, 'oh, the poor girl – is she going to make it through this ordeal?' as well as personal distress (e.g. the observer cringing and blushing when the preteen stutters).

In the example in the previous paragraph, both the target of empathy and the empathic perceiver are presumably feeling embarrassed, suggesting that personal distress resembles a form of emotional contagion (discussed earlier as a very simple form of empathy). Personal distress can, but does not necessarily, involve emotional contagion: it can also occur when feeling a *different* emotion than the target of empathy. For example, the toddler who displays anxiety and agitation in response to his depressed and withdrawn mother is showing personal distress, but not contagion. Of the two emotions, empathic concern is thought to be a more sophisticated and complex empathic response than personal distress (Eisenberg *et al.*, 1998). It emerges later developmentally (Hoffman, 1984; Zahn-Waxler *et al.*, 1992), and may require the suppression or inhibition of one's own emotions, such as personal distress (Eisenberg & Fabes, 1995). Furthermore, feeling empathic concern is considered to reflect healthy emotion regulation (Eisenberg *et al.*, 1996).

On the other side of the great empathy divide, cognitive empathy is tied to perspective taking. Sometimes called everyday mindreading or empathic accuracy (e.g. Ickes, 2003), this type of empathy requires guessing what another person is thinking or feeling. Cognitive empathy can get increasingly complex as the number of mental state inferences increases – e.g. 'She thinks that I think we're talking about how Susie quit her job, but I know that she's really upset about that disastrous incident at the club last night'. Although cognitive empathy ability can result in greater understanding and ultimately in helping other people (e.g. suggesting that a guest have a second helping when the host guesses that the guest is too polite to ask for more), there is no guarantee that 'empathic' accuracy might not be used for less charitable purposes (e.g. out-manoeuvring business rivals by guessing their game plan, or mortifying one's siblings by correctly guessing and then bringing up exactly the topic that is most embarrassing to them in front of their new date).

Such malevolent uses of empathic accuracy are rarely, if ever, considered 'empathy' in most everyday uses of the term. Outside of the laboratory, when we refer to someone who is empathic, we generally mean someone who both knows our thoughts and feelings, *and* cares about our well-being. In informal polls that we have conducted, asking people to name the most empathic person they know, mothers and best friends are most often nominated – these individuals not only have a proven record of concern about our well-being, but they also seem to know our thoughts and feelings without being explicitly told. Therapists, who are presumably also striving for this type of 'all-around' empathy, also seek to know what exactly is bothering us and then work to make it better.

However, just because both empathic concern and empathic accuracy must be present before we label someone 'empathic', this does not necessarily mean that they consistently co-occur. Although the majority of empathy researchers have chosen to focus on one aspect or the other, when both constructs are measured, they can clearly vary independently (Davis, 1983; Klein & Hodges, 2001). This suggests that the regulation of empathy may also be multifaceted, and that different strategies may be recruited for regulating the different components of empathy, and thus, in the next two sections, we will consider strategies for regulating emotional and cognitive empathy separately. However, in no way do we mean to imply that there is a split between affective and cognitive *systems* of the mind and body when either component of empathy is being regulated: emotional empathy may be regulated using cognitive strategies, and affectively charged motivators play a key role in regulating cognitive empathy.

21.3 Regulating emotional empathy

The empathic emotions, empathic concern and personal distress, are like other emotions in that they provide a signal that something needs to be attended to. Most emotions are like uninvited guests – sometimes good, often bad and only partially under our control. When we feel empathic concern for the shy kid in the kindergarten class, or personal distress while viewing the victim of a gruesome car crash, arousal of these feelings seems unintentional (e.g. see Malle & Knobe, 1997). Like other emotions, empathic concern and personal distress can be seen as serving a survival value as well (distress at a conspecific's unfortunate fate might prevent the self from suffering the same fate; concern over a kin member's fate may have prompted altruistic caring behaviours that helped save the kin member, and her related genes, or may have facilitated attachment between mother and child or romantic couples).

Like other emotions, empathic concern, and particularly personal distress, can be costly. The heightened bodily responses that accompany stressful emotions consume physiological resources at rates greater than baseline states and cannot be maintained healthily for extended periods of time (Selye, 1978). In the case of empathic emotions specifically, there are additional costs. The altruistic urges that accompany empathic concern can result in material or opportunity costs, as the empathic person may sacrifice some of his or her own resources to help another. Contemplating another's misfortune can be unpleasant (Schaller & Cialdini, 1988) and also may threaten cherished beliefs, such as the belief that the world is a safe and just place (Janoff-Bulman, 1989).

Because of these costs, generally when we talk about 'regulating emotions', it means dampening them; regulating rarely refers to amplifying a feeling. However, because the altruistic outcomes associated with empathic concern (e.g. Coke *et al.*, 1978) are widely valued, empathic concern is actually one emotion that is subject to amplification attempts. Broad categories of regulation strategies include suppression, reframing and exposure control. These strategies vary in the degree of effort involved.

Emotion suppression is an easily understood concept when applied to empathic emotion – just don't think about whatever is causing the empathic response (e.g. telling ourselves, 'Just don't think about the civilians in a war-torn city who have been injured or lost family members'). However, suppression requires a mental vigilance which may interfere with other cognitive processing (Richards & Gross, 2000) and may in fact backfire when performed under cognitive load (e.g. Wegner, 1994). Furthermore, suppression of emotions in general has recently been linked to a host of negative psychological and physical health outcomes (Butler *et al.*, 2003).

Reframing requires some cognitive effort at the front end, but may require less over time (and perhaps may even become automatic), if the 'reframer' is sufficiently convinced by his or her new story. Probably the most researched form of reframing used in regulating empathic emotions is perspective taking. Attempting to take another person's perspective generally results in increased empathic emotion. Asking perceivers to imagine things from the empathy target's point of view consistently increases empathic concern (Batson *et al.*, 1997a; Klein & Hodges, 2001; Stotland, 1969), and perhaps even more impressively, altruistic behaviour (e.g., Coke *et al.*, 1978). It is perhaps somewhat ironic that this cognitive strategy, the hallmark indicator of having achieved a Theory of Mind that is considered one of the milestones of cognitive development, consistently produces a change in affect. Of course, perspective taking produces cognitive changes too, such as increasing the degree to which representations of the self and the other overlap (e.g. Cialdini *et al.*, 1997; Davis *et al.*, 1996; Maner *et al.*, 2002).

When instructing someone to take someone else's perspective, subtle wording changes can alter the flavour of the resulting empathic emotion, specifically by affecting the mix of empathic concern and personal distress. For example, Batson *et al.* (1997a) found that when we are told of another person's plight and asked to imagine how that person feels, empathic concern is produced. However, if those instructions are varied slightly and we are asked to imagine instead how *we* would feel in the place of the other person, empathic concern is joined by personal distress. It is perhaps no accident that empathic therapists (e.g. see Rogers, 1951) are trained to restate the client's feelings from the client's perspective ('So, you're feeling betrayed by your mother's actions') rather than putting themselves in the place of the client (e.g. 'If my mother did that to me, I'd feel so betrayed!'). Such a perspective-taking strategy may keep feelings of personal distress at a minimum while still boosting empathic concern.

Other forms of reframing may be used to reduce, not increase, the intensity of empathic concern or personal distress. Just as increasing the overlap in representations of the self and other may be a key step in increasing empathic emotions, reframing strategies that help to distance the self from other people may serve to dampen empathic emotions. For example, strategies that decrease the extent to which the other person is seen as less like the self, or even inhuman, should increase the distance between the self and other. Soldiers who may initially be distressed at the idea of bombing towns, leaving hundreds to become homeless, injured and killed, are provided with the alternative frame to see these outcomes as 'collateral damage'. Derogating victims is another potential reframing strategy – referring to them with slurs may cause us to view them as worth less, and thus reduce their deservingness of our concern. We may also feel less empathic concern for people in need if we can view them as having contributed to their own bad fates (see Batson *et al.*, 1997b).

However, not all reframing strategies to reduce empathic concern are rooted in such aggressive goals: parents who would otherwise feel concern for a child who is scared of the dark still turn out the lights at bedtime. Although they normally would respond to their child's fears with behaviours designed to soothe them, not scare them, these well-intentioned parents presumably reframe 'lights out' as part of responsible parenting. Some creative reframing strategies are rooted in people's attempts to allow themselves to feel *some* empathic concern in situations where a seemingly infinite amount could be evoked. For example, while collecting anecdotes in preparation for writing this chapter, we heard about people with jobs in social service or mental health care, particularly those who might be overwhelmed by clients who evoke a great deal of empathic concern (e.g. a counsellor working with a heavy case load of child abuse victims or aids in an inpatient facility for the severely mentally ill). This potential overload sometimes led to adopting a sort of 'gallows' humour'. By using terminology for clients or procedures that mocked the seriousness of these cases, potentially counterproductive levels of emotional empathy might be defused.

More than one person we know deals with pleas from the homeless by giving money to the first person who asks for a handout each day, and then turning down all subsequent requests. We think this is a hybrid solution that blends the first two regulatory strategies. It involves reframing (seeing the contribution to the first person as being perhaps a self-imposed social service tax, in the same way that one pays money for schools or roads), plus a dose of suppression (ignoring all subsequent pleas). The combination restrains empathic concern (and the potential financial costs associated with empathic concern in this context).

The third regulatory strategy, exposure control, involves controlling exposure to factors that cause us to feel empathy. It can be used to both heighten and reduce emotional empathy. Exposure control is particularly effective for the latter (if we are never exposed to the empathy-inducing stimuli, we will not feel empathic emotions and will not have to worry about further regulation or efforts to restore ourselves to our pre-exposure states, which are often ineffective – see Wilson & Brekke, 1994). Thus, exposure control is probably the least effortful regulation strategy. However, it does require foresight, as well as meta-knowledge of the self to be effective: we have to turn the television off *before* we see the appeal to save starving children and we have to know our weakness for cute kittens well enough to stay out of homeless cat shelters.

Work by Shaw *et al.* (1994) demonstrates that people are capable of both the foresight and meta-knowledge necessary to effectively use exposure control as a means to control empathic emotion when they perceive that such emotions may cost them. In Shaw *et al.* 's study, college-aged participants were told they would hear an appeal for help from a homeless man, after which they would be given a chance to help the homeless. However, the type of help requested was varied: half the subjects heard about a low-cost form of help (addressing some letters for a few hours); the other half heard about a high-cost form of help (which entailed attending lengthy meetings over the course of several weeks). Participants were then given a choice between a high-impact appeal from the homeless man that would lead to an empathic appreciation of the man's needs, or a low-impact, objective description of his needs.

The study's results showed that when helping was costly, participants avoided choosing the high-impact appeal for help. In contrast, participants in the low-cost help condition were much less reluctant to expose themselves to the high-impact appeal, despite the fact that both groups of participants agreed at roughly equal rates that the high-impact appeal was likely to be more interesting. In sum, the study results suggest that when people think the cost of empathy will be too high, they practise exposure control, even if it means resisting their curiosity to see a compelling story.

Exposure control may be most associated with *reducing* feelings of empathic emotion, because it is such an effective strategy in this regard, but at least anecdotally, increasing one's exposure to certain stimuli can be used as a strategy to *boost* empathic concern. For example, in order to get in touch with the hardships experienced by his ancestors as they came over to the United States as slaves, Alex Haley spent time in a ship's hold (Haley, 1977). Holocaust museums and other educational memorials devoted to historically oppressed and persecuted groups serve a similar purpose on a societal level.

21.4 Regulating cognitive empathy

Whereas the majority of (but not all) attempts to regulate emotional empathy involve trying to dampen it, the majority of (but not all) attempts to regulate cognitive empathy involve trying to amplify it. Rarely are empathic accuracy levels perceived to be unpleasantly or dangerously high (e.g. when people say, 'I know just what you mean' it is generally with enthusiasm, not with trepidation). The few circumstances in which excessive cognitive empathy is problematic provide some interesting cases that we will consider at the end of this chapter, but, in general, suppression of cognitive empathy is rarely an issue. (There is evidence that people can successfully suppress taking someone else's perspective if asked to do so, as long as they have the cognitive capacity to do so, but the kinds of rebound effects and costs associated with suppressing empathic and other kinds of emotions don't seem to accompany the suppression of a cognitive perspective – see Hodges & Wegner, 1997.)

What about reframing and exposure control as cognitive regulation strategies? It could be argued that cognitive empathy is, itself, a reframing process through which individuals attempt to see the world as it is viewed and processed by another person. A case could be made for exposure control having a small role too: exposing oneself to the experiences, habits and culture of another person may facilitate taking that person's perspective accurately. Most students who do foreign exchange programmes take a big exposure control step that will affect their ability to understand people in another culture when they choose to study abroad. And just as lying in a ship's hold increased the emotions that Alex Haley felt *for* his ancestors (described above), it probably also increased his insights into what they were thinking and feeling during their heinous transport. If nothing else, the Haley example should remind us that emotional and cognitive empathy routinely (but do not always) co-occur in everyday human experiences.

There is a certain all-or-nothing quality to emotional empathy that does not apply to cognitive empathy: although we can feel more or less empathic concern or personal distress, there is a minimal threshold that must be crossed in order for us to note feeling anything at all. In contrast, when it comes to taking someone's perspective, there is a theoretical continuum of empathic accuracy all the way from zero (absolutely no idea what the other person is thinking or feeling) to some maximum bounded only by an asymptote associated with the 'other minds problem' (i.e. we can never really get into another person's head and know what he or she is thinking).

A variety of factors determine empathic accuracy, and several of these are beyond the control of the empathic perceiver. For example, some targets of empathic accuracy attempts are simply more transparent than others, making them easier to read accurately (e.g. Simpson *et al.*, 1995). In addition, individual differences in empathic accuracy (e.g. Marangoni *et al.*, 1995) may be the result of personality characteristics that are hard or even impossible to tinker with (but see also Ickes *et al.*, 2000). However, a big chunk of the variance in empathic accuracy performance can be regulated directly by how hard the empathic perceiver works at it. Thus, what most clearly categorizes attempts to use both reframing and exposure control towards a goal of cognitive empathy is the direct relationship between effort and success at this goal.

There's no two ways around it – trying to guess what someone else is thinking is hard and soaks up limited cognitive resources (Hodges & Wegner, 1997; Rossnagel, 2000; Sabbagh & Taylor, 2000). People's usual guesses about what another person is thinking in empathic accuracy studies are often far from the bull's eye (e.g. Klein & Hodges, 2001; Marangoni et al., 1995; Stinson & Ickes, 1992). At the same time, people's attempts at empathic accuracy yield a range of scores with a mean well above that which would be achieved by chance.

Because of the effort required to achieve cognitive empathy, motivation is key. Sometimes that motivation may stem from a simple interest in the target of empathy. For example, Ickes et al. (1990) found that college students performed better at reading the thoughts and feelings of strangers when those strangers were physically attractive. At other times, motivation may stem from the anticipation of rewards associated with accuracy. For example, the investor who can accurately guess a CEO's future plans may stand to win big if such empathic accuracy guides that investor to buy or sell at the right moment. When Klein and Hodges (2001) translated empathic accuracy performance into concrete monetary rewards by promising research participants greater payoffs for greater accuracy, these participants achieved significantly greater empathic accuracy than participants not promised monetary payoffs.

Although money may be a nearly universal motivator, it is important to remember that motivation occurs within a social context. Desire to behave in a manner consistent with gender roles may also motivate greater accuracy (Klein & Hodges, 2001). In Western culture at least, women are expected to be more empathic than men (Eisenberg & Lennon, 1983). Because empathy is a component of the female gender role, Klein and Hodges (2001) hypothesized that when the empathic nature of a task is highlighted, women, but not men, will be motivated to try harder. Consistent with their predictions, when participants were first asked how much empathic concern they felt for a target, prior to trying to guess what that target was thinking and feeling, women scored higher than men on empathic accuracy. When the empathic concern scale was given *after* measuring empathic accuracy, men's and women's empathic accuracy scores were comparable. (Interestingly, the monetary motivators described above overrode the manipulations designed to create sex differences in empathic accuracy!)

Although certain social roles appear to enhance empathic accuracy, conversely, there may be other roles or social situations that *dampen* the motivation to be accurate, or even lead people to be *inaccurate*. Simpson and Ickes (e.g. Simpson et al., 1995, 2003) have outlined a model of this kind of motivated empathic inaccuracy in the context of romantic relationships. When the empathic accuracy task involved asking heterosexual dating couples to guess how their partners felt about members of the opposite sex (a situation in which accuracy might reveal unpleasant information about their partners' interest in other people), the participants who showed the least accuracy were those whose relationship would be most threatened by their partners' potential interest in the other people: those whose partners were asked about very attractive opposite-sex people, those who reported greater interdependence with their partners, and those who reported higher levels of uncertainty about the future prospects of the relationship (Simpson *et al.*, 1995).

Later work by Simpson *et al.* (2003) shows that the intuitions of the couples about the costs of accuracy in the 1995 sample were correct. The 2003 study looked at married couples who were asked to infer their spouses' thoughts and feelings. When these thoughts and feelings were non-threatening to the relationship, greater empathic accuracy led to feelings of greater closeness. However, when the spouses were thinking thoughts that were threatening to the relationship, greater accuracy had its costs, leading to reduced feelings of closeness. Thus, just as in Shaw *et al.*'s (1994) study involving a homeless man, where research participants knew when empathic *concern* would cost them, Simpson *et al.*'s (1995) dating couples seemed to know when empathic *accuracy* would cost them. However, unlike Shaw *et al.*'s study, where participants took a fairly dramatic form of exposure control, Simpson *et al.*'s (1995) subjects seemed to 'blur' their exposure, rather than avoid it altogether.

The combined results of these two studies have led Simpson and Ickes to develop a model of regulating the costs of empathic accuracy in romantic relationships (Ickes *et al.*, 2005). According to this model, as long as a partner's potentially threatening thoughts are ambiguous, the other partner can go to the root of motivated inaccuracy. However, when the threatening thoughts are clearly unambiguous, the other partner is forced to see the truth and to pay a price for it in terms of relationship closeness; the cost of this truth varies according to just how threatening the thoughts are, how important the relationship is, and how much stress the relationship can withstand.

21.5 Shortcuts to cognitive empathy

One of the things that makes empathic accuracy so hard to achieve is that it is an idiosyncratic task – each target's thoughts are unique. However, there may be some similarity across targets with similar demographic or personality characteristics, or across targets who are in similar situations. Thus, just as humans are likely to develop heuristics and shortcuts in order to reduce the load associated with cognitively taxing tasks (Payne *et al.*, 1993), an empathic perceiver inferring another person's thoughts may use theories, stereotypes and schemas to help guess the content of those thoughts.

One highly accessible schema that is frequently employed in perspective taking is the self: often, our guesses about what other people are thinking are strongly influenced by what we ourselves are thinking (e.g. Hodges *et al.*, 2002; Krueger, 2002; Nickerson, 1999; Van Boven & Loewenstein, 2003). In the absence of other sources of information, this strategy is defensible (Dawes, 1990). However, projecting from the self is often misleading, because people do not take into account other relevant information about the target person, because they are unaware of biasing influences on their own state of mind (Van Boven & Loewenstein, 2003), or even because they make incorrect predictions about their own state of mind under similar circumstances and project these incorrect states on to others (Van Boven *et al.*, 2000). Furthermore, although there is a pervasive belief that having experienced a life event oneself will give one insight into another person's similar life experience, this belief may be unmerited (Hodges, 2005). Thus, seeking out similar experiences (a form of exposure control) as a means of increasing empathic accuracy may be of questionable worth.

Like other effortful tasks, there is also the potential for aspects of perspective taking to become automatic with repeated practice over time (e.g. see Dreyfus & Dreyfus, 1986). For example, Baldwin *et al.* (1990) found that subliminally priming participants with people who played a significant role in their lives resulted in those participants making judgements that appeared to be influenced by the significant others' opinions. It was as if the significant others' perspectives were being automatically consulted and integrated into the participants' judgements. Similarly, Taylor *et al.* (2003) found that fiction writers – who spend a lot of time imagining their fictional characters' point of view – often experienced a strange phenomenon whereby their characters seemed to come to life, providing dialogue and action for the story without any perceived effort on the part of the author.

21.6 The dark side of empathy ... the costs of poor regulation

We opened this chapter with examples demonstrating how much empathy is valued, but alluded to the idea that, desirable as it is, too much empathy can be costly. Now that we have summarized some of the known mechanisms of regulating both emotional and cognitive empathy, we will explore examples of regulation gone awry – problems with hitting the ideal level of empathy both due to undershooting (too little empathy) and overshooting (too much). Because of asymmetries in regulating emotional and cognitive empathy, regulatory problems are not evenly distributed across the two-by-two matrix that would be created by crossing

Table 21.1: Breakdown of regulatory problems by type of empathy

Regulatory problem	Type of empathy	
	Emotional Empathy	Cognitive Empathy
Undershooting	Callousness, insensitivity (fairly common)	Egocentrism (very common)
Overshooting	Personal distress (somewhat common)	Loss of self (somewhat rare)

'type of regulatory problem' (over/under shooting) with 'type of empathy' (cognitive/ emotional – see Table 21.1). Problems in regulating cognitive empathy most commonly arise from undershooting (too little cognitive empathy), whereas problems in regulating emotional empathy perhaps more often come from over-shooting (feeling too much emotional empathy), but also come from undershoot-ing. Regulatory problems can also emerge when learned or practised strategies that were potentially adaptive in one context are maladaptive in another context.

21.7 Undershooting emotional empathy

With empathy as a valued commodity, not demonstrating enough of it, especially not enough emotional empathy, can create serious problems. Several of the other chapters in this book address psychological disorders that result in such emotional empathy deficits. However, rather than focus on the plight of individuals whose capacity to feel empathy is damaged or even prevented by mental illness, we will instead present an example of what happens when someone with a normal empathic capacity for empathy adapts to an abnormal environment. Lt. Col. Dave Grossman's landmark book, *On Killing* (1995), explores the psychological process that humans go through when killing – and in particular, shooting – another human being. Grossman's main focus is soldiers, and, among other things, he points to an interesting historical shift in the number of soldiers who successfully fire their guns and actual kill enemy soldiers. For example, estimates of the percentage of soldiers not firing their guns in World War II are around 75–80%, whereas estimates are about 5% in the Vietnam War. Why the difference?

Grossman systematically enumerates the changes in armies and training (among other factors) that he thinks have made the difference: weapon innovations that allowed soldiers to hit their targets without being able to see distinctive (and humanizing) features of their targets; classical conditioning (including the use of more lifelike targets in target practice, so that soldiers practise hitting a human-like figure, rather than an abstract bull's eye); and the use of euphemistic terms for the act of killing (such as 'engaging the target'). Essentially, much of this training constitutes the reframing strategy discussed earlier as a strategy for reducing empathic concern. (Aspects of this training have been perhaps unintentionally integrated into many young peoples' 'education' as well, as it has been found that violent video games may provide similar desensitization – Funk *et al.*, 2003.)

The increased shoot percentages and kill numbers from army statistics suggest that the military training is an effective strategy for overcoming natural tendencies to feel concern for the enemy. Alas, the training is perhaps *too* effective in destroying any kind of concern for those who may be seen as enemies, as behaviour by American soldiers at the Abu Ghraib prison in Iraq and numerous other examples of wartime atrocities suggest. The reframing also appears to have a limited shelf life, working effectively only in the context that supports it (e.g. a combat situation). When restored to 'normal' human environments, which generally discourage killing others, soldiers who killed others at close range in battle tend to suffer more severe post-war distress than those who either did not kill, or killed from a distance (Grossman, 1995).

Suppression of emotional concern may also lead to long-term problems, particularly for groups of people whose jobs or lives entail spending a lot of time working with others who evoke empathic concern (e.g. medical personnel on intensive care units, counsellors of abuse victims, teachers of severely disabled children). In the short term, additional resources can be mobilized to regulate the response to an emotion trigger, such as suppressing thoughts about burn or incest victims. However, the circumstances that shaped the evolution of emotions as an adaptive response have created optimal operation among humans encountering the occasional other person in distress, not among modern-day care providers whose whole days are filled with interactions with such individuals. Eventually, the strain on caregivers can take the form of 'compassion fatigue', – the term given to the experience of therapists who get burned out from constant work with clients undergoing distressing experiences (Figley, 2002). We suspect that caregivers are particularly susceptible to 'compassion fatigue' when other routes to regulation are blocked – when, for example, work pressures require few breaks from victims (which would provide relief in the form of exposure control), or when reframing is difficult (for example, when the prospect of the victims making any progress is dim, or when the caregivers are unable to see their work as having any impact or meaning). This view is supported by empirical models of burnout among social service workers (Miller *et al.*, 1995).

A special group of people who might experience unique problems undershooting the ideal level of empathic concern are those who regularly interact with others who are likely to evoke sympathy for the purpose of exploiting it. Parole officers, guards (military or civilian) and therapists who work with sociopaths fall into this category. Becoming too empathically concerned (and the accompanying desire to help that accompanies empathic concern) could quite literally be a matter of life and death for these people, which suggests that they may learn to set the default level of empathic concern quite low. Furthermore, their tendency to feel empathic concern may be generally dampened due to the fact that they encounter a much higher base rate of people who seem unworthy of empathic concern (i.e. these individuals develop a more cynical view of humanity). Together, these biases may also explain why abuses of power are closely associated with some of these positions (again, consider the Abu Ghraib scandal in Iraq).

21.8 Overshooting emotional empathy

Personal distress is one outcome that occurs when people fail to rein in emotional empathy. This 'evil twin' emotion often accompanies empathic concern, but focuses more on the perceiver's own feelings of distress while encountering another person, rather than feeling *for* the other person. The quintessential example of this phenomenon is the bystander who witnesses a gruesome accident and can only stand by, gasping and shrieking, rather than comforting the victim or going for help. Merely ramping up levels of empathic concern will not necessarily kick perceivers into the reaches of personal distress, but psychologists have suggested that the development of emotional regulatory processes is what allows humans to feel empathic concern (which is associated with desirable pro-social behaviours) instead of just personal distress (Hoffman, 1984; Zahn-Waxler *et al.*, 1992).

21.9 Undershooting cognitive empathy

A cynical, but not entirely inaccurate view of human nature would posit that humans' tendency toward egocentrism causes us to *consistently* undershoot cognitive empathy. Widespread and well-documented examples of human egocentrism abound (see Nickerson, 1999). Performance on simple perspective-taking tasks (Keysar *et al.*, 1998) can be embarrassingly poor. However, to be fair, at least part of the problem is not regulatory in nature, but simply due to limits on ability and mental capacity. (As an analogy, if the average woman were trying to outrun Olympic sprinter Gail Devers and lost, we would be unlikely to chalk the loss up to regulatory problems!)

Just because studies have demonstrated that cognitive empathy (when measured in the form of empathic accuracy) increases in the presence of motivators (Klein & Hodges, 2001), these results do not necessarily imply poor regulation of cognitive empathy. They may instead reflect a well-calibrated optimizer that expends effort only to the degree that it is worth it. Even if we can bring to mind a few spectacular interpersonal disasters brought about by the failure to take another person's perspective, it is still unclear whether routinely exerting greater effort would pay off, even if it did allow us to avoid the rare egocentric incidents that were truly damaging. In order to find an example of a true regulatory 'error' in undershooting cognitive empathy, it would be necessary to demonstrate that the advantages of greater empathic accuracy outweighed the costs of expending greater cognitive effort. All this said, there are clearly times when abandoning our egocentrism would not only be fairly easy, but also to our advantage, and yet we still seem reluctant to do so.

21.10 Overshooting cognitive empathy

Greater cognitive empathy generally requires greater effort, therefore regulatory problems that result in cognitive empathy levels that are higher than ideal may seem counterintuitive, but such instances can occur. One possible route to cognitive over-empathizing may be through practice: perspective taking might be like other processes that are controlled at first and become automatic. For example, learning to knit or play a musical instrument requires a great deal of concentration at first, but with time, aspects of these activities can become so automatic that they can be done while simultaneously performing other activities (Bargh, 1989; Dreyfus & Dreyfus, 1986).

If (as we cynically suggested earlier) humans' egocentrism is a potential design flaw, then it may be hard to see the development of automatic perspective taking as leading to an 'overshoot' in cognitive empathy. Instead, it might be perceived as leading to more *optimal* levels of perspective taking. Indeed, we would like to go down on record as saying that routinely considering other people's points of view would generally provide a huge benefit to humanity. However, under some circumstances, particularly in close relationships, automatically taking the other person's perspective may come at the expense of the self. For example, Dana Jack (1987) describes the phenomenon of 'silencing the self', which is noted as being particularly prevalent in women who are mothers and wives. Attempts to satisfy others' desires take the forefront, while self needs go unmet (hence, the self is 'silenced').

Another example of potentially overshooting cognitive empathy is when people (often women) in abusive relationships devote a great deal of time and effort to figuring out what will trigger their partner's rage and working to prevent it. Rather than recognizing that the more effective strategy would be to exit or change the relationship, these individuals instead try to adopt a destructive perspective within it. Both of the previous examples suggest that women may be disproportionately likely to experience cognitive empathy overshoots, raising an interesting issue for future research.

21.11 Closing thoughts

We hope this chapter challenges the notion that more empathy is always good, while at the same time acknowledging that more empathy is *often* good. We have presented general strategies humans use for regulating both cognitive and emotional empathy, and discussed the merits and weaknesses of suppression, reframing and exposure control. We have tried to 'bring to life' instances where one or the other broad categories of empathy (cognitive or emotional) shows evidence of poor regulation – resulting in empathy levels that are either greater or less than ideal in a particular set of circumstances.

In closing, we hope that we have demonstrated the remarkable flexibility and creativity present in the specific techniques that humans use for regulating empathy. Some of these strategies are intentional; others occur without us consciously monitoring or adjusting our empathy levels. Some strategies are used routinely, every day or even every hour; others get called into play only to deal with special occasions. We concede that there may be several strategies not covered this chapter, and that these strategies may fail to fit neatly into the taxonomy we have presented. We welcome these challenging cases as providing possible future directions for studying the regulation of empathy, and ultimately how the effective regulation of empathy translates into changes in human behaviour and interactions. Like fire, empathy is a powerful and valuable tool available to our species, made infinitely more useful when we know how to manage it.

Acknowledgements

The authors wish to thank Mike Myers for his helpful comments on a draft of the chapter. They would also like to thank Devika Bakshai and Josie Casey Witte for sharing their creative ideas about concepts discussed in this chapter.

REFERENCES

Baldwin, M. W., Carrell, S. E., & Lopez, D. E. (1990). Priming relationship schemas: my advisor and the pope are watching me from the back of my mind. *Journal of Experimental Social Psychology*, **26**, 435–454.

Bargh, J. A. (1989). Conditional automaticity: varieties of automatic influence in social perception and cognition. In J. S. Uleman, & J. A. Bargh (eds.), *Unintended Thought* (pp. 3–51). New York: Guilford Press.

Batson, C. D., Early, S., & Salvarani, G. (1997a). Perspective taking: imagining how another feels versus imagining how you would feel. *Personality and Social Psychology Bulletin*, **23**, 751–758.

Batson, D. C., Polycarpou, M. P., Harmon-Jones, E., *et al.* (1997b). Empathy and attitudes: can feeling for a member of a stigmatized group improve feelings toward the group? *Journal of Personality and Social Psychology*, **72**, 105–118.

Butler, E. A., Egloff, B., Wilhelm, F. H., Smith, N. C., Erickson, E. A., & Gross, J. J. (2003). The social consequences of expressive suppression. *Emotion*, **3**, 48–67.

Chlopan, B. E., McCain, M. L., Carbonell, J. L., & Hagen, R. L. (1985). Empathy: review of available measures. *Journal of Personality and Social Psychology*, **48**, 635–653.

Cialdini, R. B., Brown, S. L., Lewis, B. P., Luce, C., & Neuberg, S. L. (1997). Reinterpreting the empathy-altruism relationship: when one into one equals oneness. *Journal of Personality and Social Psychology*, **73**, 481–494.

Coke, J. S., Batson, C. D., & McDavis, K. (1978). Empathic mediation of helping: a two-stage model. *Journal of Personality and Social Psychology*, **36**, 752–766.

Davis, M. H. (1983). Measuring individual differences in empathy: evidence for a multidimensional approach. *Journal of Personality and Social Psychology*, **44**, 113–126.

Davis, M. H., Conklin, L., Smith, A., & Luce, C. (1996). Effect of perspective taking on the cognitive representations of persons: a merging of self and other. *Journal of Personality and Social Psychology*, **70**, 713–726.

Dawes, R. M. (1990). The potential nonfalsity of the false consensus effect. In R. M. Hogarth (ed.), *Insights in Decision Making: A Tribute to Hillel J. Einhorn* (pp. 179–199). Chicago, Ill.: University of Chicago Press.

Dreyfus, H. L., & Dreyfus, S. E. (1986). *Mind over Machine*. New York: The Free Press.

Eisenberg, N., & Fabes, R. A. (1995). The relation of young children's vicarious emotional responding to social competence, regulation, and emotionality. *Cognition and Emotion*, **9**, 203–228.

Eisenberg, N., Fabes, R. A., Murphy, B., *et al.* (1996). The relations of children's dispositional empathy-related responding to their emotionality, regulation, and social functioning. *Developmental Psychology*, **32**, 195–209.

Eisenberg, N., & Lennon, R. (1983). Sex differences in empathy and related capacities. *Psychological Bulletin*, **94**, 100–131.

Eisenberg, N., Wentzel, M., & Harris, J. D. (1998). The role of emotionality and regulation in empathy-related responding. *School Psychology Review*, **27**, 505–521.

Figley, C. R. (2002). Compassion fatigue: psychotherapists' chronic lack of self-care. *Journal of Clinical Psychology*, **58**, 1433–1441.

Funk, J. B., Buchman, D. D., Jenks, J., & Bechtoldt, H. (2003). Playing violent video games, desensitization, and moral evaluation in children. *Journal of Applied Developmental Psychology*, **4**, 413–436.

Grossman, D. (1995). *On Killing*. Boston, Mass.: Little, Brown and Company.

Haley, A. (1977). *The Search for Roots*. [Video recording]. Princeton, N. J.: Films for the humanities.

Hatfield, E., Cacioppo, J. T., & Rapson, R. L. (1993). Emotional contagion. *Current Directions in Psychological Science*, **2**, 96–99.

Hodges, S. D. (2005). Is how much you understand me in your head or mine? In B. F. Malle, & S. D. Hodges (eds.), *Other Minds*. New York: Guilford Press.

Hodges, S. D., Johnsen, A. T., & Scott, N. S. (2002). You're like me, no matter what you say: self projection in self-other comparisons. *Psychologica Belgica*, **42**, 107–112.

Hodges, S. D., & Wegner, D. M. (1997). The mental control of empathic accuracy. In W. Ickes (ed.), *Empathic Accuracy* (pp. 311–339). New York: Guilford.

Hoffman, M. L. (1984). Interaction of affect and cognition in empathy. In C. E. Izard, J. Kagan, & R. B. Zajonc (eds.), *Emotions, Cognition, and Behavior* (pp. 103–131). Cambridge: Cambridge University Press.

Hogan, R. (1969). Development of an empathy scale. *Journal of Consulting and Clinical Psychology*, **33**, 307–316.

Jack, D. (1987). Silencing the self: the power of social imperatives in female depression. In R. Formanek, & A. Gurian (eds.), *Women and Depression: A Lifespan Perspective* (pp. 161–181). New York: Springer Publishing Company.

Ickes, W. (2003). *Everyday Mind Reading*. Amherst, N. Y.: Prometheus Books.

Ickes, W., Buysse, A., Pham, H., *et al.* (2000). On the difficulty in distinguishing 'good' and 'poor' perceivers: a social relations model of empathic accuracy data. *Personal Relationships*, **7**, 219–234.

Ickes, W., Simpson, J. A., & Oriña, M. M. (2005). Empathic accuracy and inaccuracy in close relationships. In B. F. Malle, & S. D. Hodges (eds.), *Other Minds*. New York: Guilford Press.

Ickes, W., Stinson, L., Bissonnette, V., & Garcia, S. (1990). Naturalistic social cognition: empathic accuracy in mixed-sex dyads. *Journal of Personality and Social Psychology*, **59**, 730–742.

Janoff-Bulman, R. (1989). Assumptive worlds and the stress of traumatic events: applications of the schema construct. *Social Cognition*, **7**, 113–136.

Keysar, B., Barr, D. J., & Horton, W. S. (1998). The egocentric basis of language use: insights from a processing approach. *Current Directions in Psychological Science*, **7**, 46–50.

Klein, K. J. K., & Hodges, S. D. (2001). Gender differences, motivation and empathic accuracy: when it pays to understand. *Personality and Social Psychology Bulletin*, **27**, 720–730.

Krueger, J. I. (2002). On the reduction of self-other asymmetries: benefits, pitfalls, and other correlates of social projection. *Psychologica Belgica*, **42**, 23–41.

Malle, B. F., & Knobe, J. (1997). The folk concept of intentionality. *Journal of Experimental Social Psychology*, **33**, 101–121.

Maner, J. K., Luce, C. L., Neuberg, S. L., *et al.* (2002). The effects of perspective taking on motivations for helping: still no evidence for altruism. *Personality and Social Psychology Bulletin*, **28**, 1601–1610.

Marangoni, C., Garcia, S., Ickes, W., & Teng, G. (1995). Empathic accuracy in a clinically relevant setting. *Journal of Personality and Social Psychology*, **68**, 854–869.

Meltzoff, A. N., & Moore, M. K. (1983). Newborn infants imitate adult facial gestures. *Child Development*, **54**, 702–709.

Miller, K., Birkholt, M., Scott, C., & Stage, C. (1995). Empathy and burnout in human service work: an extension of a communication model. *Communication Research*, **22**, 123–147.

Nickerson, R. S. (1999). How we know – and sometimes misjudge – what others know: imputing one's own knowledge to others. *Psychological Bulletin*, **125**, 737–759.

Norman, W. T. (1967). 2800 personality trait descriptors: normative operating characteristics for a university population. Unpublished Technical Report, Department of Psychology, University of Michigan, Ann Arbor, Mich.

Payne, J. W., Bettman, J. R., & Johnson, E. J. (1993). *The Adaptive Decision Maker*. Cambridge: Cambridge University Press.

Pithers, W. D. (1994). Process evaluation of a group therapy component designed to enhance sex offenders' empathy for abuse survivors. *Behavior Research and Therapy*, **32**, 565–570.

Richards, J. M., & Gross, J. J. (2000). Emotion regulation and memory: the cognitive costs of keeping one's cool. *Journal of Personality and Social Psychology*, **79**, 410–424.

Rizzolatti, G., Fadiga, L., Fogassi, L., & Gallese, V. (2002). From mirror neurons to imitation: facts and speculations. In A. N. Meltzoff, & W. Prinz (eds.), *The Imitative Mind: Development, Evolution, and Brain Bases* (pp. 247–266). New York: Cambridge University Press.

Rogers, C. R. (1951). *Client Centered Therapy*. Boston, Mass.: Houghton Mifflin.

Rossnagel, C. (2000). Cognitive load and perspective-taking: applying the automatic-controlled distinction to verbal communication. *European Journal of Social Psychology*, **30**, 429–445.

Sabbagh, M., & Taylor, M. (2000). Neural correlates of 'theory of mind' reasoning: an event-related potential study. *Psychological Science*, **11**, 46–50.

Schaller, M., & Cialdini, R. B. (1988). The economics of helping: support for a mood management motive. *Journal of Experimental Social Psychology*, **24**, 163–181.

Selye, H. (1978). *The Stress of Life*. New York: McGraw Hill.

Shaw, L. L., Batson, C. D., & Todd, R. M. (1994). Empathy avoidance: forestalling feeling for another in order to escape the motivational consequences. *Journal of Personality and Social Psychology*, **67**, 879–887.

Simpson, J. A., Ickes, W., & Blackstone, T. (1995). When the head protects the heart: empathic accuracy in dating relationships. *Journal of Personality and Social Psychology*, **69**, 629–641.

Simpson, J. A., Oriña, M. M., & Ickes, W. (2003). When accuracy hurts, and when it helps: a test of the empathic accuracy model in marital interactions. *Journal of Personality and Social Psychology*, **85**, 881–893.

Stinson, L., & Ickes, W. (1992). Empathic accuracy in the interactions of male friends versus male strangers. *Journal of Personality and Social Psychology*, **62**, 787–797.

Stotland, E. (1969). Exploratory investigations in empathy. In L. Berkowitz (ed.), *Advances in Experimental Social Psychology* (Vol. 4) (pp. 271–314). New York: Academic Press.

Taylor, M., Hodges, S. D., & Kohányi, A. (2003). The illusion of independent agency: do adult fiction writers experiences their characters as having minds of their own? *Imagination, Cognition, and Personality*, **22**, 361–380.

Van Boven, L., Dunning, D., & Loewenstein, G. (2000). Egocentric empathy gaps between owners and buyers: misperceptions of the endowment effect. *Journal of Personality & Social Psychology*, **79**, 66–76.

Van Boven, L., & Loewenstein, G. (2003). Social projection of transient drive states. *Personality and Social Psychology Bulletin*, **29**, 1159–1168.

Wegner, D. M. (1994). Ironic processes of mental control. *Psychological Review*, **101**, 34–52.

Wilson, T. D., & Brekke, N. (1994). Mental contamination and mental correction: unwanted influences on judgments and evaluations. *Psychological Bulletin*, **116**, 117–142.

Zahn-Waxler, C., Radke-Yarrow, M., Wagner, E., & Chapman, M. (1992). Development of concern for others. *Developmental Psychology*, **28**, 126–136.

Empathic accuracy: measurement and potential clinical applications

Marianne Schmid Mast[1] and William Ickes[2]

[1]Social and Health Psychology, University of Zurich
[2]Department of Psychology, University of Texas at Arlington

22.1 Introduction

Empathic inference is the 'everyday mind reading' that people do whenever they attempt to infer other people's thoughts and feelings. *Empathic accuracy* is the extent to which such everyday mind reading attempts are successful (Ickes, 1997, 2003). To put it simply, empathically accurate perceivers are those who are good at 'reading' other people's thoughts and feelings.

Empathic accuracy is a quintessential (indeed, perhaps *the* quintessential) aspect of emotional intelligence (Goleman, 1995; Ickes, 1997, 2003; Salovey & Mayer, 1989). The ability to accurately 'read' other people's thoughts and feelings is a fundamental skill that affects people's social adjustment in many different domains of their lives (Goleman, 1995). For example, Crosby (2002) found that mothers who were more accurate in inferring their own child's thoughts and feelings had children with more positive self-concepts as family members. And with regard to people's dating and marriage relationships, Simpson *et al.* (2001) found evidence that accurately 'reading' your partner in order to anticipate a need, avert a conflict, or keep a small problem from escalating into a large one is likely to be healthy and adaptive (Ickes *et al.*, 2005; Simpson *et al.*, 2001, 2003).

Empathic accuracy is a subarea of interpersonal perception research – a field of study that has a long tradition in psychology (Heider, 1944; Taft, 1955). In the early days of its study, researchers tended to focus on bias, error and inaccurate person perception rather than on accuracy. But even the earliest work in this area received a very tough critical appraisal. Most notably, Cronbach (1955) published an influential article detailing the various measurement artefacts that could compromise researchers' efforts to assess the accurate social perception of others.

Empathy in Mental Illness, eds. Tom F. D. Farrow and Peter W. R. Woodruff. Published by Cambridge University Press. © Cambridge University Press 2007.

This article had the unfortunate effect of initiating an immediate and precipitous decline in the study of accurate person perception. To make matters worse, the early research in this area often yielded disappointing or inconsistent results (Funder 1995; Funder & West, 1993).

For both of these reasons, the research on accuracy in person perception lay dormant for most of the next three decades. Fortunately, however, a renewed interest in the topic arose during the l980s and has gathered strength since then (for an overview, see Hall & Bernieri, 2001). This interest is probably due in part to the transition within the field of psychology from a focus on pathology to a focus on positive psychology (Seligman & Csikszentmihalyi, 2000), in which the concept of empathy has come to play a central role.

As a broad generalization, it can be argued that interpersonal perception research began with the study of accuracy regarding stable and enduring dispositions and then gradually turned to the study of accuracy regarding more unstable and transient dispositions. The first and longest-studied area within the accuracy tradition focuses on perceivers' accuracy in judging other people's personality traits (e.g. Asch, 1946; Cronbach, 1955; Funder & Colvin, 1988; McCrae, 1982). The second and next longest studied area focuses on dyad members' accurate perceptions or understanding of each other's attitudes, values and self-conceptions (e.g. Knudson *et al.*, 1980; Laing *et al.*, 1966; Rogers & Dymond, 1954). The third and more recent area focuses on perceivers' affective sensitivity in inferring the emotional state(s) of one or more target persons (e.g. Costanzo & Archer, 1989; Ekman & Friesen, 1975; Hall, 1984; Noller, 1980, 1981; Rosenthal *et al.*, 1979). The fourth and most recent area concerns perceivers' empathic accuracy – the focus of the present chapter (e.g. Ickes, 1997, 2003; Ickes *et al.*, 1990b; Levenson & Ruef, 1992; Marangoni *et al.*, 1995; Simpson *et al.*, 1995; Stinson & Ickes, 1992).

22.2 Assessment: the empathic accuracy paradigm

The essential feature of the empathic accuracy paradigm is that a perceiver infers a target person's thoughts or feelings from either a videotaped record of their spontaneous interaction together (the *unstructured dyadic interaction paradigm*; Ickes & Tooke, 1988; Ickes *et al.*, 1990a; Stinson & Ickes, 1992) or a standard set of videotaped interactions of multiple targets (the *standard stimulus paradigm*, Gesn & Ickes, 1999; Marangoni *et al.*, 1995). In each case, the target individuals have previously reported the actual thoughts and feelings they had at specific points during the videotaped interaction, thereby enabling the researcher to compare the perceiver's inferred thoughts and feelings with the target person's actual thoughts and feelings in order to assess the perceiver's empathic accuracy.

22.2.1 The unstructured dyadic interaction paradigm

The dyadic interaction paradigm is used in studies of dyad members' ability to infer the specific content of each other's thoughts and feelings during a brief, unstructured interaction period. A typical dyadic interaction study begins when the participants have been recruited for a given session. The experimenter escorts the two participants into the observation room and asks them to take a seat on a couch. The room is equipped with a concealed wireless microphone, and a video camera is also concealed in a way that enables the dyad members' interaction to be unobtrusively videotaped.

Once both participants have been seated in the observation room, the experimenter 'discovers' a reason for having to run a quick errand (either to retrieve additional consent forms or to replace a slide projector bulb that has apparently just burned out), and leaves the participants alone together. At that point, a research assistant in the control room activates the video equipment to begin taping the dyad members' unstructured interaction. Exactly 6 min later, at the end of the observation period, the experimenter returns to the observation room and the videotaping is terminated.

After probing for any evidence of suspicion, the experimenter conducts a partial debriefing. The participants are told that they have been videotaped for the purpose of studying their naturally occurring interaction behaviour. If either one or both of the participants object to having been videotaped without their permission, they may exercise their right to have the tape erased immediately. If both participants agree to release their taped interaction as a source of data, they are asked to read and sign a consent form indicating their willingness to do so.

In the next phase of the experiment, the participants are asked to view the tape of the interaction in which they have just participated and provide written records of their own thoughts and feelings during the interaction. To accomplish this task, the participants are seated in separate but identical cubicles where they each view a separate copy of the videotape. They are asked to report all of the thoughts and feelings they distinctly remember having had during the interaction, but *not* to report any thoughts or feelings that they experience for the first time while viewing the videotape. The participants view the entire interaction and stop the tape at each of those points at which they distinctly remember having had a specific thought or feeling. At each of these 'tape stops', the participants use a coding form to record: (1) the time the thought or feeling occurred (available from a time-counter overlay that is superimposed on the video image), (2) whether they were experiencing a thought or a feeling at that time, and (3) the specific content of the thought or feeling, expressed in sentence form. This procedure is repeated until both dyad members have independently recorded all of their actual thoughts and feelings during the videotaped interaction sequence.

The participants are then asked to view the tape a second time, this time for the purpose of inferring the specific thoughts and feelings that their interaction partner reported having had at each of his or her tape stops. The research assistant who is seated in the control room pauses the tape at each of the times the participant's interaction partner reported having had a specific thought or feeling (i.e. each perceiver has a different set of tape stops that occur at the times when that perceiver's partner reported having had a specific thought or feeling). The participants write down their thought/feeling inferences at each of these tape stops.

22.2.2 The standard stimulus paradigm

The prototype of the standard stimulus paradigm was developed by Marangoni *et al.* (1995). These investigators studied empathic accuracy in a clinically relevant setting. In separate videotaped therapy sessions, three female clients discussed a genuine personal problem with a male, client-centred therapist. Each client knew beforehand that her therapy session would be videotaped for use in future research, and had signed a consent form granting her permission for the tape to be used for this purpose. Though simulated for research purposes, the psycho-therapy sessions were videotaped 'live' without any rehearsal, and the genuineness and spontaneity of the sessions were evident in the clients' range of emotional expressions.

Immediately after their respective sessions with the therapist were completed, each client was debriefed and asked to sign a second consent form indicating her willingness to participate in an assessment of the specific thoughts and feelings she had experienced during the videotaped session. She was then seated in a cubicle, where she made a complete, video-cued record of all her thoughts and feelings during the interaction using the same thought/feeling assessment procedure described above. Edited versions of these three psychotherapy tapes were later used as 'standard stimulus tapes' that naive participants viewed for the purpose of attempting to infer the actual thoughts and feelings reported by each of the client target persons.

Other kinds of standard stimulus tapes have been developed as well. For example, in a study investigating how different levels of power affect empathic accuracy, Schmid Mast *et al.* (2006) used videotaped competitive interactions between strangers as their standard stimulus tapes. But this is only one of many possible examples. Videotapes of the unstructured interactions of strangers, friends, dating partners, marriage partners, parent–child, teacher–student, supervisor–employee, salesperson–customer pairs, etc., could all be used as the standard stimuli, depending on the goals of the particular research project in which the tapes are presented.

22.2.3 Obtaining a measure of empathic accuracy

To obtain a measure of empathic accuracy, we need to assess the degree to which the content of each of the perceiver's empathic inferences matches the content of the corresponding thought or feeling that the target person actually reported. This is done by having independent raters make subjective judgements about the similarity between the content of each *actual* thought or feeling and the content of the corresponding *inferred* thought or feeling (Ickes & Trued, 1985; Ickes *et al.*, 1990a). The raters' task is to compare each inferred thought or feeling with the actual thought or feeling and to judge how similar they are on a scale from 0 to 2. A rating of 0 is assigned if there is no apparent similarity in the content of the inferred thought/feeling compared to the actual thought/feeling; a rating of 2 is assigned if the same content is evident (though paraphrased or expressed in different words); and a score of 1 is assigned to all of the 'grey area' cases in between.

For each inference, the similarity ratings of all of the independent raters are averaged. In a next step, those averaged ratings are summed up across all inferences to compute the 'total accuracy points' earned by each perceiver. It is important to recognize that the 'total accuracy points' will be greater for perceivers who make many inferences than for those who make few inferences. Therefore, each perceiver's 'total accuracy points' is divided by the maximum number of possible accuracy points (number of inferences times the maximum score per inference) and multiplied by 100 to obtain a percent-correct empathic accuracy measure that has a potential range of 0 to 100. This percentage measure of empathic accuracy is conveniently scaled, easy to interpret and corrects reasonably well for differences in the total number of inferences made.

22.2.4 Reliability

Since several raters assess the degree of similarity between the perceiver's empathic inferences and the corresponding thoughts or feelings that the target person actually reported, one can assess *interrater reliability*. Interrater reliability in empathic accuracy studies has consistently been quite high (Cronbach's alpha), ranging from a low of 0.85 in a study in which only four raters were used to a high of 0.98 in two studies in which either seven or eight raters were used. Across all of the studies conducted to date, the average interrater reliability has been about 0.90 (Ickes, 2001).

A second way to assess the reliability of the empathic accuracy measure is in terms of *cross-target consistency*. This aspect of the measure's reliability is applicable only in the standard stimulus paradigm – that is, only in designs in which individual perceivers infer the thoughts and feelings of the same set of multiple target persons. Cross-target consistency in the first standard stimulus study conducted by Marangoni *et al.* (1995) was 0.86 (Cronbach's alpha) across the three target tapes used. In a more recent study using highly edited versions of the same three tapes, Gesn and Ickes (1999) reported an alpha of 0.91. These high alpha values might be partly attributable to homogeneity in the set of target persons (all three were middle-class, college-educated, Anglo-American women) and in the problems they discussed (marital relationship issues). Still, the data are compelling in their implication that the empathic accuracy measure reflects a stable and reliably assessed social skill that perceivers can apply to different target persons with a striking degree of cross-target consistency (Gesn & Ickes, 1999).

22.2.5 Validity

A number of *predictive validity* studies have been conducted to date. One of the first predictions tested was straightforward and commonsensical: if the procedure for assessing empathic accuracy was indeed valid, close friends should display higher levels of accuracy than strangers when inferring the content of each other's thoughts and feelings. This prediction was confirmed in studies by Stinson and Ickes (1992) and Graham (1994), which revealed that, on average, the empathic accuracy scores of close, same-sex friends were about 50% higher than those of same-sex strangers – a statistically significant difference in both studies.

In the clinically relevant study conducted by Marangoni *et al.* (1995), the predictive validity of the empathic accuracy measure was further tested with respect to two hypotheses. First, perceivers' empathic scores should be significantly greater at the end of the psychotherapy tapes than at the beginning, reflecting their greater acquaintance with the clients and their problems. Second, perceivers who receive immediate feedback about the clients' actual thoughts and feelings during the middle portion of each tape should subsequently achieve better empathic accuracy scores by the end of the tape than perceivers who do not receive such feedback. Statistically significant support for both of these hypotheses was obtained.

Establishing the *convergent and discriminant validity* of the empathic accuracy measure has proven to be more difficult and complicated. Davis and Kraus (1997) found that self-report measures of empathically relevant dispositions generally fail to predict performance on interpersonal accuracy/sensitivity tests, suggesting that it might be difficult to find self-report measures that reliably correlate with the performance measure of empathic accuracy. Similarly, Mortimer (1996) failed to find a predicted relationship between participants' scores on a cross-target measure of empathic accuracy [based on the Marangoni *et al.* (1995) tapes] and their scores on Costanzo and Archer's (1989) interpersonal perception task – the interpersonal sensitivity measure that (superficially, at least) most resembles the empathic accuracy measure in its stimulus materials and available channels of information. The correlation that Mortimer (1996) obtained was not significantly different from zero ($r = 0.06$).

This null result is similar to that reported by other investigators who have attempted to correlate different performance measures of interpersonal sensitivity with each other (Hall, 2001). The explanation for these null findings is not yet clear. It is possible that different types of interpersonal sensitivity exist that are not necessarily related to each other. At any rate, if the convergent validity of such measures cannot be established with respect to either conceptually relevant self-report measures or conceptually relevant performance-based measures, then establishing the discriminant validity of such measures becomes equally problematic, and other validity criteria (in particular, predictive validity) must be relied upon instead.

22.3 Clinical implications of empathic accuracy research

Writing nearly 50 years ago, Carl Rogers identified *accurate empathy* as one of the three 'necessary and sufficient facilitative core conditions' for therapeutic change – the other two conditions being the therapist's genuineness and non-judgemental caring for the client. The available research findings support the belief of clinical researchers and practitioners by showing that client perceptions of the therapist's empathy play an important role in successful psychotherapy outcomes (Greenberg *et al.*, 2001). However, appearing empathic is one thing and being empathically accurate is quite another. It is important to know whether the actual empathic accuracy of clinicians and counsellors is related to successful therapy outcomes. It is also important to know what practical implications the research on empathic accuracy might have for improving the performance of psychotherapists.

As Ickes (2003) has suggested, the most general implications involve ways to improve the selection and training of psychotherapists. More specific implications concern the kinds of cues that therapists should attend to most closely during their therapy sessions, and the kinds of pitfalls they should avoid in working with particular patient types – for example, distressed relationship partners, autistic individuals and patients with borderline personality disorder.

22.3.1 Individual differences in empathic accuracy

The most important practical implication of the research on empathic accuracy is that it provides a reliable and objective method for measuring people's performance as everyday mind readers. Some of the most compelling evidence for this claim is found in the results of the previously mentioned study in which 80 undergraduate men and women attempted to infer the actual thoughts and feelings reported by each of three female clients who had been videotaped during their respective sessions with a male, client-centred therapist (Marangoni *et al.*, 1995). The results of this study showed that there were reliable individual differences in the perceivers' empathic accuracy – with some perceivers being consistently good, other perceivers being consistently average, and still other perceivers being consistently poor at inferring the specific thoughts and feelings of the female clients. Indeed, the average inter-target correlation of the perceivers' empathic accuracy scores (0.60) was impressively high in this study.

Selecting for empathic accuracy

In practical terms, this finding means that it is possible to distinguish people who are empathically skilled from those who are empathically challenged, and to then use this information as a selection criterion. So instead of selecting aspiring psychotherapists (students who have applied for advanced training as clinical psychologists, counselling psychologists, or psychiatrists) solely on the basis of their undergraduate grade-point averages (GPA) and their scores on the Graduate Record Exam (GRE), the applicants could also be required to complete a standard empathic accuracy performance test. The results of this test could then be used, along with the GPA and GRE data, to help selection committees decide which students to admit to graduate schools and other professional programmes that train aspiring counsellors and psychotherapists.

There are at least two good reasons for believing that the candidates' empathic accuracy might prove to be a uniquely valid predictor of their future 'on-the-job' performance as practising psychotherapists. First, empathic accuracy has long been regarded as one of the most important criteria for success as a psychotherapist (Rogers, 1957). Second, the available research findings suggest that the therapist's actual empathy (in addition to clients' perceptions of the therapist's empathy) really does play an important role in successful psychotherapy outcomes (Greenberg *et al.*, 2001). Clearly, a major advantage of the empathic accuracy research is that it offers a truly objective way to measure the therapist's empathy – i.e. by assessing how accurately the therapist can infer the actual, reported thoughts and feelings of clients who appear in a set of standard videotapes. Even better, there is evidence that such tapes can be used not only to *assess* people's empathic accuracy but also to *train* them to become more empathically accurate.

Training empathic accuracy

Evidence for the effectiveness of empathic accuracy training comes from the previously described study by Marangoni *et al.* (1995). Recall that the 'amateur therapists' in this study attempted to infer the actual thoughts and feelings of the three female clients who appeared in the standard stimulus tapes. To see if immediate, veridical feedback about the clients' actual thoughts and feelings could be used to train the participants to be more empathically accurate, Marangoni and her colleagues randomly assigned half of the participants to a feedback condition in which they saw the client's actual thought or feeling immediately after they had written down their inferred thought or feeling. Compared to their counterparts in the no-feedback condition, the participants who received the feedback during the middle portion of each tape were significantly more accurate in their subsequent empathic inferences. This finding suggests that empathic accuracy can be significantly enhanced through feedback training, even over the course of a single experimental session.

To improve the effects of 'empathy training' even more, it would be useful to know what kinds of cues perceivers rely on when inferring other people's thoughts and feelings. To this end, Gesn and Ickes (1999) systematically varied the information channels that participants had available to them when they tried to infer the thoughts and feelings of the clients in the Marangoni *et al.* (1995) videotapes. By editing these tapes with the aid of an audio/video mixing board, they created three versions of the tapes – one for each of three information channel conditions. First, there was a video-and-audio condition, in which the clients on the tapes could be both clearly seen and clearly heard. Second, there was a video-and-filtered-audio condition, in which the clients could be seen but their words could not be understood because their speech had been electronically filtered so that only the paralinguistic cues (inflection, tone of voice, loudness, etc.) remained. Third, there was an audio-only condition in which the clients' video images did not appear on the blank TV monitor but their conversation with the therapist was clearly audible.

Results comparing the performance of participants who were randomly assigned to each of the three information-channel conditions showed that empathic accuracy was best in the video-and-audio condition. By comparison, there was only a small (i.e. negligible) drop in empathic accuracy in the audio-only condition. However, when the clients' words were rendered unintelligible in the video-and-filtered-audio condition but the client–therapist interaction could be clearly seen, the perceivers' average empathic accuracy was substantially worse than in both of the other conditions. These findings suggest that although both verbal and non-verbal information can be important, therapists should in most cases pay more attention to what their clients say than to their non-verbal behaviour if they want to accurately infer the specific content of the clients' thoughts and feelings.

22.3.2 Empathic accuracy and couples' therapy

Being able to predict the relation between empathic accuracy and relationship satisfaction and stability is the goal of Ickes and Simpson's *empathic accuracy model* (Ickes & Simpson, 1997, 2001). This model posits a general rule along with two major exceptions. As a general rule, it is presumed that greater empathic accuracy tends to be good for close relationships. For most everyday interactions, knowledge of a partner's thoughts and feelings should promote the kind of mutual understanding that enables partners to coordinate their individual and shared goals and actions and thereby maintain a more satisfying and stable relationship.

There are, however, two important exceptions to this rule. First, in situations in which one or both partners recognize that greater empathic accuracy has the potential to damage their relationship by revealing their partner's relationship-threatening thoughts and feelings, they can use *motivated inaccuracy* to help buffer the relationship from the dissatisfaction and instability that might otherwise occur. Second, despite realizing that greater empathic accuracy might sometimes damage the relationship, one or both of the partners can have such a strong motive to 'know the truth' that they become hypervigilant and display *motivated accuracy* with respect to their partner's unexpressed thoughts and feelings. This second exception is pertinent to individuals with insecure attachment styles (Simpson *et al.*, 1999) and/or those with 'suspicious minds' (Ickes *et al.*, 2003).

Motivated inaccuracy

A study illustrating the first exception to the rule (i.e. that there are times when motivated *inaccuracy* can help the partners' relationship) was conducted by Simpson *et al.* (1995). In this study, heterosexual dating partners individually reported their level of interdependence and insecurity within the relationship, and were then put in a situation in which each dating partner audibly rated photographs of members of the opposite sex on the dimensions of physical attractiveness and sexual appeal while the other partner was present. In addition, the dating partners were assigned to either a high-threat condition (in which all the photographs depicted very attractive individuals) or to the low-threat condition (in which all the photographs depicted individuals who were below average in their physical attractiveness).

After the rating task, the dating partners were informed that their rating session had been covertly videotaped. After separating the partners and giving them their own copy of the tape to view, they were asked to record their own thoughts and feelings during a first viewing of the tape, and then to infer their dating partner's thoughts and feelings during a second viewing. It was expected that the partners in the high-threat condition (who had reason to feel more threatened by each other's perceptions) would be less accurate in their attempts to infer each other's thoughts and feelings from the videotape than the partners in the low-threat condition. The results confirmed this effect, which was particularly evident for the insecure yet mutually dependent couples who had been in the high-threat condition. These couples not only felt the most threatened during the rating session, but their average level of empathic accuracy was significantly worse than that of total strangers and not significantly greater than chance. In contrast, the least threat-ened couples were those who had been in the low-threat condition, and who also described their relationship as secure and not fostering a high level of mutual dependency. Interestingly, these couples were the most empathically accurate.

But can *motivated inaccuracy* really help to buffer close relationships from the instability that would result if the partners had accurately inferred each other's relationship-threatening thoughts and feelings? To find out, Simpson *et al.* (1995) contacted the dating partners individually 4 months after they had participated in the study to determine whether they were still dating each other. The results showed that, for the group of couples in which motivated inaccuracy had been most evident, none of the couples had broken up. On the other hand, there was a nearly 30% break-up rate among the remaining couples in the study. These findings suggest that there are indeed circumstances in which partners' motivated inaccuracy can help to protect and preserve their relationships from the potentially destructive effects of a temporary threat.

What implications do these findings have for relationship therapy? According to Ickes (2003), therapists should accept the fact that the stability of many relation-ships is predicated on the partners' routine *avoidance* of each other's relationship-threatening thoughts and feelings.

For many couples, the implicit agreement to follow the policy of 'don't ask, don't tell' may be the primary reason why their relationship has worked as well as it has. If the therapist fails to appreciate this fact, more harm than good can be accomplished when the partners are pressed to confront their most relationship-threatening issues before they feel capable of doing so. And the risk of this harm (the therapist's intervention evoking the kinds of volatile feelings that could precipitate greater conflict or even divorce) may further increase when the therapist feels obliged to treat the couple within the accelerated timeframe of a few brief sessions that have been authorized by the bureaucracy of a managed care organization. To help minimize this risk, the therapist who wants to foster greater empathy in one or both partners should begin by having them discuss relatively benign, non-threatening issues, and then gradually introduce more relationship-threatening issues only when the partners themselves feel ready to confront them.

Motivated accuracy

Although motivated inaccuracy is a common defence against having to confront a relationship partner's potentially relationship-threatening thoughts and feelings, some people actually seek, rather than avoid, such confrontations. As Simpson *et al.* (1999) and Dugosh (1998, 2001) have discovered, women with an anxious attachment style become hypervigilant in relationship-threatening situations, and their hypervigilance takes the form of increased empathic accuracy. When anxious individuals are faced with an imminent threat to their relationship, they apparently try to 'get into the other person's head' to see how big a threat they are actually facing and what, if anything, might be done about it. Instead of being motivated to inaccurately infer the partner's potentially threatening thoughts and feelings, these highly anxious partners seem to be motivated to infer their partner's thoughts and feelings more accurately.

In the Simpson *et al.* (1999) study, the more anxiously attached women behaved as if they were compelled to know, at the first sign of threat, what their male dating partners were thinking and feeling in the relationship-threatening situation. Although their hypervigilance may have enabled them to gauge the severity of a threat more accurately, by giving them clearer insights into their partner's thoughts and feelings, it also carried a high price in terms of the corresponding emotional and relational distress it engendered. For when these women were asked about their feelings at the end of the session, they were particularly likely to report feeling jealous and threatened in the relationship-threatening situation, and to feel less close to their partner than they had at the start of the session.

More recently, a series of studies by Ickes *et al.* (2003) has focused on individual differences in the motivation to acquire relationship-threatening information. Ickes and his colleagues developed a self-report measure of the motivation to acquire relationship-threatening information (MARTI). They found that dating partners with high MARTI scores were lower in relational trust and reported engaging in more 'suspicion behaviours' such as eavesdropping on a partner's private phone conversation or calling to see if a partner was where he or she was supposed to be. Moreover, dating partners with higher MARTI scores were more likely to break up within 5 months.

What implications do such findings have for relationship therapy? According to Ickes (2003):

The therapist must realize that some people are predisposed to 'look for trouble' in their intimate relationships, and that their readiness to confront relationship-threatening issues may be part of the problem rather than part of the solution. People in this category can include women with an anxious attachment orientation, who act as if they are compelled to know their husbands' relationship-threatening thoughts and feelings, and suspicious partners who have a strong motive to acquire relationship-threatening information. Although different interventions may be required in each case, the therapist should learn to recognize these predispositions to 'look for trouble' and make them a focus of the therapy.

Motivated attributional bias

Recently, researchers have used the empathic accuracy paradigm in conjunction with signal detection analyses to explore the kinds of attributional biases that contribute to interpersonal conflicts (Schmid Mast *et al.*, 2006; Schweinle *et al.*, 2002; Schweinle & Ickes, 2006). For example, Schmid Mast and her colleagues have found that men who seek a dominant role are more likely to attribute power-related thoughts and feelings to others than are men who prefer a subordinate position (Schmid Mast *et al.*, 2006). Similarly, Schweinle and his colleagues have found that men who report abusing their own female partners are more likely than non-abusive men to presume that women are harbouring critical and rejecting thoughts and feelings about their male partners. Presented with the task to infer the thoughts and feelings of the three female clients who appear in the standard stimulus tapes, the abusive men 'saw' criticism and rejection significantly more often than it actually occurred.

So far, at least, motivated attributional biases appear to be domain-specific, applying to specific aspects of one's relationships. For example, the attributional bias of abusive men applies specifically to inferences about the potentially critical and rejecting thoughts and feelings harboured by women, whereas the attributional bias of men who prefer a dominant role applies specifically to inferences about the potentially dominance-related thoughts and feelings of others. Attributional biases can be understood as lenses through which one perceives the world, and we believe that they are 'motivated' to the extent that they serve the purpose of legitimizing the perceiver's own behaviour (e.g. abusing one's spouse is perceived as justified *because* the spouse harbours critical and rejecting thoughts and feelings).

In general, we are relatively unaware of our own attributional biases when we interact with others because they take the form of overlearned 'schemas' that operate automatically, at a low level of conscious awareness. For this reason, therapeutic attempts to correct such biases must begin by bringing them to the client's attention and then helping the client to adopt a more realistic view in order to facilitate subsequent behavioural change. Because such biases often are responsible for initiating and sustaining interpersonal conflicts (e.g. by motivating power-oriented men to dominate others and by motivating ego-threatened men to intimidate and abuse their female partners), clinical interventions designed to correct such biases could potentially reduce much of the interpersonal conflict that couples and individual patients report.

22.3.3 Empathic accuracy and autism

Baron-Cohen and his colleagues (e.g. Baron-Cohen, 1995, 2003; Baron-Cohen *et al.*, 2001) have posited a strong link between empathic accuracy and autism, arguing that severe autism can be characterized as *mindblindness* – an inability to accurately infer, or perhaps even to recognize the existence of, other people's thoughts and feelings. Extending this claim, they have argued that the degree of autism varies across a spectrum that connects profoundly autistic individuals with normally developing individuals (Baron-Cohen *et al.*, 2001). More recently, Baron-Cohen (2003) has further claimed that men, on average, are more autistic-like and less empathically accurate than women.

Curiously, the last of the claims seems to have been made without regard to the relevant empathic accuracy research, which has revealed no evidence of a reliable gender difference in empathic *ability* for participants in the mostly normally developing college student samples that have been used in this research (see Ickes *et al.*, 2000). On the other hand, the empathic accuracy literature has revealed some preliminary evidence for a reliable gender difference in empathic *motivation*, suggesting that women may be more easily motivated than men to do their best on empathy-related tasks (see chapter 6 of Ickes, 2003; Klein & Hodges, 2001). There is no doubt, however, that when autism is profound enough to be recognized and diagnosed, its victims are much more likely to be male than female, with a sex ratio of four to five autistic men for every autistic woman (Baron-Cohen, 1995).

With regard to the first two claims by Baron-Cohen and his colleagues, it is beginning to appear that the degree of 'autistic-like behaviour', as assessed by their autism spectrum measure (Baron-Cohen *et al.*, 2001), is not linked to empathic accuracy. In recent studies conducted in Belgium with young adults (Ponnet, 2004) and in the United States with early adolescents (Gleason *et al.*, 2004), the participants' scores on the autism spectrum measure were not significantly correlated with their global empathic accuracy scores. Moreover, in Gleason *et al.*'s (2004) study, the two variables were found to make *independent* contributions to social adjustment, such that the poorest adjustment was evident in the adolescents who had low empathic accuracy and high levels of autistic-like behaviour.

The implication of these findings for therapists who work with autistic individuals is that they should resist the temptation to equate autistic-like behaviours with impaired empathic accuracy, as these two characteristics seem to vary independently of each other within the upper (i.e. more normal) range of the autism spectrum. On the other hand, individuals who display both low empathic accuracy and high levels of autistic-like behaviour appear to be particularly at risk for problems in their social development, and early intervention may be needed in order to minimize the negative consequences of these attributes.

22.3.4 Empathic accuracy and borderline personality disorder

With regard to therapy involving patients with borderline personality disorder (BPD), the results of a study by Flury and Ickes (2006) appeared, at first glance, to confirm what clinical practitioners have long suspected: that BPD patients are above average in their ability to infer other people's thoughts and feelings. In this study, same-sex dyads were created in which one of the members scored high on a measure of BPD symptomology, whereas the other member scored low. Although the higher-BPD members were more accurate in 'reading' the thoughts and feelings of the lower-BPD members than vice versa, this effect was no longer significant when the authors controlled for a corresponding difference in the inferential difficulty of the dyad members' reported thoughts and feelings. The authors concluded from this pattern of results that people with BPB symptoms are not, on average, more empathically accurate than those without. They do, however, enjoy an empathic advantage over their conversation partners because their own reported thoughts and feelings are atypical and quite difficult to 'read' in comparison to those reported by their non-BPD interaction partners.

The implication of this finding for therapists is that they should guard against presuming that they can accurately infer the thoughts and feelings of their BPD patients. Instead, they should assertively and continually question these patients about the contents of their thoughts and feelings, which are likely to offer repeated surprises and unexpected insights. Indeed, including atypical, hard-to-infer thoughts and feelings as one of the characteristics of BPD in future versions of the *Diagnostic and Statistical Manual of Mental Disorders* might help to spread the word about this newly identified aspect of BPD.

22.4 Summary

Empathic accuracy is a skill in which individuals differ greatly: some people are good, others are average, and still others are poor at correctly inferring the specific content of other people's thoughts and feelings. Despite these pre-existing individual differences, there is evidence that individuals can be trained to achieve a significantly higher level of empathic accuracy within a relatively short period of time. The empathic accuracy paradigm described in this chapter provides an objective measure of empathic accuracy and a related set of methods that can be used to train people to improve their skills in 'everyday mind reading'.

Empathic accuracy is also a key element for clients who wish to effect change in distressed social relationships. Relationship problems are ubiquitous in therapy and counselling situations, and the role that empathic accuracy plays in relationship dynamics is particularly important to understand. In couples, knowing what the partner thinks or feels is generally desirable and should be encouraged by therapists. However, there are circumstances in which *not* knowing what the partner thinks or feels can help to protect and preserve vulnerable relationships from destabilizing threats. Research suggests that the buffering effect of *motivated inaccuracy* is most pronounced in insecure and mutually dependent partners who find themselves in circumstances in which their relationship is threatened. For these individuals, 'not knowing' their partner's thoughts and feelings is sufficiently adaptive that the therapist must proceed with extreme caution, and encourage self-disclosure about relationship-threatening issues only gradually.

On the other hand, there are individuals who are so obsessed about wanting to know their partner's potentially relationship-threatening thoughts and feelings that they display *motivated accuracy* instead. Women with an anxious attachment style and suspicious men and women are particularly likely to display motivated accuracy. By trying to 'get into their partner's head' and anticipate their partner's every move, these people experience considerable jealousy and distress, and they may paradoxically jeopardize the very relationship that they so desperately want to save. Therapeutic intervention in this case should emphasize the virtue of cultivating a sense of *discretion*, i.e. of knowing when to get inside one's partner's head and when to stay out of it.

When perceivers consistently misread other people's thoughts and feelings as if through a distorted lens, there is reason to suspect the operation of a *motivated attributional bias*. For example, abusive men overestimate the degree to which women harbour critical or rejecting thoughts and feelings about their male partners. This bias can damage a relationship in that abusive men often use it to legitimize their own abusive behaviour. Therapeutic intervention aimed at correcting such distorted views is particularly important in this case because many abusive men appear to be unaware that their perceptions are biased at all. Beyond this example, there likely exist other domains of motivated attributional biases that are characteristic of specific psychological disorders (e.g. the tendency of schizophrenics to overattribute controlling thoughts and feelings to others).

Therapists and clinicians need to be put on guard against clinical stereotypes which suggest that people with certain disorders are particularly good (or bad) in their empathic accuracy. For example, it has been proposed that autistic individuals are particularly poor and that individuals with borderline personality disorder (BPD) are particularly good at inferring other people's thoughts and feelings. The relevant empirical evidence has not confirmed these simple claims, but has instead revealed that more complicated and refined views are needed.

First, apart from the most extreme and obvious cases, individuals throughout much of the 'autism spectrum' seem to vary substantially in their empathic accuracy skills. Nevertheless, when pronounced autistic symptoms are paired with low empathic accuracy, social development and adjustment are substantially impaired.

Second, countering another clinical stereotype, individuals with BPD are generally no better (or worse) than others when it comes to inferring other people's thoughts and feelings. However, people with BPD are particularly hard to 'read' because their thoughts and feelings are so atypical. In general, it would be helpful for therapists to know how hard (or easy) it is to infer a patient's thoughts and feelings depending on the specific disorder the patient is diagnosed with. This information could help therapists determine how much they can trust their own intuition and how much careful and unbiased questioning may be needed to form an accurate impression of the patient.

REFERENCES

Asch, S. E. (1946). Forming impressions of personality. *Journal of Abnormal and Social Psychology*, **41**, 258–290.

Baron-Cohen, S. (1995). *Mindblindness: An Essay on Autism and Theory of Mind*. Cambridge, Mass.: MIT Press.

Baron-Cohen, S. (2003). *The Essential Difference: The Truth about the Male and Female Brain*. New York: Basic Books.

Baron-Cohen, S., Wheelwright, S., Skinner, R., Martin, J., & Clubley, E. (2001). The Autism-Spectrum Quotient (AQ): evidence from Asperger Syndrome/high-functioning autism, males and females, scientists and mathematicians. *Journal of Autism and Communication Disorders*, **31**, 5–17.

Costanzo, M., & Archer, D. (1989). Interpreting the expressive behavior of others: the Interpersonal Perception Task. *Journal of Nonverbal Behavior*, **13**, 225–245.

Cronbach, L. J. (1955). Processes affecting scores on 'understanding of others' and 'assumed similarity'. *Psychological Bulletin*, **52**, 177–193.

Crosby, L. (2002). The relation of maternal empathic accuracy to the development of self concept. Unpublished doctoral thesis, The Fielding Institute, Santa Barbara, California.

Davis, M. H., & Kraus, L. A. (1997). Personality and empathic accuracy. In W. Ickes (ed.), *Empathic Accuracy* (pp. 144–168). New York: Guilford.

Dugosh, J. W. (1998). Adult attachment style influences on the empathic accuracy of female dating partners. Unpublished master's thesis, University of Texas, Arlington.

Dugosh, J. W. (2001). Effects of relationship threat and ambiguity on empathic accuracy in dating couples. Unpublished doctoral thesis, University of Texas, Arlington.

Ekman, P., & Friesen, W. V. (1975). Unmasking the face. A guide to recognizing emotions from facial clues. Palo Alto, Calif.: Consulting Psychologists Press.

Flury, J., & Ickes, W. (2006). Emotional intelligence and empathic accuracy. In J. Ciarrochi, J. Forgas, & J. Mayer (eds.), *Emotional Intelligence in Everyday Life: A Scientific Inquiry*, 2nd edn. (pp. 140–165). New York: Psychology Press.

Funder, D. C. (1995). On the accuracy of personality judgment: a realistic approach. *Psychological Review*, **102**, 652–670.

Funder, D. C., & Colvin, C. R. (1988). Friends and strangers: acquaintanceship, agreement, and the accuracy of personality judgment. *Journal of Personality and Social Psychology*, **55**, 149–158.

Funder, D. C., & West, S. G. (1993). Consensus, self-other agreement, and accuracy in personality judgment: an introduction. *Journal of Personality*, **61**, 457–476.

Gesn, P. R., & Ickes, W. (1999). The development of meaning contexts for empathic accuracy: channel and sequence effects. *Journal of Personality and Social Psychology*, **77**, 746–761.

Gleason, K., Johnson, B., Ickes, W., & Jensen-Campbell, L. (2004). Autistic characteristics, empathic accuracy, and prosocial skills in adolescents. Poster presentation given at the Annual Conference of the Society for Personality and Social Psychology, Austin, Texas, 20 January, 2004.

Goleman, D. (1995). *Emotional Intelligence*. New York: Bantam Books, Inc.

Graham, T. (1994). Gender, relationship, and target differences in empathic accuracy. Master's Thesis, University of Texas, Arlington.

Greenberg, L. S., Watson, J. C., Elliot, R., & Bohart, A. C. (2001). Empathy. *Psychotherapy: Theory, Research, Practice, Training*, **38**, 380–384.

Hall, J. A. (1984). *Nonverbal Sex Differences: Communication Accuracy and Expressive Style*. Baltimore, Md.: Johns Hopkins University Press.

Hall, J. A. (2001). The PONS Test and the psychometric approach to measuring interpersonal sensitivity. In J. A. Hall, & F. J. Bernieri (eds.), *Interpersonal Sensitivity: Theory and Measurement* (pp. 143–160). Mahwah, N.J.: Erlbaum.

Hall, J. A., & Bernieri, F. J. (eds.). (2001). *Interpersonal Sensitivity: Theory and Measurement*. Mahwah, N.J.: Lawrence Erlbaum Associates.

Heider, F. (1944). Social perception and phenomenal causality. *Psychological Review*, **51**, 358–374.

Ickes, W. J. (ed.). (1997). *Empathic Accuracy*. New York: Guilford Press.

Ickes, W. (2001). Measuring empathic accuracy. In J. A. Hall, & F. J. Bernieri (eds.), *Interpersonal Sensitivity: Theory and Measurement. The LEA Series in Personality and Clinical Psychology* (pp. 219–241). Mahwah, N.J.: Lawrence Erlbaum Associates.

Ickes, W. (2003). *Everyday Mind Reading: Understanding What Other People Think and Feel*. Amherst, N.Y.: Prometheus Books.

Ickes, W., Bissonnette, V., Garcia, S., & Stinson, L. L. (1990a). Implementing and using the dyadic interaction paradigm. In C. Hendrick, & M. S. Clark (eds.), *Research Methods in Personality and Social Psychology. Review of Personality and Social Psychology* (Vol. 11) (pp. 16–44). Thousand Oaks, Calif.: Sage Publications, Inc.

Ickes, W., Dugosh, J. W., Simpson, J. A., & Wilson, C. L. (2003). Suspicious minds: the motive to acquire relationship-threatening information. *Personal Relationships*, **10**, 131–148.

Ickes, W., Gesn, P. R., & Graham, T. (2000). Gender differences in empathic accuracy: differential ability or differential motivation? *Personal Relationships*, **7**, 95–109.

Ickes, W., & Simpson, J. A. (1997). Managing empathic accuracy in close relationships. In W. J. Ickes (ed.), *Empathic Accuracy*. (pp. 218–250). New York, N.Y.: Guilford Press.

Ickes, W., & Simpson, J. A. (2001). *Motivational Aspects of Blackwell Handbook of Social Psychology: Interpersonal Processes* (pp. 229–249). Oxford: Blackwell.

Ickes, W., Simpson, J. A., & Oriña, M. (2005). Empathic accuracy and inaccuracy in close relationships. In B. Malle, & S. Hodges (eds.), *Other Minds*. New York: Guilford Press.

Ickes, W., Stinson, L., Bissonnette, V., & Garcia, S. (1990b). Naturalistic social cognition: empathic accuracy in mixed-sex dyads. *Journal of Personality and Social Psychology*, **59**, 730–742.

Ickes, W., & Tooke, W. (1988). The observational method: studying the interactions of minds and bodies. In S. Duck, D. F. Hay, S. E. Hobfoll, W. Ickes, & B. Montgomery (eds.), *Handbook of Personal Relationships: Theory, Research, and Interventions* (pp. 79–97). Chichester: Wiley.

Ickes, W., & Trued, S. (1985). A system for collecting dyadic interaction data on the Apple II. Electronic Social Psychology. [Online serial], 1, Article no. 8501012.

Klein, K. J. K., & Hodges, S. D. (2001). Gender differences, motivation, and empathic accuracy: when it pays to understand. *Personality and Social Psychology Bulletin*, **27**, 720–730.

Knudson, R. M., Sommers, A. A., & Golding, S. L. (1980). Interpersonal perception and mode of resolution in marital conflict. *Journal of Personality and Social Psychology*, **38**, 751–763.

Laing, R. D., Phillipson, H., & Lee, A. R. (1966). *Interpersonal Perception: A Theory and a Method of Research*. New York: Springer.

Levenson, R. W., & Ruef, A. M. (1992). Empathy: a physiological substrate. *Journal of Personality and Social Psychology*, **63**, 234–246.

Marangoni, C., Garcia, S., Ickes, W., & Teng, G. (1995). Empathic accuracy in a clinically relevant setting. *Journal of Personality and Social Psychology*, **68**, 854–869.

McCrae, R. R. (1982). Consensual validation of personality traits: evidence from self-reports and ratings. *Journal of Personality and Social Psychology*, **43**, 293–303.

Mortimer, D. C. (1996). 'Reading' ourselves 'reading' others: Actual versus self-estimated empathic accuracy. Unpublished master's thesis, University of Texas, Arlington.

Noller, P. (1980). Misunderstanding in marital communication: a study of couples' nonverbal communication. *Journal of Personality and Social Psychology*, **39**, 1135–1148.

Noller, P. (1981). Gender and marital adjustment level differences in decoding messages from spouses and strangers. *Journal of Personality and Social Psychology*, **41**, 272–278.

Ponnet, K. (2004). Mind-reading in adolescents and adults with a pervasive developmental disorder. PhD thesis, University of Ghent, Belgium.

Rogers, C. R. (1957). The necessary and sufficient conditions of therapeutic personality change. *Journal of Consulting Psychology*, **21**, 95–103.

Rogers, C. R., & Dymond, R. F. (1954). *Psychotherapy and Personality Change*. Chicago, Ill.: University of Chicago Press.

Rosenthal, R., Hall, J. A., DiMatteo, M. R., Rogers, P. L., & Archer, D. (1979). *Sensitivity to Nonverbal Communication: The PONS Test*. Baltimore, Md.: The Johns Hopkins University Press.

Salovey, P., & Mayer, J. D. (1989). Emotional intelligence. *Imagination, Cognition and Personality*, **9**, 185–211.

Schmid Mast, M., Hall, J. A., & Ickes, W. (2006). Inferring power-related thoughts and feelings in others: a signal detection analysis. *European Journal of Social Psychology*, **36**, 1–10.

Schweinle, W. E., & Ickes, W. (2006). The role of men's critical/rejecting overattribution bias, affect, and attentional disengagement in marital aggression. In press.

Schweinle, W. E., Ickes, W., & Bernstein, I. H. (2002). Empathic inaccuracy in husband to wife aggression: the overattribution bias. *Personal Relationships*, **9**, 141–158.

Seligman, M. E. P., & Csikszentmihalyi, M. (2000). Positive psychology: an introduction. *American Psychologist*, **55**, 5–14.

Simpson, J. A., Ickes, W., & Blackstone, T. (1995). When the head protects the heart: empathic accuracy in dating relationships. *Journal of Personality and Social Psychology*, **69**, 629–641.

Simpson, J. A., Ickes, W., & Grich, J. (1999). When accuracy hurts: reactions of anxious-ambivalent dating partners to a relationship-threatening situation. *Journal of Personality and Social Psychology*, **76**, 754–769.

Simpson, J. A., Ickes, W., & Oriña, M. (2001). Empathic accuracy and preemptive relationship maintenance. In J. Harvey, & A. Wenzel (eds.), *Close Romantic Relationships: Maintenance and Enhancement* (pp. 27–46). Mahwah, N.J.: Lawrence Erlbaum Associates.

Simpson, J. A., Oriña, M. M., & Ickes, W. (2003). When accuracy hurts, and when it helps: a test of the empathic accuracy model in marital interactions. *Journal of Personality and Social Psychology*, **85**, 881–893.

Stinson, L., & Ickes, W. (1992). Empathic accuracy in the interactions of male friends versus male strangers. *Journal of Personality and Social Psychology*, **62**, 787–797.

Taft, R. (1955). The ability to judge people. *Psychological Bulletin*, **52**, 1–23.

A perception-action model for empathy

Stephanie D. Preston

Department of Psychology, University of Michigan

You can only understand people if you feel them in yourself

John Steinbeck (1952/2002), *East of Eden*, p. 444

23.1 Introduction

This chapter describes and augments the perception-action model (PAM) of empathy, first detailed in Preston and de Waal (2002b). Empathy, ironically, is a term that means different things to different people. It has been difficult to distinguish empathy from sympathy because they both involve the emotional state of one related to the state of another. This problem was compounded by the fact that the mapping of the terms has recently reversed: what is now commonly called empathy was referred to before the middle of the twentieth century as sympathy (see Wispé, 1986 for a full discussion) and some researchers still use the old connotations (e.g. Batson, 1997).

According to a PAM, empathy is defined as a *shared emotional experience* occurring when one person (the subject) comes to feel a *similar emotion* to another (the object) as a result of *perceiving* the other's state. This process results from the fact that the subject's *representations* of the emotional state are *automatically* activated when the subject pays *attention* to the emotional state of the object. The *neural mechanism* assumes that brain areas have processing domains based on their cellular composition and connectivity; as such, there is no 'empathy area' and brain areas are recruited when the relevant domain is required by the task. This definition contains much information, so the model will be detailed in this chapter by deconstructing the definition, focusing on the italicized words.

23.2 Breaking down the PAM

23.2.1 Perception Action

This model is called the *perception-action model* because it is based on tenants of motor behaviour by the same name. In motor behaviour, the term *perception-action*

Empathy in Mental Illness, eds. Tom F. D. Farrow and Peter W. R. Woodruff. Published by Cambridge University Press. © Cambridge University Press 2007.

describes the fact that there are shared representations for perceiving and generating action. For example, if the subject witnesses the object swinging a hammer, then the part of the subject's brain that is used to swing a hammer is activated (e.g. the hand and arm region of the primary motor cortex). Naming and observing common tools activates the representation for the related motor act in the left premotor cortex (Grafton *et al.*, 1997) and even imagined movements activate the shared representations for perception and action (e.g. Jeannerod & Frak, 1999). In this way, the *perception* of *perception-action* in motor behaviour refers to direct perception as well as imagery or imagination and *action* refers to overt acts, imagined acts and even relatively abstract cognitive affordances.

A shared representation between perception and action was proposed in 1903 (Lipps, 1903), was emphasized in *Phenomenology of Perception* (Merleau-Ponty, 1962/1970), and defined the theories of Wolfgang Prinz (1992), Alan Allport (1987), and Michael Turvey (1992), but 1992 was a watershed year in the development of perception-action models. Searching for the keyword/term 'perception-action' in the database PsychInfo (November, 2004), there were 91 articles written on the topic between 1872 and 1992 (0.76 per year), 16 in 1992 alone (16 per year) and 408 since 1992 (34 per year). In 1992, some of the most important theoretical papers were published on the topic (e.g. Prinz, 1992) and the Rizzolatti group in Parma, Italy discovered 'mirror neurones' in the rostral-most part of the left premotor area that responded when a monkey observed and performed a grasping movement (di Pellegrino *et al.*, 1992). This latter finding made international headlines and, since then, neurones with similar properties have also been found in the rostral-most part of the right superior parietal lobule (Decety *et al.*, 1997; Iacoboni *et al.*, 1999).

As with motor behaviour, the stimuli for the PAM of empathy can be another person, animal, or even an entity such as 'the earth' or 'New York City', and the *perception* of the PAM can arise from situations where the subject directly perceives the object as well as situations where the subject imagines the state of the object (often called 'cognitive empathy', e.g. Povinelli *et al.*, 1992). Because the PAM is embedded in an evolutionary framework (Preston, 2004a; Preston & de Waal, 2002a, 2002b), we assume that the system evolved to handle live interactions with other individuals and so live objects drive the system better than imagined objects, resulting in more intense forms of empathy. In terms of the neural mechanism, this more cognitive form of empathy would probably not engage the amygdala, which usually responds to ephemeral stimuli requiring an immediate response, but would require the dorsolateral prefrontal cortex to maintain information about the object in working memory. In imagination, while additional activation is required to bring the state of the object into mind, once the subject succeeds in feeling the state of the object, the activation for the state would be the same as that arrived at through direct perception. However, the strength of activation in imagined empathy is rarely as high as in direct empathy because of the increased difficulty in attending to internal over external stimuli.

23.2.2 Representations

The term *representation* has been used in psychology in many different contexts. In this case, a representation is a pattern of activation in the brain and body corresponding to a particular state so repeated instances of the same event reliably activate the same pattern. This is similar to a neural network (McClelland & Rumelhart, 1985), but here representation applies broadly to central and peripheral processes including autonomic arousal and endocrine responses – to all of the concomitants of the subject's subjective state. The term *representation* is used in this way to underscore that the brain and body give rise to complex emotion. For example, the temporal lobe is known to store long-term memories of people, places and objects, with the fusiform 'face' area specializing in face and eye-gaze information. The somatosensory-related areas store representations of feeling states with somatosensory cortex storing sensations and the cingulate cortex storing subjective reactions to the sensations. According to the PAM, these areas are necessary to the extent that the experience of the object involves these particular representations.

23.2.3 Shared emotional experience and similar emotion

Of course, a *shared emotional experience* is the sine qua non of empathy; by definition, empathy results when the subject feels the emotion of the object. In contrast to theories of empathy where the subject's state must match (e.g. Feshbach & Roe, 1968) or accurately portray (e.g. Levenson & Reuf, 1992) the state of the object, with the PAM the subject's state must be *similar to* that of the object. Accuracy and state matching are not discrete variables but rather exist in a continuum. It is improbable that the subject's and object's state will ever match exactly, and even if they did there would be no way to demonstrate it empirically. The PAM emphasizes degrees of matching between the subject and object because it relies on representations; the subject can only match or resonate with the state of the object to the degree that the subject has existing representations for the state of the object. This makes empathy itself a continuum.

Supporting the importance of similar representations in the PAM, empathy increases with past experience, similarity and familiarity. For example, subjects with highly distressing childhood experiences have more trait empathy and report more empathy for a patient in a video (Barnett & McCoy, 1989), presumably because they have ready access to representations of distress that are similar to those of the patient. Thus, the more similar the object's emotion is to something the subject has experienced in the past, the more the subject's representations will match the object's and the more their states will resonate. Similar past experiences also make the subject more accurate, more helpful, and more likely to be characterized as empathizing. In contrast, less similar past experiences will make the subject less accurate, less helpful and more likely to be characterized as 'projecting' (putting his emotions onto the object). This feature of the model explains the layperson's definition of empathy whereby the subject can only say that they empathize with the object if they have actually had the same experience. For example, it is considered inappropriate, and sometimes even offensive, for a man to say that he empathizes with a woman's pain from childbirth or for a child to say that they empathize with the parent's distress from aging.

The role of representations can also eliminate the need to distinguish empathy from 'projection'. In empathy, the subject feels the object's state; in projection, the subject assumes his or her own state to be that of the object. Projection is thought to be inconsistent with empathy, because the mapping goes from subject to object rather than object to subject (Eisenberg & Strayer, 1987) and human interpretations of animal behaviour are often criticized for resulting from projection rather than perception (Mitchell *et al.*, 1997). With the PAM, the process is the same for both empathy and projection because in both cases the subject's representations are activated by perception of the object. Whether the subject is empathizing or projecting depends upon whether the subject's representations are similar enough to those of the object to convince the object that s/he is understood, or to convince observers that the object is understood. In a way there is no empathy that is *not* projection since the subject always uses his or her own representations to understand the object, but because of the intersubjectivity problem, this fact only becomes apparent when the subject says or does something inconsistent with the object's state.

Recognizing the overlap between empathy and projection, Hume noted 'a very remarkable inclination in human nature, to bestow on external objects the same emotions, which it observes in itself; and to find every where those ideas, which are most present to it' (1739–1740/1990; p. 224). A high-functioning autistic adult similarly believes that people do not think he can empathize simply because his way of experiencing the world differs from that of others and so his projections do not match their experiences and vice versa. He states, 'It is ... much easier to empathize with someone whose ways of experiencing the world are similar to one's own than to understand someone whose perceptions are very different' (Cesaroni & Garber, 1991).

Hume also noted that it is easier to sympathize with someone if you have something in common with that person (1739–1740/1990). This refers not only to commonalities due to similar past experiences, but also to similarities due to things such as personality, temperament and socioeconomic status because they predict overlap between the representations of the subject and object. In experiments with adult humans, subjects who witness the electric shock of an object offer to take the shocks for the object if their similarity is manipulated with demographic descriptions. If they do not feel similar, they only offer to take the shocks if they have to watch the object receive the remaining shocks (e.g. Batson *et al.*, 1981). In another paradigm, male subjects who were made to feel similar to an object who won money or was shocked showed more of a physiological response, identified with the object more, reported more distress to the shock and helped more (Krebs, 1975). Preadolescent boys imitate the actions of a model more in a war strategy game when manipulated to feel similar to the model (Rosekrans, 1967). In general, children prefer to play with children of the same age and sex (Smith, 1988) and have more empathy for objects that are the same sex (Feshbach & Roe, 1968). At the University of Iowa, subjects reported feeling the same emotion as they observed in an actor (but to a lesser degree), and the more similar they felt to the actors, the more intense ratings they gave of the actor's emotion (Preston *et al.*, 2003).

Familiarity with the object also increases empathy in the subject with the PAM for three main reasons, the first two being extensions of past experience and similarity. First, familiar individuals share past experiences, increasing the likelihood that they have representations in common. Second, people are usually closest to others of like age, gender, class and culture (e.g. Feshbach & Roe, 1968). Third, when the subject is familiar with the object, the subject has developed, over time, an internal model of the object. This model takes the form of a representation of the object in the subject, so when the subject perceives the object, this representation is activated, allowing the subject to be empathic even when the subject has not had a similar past experience. For example, a man may not share with his wife the fear of making a social blunder or the joy at fitting into a pair of jeans; however, because of their shared experience, the man can predict, understand and respond appropriately to his wife's state: he can be empathic.

Familiarity can even supplant absolute similarity, especially when emotional attachment is involved. In home tests of empathy with children, the family pet often responds with consolation to the adult feigning distress (Zahn-Waxler *et al.*, 1984). Lucy, a chimpanzee raised by a human family, is anecdotally described as exhibiting efforts to break up conflicts, running to comfort the wife when ill, exhibiting 'protectiveness toward her, bringing her food, sharing her own food, or ... attempting to comfort by stroking and grooming her' (Temerlin, 1975, p. 165). There are also anecdotal reports of apes helping unfamiliar birds and humans, sometimes even incurring great risk to do so (e.g. O'Connell, 1995). It is likely that the feeling of familiarity itself results from a facile mapping of object onto subject, which can result from overt similarity (e.g. 'I felt like I have known him all my life') or from practice mapping the object onto the subject through shared experience. This explains how a subject that is dissimilar from the object can nonetheless identify with the object, such as a human owner and its pet, a chimpanzee and its caretaker, or a babysitter with its baby charge.

23.2.4 Automatically

According to the PAM, when the subject attends to the state of the object, the relevant representations will automatically activate. As an example, if the object displays a facial expression or a body posture indicating sadness, the areas in the subject's brain that represent those movements and that feeling are automatically activated. This fact about emotion perception is most noticeable when the object's state is particularly salient to the subject, such as the jerking of a leg in a soccer fan before the big kick or the drawn facial expressions of movie-goers in an intense moment. In these cases, a brief, truncated version of the movement is produced – an 'ideo-motor action' (c.f. Carpenter, 1874; Prinz, 1987). These 'leaks' occur when the subject is particularly engrossed in the state of the object, attending to the state of the object and not attempting to control his or her reaction.

This phenomenon is the result of processes in the cerebellum and the frontal lobes. The frontal lobe normally inhibits behaviour centrally while the cerebellum inhibits behaviour peripherally (through projections to the pons where it inhibits motor neurones descending to the dorsal root ganglion). But in 'feed-forward models' (Wolpert et al., 1998), projections from the cerebellum determine if the subject's actions are executed as planned; if the expected response is not detected, an error signal is generated that reduces inhibitory processes in the frontal lobes and spinal cord. In *the subject*, this is probably adaptive because the reduced inhibition facilitates the expected action, but if the subject is instead modelling the state of *the object*, then reduced inhibition would cause the subject to enact the expected behaviour of *the object*, thus accounting for ideomotor actions. For example, if a soccer fan watches a wing run down the field toward the goal and stop, the expected action is to kick the ball toward the goal. If this action is not taken by the object, an error signal is generated in the subject, reducing motor inhibition and resulting in an actual kicking movement in the subject. Such reduced inhibition also explains large, non-functional acts that are generated when a subject is surprised, such as arms flailing and shouting.

As with the PAM itself, these concepts from motor behaviour can be applied to explain phenomena in empathy. During *direct* forms of empathy, the forward model generates in the subject a prediction regarding the affect of the object, which can out as a contagious display when inhibition is reduced. During *indirect* forms of empathy, the forward model generates a sensation for how the object must feel, even though the object is not present, and uses this information to respond appropriately. In this cognitive form of empathy, subjects could take the spatial perspective of the object (as proposed by perspective-taking models of empathy, e.g. Decety & Chaminade, 2003), but more often subjects probably just imagine themselves to be the object. In this process, the orbitofrontal cortex is needed as a 'convergence/divergence zone', to link the constructed feeling state of the object with an appropriate response (Bechara *et al.*, 2000). Disorders of empathy and functional imaging studies of empathy (discussed below) support this proposed role for the cerebellum and frontal lobes in empathy.

23.2.5 Attention

Even though activation of the subject's representations is automatic, this does not mean that one should expect to see contagious behaviour whenever a subject perceives an object. Subjects' responses are not predetermined, unavoidable, or beyond the ken of conscious will, primarily because the subject must *attend to* the state of the object; oftentimes the subject does not attend to the object fully. Because of the PAM, it is inherently distressing to attend to the distress of another, so subjects allocate attention to control the extent to which they are drawn into the object's situation. For example, people turn their heads away from the homeless man and change the channel in response to a plea for aid for impoverished children. However, even when the subject attempts to look away from the object to control his or her reaction, a covert response may still occur. For example, in orienting studies with infants, even though overt distress can be decreased by distracting the baby, distress returns to almost equal levels when the distraction is removed, and the hormonal stress response remains throughout (reviewed in Rothbart *et al.*, 1994). This internal 'distress keeper' may be the mechanism for negative feelings such as guilt and remorse that pervade even when attention is shifted. As evidence, trait sympathy is correlated with the probability for entering situations of distress and the susceptibility for guilt and shame after refusing to help (reviewed by Smith, 1992).

The cerebellum (and its interconnections with the frontal lobe) is necessary to learn and execute such attentional shifts, to track the state of the object, and to avoid attending to the object when doing so would be unnecessarily distressing. This structure is probably more necessary for more subtle events (e.g. the object darts his eyes at the mention of a sensitive topic), which require attention, tracking and processing speed involving connections between the cerebellum and the frontal eye fields; larger displays (e.g. crying and smiling) can be understood explicitly.

Despite attention, an automatic response may not be observable; the subject might not even feel it. There are degrees of emotion in the object, degrees of attention to the object and, thus, degrees of activation. Thus, the activation of the relevant representations in the subject may not be strong enough to reach the threshold for generating a response or for reaching conscious awareness. Mere comprehension of the object's state by the subject is evidence that the relevant representations were activated to a degree; this can be demonstrated with functional magnetic or PET imaging (see studies below), with EEG, MEG or TMS, and with behavioural paradigms that use reaction time. For example, in our own laboratory we have shown that people automatically process the emotion in faces (using Ekman's face stimuli), even when they are attending and responding to superimposed words. Subjects also may not exhibit a matching response to the object because of mechanisms to inhibit such responses (discussed above). The fact that these inhibitory processes develop over the course of a lifetime explains the developmental sequence of empathy from emotional contagion to mixtures of contagion and helping to 'true empathy' (Ungerer, 1990). For example, infants' attention towards and imitation of a model decreases between 2 and 6 months (Field *et al.*, 1986).

A benefit of the PAM is that it can predict when a subject will attend to the object. Subjects will attend more to salient stimuli such as loud displays of distress and releasing stimuli such as crying (Colby & Goldberg, 1999; Taylor & Stein, 1999). In my ongoing investigation into subjects' responses to the distress of patients with chronic or terminal illness, subjects' responses bifurcate at the highest levels of distress. Half of the subjects report empathy levels that increase linearly with the level of distress of the patient, while the other half report empathy levels that drop off at the highest levels of distress (Preston, 2004b). The latter subjects may decrease responding because they are overwhelmed and thus divert attention away from the films or because they perceive the patient's display of distress to be disproportional to the need (i.e. 'neediness'). Subjects tend to offer more help when the level of need or potential benefit to the object is higher (e.g. Staub & Baer, 1974), so they may not feel empathic towards objects who do not appear to have a legitimate need. A current fMRI study is investigating this further (Neo *et al.*, 2006).

Because of the shared representations of perception and action in the PAM, subjects are predicted to attend to objects that require a response. In group-living species, objects who require a response are those that the subject relies upon to attain personal goals, usually friends and relatives. This interdependence can be temporary and superficial, like when the subject and object must cooperate for a local goal or when the object's distress blocks a goal of the subject. For example, human children are more motivated to help when they have a responsibility for the object's distress (Chapman *et al.*, 1987) and monkeys that are trained to cooperate for food dramatically increase conciliation (Cords & Thurnheer, 1993). Interdependence can also be long lasting and deep, for example the interdependence of family members or spouses who must cooperate for long-term goals spanning a lifetime. For example, species with cooperative kin relationships show higher levels of reconciliation between related individuals than non-related individuals (e.g. Aureli *et al.*, 1992) and in chimpanzees, where male alliances are very important, reconciliation is higher among males than among females (e.g. de Waal, 1986). In general, the more interdependent the subject and object, the more the subject will attend to the object, the more their similar representations will be activated, and the more likely a response.

Once the subject attends to the state of the object, emotion-perception areas such as the limbic system will be activated. The amygdala projects directly to brainstem areas that control autonomic states and code for learned emotional associations, and projects indirectly to hypothalamic nuclei that control endocrine responses and maintain homeostasis. The limbic circuit also projects to the cingulate cortex, which stores representations of affective states, and to the orbitofrontal cortex, which helps regulate emotion (preventing overarousal), links the event to stored representations in long-term memory and generates an adaptive response (Bechara *et al.*, 1994).

Most of the examples in this chapter are for negative emotional states such as distress, and indeed distress is the typical emotion of the object when the term empathy is used colloquially or in the literature. However, the model also applies to positive emotions and is likely to be particularly apparent in emotions such as joy and excitement. It is often postulated that negative emotions are more biologically relevant because they are more crucial for survival (e.g. Adolphs *et al.*, 1995; Ekman *et al.*, 1983), as in the proverbial case of the man running from the tiger in the savannah. This is unlikely to be the case since positive reward states associated with eating, mating and care of offspring are at least as important for survival as the fear of predators. However, these positive states are usually classified as drive states or motivations rather than emotions and so have not entered the dialogue into positive emotions although they surely qualify. Another possible reason why the literature focuses on negative states is that neuroscientific research often studies animals and it is considered more difficult to research the origins of positive emotions in animals. However, this is probably only true for more abstract positive emotions (which are also difficult to study in humans) and positive emotions such as excitement are palpable in many animal displays, for example the pacing of rats before a food reward or the jumping of sled dogs before a race. According to the PAM, negative states are not actually more entrenched or easy to study, but they are more salient to researchers because they require a response. Distress requires alleviation and psychological disorders require a cure, but joy is a state for which we should just be grateful. Cross-cultural research is needed to determine whether our focus on eliminating negative states rather than preventing them or striving for positive states is a product of the nervous system or is just a characteristic of Western culture.

23.3 Recent neuroscientific evidence

Recent imaging research supports the PAM because evidence supports the existence of shared representations for perception and production of emotional states and the exact structures engaged depend on the type of task. Tasks where the subjects must observe the emotional state of the object such as pictures of basic emotions (Carr *et al.*, 2003), videos of actors telling sad stories (Decety & Chaminade, 2003), visual cues that a loved one is in pain (Singer *et al.*, 2004), videos of objects displaying disgust (Wicker *et al.*, 2003a) and pictures of an object's bodily state of fear (de Gelder *et al.*, 2004) engage areas known to be related to the representation of one's own feeling state such as the anterior insula and cingulate cortex. Supporting the PAM, experiencing pain and being cued that another is experiencing pain both activate the anterior insula, rostral anterior cingulate, brainstem and cerebellum, and the activation in the insula and cingulate correlates with trait empathy. When subjects view static pictures of body postures during neutral gestures versus gestures of fear and happiness, the emotion-representation areas are activated (orbitofrontal cortex, posterior cingulate, anterior insula, nucleus accumbens, amygdala) as well as areas that represent action [inferior frontal gyrus, the supplementary motor area (SMA), inferior parietal lobule, precentral gyrus] (de Gelder *et al.*, 2004). The authors interpreted the motor activation as evidence for response preparation to a fearful stimulus, but more research is required to separate matching or imitative activation of the object from activation related to the subject's response. For example, the activation in this study was in pre-SMA and previous research found anterior SMA activity to be associated with grasp observation and imitation and posterior SMA activity with grasp performance (Grafton *et al.*, 1996a). Tasks where the subject must take the perspective of the object have found consistent engagement of right inferior parietal (thought to suppress the subject's own perspective) and medial prefrontal and frontal pole (thought to inhibit the subject's self-processes) (Decety & Chaminade, 2003; Decety *et al.*, 2002; Ruby & Decety, 2001). In a task where objects directed their emotion toward the subject (as opposed to away from the subject), the anterior portion of the superior temporal lobe was selectively activated (Wicker *et al.*, 2003b). Observation of an object being touched activates the secondary sensory area (SII), the brain area that represents the sensation of touch (Keysers *et al.*, 2004).

In our own investigation of cognitive empathy (Preston *et al.*, 2002), subjects imagined events of fear or anger either from their own past or from the past of another subject (to which they could relate or not). There were no differences in activation or arousal between personal and empathic imagery when the subject *could* relate to the situation of the object, presumably because subjects simply activated their own existing representations. However, when the subject *could not* relate to the situation of the object, there was less autonomic arousal and more neural activation in the left fusiform gyrus and the left cerebellum, presumably because they did not have a similar representation and had to create an image online by activating high-level visual association cortex and posterio-lateral cerebellum, which is more associated with imagined movement (though usually on the right; Allen *et al.*, 1997; Grafton *et al.*, 1996b; Hanakawa *et al.*, 2003). This same portion of the cerebellum was activated in the Singer *et al.* study (2004) both when subjects experienced pain and were cued to the pain of a loved one. Taken together, the results support the idea that empathy is a distributed process that recruits different brain structures depending on the nature of the task, rather than localized to a single location in the brain, such as the right prefrontal cortex (c.f., Gallup & Platek, 2002).

Not all brain areas are in common between perception and action or between perception and imagination. For example, performing, imagining and observing a grasping movement all activate SMA, but performing activates the caudal portion of SMA-proper while imagining (and to a lesser extent, observing) activates the rostral portion of SMA-proper. The anterior cerebellar cortex is active for performing, while different portions of the right posterior cerebellum are active for imagining and observing. Effects are often seen in hemispheric differences, such as the activation of dorsal premotor cortex on the right for observation and the left for imagination (Grafton *et al.*, 1996a). Similarly, experiencing pain and imagining the pain of another both activate areas that represent the affective quality of the pain stimulus such as the anterior insular cortex and the rostral anterior cingulate cortex. In contrast, only experiencing pain directly activated the areas that represent the sensory quality of the pain stimulus such as the posterior insula, caudal anterior cingulate cortex, SII and SI (Singer *et al.*, 2004). These shifts in location within a brain area or non-overlapping activations between perception and action are to be expected because, after all, different qualitative experiences cannot occur without some different biological substrates, but the PAM is bolstered by findings of overlap in the representations.

23.4 Disorders of empathy

Empathy disorders are characterized by impairments in the conception of mental states, expression of emotions and verbalization of feeling states due to dysfunction in the brain areas that subserve empathy (c.f., Baron-Cohen, 1993). Because the PAM characterizes empathy as a process with multiple necessary phases, it can account for disorders of empathy that have different aetiologies. In order to achieve empathy, subjects must be motivated to and capable of attending to the state of the object, they must be able to activate personal representations of a similar state, and to generate an emotional response. Thus impairment in any of these phases will create an impairment of empathy.

23.4.1 Autism

Individuals with autism show impairments in expression, imitation and recognition of expressions and gestures, making it likely that autism is characterized by an impairment early on in the perception-action pathway, such as in attending to the relevant stimuli in order to perceive and learn from the emotional states of others (see also Williams *et al.*, 2001). There is also evidence for impairment in autism in multiple brain areas including the frontal lobe, amygdala and cerebellum (Harris *et al.*, 1999).

23.4.2 Psychopathy

Individuals with psychopathy do not generate appropriate psychophysiological responses to emotional stimuli (Blair, 1999; Blair *et al.*, 1997). Thus, in the context of the PAM, these people have an impairment of empathy because they cannot link the distress of the object to their own feeling states. There is reduced prefrontal grey matter in men with psychopathy compared to multiple control groups and the individuals with smaller volumes also have reduced skin conductance responses on a social stressor (Raine *et al.*, 2000). Individuals with psychopathy also have abnormalities in the corpus callosum (Raine *et al.*, 2003), amygdala (Blair & Frith, 2000), anterior temporal lobe and lateral frontal lobe, and in functional imaging studies, there are differences in activation in multiple brain areas suggesting that psychopaths process emotional as well as non-emotional stimuli differently than controls (Kiehl, 2000; Kiehl *et al.*, 2004).

23.4.3 Frontal lobe damage

The frontal lobes are often implicated in disorders of empathy for multiple reasons. Theoretically, the frontal lobes are thought necessary to focus on the state of the object, to link the object's state to the subject's own feeling states and memories, and to inhibit contagious and imitative responses. There are documented impairments in empathy in subjects with acquired damage to the frontal lobes (Eslinger, 1998) and individuals with early, developmental damage to the frontal lobe have a syndrome that presents similarly to psychopathy with decision-making problems and emotional insensitivity (Anderson *et al.*, 1999). Empathy impairments in sociopathy as well as autism are thought to be partially due to a disruption in the prefrontal system because both disorders have abnormalities in the frontal lobes (above) and involve deficiencies in planning, attention and inhibition (e.g. Gillberg, 1999). Even if frontal patients may imitate the object's actions (Lhermitte *et al.*, 1986) they cannot share in the state of the object because they can no longer link the state of the object to the representations of feelings and, thus, cannot experience empathy.

The fact that the frontal lobes are necessary for empathy does not mean that it is a putative 'empathy area' since many other areas are activated in functional imaging studies of empathy and are damaged in disorders of empathy (e.g. cerebellum). Moreover, the effect of brain abnormalities on empathy depends on an interaction between location and the time of damage. For example, early damage to the amygdala would preclude the development of appropriate emotional responses while late damage to the amygdala would prevent new emotional experiences from being processed, but would leave cortical representations intact and accessible through frontal connections (e.g. LeDoux, 1996/1998).

23.4.4 Depression

The PAM predicts that individuals with depression would have an empathy impairment due to an excessive focus on the self, precluding the necessary interest in and attention to the state of the object. There seems to be a paucity of research on this topic – the majority of research is aimed at using empathy to *help* individuals with depression, or looks at effects of maternal depression on empathy in offspring. An inverse relationship between empathy and depression has been supported (Andersen, 2001), but surprisingly, multiple investigations have also found positive relationships between empathy and depression (Forgus, 1995; Gawronski & Privette, 1997; Horne, 1999; McLaughlin, 1996; O'Connor *et al.*, 2002; Zahn-Waxler *et al.*, 1991). Discrepancies are both theoretical and definitional. Theoretically, empathy and depression may be inversely correlated within an individual, but it is thought that some exposure to maternal depression may sensitize children to the emotions of others, making them more empathic (but see Jones *et al.*, 2000). Effects also depend on the type of depression and the type of empathy because while major depression may decrease the likelihood of empathy, it increases the likelihood of empathic distress (O'Connor *et al.*, 2002). Cognitive empathy decreases the chances of reactive depression in caregivers while emotional empathy increases the chances (Gawronski & Privette, 1997). Faced with a depressed parent, children who were actively empathic were less depressed while those who were emotionally overinvolved were more depressed (Solantaus-Simula *et al.*, 2002).

The different relationships found in these studies point to the importance of a non-linear relationship between arousal and empathy, with the highest levels of empathy occurring at intermediate levels of arousal. Eisenberg and colleagues have repeatedly found that empathy is best predicted by the combination of high emotionality and high emotional regulation because subjects without the ability to regulate emotion tend to become personally distressed and thus self-focused in the face of the object's distress (Eisenberg *et al.*, 1998).

23.5 Summary

The perception-action model of empathy was originally based on the shared representations of perception and action in motor behaviour, because such shared representations could easily explain how a subject could come to feel the emotional state of an object. Much behavioural evidence in empathy, in humans and animals, points to the fact that subjects use their own representations in order to understand and feel the state of the object, such as increases in empathy with shared past experiences, similarity and familiarity. Since the model was conceived, additional neuroscientific evidence for the PAM has emerged, demonstrating that the neural substrates for experiencing an emotion overlap with the substrates for perceiving that emotion. Evidence from neuroscience as well as from disorders of empathy support the PAM because appropriate empathic responding requires a distributed neural circuit that allows for all phases of the empathic process. The subject must be able to attend to the object, experience a similar emotional state as the object, and respond appropriately to the object all while inhibiting contagious distress and maintaining focus on the object. If the integrity of any of these processes is undermined, so is the subject's ability to empathize.

There are still many things to discover about empathy. For example, it is currently unknown if there are qualitative differences between empathy for positive and negative states or between empathizing in order to help a loved one versus hurt an enemy. We also need to distinguish among the various models and types of empathy such as between descriptions where the subject imagines he or she *is* the object versus imagines what it would be like to *be* the object. The neurosciences also need to make tests of shared-representation theories more falsifiable and to contrast among empathic states rather than between empathic and neutral states. Tools with good temporal resolution (EEG, MEG, event-related fMRI) should also be used to look at changes over the time-course of the empathic process. For example, the initial process of effortfully trying to empathize can be compared with the subsequent feeling of empathy or the initial process of resonating *with* the object can be compared with the subsequent response *to* the object. There is much work to be done, but by employing strong inference to resolve specific questions in the literature, agreement can be reached.

REFERENCES

Adolphs, R., Tranel, D., Damasio, H., & Damasio, A. R. (1995). Fear and the human amygdala. *Journal of Neuroscience*, **15(9)**, 5879–5891.

Allen, G., Buxton, R. B., Wong, E. C., & Courchesne, E. (1997). Attentional activation of the cerebellum independent of motor involvement. *Science*, **275(5308)**, 1940–1943.

Allport, A. (1987). Selection for action: some behavioral and neurophysiological considerations of attention and action. In H. Heuer, & A. F. Sanders (eds.), *Perspectives on Perception and Action* (pp. 395–419). Mahwah, N.J.: Lawrence Erlbaum Associates, Inc.

Andersen, D. T. (2001). Empathy, attachment, mediation, and mental health. *Dissertation Abstracts International: Section B: The Sciences & Engineering*, **61(10–B)**, 5549.

Anderson, S. W., Bechara, A., Damasio, H., Tranel, D., & Damasio, A. R. (1999). Impairment of social and moral behavior related to early damage in human prefrontal cortex. *Nature Neuroscience*, **2(11)**, 1032–1037.

Aureli, F., Das, M., & Veenema, H. C. (1992). Interspecific differences in the effect of kinship on reconciliation frequency in macaques. Abstracts of the 30th Annual Meeting of the Animal Behavior Society, 5.

Barnett, M. A., & McCoy, S. J. (1989). The relation of distressful childhood experiences and empathy in college undergraduates. *The Journal of Genetic Psychology; Child Behavior, Animal Behavior, and Comparative Psychology*, **150(4)**, 417–426.

Baron-Cohen, S. (1993). From attention-goal psychology to belief-desire psychology: the development of a theory of mind and its dysfunction. In S. Baron-Cohen, H. Tager-Flusberg, & D. Cohen (eds.), *Understanding Other Minds: Perspectives from Autism* (pp. 59–82). Oxford: Oxford University Press.

Batson, C. D. (1997). Self-other merging and the empathy-altruism hypothesis: reply to Neuberg *et al.* (1997). *Journal of Personality and Social Psychology*, **73(3)**, 517–522.

Batson, C. D., Duncan, B. D., Ackerman, P., Buckley, T., & Birch, K. (1981). Is empathic emotion a source of altruistic motivation? *Journal of Personality and Social Psychology*, **40(2)**, 290–302.

Bechara, A., Damasio, H., & Damasio, A. R. (2000). Emotion, decision making and the orbito-frontal cortex. *Cerebral Cortex*, **10(3)**, 295–307.

Bechara, A., Damasio, A. R., Damasio, H., & Anderson, S. W. (1994). Insensitivity to future consequences following damage to human prefrontal cortex. *Cognition*, **50(1–3)**, 7–15.

Blair, J., & Frith, U. (2000). Neurocognitive explanations of the antisocial personality disorders. *Criminal Behaviour & Mental Health*, **10**, S66–S81.

Blair, R. J. R. (1999). Psychophysiological responsiveness to the distress of others in children with autism. *Personality & Individual Differences*, **26(3)**, 477–485.

Blair, R. J. R., Jones, L., Clark, F., & Smith, M. (1997). The psychopathic individual: a lack of responsiveness to distress cues? *Psychophysiology*, **34(2)**, 192–198.

Carpenter, W. B. (1874). *Principles of Mental Physiology, with their Applications to the Training and Discipline of the Mind and the Study of its Morbid Conditions*. New York: Appleton.

Carr, L., Iacoboni, M., Dubeau, M. C., Mazziotta, J. C., & Lenzi, G. L. (2003). Neural mechanisms of empathy in humans: a relay from neural systems for imitation to limbic areas. *Proceedings from the National Academy of Sciences of the USA*, **100(9)**, 5497–5502.

Cesaroni, L., & Garber, M. (1991). Exploring the experience of autism through firsthand accounts. *Journal of Autism & Developmental Disorders*, **21(3)**, 303–313.

Chapman, M., Zahn-Waxler, C., Cooperman, G., & Iannotti, R. (1987). Empathy and responsibility in the motivation of children's helping. *Developmental Psychology*, **23(1)**, 140–145.

Colby, C. L., & Goldberg, M. E. (1999). Space and attention in parietal cortex. *Annual Review of Neuroscience*, **22**, 319–349.

Cords, M., & Thurnheer, S. (1993). Reconciling with valuable partners by long-tailed macaques. *Ethology*, **93**, 315–325.

de Gelder, B., Snyder, J., Greve, D., Gerard, G., & Hadjikhani, N. (2004). Fear fosters flight: a mechanism for fear contagion when perceiving emotion expressed by a whole body. *Proceedings of the National Academy of Sciences*, **101(47)**, 16701–16706.

de Waal, F. B. M. (1986). Integration of dominance and social bonding in primates. *Quarterly Review of Biology*, **61**, 459–479.

Decety, J., & Chaminade, T. (2003). Neural correlates of feeling sympathy. *Neuropsychologia*, **41(2)**, 127–138.

Decety, J., Chaminade, T., Grèzes, J., & Meltzoff, A. N. (2002). A PET exploration of the neural mechanisms involved in reciprocal imitation. *NeuroImage*, **15**, 265–272.

Decety, J., Grezes, J., Costes, N., *et al.* (1997). Brain activity during observation of actions: influence of action content and subject's strategy. *Brain*, **120(10)**, 1763–1777.

di Pellegrino, G., Fadiga, L., Fogassi, L., Gallese, V., & Rizzolatti, G. (1992). Understanding motor events: a neurophysiological study. *Experimental Brain Research*, **91**, 176–180.

Eisenberg, N., & Strayer, J. (eds.). (1987). *Empathy and its Development*. New York: Cambridge University Press.

Eisenberg, N., Wentzel, M., & Harris, J. D. (1998). The role of emotionality and regulation in empathy-related responding. *School Psychology Review*, **27(4)**, 506–521.

Ekman, P., Levenson, R. W., & Friesen, W. V. (1983). Autonomic nervous system activity distinguishes among emotions. *Science*, **221(4616)**, 1208–1210.

Eslinger, P. J. (1998). Neurological and neuropsychological bases of empathy. *European Neurology*, **39(4)**, 193–199.

Feshbach, N. D., & Roe, K. (1968). Empathy in six- and seven-year-olds. *Child Development*, **39(1)**, 133–145.

Field, T., Goldstein, S., Vega-Lahr, N., & Porter, K. (1986). Changes in imitative behavior during early infancy. *Infant Behavior & Development*, **9(4)**, 415–421.

Forgus, J. K. (1995). Empathy and prosocial behaviour in young children. *Dissertation Abstracts International: Section B: The Sciences & Engineering*, **55(10–B)**, 4621.

Gallup, G. G. J., & Platek, S. M. (2002). Cognitive empathy presupposes self-awareness: evidence from phylogeny, ontogeny, neuropsychology and mental illness. *Behavioral and Brain Sciences*, **25(1)**, 36–37.

Gawronski, I., & Privette, G. (1997). Empathy and reactive depression. *Psychological Reports*, **80(3, Pt 1)**, 1043–1049.

Gillberg, C. (1999). Neurodevelopmental processes and psychological functioning in autism. *Development & Psychopathology*, **11(3)**, 567–587.

Grafton, S. T., Arbib, M. A., Fadiga, L., & Rizzolatti, G. (1996a). Localization of grasp representations in humans by positron emission tomography: observation compared with imagination. *Experimental Brain Research*, **112(1)**, 103–111.

Grafton, S. T., Fadiga, L., Arbib, M. A., & Rizzolatti, G. (1997). Premotor cortex activation during observation and naming of familiar tools. *Neuroimage*, **6**, 231–236.

Grafton, S. T., Fagg, A. H., Woods, R. P., & Arbib, M. A. (1996b). Functional anatomy of pointing and grasping in humans. *Cerebral Cortex*, **6(2)**, 226–237.

Hanakawa, T., Immisch, I., Toma, K., *et al.* (2003). Functional properties of brain areas associated with motor execution and imagery. *Journal of Neurophysiology*, **89**, 989–1002.

Harris, N. S., Courchesne, E., Townsend, J., Carper, R. A., & Lord, C. (1999). Neuroanatomic contributions to slowed orienting of attention in children with autism. *Cognitive Brain Research*, **8**, 61–71.

Horne, S. G. (1999). The role of parental narcissism and depression in predicting adolescent empathy, narcissism, self-esteem, pleasing others, and peer conflict. *Dissertation Abstracts International Section A: Humanities & Social Sciences*, **59(10–A)**, 3745.

Hume, D. (1739–1740/1990). *A Treatise of Human Nature* (7th impression of 2nd edn.). Oxford: Clarendon Press.

Iacoboni, M., Woods, R. P., Brass, M., *et al.* (1999). Cortical mechanisms of imitation. *Science*, **286**, 2526–2528.

Jeannerod, M., & Frak, V. (1999). Mental imaging of motor activity in humans. *Current Opinion in Neurobiology*, **9(6)**, 735–739.

Jones, N. A., Field, T., & Davalos, M. (2000). Right frontal EEG asymmetry and lack of empathy in preschool children of depressed mothers. *Child Psychiatry & Human Development*, **30(3)**, 189–204.

Keysers, C., Wicker, B., Gazzola, V., *et al.* (2004). A touching sight: SII/PV activation during the observation and experience of touch. *Neuron*, **42**, 335–346.

Kiehl, K. A. (2000). A neuroimaging investigation of affective, cognitive, and language functions in psychopathy. Unpublished Dissertation, University of British Columbia, Vancouver.

Kiehl, K. A., Smith, A. M., Mendrek, A., *et al.* (2004). Temporal lobe abnormalities in semantic processing by criminal psychopaths as revealed by functional magnetic resonance imaging. *Psychiatry Research: Neuroimaging*, **130(1)**, 27–42.

Krebs, D. (1975). Empathy and altruism. *Journal of Personality and Social Psychology*, **32**, 1134–1146.

LeDoux, J. E. (1996/1998). *The Emotional Brain: The Mysterious Underpinnings of Emotional Life* (1st Touchstone edn.). New York: Touchstone/Simon & Schuster.

Levenson, R. W., & Reuf, A. M. (1992). Empathy: a physiological substrate. *Journal of Personality and Social Psychology*, **63(2)**, 234–246.

Lhermitte, F., Pillon, B., & Serdaru, M. (1986). Human autonomy and the frontal lobes: Part I. Imitation and utilization behavior: a neuropsychological study of 75 patients. *Annals of Neurology*, **19**(4), 326–334.

Lipps, T. (1903). Einfühlung, innere Nachahmung und Organempfindung. *Archiv für die Gesamte Psychologie*, **1**, 465–519.

McClelland, J. L., & Rumelhart, D. E. (1985). Distributed memory and the representation of general and specific information. *Journal of Experimental Psychology: General*, **114**(2), 159–188.

McLaughlin, K. P. (1996). High-risk binge eating and drug use among secondary and university students on measures of empathy, intimacy, body image, alexithymia, depression and family environment. *Dissertation Abstracts International: Section B: The Sciences & Engineering*, **56**(9–B), 5177.

Merleau-Ponty, M. (1962/1970). *Phenomenology of Perception*, 5th edn. London/New York: Routledge & Kegan Paul/The Humanities Press.

Mitchell, R. W., Thompson, N. S., & Miles, H. L. (eds.). (1997). *Anthropomorphism, Anecdotes, and Animals*. New York: State University of New York Press.

Neo, W. S., Grabowski, T. J., Magnotta, V. A., *et al.* (2006). The neural correlates of empathy and helping: responses to patient accounts of serious illness. *Journal of Cognitive Neuroscience*. April Supplement, **180**.

O'Connell, S. M. (1995). Empathy in chimpanzees: evidence for theory of mind? *Primates*, **36**(3), 397–410.

O'Connor, L. E., Berry, J. W., Weiss, J., & Gilbert, P. (2002). Guilt, fear, submission, and empathy in depression. *Journal of Affective Disorders*, **71**(1–3), 19–27.

Povinelli, D. J., Nelson, K. E., & Boysen, S. T. (1992). Comprehension of role reversal in chimpanzees: evidence of empathy? *Animal Behaviour*, **43**(4), 633–640.

Preston, S. D. (2004a). Empathy. In M. Bekoff (ed.), *Encyclopedia of Animal Behavior*. Westport, Conn.: Greenwood Publishing Group.

Preston, S. D. (2004b). *The Physiology of Love: Empathic Responding to Emotional Reactions*. Paper presented at the Compassionate Love Research Conference, 21–23 May, Washington, D.C.

Preston, S. D., Bechara, A., Damasio, H., & Damasio, A. (2003). *The Substrates of Emapthy: Behavioral and Psychophysiological Responses to Emotional Social Interactions*. Paper presented at the Cognitive Neuroscience Society, New York, N.Y.

Preston, S. D., Bechara, A., Grabowski, T. J., Damasio, H., & Damasio, A. R. (2002). Functional anatomy of emotional imagery: positron emission tomography of personal and hypothetical experiences. *Journal of Cognitive Neuroscience* (April Supplement), 126.

Preston, S. D., & de Waal, F. B. M. (2002a). The communication of emotions and the possibility of empathy in animals. In S. Post, L. G. Underwood, J. P. Schloss, & W. B. Hurlburt (eds.), *Altrusim and Altruistic Love: Science, Philosophy, and Religion in Dialogue* (pp. 284–308). Oxford: Oxford University Press.

Preston, S. D., & de Waal, F. B. M. (2002b). Empathy: its ultimate and proximate bases. *Behavioral and Brain Sciences*, **25**(1), 1–71.

Prinz, W. (1987). Ideo-motor action. In H. Heuer, & A. F. Sanders (eds.), *Perspectives on Perception and Action* (pp. 47–76). Hillsdale, N.J.: Lawrence Erlbaum Associates, Inc.

Prinz, W. (1992). Why don't we perceive our brain states? *European Journal of Cognitive Psychology*, **4(1)**, 1–20.

Raine, A., Lencz, T., Bihrle, S., LaCasse, L., & Colletti, P. (2000). Reduced prefrontal gray matter volume and reduced autonomic activity in antisocial personality disorder. *Archives of General Psychiatry*, **57(2)**, 119–127.

Raine, A., Lencz, T., Taylor, K., *et al.* (2003). Corpus callosum abnormalities in psychopathic antisocial individuals. *Archives of General Psychiatry*, **60(11)**, 1134–1142.

Rosekrans, M. A. (1967). Imitation in children as a function of perceived similarity to a social model and vicarious reinforcement. *Journal of Personality and Social Psychology*, **7(3)**, 307–315.

Rothbart, M. K., Posner, M. I., & Rosicky, J. (1994). Orienting in normal and pathological development. *Development and Psychopathology*, **6**, 635–652.

Ruby, P., & Decety, J. (2001). Effect of subjective perspective taking during simulation of action: a PET investigation of agency. *Nature Neuroscience*, **4(5)**, 546–550.

Singer, T., Seymour, B., O'Doherty, J., *et al.* (2004). Empathy for pain involves the affective but not sensory components of pain. *Science*, **303**, 1157–1162.

Smith, K. D. (1992). Trait sympathy and perceived control as predictors of entering sympathy-arousing situations. *Personality and Social Psychology Bulletin*, **18(2)**, 207–216.

Smith, P. K. (1988). The cognitive demands of children's social interactions with peers. In R. W. Byrne, & A. Whiten (eds.), *Machiavellian Intelligence: Social Expertise and the Evolution of Intellect in Monkeys, Apes, and Humans*. Oxford/New York: Clarendon Press/Oxford University Press.

Solantaus-Simula, T., Punamaeki, R.-L., & Beardslee, W. R. (2002). Children's responses to low parental mood: I. Balancing between active empathy, overinvolvement, indifference and avoidance. *Journal of the American Academy of Child & Adolescent Psychiatry*, **41(3)**, 278–286.

Staub, E., & Baer, R. S. (1974). Stimulus characteristics of a sufferer and difficulty of escape as determinants of helping. *Journal of Personality & Social Psychology*, **30(2)**, 279–284.

Steinbeck, J. (1952/2002). *East of Eden* (John Steinbeck Centennial edition). New York: Penguin Books.

Taylor, K., & Stein, J. (1999). Attention, intention and salience in the posterior parietal cortex. *Neurocomputing: An International Journal*, **26**, 901–910.

Temerlin, M. K. (1975). *Lucy: Growing up Human*. Palo Alto, Calif.: Science and Behavior Books.

Turvey, M. T. (1992). Ecological foundations of cognition: invariants of perception and action. In H. L. J. Pick, P. W. van den Broek, & D. C. Knill (eds.), *Cognition: Conceptual and Methodological Issues* (Vol. xiv) (pp. 85–117). Washington, D.C.: American Psychological Association.

Ungerer, J. A. (1990). The early development of empathy: self-regulation and individual differences in the first year. *Motivation and Emotion*, **14(2)**, 93–106.

Wicker, B., Keysers, C., Plailly, J., *et al.* (2003a). Both of us disgusted in *my* insula: the common neural basis of seeing and feeling disgust. *Neuron*, **40**, 655–664.

Wicker, B., Perrett, D. I., Baron-Cohen, S., & Decety, J. (2003b). Being the target of another's emotion: A PET study. *Neuropsychologia*, **41(2)**, 139–146.

Williams, J. H. G., Whiten, A., Suddendorf, T., & Perrett, D. I. (2001). Imitation, mirror neurons and autism. *Neuroscience & Biobehavioral Reviews*, **25**(4), 287–295.

Wispé, L. (1986). The distinction between sympathy and empathy: to call forth a concept, a word is needed. *Journal of Personality & Social Psychology*, **50**(2), 314–321.

Wolpert, D. M., Mial, R. C., & Kawato, M. (1998). Internal models in the cerebellum. *Trends in the Cognitive Sciences*, **2**, 338–347.

Zahn-Waxler, C., Cole, P. M., & Barrett, K. C. (1991). Guilt and empathy: sex differences and implications for the development of depression. In J. Garber, & K. A. Dodge (eds.), *The Development of Emotion Regulation and Dysregulation* (Vol. xii) (pp. 243–272). New York: Cambridge University Press.

Zahn-Waxler, C., Hollenbeck, B., & Radke-Yarrow, M. (1984). The origins of empathy and altruism. In M. W. Fox, & L. D. Mickley (eds.), *Advances in Animal Welfare Science* (pp. 21–39). Washington, D. C.: Humane Society of the United States.

The Shared Manifold Hypothesis: embodied simulation and its role in empathy and social cognition

Vittorio Gallese

Dipartimento dü Neuroscienze – Sezione di Fisiologia, Universita' di Parma

24.1 Introduction

Our social mental skills enable us to successfully retrieve the mental contents of others. Sometimes we misrepresent them, henceforth misunderstanding others. Most of the time, though, we are pretty good at understanding what is the goal of others' behaviour, why the goal was set, and on the basis of which previous elements it was set as such. We are doing it effortlessly and continuously during our daily social interactions. How is that accomplished? The dominant view in cognitive science is to put most efforts into clarifying the formal rules structuring a solipsistic mind. Much less investigated is what triggers the sense of social identity that we experience with the multiplicity of 'other selves' populating our social world. Is the solipsistic type of analysis inspired by folk-psychology the best explanatory approach? In particular, is it doing full justice to the phenomenal aspects of our social intentional relations?

As human beings, we do not only mentally entertain an 'objective' account of the behaviours constituting the social world in which we live. Beyond phenomenally experiencing the external, objective nature of an observed action, and viewing it as something displayed and acted by an external biological object with distinct qualities, we also experience its goal-directedness or intentional character, similarly to when we experience ourselves as the willful conscious agents of our ongoing behaviour. From a first-person perspective, our dynamic social environment appears being populated by volitional agents capable of entertaining, similarly to us, an agentive intentional relation to the world. We experience ourselves as being 'intentionally attuned' to other individuals. This 'intentional attunement' allows us to experience others as *directed* to certain target states or objects, similarly to how we experience ourselves when doing so.

Empathy in Mental Illness, eds. Tom F. D. Farrow and Peter W. R. Woodruff. Published by Cambridge University Press. © Cambridge University Press 2007.

The same dual perspective is at work when witnessing the emotions and sensations experienced by others. We can provide an 'objective' description of these emotions or sensations. When explicitly asked to recognize, discriminate, parameterize, or categorize the emotions or sensations displayed by others, we exert our cognitive operations by adopting a third-person perspective, aimed exactly at *objectifying* the content of our perceptions. The overall goal of these cognitive operations is the deliberate categorization of an external state of affairs.

Though, when we are involved online with social transactions, we experience a totally different attitude toward the objects of our social perceptions. There is actually a shift of the object of our intentional relation. We are no longer directed to the content of a perception in order to categorize it. We are just *attuned to the intentional relation displayed by someone else*. At odds with Mr. Spock, the famous character of the Star Trek saga, our social mental skills are not confined to a declarative third-person perspective. We are not alienated from the actions, emotions and sensations of others, because we entertain a much richer and affectively nuanced perspective of what other individuals do, experience and feel. What makes this possible is the fact that *we own* those same actions, emotions and sensations.

To naturalize social intentionality we should therefore follow an alternative route. The alternative strategy I suggest here is a bottom-up characterization of the non-declarative and non-propositional contents of social cognition. It consists of investigating the neural basis of our capacity to be attuned to the intentions of others. By means of *intentional attunement*, 'the other' is much more than a different representational system; it becomes a *person*, like us. The advantage of this epistemological approach is that it generates predictions about the intrinsic functional nature of our social cognitive operations that cut across, and neither necessarily depend on, nor are subordinate to any specific cognitive mind ontology, folk psychology included.

Neuroscientific research has unveiled the neural mechanisms mediating between the personal experiential knowledge we hold of our lived body, and the implicit certainties we simultaneously hold about others' experiences. Such personal body-related experiential knowledge enables our intentional attunement with others, which in turn constitutes a shared manifold of intersubjectivity. This we-centric space allows us to directly experience the meaning of the actions performed by others, and to decode the emotions and sensations they experience. An implicit form of 'experiential understanding' is achieved by modelling the behaviour of other individuals as intentional experiences on the basis of the equivalence between what the others do and feel and what we do and feel. This modelling mechanism is embodied simulation. Mirror neurones are likely the neural correlate of this mechanism.

The paper will be structured as follows. After having clarified the sense and the use made here of the notion of embodied simulation, recent neuroscientific results are presented on how the execution of actions and their observation when executed by others are neurally mapped. The second part focuses on the first- and third-person experience of emotions and sensations, and their neural underpinnings. I show that the same neural circuits involved in the first-person experience of emotions and sensations are also active when witnessing the same emotions and sensations of others. It will be concluded that the functional mechanism at the basis of the double activation pattern of those neural circuits is embodied simulation.

In the last part of the paper I discuss the possible relevance of my approach to psychopathology, with a particular emphasis on schizophrenia and autism.

24.2 Embodied simulation

The notion of simulation is at present employed in many different domains, often with different, not necessarily overlapping, meanings. Simulation is a functional process possessing a certain content, typically focusing on possible states of its target object. For example, an authoritative view on motor control characterizes simulation as the mechanism employed by forward models to predict the sensory consequences of impending actions. According to this view, the predicted consequences are the simulated ones.

In philosophy of mind, on the other hand, the notion of simulation has been used by the proponents of Simulation Theory of mind reading to characterize the pretend state adopted by the attributer in order to understand others' behavior (see Goldman, 1989, 1992a, b, 1993a, b, 2000; Gordon, 1986, 1995, 1996, 2005).

The Oxford English Dictionary provides three different definitions of 'simulation':
1. The action or practice of simulating, with intent to deceive; false pretence, deceitful profession.
2. A false assumption or display, a surface resemblance or imitation, of something.
3. The technique of imitating the behaviour of some situation or process (whether economic, military, mechanical, etc.) by means of a suitably analogous situation or apparatus, esp. for the purpose of study or personnel training.

The first two definitions convey the idea of simulation as something fake, something supposedly aimed to deceive, by *pretending to be similar* to what really differs under many respects. The third definition conveys a different meaning; namely, it characterizes simulation as a process meant to produce a better understanding of a given situation or state of affairs, by means of modelling it.

The third definition of simulation appears to be closer than the previous ones to the etymology of the word. Indeed 'to simulate' comes from the Latin *simulare*, which in turn derives from *similis*, which means 'like', 'similar to'. The third definition of simulation, incidentally, also defines the prevalent epistemic approach of the classic Greek–Roman western world: knowledge is conceived of as a process in which the knower *assimilates* what he/she is supposed to know (e.g. see the Latin expression *similia similibus, or* the Greek verb *homologhêin*).

I will use the term *embodied simulation* in a way that is close to the third definition given above; that is, as an obligatory, unconscious and non-propositional functional mechanism, whose function is the modelling of objects, agents and events to be controlled. Embodied simulation, as conceived of in the present paper, is therefore not necessarily the result of a willed and conscious cognitive effort, aimed at interpreting the intentions hidden in the overt behaviour of others, but rather a basic functional mechanism of our brain. However, because it also generates representational content, this functional mechanism plays a major role in our epistemic approach to the world. It represents the outcome of a possible action, emotion, or sensation one could take or experience, and serves to attribute this outcome to another organism as a real goal-state it tries to bring about, or as a real emotion or sensation it is experiencing.

Successful perception requires the capacity of predicting upcoming sensory events. Similarly, successful action requires the capacity to predict the expected consequences of action. As suggested by an impressive and coherent amount of neuroscientific data (for a review, see Gallese, 2003a; see also Gallese & Lakoff, 2005), both types of predictions seem to depend on the results of unconscious and automatically driven neural states, functionally describable as simulation processes. According to the use I will make of this notion in the present paper, embodied simulation is not conceived of as being confined to the domain of motor control, but rather as a more general and basic endowment of our brain. It is mental because it has content, but it is sensory-motor because its function is realized by the sensory-motor system. I call it 'embodied' – not only because it is neurally realized, but also because it uses a pre-existing model of the body in the brain, and therefore involves a non-propositional form of self-other representation.

In this context, embodied simulation in social cognition can also be seen as an exaptation. It is possible that there has never been any 'special design' for the function I describe here. It might be an extended functionality later co-opted from a distinct original adaptational functionality; namely, sensory-motor integration for body-control purposes.

24.3 Action understanding

Our social world is inhabited by a multiplicity of acting individuals. Much of our social competence depends on our capacity to understand the meaning of the actions we witness. These actions basically pertain to two broad categories. The first is the category of transitive, object-related actions, such as grasping a coffee mug, picking up a phone, biting an apple, or kicking a football. The second category of social actions is that of intransitive, expressive or deictic actions, such as sending kisses, uttering words, or pointing to a person or location in space. What makes our perception of both types of actions different from our perception of the inanimate world is the fact that there is something shared between the first- and third-person perspective of the former events; the observer and the observed are both human beings endowed with a similar brain-body system making them act and perceive alike (Gallese, 2001).

The discovery of mirror neurones has triggered new perspectives on the neural mechanisms at the basis of action understanding. I deal first with transitive actions.

24.3.1 The understanding of object-related actions

About 10 years ago we discovered in the macaque monkey brain a class of premotor neurones that discharge not only when the monkey executes goal-related hand actions such as grasping objects, but also when observing other individuals (monkeys or humans) executing similar actions. We called them 'mirror neurones' (Gallese *et al.*, 1996; Rizzolatti *et al.*, 1996a; see also Gallese, 2000, 2001, 2003a, b, 2005). Neurones with similar properties were later discovered in a sector of the posterior parietal cortex reciprocally connected with area F5 (PF mirror neurones, see Gallese *et al.*, 2002).

The observation of an object-related action leads to the activation of the same neural network that is active during its actual execution. Action observation causes in the observer the automatic simulated re-enactment of the same action. We proposed that this mechanism could be at the basis of a direct form of action understanding (Gallese *et al.*, 1996; Rizzolatti *et al.*, 1996a; see also Gallese, 2000, 2003b; Gallese *et al.*, 2002).

The relationship between action understanding and action simulation is even more evident in the light of the results of two more recent studies carried out in our laboratory. In the first series of experiments, F5 mirror neurones were tested in two conditions. In the first condition the monkey could see the entire action (e.g. a hand grasping action); in the second condition, the same action was presented, but its final critical part, that is the hand–object interaction, was hidden. Therefore, in the hidden condition the monkey only 'knew' that the target object was present behind the occluder. The results showed that more than half of the recorded neurones responded also in the hidden condition (Umiltà *et al.*, 2001).

These results seem to suggest that predictions – or, to use a mentalistic term, inferences – about the goals of the behaviour of others appear to be mediated by the activity of motor neurones coding the goal of the same actions in the observer's brain. Out of sight is not 'out of mind' just because, by simulating the action, the gap can be filled.

Some transitive actions are characteristically accompanied by a specific sound. Often this particular sound enables us to understand what is going on even without any visual information about the action producing the sound. The perceived sound has the capacity to make an invisible action inferred, and therefore present and understood.

We showed that a particular class of F5 mirror neurones, 'audio-visual mirror neurones', discharges not only when the monkey executes or observes a particular type of noisy action (e.g. breaking a peanut), but also when it just listens to the sound produced by the action (see Kohler *et al.*, 2002).

These 'audio-visual mirror neurones' not only respond to the sound of actions, but also discriminate between the sounds of different actions. The actions, whose sounds maximally trigger the neurones' discharge when heard, are those also producing the strongest response when observed or executed. The activation of the premotor neural network normally controlling the execution of action 'A' by sensory information related to the same action 'A', be it visual or auditory, can be characterized as simulating action 'A'.

The multi-modally driven simulation of action goals instantiated by neurones situated in the ventral premotor cortex of the monkey, instantiates properties that are strikingly similar to the symbolic properties characteristic of human thought. The similarity with conceptual content is quite appealing: the same conceptual content ('the goal of action A') results from a multiplicity of states subsuming it, such as sounds, or observed and executed actions. These states, in turn, are subsumed by differently triggered patterns of activations within a population of 'audio-visual mirror neurones'.

The *action simulation* embodied by audiovisual mirror neurones is indeed reminiscent of the use of predicates. The verb 'to break' is used to convey a meaning that can be used in different contexts: 'Seeing someone breaking a peanut', 'Hearing someone breaking a peanut', 'Breaking a peanut'. The predicate, similar to the responses in audiovisual mirror neurones, does not change depending on either the context to which it applies, or the subject/agent performing the action. All that changes is the context to which the predicate refers (Gallese, 2003c; Gallese & Lakoff, 2005).

The general picture conveyed by these results is that the sensory-motor integration, supported by the premotor-parietal F5-PF mirror matching system, instantiates simulations of transitive actions utilized not only to generate and control goal-related behaviours, but also to map the goals and purposes of others' actions, by means of their simulation. This account does not entail an explicit declarative format. It is meaningful, implicit and direct.

What is the importance of these data for our understanding of *human* social cognition? Several studies using different experimental methodologies and techniques have demonstrated in humans also the existence of a similar mirror system, matching action perception and execution (see Buccino *et al.*, 2001; Cochin *et al.*, 1998; Decety *et al.*, 1997; Fadiga *et al.*, 1995; Grafton *et al.*, 1996; Hari *et al.*, 1998; Iacoboni *et al.*, 1999; Rizzolatti *et al.*, 1996b). In particular, it is interesting to note that brain imaging experiments in humans have shown that during action observation there is a strong activation of premotor and parietal areas, the likely human homologue of the monkey areas in which mirror neurones were originally described (Buccino *et al.*, 2001; Decety & Grèzes, 1999; Decety *et al.*, 1997; Grafton *et al.*, 1996; Iacoboni *et al.*, 1999; Rizzolatti *et al.*, 1996b).

24.3.2 The understanding of intransitive actions

The macaque monkey ventral premotor area F5 also contains neurones related to mouth actions. These neurones largely overlap with hand-related neurones; however, in the most lateral part of F5, mouth-related neurones tend to be prevalent. We recently explored the most lateral part of area F5, in which we described a population of mirror neurones mostly related to the execution/observation of mouth-related actions (Ferrari *et al.*, 2003). The majority of these neurones discharge when the monkey executes and observes transitive object-related ingestive actions, such as grasping, biting, or licking. However, a small percentage of mouth-related mirror neurones discharge during the observation of intransitive, communicative facial actions performed by the experimenter in front of the monkey ('communicative mirror neurones', Ferrari *et al.*, 2003). These actions are lip-smacking, lips or tongue protrusion. A behavioural study showed that the observing monkeys correctly decoded these and other communicative gestures performed by the experimenter in front of them, because they elicited congruent expressive reactions (Ferrari *et al.*, 2003). It is therefore plausible to propose that communicative mirror neurones might constitute a further instantiation of a simulation-based social heuristic.

A recent brain imaging study, in which human participants observed mouth actions performed by humans, monkeys and dogs (Buccino *et al.*, 2004), further corroborates this hypothesis. The observed mouth actions could be either transitive, object-directed actions, such as a human, a monkey, or a dog biting a piece of food, or intransitive communicative actions, for example human silent speech, monkey lip-smacking and dog barking. The results showed that the observation of all biting actions led to the activation of the mirror circuit, encompassing the posterior parietal and ventral premotor cortex (Buccino *et al.*, 2004).

Interestingly, the observation of communicative mouth actions led to the activation of different cortical foci according to the different observed species.

The observation of human silent speech activated the pars opercularis of the left inferior frontal gyrus, the premotor sector of Broca's region. The observation of monkey lip-smacking activated a smaller part of the same region bilaterally. Finally, the observation of the barking dog activated only extrastriate visual areas. Actions belonging to the motor repertoire of the observer (e.g. biting and speech reading) or very closely related to it (e.g. monkey's lip-smacking) are mapped on the observer's motor system. Actions that do not belong to this repertoire (e.g. barking) are mapped and henceforth categorized on the basis of their visual properties.

The involvement of the motor system during observation of communicative mouth actions is also testified by the results of a TMS study by Watkins *et al.* (2003), in which they showed that the observation of silent speech-related lip movements enhanced the size of the motor-evoked potential in lip muscles. This effect was lateralized to the left hemisphere. Consistent with the brain imaging data of Buccino *et al.* (2004), the results of Watkins *et al.* (2003) show that the observation of communicative, speech-related mouth actions facilitates the excitability of the motor system involved in the production of the same actions. Again, we have evidence that embodied simulation mediates the decoding of social, meaningful actions.

24.4 Experiencing the actions of others as embodied action simulation

When a given action is planned, its expected motor consequences are forecast. This means that when we are going to execute a given action we can also predict its consequences. This prediction is the computational result of the action model. Through a process of 'equivalence' between what is acted and what is perceived, given its shared and overlapping sub-personal neural mapping, this information can also be used to predict the consequences of actions performed by others. This equivalence – underpinned by the activity of mirror neurones – is made possible by the fact that both predictions (of our actions and of others' actions) are simulation (modelling) processes. The same functional logic that presides over self-modelling is employed also to model the behaviour of others: to perceive an action is equivalent to internally simulating it. This enables the observer to use her/his own resources to penetrate the world of the other by means of an implicit, automatic and unconscious process of motor simulation. Such a simulation process establishes a direct link between agent and observer, in that both are mapped in a neutral fashion. The agent parameter is specified, but not its specific filler, which is indeterminate. Mirror neurones constitutively map an agentive relation; the mere observation of an object not acted upon indeed does not evoke any response. It is just the agentive relational specification to trigger the mirror neurones' response. The fact that a *specific agent* is not mapped does not entail that an agentive relation be not mapped, but simply that the agent parameter can either be oneself or the other.

As we have seen, in humans as in monkeys, action observation constitutes a form of embodied action simulation. This kind of simulation, however, is different from the simulation processes occurring during visual and motor imagery. Action observation *automatically triggers action simulation*, while in mental imagery the simulation process is triggered by a deliberate act; one purposely decides to imagine observing something or doing something. An empirical validation of this difference comes from brain imaging experiments carried out on healthy human participants. By comparing the motor centres activated by action observation with those activated during voluntary mental motor imagery, it emerges that only the latter leads to the activation of pre-SMA and of the primary motor cortex (see Ehrsson *et al.*, 2003).

That said it appears nonetheless that both mental imagery and action observation are kinds of simulation. The main difference is what triggers the simulation process: an internal event, in the case of mental imagery, and an external event, in the case of action observation. This difference leads to slightly different patterns of brain activation. However, both conditions share a common mechanism: the simulation of actions by means of the activation of parietal–premotor cortical networks. I submit that this process of automatic simulation also constitutes a basic level of experiential understanding, a level that does not entail the explicit use of any theory or propositional representation (see also Gallese & Goldman, 1998).

24.5 The body of emotions

Emotions constitute one of the earliest ways available to the individual to acquire knowledge about its own state, thus enabling her/him to reorganize this knowledge on the basis of the outcome of the relations entertained with others. This points to a strong interaction between emotion and action. We dislike things that we seldom touch, look at or smell. We do not 'translate' these things into motor schemas suitable for interacting with them, which are likely 'tagged' with positive affective-hedonic values, but rather into aversive motor schemas, likely 'tagged' with negative affective-hedonic connotations.

The coordinated activity of sensory-motor and affective neural systems results in the simplification and automatization of the behavioural responses that living organisms are supposed to produce in order to survive. The strict coupling between affect and sensory-motor integration appears to be one of the most powerful drives leading the developing individual to the achievement of progressively more 'distal' and abstract goals (see Gallese & Metzinger, 2003; Metzinger & Gallese, 2003).

Such a coupling between emotion and action is indeed highlighted by a study of Adolphs *et al.* (2000), where over 100 brain-damaged patients were reviewed. This study showed that the patients who suffered damage to the sensory-motor cortexes were also those who scored worst when asked to rate or name facial emotions displayed by human faces. As emphasized by Adolphs (2002, 2003), the integrity of the sensory-motor system appears to be critical for the recognition of emotions displayed by others, because the sensory-motor system appears to support the reconstruction of what it would feel like to be in a particular emotion, by means of simulation of the related body state.

Before addressing the role of embodied simulation in the understanding of emotions, it is necessary to clarify what exactly we refer to when we speak of emotions. There are many different ways to experience an emotion. Emotion is a word that designates and refers to a multidimensional aspect of our life. To experience an emotion can be described as subjectively experiencing 'inner body states' of varied intensity and amplitude that can surface, with a variety of degrees of explicitness, as ostensive behaviours, often localized to specific body parts, such as the face.

Under both first- and third-person perspectives of emotion experience, a complex state of the organism is accompanied by variable degrees of awareness and meta-awareness, variously indicated as 'appraisal'. It is a common experience to be asked by people we know questions such as: 'Why are you so angry at me?' without having realized until the very moment in which the question was asked that we were indeed expressing the emotion of anger. We can be in a given emotional state, and express it ostensibly with our body, without fully experiencing its content as that of a particular emotion. Lambie and Marcel (2002) have distinguished two levels of emotion appraisal: a first-order phenomenal state, what they call 'first-order emotion experience', and conscious second-order awareness. Both states can be either self-directed (first-person perspective) or world-directed (third-person perspective). The content of the first-order phenomenal state is physical, centred on one's body state. The content of second-order conscious awareness can be either propositional or non-propositional.

It should be emphasized that it is indeed possible to witness the expression of a given emotional state displayed by someone else without explicitly relying on the propositional description of that state. It is precisely this unmediated, direct form of emotion understanding that I will be addressing here. More specifically, I will characterize the neural underpinnings of a simulation-based type of basic social emotion understanding.

A recent empirical support to a tight link between embodied simulation and our perception of the emotions of others as displayed by their facial expressions comes from an fMRI study on healthy participants by Carr *et al.* (2003). This study shows that both observation and imitation of the facial expression of emotions activate the same restricted group of brain structures, including the ventral premotor cortex, the insula and the amygdala. These data show that the perception and production of emotion-related facial expressions both impinge upon common neural structures whose function could be characterized as that of a neural mirror matching mechanism. However, one might argue that pretence, the purposive enactment of the overt body expression of an emotion, does not grant its characteristic phenomenal awareness. Imitating the expression of emotions does not necessarily produce the first-person experience of the emotion one is imitating.

In a recently published fMRI study carried out on healthy human participants, we specifically addressed the issue of whether the first- and third-person experience of a particular emotion are mapped by a shared neural representation. To that purpose, we scanned the brain activity of healthy participants during the phenomenal experience of disgust, by having them inhaling disgusting odorants, and during the observation of the same emotion as displayed by video clips of other individuals dynamically expressing it with their facial expression. The results of this study showed that witnessing the facial expression of disgust of others activates the left anterior insula at the same overlapping location activated by the first-person subjective experience of disgust (Wicker *et al.*, 2003).

The anterior sector of the insula receives rich connections from olfactory and gustatory structures and from the anterior sectors of the ventral bank of the superior temporal sulcus, where cells have been found in the monkey to respond to the sight of faces (Bruce *et al.*, 1981; Perrett *et al.*, 1982). The anterior insula thus appears to link gustatory, olfactory and visual stimuli with visceral sensations and the related autonomic and viscero-motor responses (see also Gallese *et al.*, 2004). Penfield and Faulk (1955) electrically stimulated the anterior insula in humans undergoing neurosurgery. During the stimulation the patients reported feeling nauseous and sick. More recently, Krolak-Salmon *et al.* (2003), using shorter and weaker stimulation parameters, evoked unpleasant sensations in the throat and mouth. These findings support the link between the anterior viscero-motor insula and the experience of disgust or related aversive visceral sensations and viscero-motor reactions.

Few clinical cases also show that when the anterior insula is damaged, both the subjective experience of disgust and the capacity to recognize this emotion in others are seriously impaired. Calder *et al.* (2000) report the case of the patient N. K., who after lesions of the left insula and neighbouring structures was selectively impaired in recognizing disgust in the facial expressions of others. This incapacity to perceive disgust extended to the auditory modality: he did not recognize the emotional valence of sounds typical for disgust, such as retching, while easily recognizing that of sounds characteristic of other emotions such as laughter. His recognition of the facial expression of other emotions, including that of fear, was normal. What is most interesting for our discussion is the fact that the multimodal perceptual deficit for disgust of N. K. was mirrored by an equivalent deficit in N.K.'s first-person experience of the same emotion. He reported having a reduced sensation of disgust, ranking almost two standard deviations below the normal score in a questionnaire measuring the emotional experience of disgust. His experience of other emotions, though, was fairly normal.

A similar pattern of deficits was reported by Adolphs *et al.* (2003). They described the patient B. who, following bilateral damage to the insula, showed substantial deficits in recognizing the facial expression of disgust, while preserving his recognition of other facial expressions. Patient B.'s incapacity to experience disgust is evident from the fact that he ingests food indiscriminately, including inedible items, and fails to feel disgust when presented with stimuli representing disgusting food items.

Experiencing disgust and witnessing the same emotion expressed by the facial mimicry of someone else both activate the same neural structure, the anterior insula. The damage of this structure impairs both the capacity to experience disgust and that of recognizing it in others. This suggests, at least for the emotion of disgust, that the first- and third-person experience of a given emotion is underpinned by the activity of a shared neural substrate. When I see a given facial expression, and this perception leads me to understand that expression as characterized by a particular affective state, I do not accomplish this type of understanding through an argument by analogy. The other's emotion is constituted and experienced, hence directly understood by means of an embodied simulation producing a shared body state. It is the body state shared by the observer and the observed that enables direct understanding. A similar simulation-based mechanism has been proposed by Goldman and Sripada (2005) as 'unmediated resonance'.

24.6 Being 'in touch'

In the second book of his posthumous Ideas (1989), Husserl points out that the alive body (Leib) is the constitutive foundation of any perception, the perception of others included. Were we adopting a similar perspective to frame social cognition, we could say that the self-modelling functional architecture of the alive body scaffolds the modelling of the intentional relations of other individuals. The multimodal dynamic model of our body as of a goal-seeking organism brings about the basic representational architecture for the mapping of intentional relations. The empirical evidence so far reviewed on action and emotion perception seems to support this line of thought. Let us focus now on tactile sensations as the target of our social perception.

Touch has a privileged status in making possible the social attribution of alive personhood to others. 'Let's be in touch' is a common clause in everyday language, which metaphorically describes the wish to keep on being related, being in contact with someone else. Such examples show how the tactile dimension is intimately related to the interpersonal dimension. In a recent fMRI experiment we have shown that the first-person subjective experience of being touched on one's body activates the same neural networks that are activated by observing the body of someone else being touched (Keysers *et al.*, 2004). Within SII-PV, a multimodal cortical region perhaps exceeding the limits of the traditional unimodal second somatosensory area, there is a localized neural network similarly activated by the self-experienced sensation of being touched, and the perception of an external tactile relation.

Such an activation, obtained during the perception of another body being touched, could perhaps be more parsimoniously interpreted as the outcome of the prediction of a body impact on the observer's own body. However, in sharp contrast with what this interpretation would have predicted, the manipulation of the perspective (subjective versus objective) under which the observed tactile stimulation was presented to participants did not modify the degree of activation of the same overlapping region within SII-PV. Thus, visual stimuli activate SII/PV in a way that is unaffected by how easily they can be integrated into our body schema.

In a second experiment, we replaced the legs of the actors in the movies by inanimate objects: rolls of paper towels and binders. Results indicated that even seeing an object getting touched produced a significantly larger activation of SII/PV compared to seeing the object being only approached (see Keysers *et al.*, 2004). The touching of two surfaces in the outside world is something in principle very abstract, if only visually mapped. Mapping it onto what we feel when one of the surfaces being touched is our own body fills this abstract visual event with a very personal meaning: what it feels like to be touched.

It appears therefore that the critical stimulus for SII/PV activation is the perception of touch; be it the touch of an object, another human being, or our own legs. This double pattern of activation of the same brain region seems to suggest that both our capacity to recognize and implicitly understand the tactile experience of others, and a more abstract notion of touch (as in the case of object touch) could be mediated by embodied simulation.

It is interesting to note that Husserl (1989) wrote that every thing we see, we simultaneously also see as a tactile object, as something which is directly related to the alive body, but not by virtue of its visibility. The 'tactile lived body', in particular, provides the constitutive foundation of our cognitive and epistemic self-referentiality. The perspectival spatial location of our body provides the essential foundation to our determination of reality.

24.7 The shared manifold and empathy

The establishment of self-other identity is a driving force for the cognitive development of more articulated and sophisticated forms of intersubjective relations. I have proposed that the mirror matching system could be involved in enabling the constitution of this identity (Gallese, 2001, 2003a, 2005). I think that the concept of 'empathy' should be extended in order to accommodate and account for all different aspects of expressive behaviour enabling us to establish a meaningful link between others and ourselves. This 'enlarged' notion of empathy opens up the possibility of unifying under the same account the multiple aspects and possible levels of description of intersubjective relations.

As we have seen, when we enter in to a relation with others there is a multiplicity of states that we share with them. We share emotions, our body schema, and our being subject to somatic sensations such as touch, pain, etc. A comprehensive account of the richness of content we share with others should rest upon a conceptual tool capable of being applied to all these different levels of description, while simultaneously providing their functional and subpersonal characterization.

I introduced this conceptual tool as the *shared manifold* of intersubjectivity (see Gallese, 2001, 2003a, b). I posit that it is by means of this shared manifold that we directly experience other human beings as similar to us. It is just because of this shared manifold that intersubjective communication, social imitation and mind reading become possible (Gallese, 2003a, 2005). The shared manifold can be operationalized at three different levels: a phenomenological level, a functional level, a subpersonal level.

The phenomenological level is the one responsible for the sense of similarity, of being individuals within a larger social community of persons like us that we experience every time we meet other human beings. It could be defined also as the *empathic* level, provided that empathy is characterized in the 'enlarged' way I am advocating here. Actions, emotions and sensations experienced by others become *experientially* meaningful to us because we can *share* them with others.

The functional level can be characterized in terms of *as if* modes of interaction enabling models of self/other to be created. The same functional logic is at work during both self-modelling and the understanding of others' behaviour. Both are models of interaction, which map their referents to identical relational functional nodes. All modes of interaction share a relational character. At the functional level of description, the relational logic of operation produces the self/other identity by enabling the system to detect coherence, regularity and predictability, independently from their situated source. This view is similar to that proposed by Damasio and Adolphs on the understanding of emotions (Adolphs, 2003; Damasio, 1994, 1999). There is, however, an important difference between the 'as if' view proposed here and that of Damasio, as far as the underlying neural mechanism is concerned. According to the present proposal (see also Gallese *et al.*, 2004), crucial for both first- and third-person experiential understanding of social behaviour is the activation of the cortical sensori-motor or viscero-motor centres whose outcome, when activating downstream centres, determines a specific 'behaviour', be it an action or an emotional state. When only the cortical centres, decoupled from their peripheral effects, are active, the observed actions, emotions, or sensations are 'simulated' and thereby understood.

The subpersonal level is instantiated as the level of activity of a series of mirror matching neural circuits. The activity of these neural circuits is, in turn, tightly coupled with multi-level changes within body states. We have seen that mirror neurones instantiate a multimodal intentional shared space. My hypothesis is that analogous neural networks are at work to generate multimodal emotional and sensitive shared spaces (see Gallese, 2001, 2003a, b; Gallese *et al.*, 2004; Goldman & Gallese, 2000). These are the shared spaces that allow us to directly experience and understand the emotions and the sensations we take others to experience. The neuroscientific results reviewed in the previous sections seem to suggest that my hypothesis might be not so ill founded.

24.8 Psychopathological implications of intentional attunement: schizophrenia

All of our social transactions depend on mutual understanding. Simultaneously, however, interpersonal intelligibility is sided by the capacity to establish clear-cut boundaries, carving out a 'self' from the 'outside world'. Being 'oneself' is experienced as being similar to other selves, while simultaneously experiencing its unique character.

In schizophrenia, self and other are no longer mutually interrelated, but they tend to diverge and crystallize into segregated, incomprehensible and impenetrable realms. In spite of this lack of interpersonal relatedness, the self can experience dramatic loss of its boundaries (Schneider, 1955), as epitomized by Schneiderian-positive symptoms such as thought-insertion, auditory hallucinations and delusion of action control. Social and personal identity are both disrupted. The problem of psychopathology is therefore to reconcile all these different psychotic articulations within a coherent explanatory frame.

Schizophrenia, as pointed out by Terenius (2000), has been so far an elusive target for research. Furthermore, the current DSM-IV-inspired operational diagnostic criteria provide a much clearer picture of what schizophrenia *is not* than of what *it is*. A possible reason accounting for this elusiveness could be the fact that a comprehensive account of schizophrenia – but the same could be said of all psychoses – implies a global understanding of the human mind. Any serious attempt to understand cognition, emotions and language, devoid of a 'global perspective', is doomed to failure. This challenging enterprise requires an integrative approach. I believe the same to hold true for schizophrenia. From that follows that a global approach to schizophrenia cannot but incorporate the same multiple levels of explanation that we adopt when trying to build a coherent account of cognition, language and affective behaviour.

However, this is by no means a new idea. In his seminal monograph '*La Schizophrénie*' (1927), Minkowski wrote that we cannot fully understand schizophrenia unless we are able to frame it within a thorough account of the structure of subjectivity. According to Minkowski (1927), autism, the incapacity to be attuned with the world, constitutes the basic clinical essence of schizophrenia. Minkowski developed an original intuition of his mentor Bleuler, who wrote that schizophrenics cut themselves off from any contact with the external world (see Bleuler, 1911). The core problem of schizophrenics is, accordingly, their lack of 'vital contact with reality' (Minkowski, 1927, p. 98), viewed as an incapacity to 'resonate with the world', to establish meaningful bonds with other individuals. The contact with reality is loosened or completely lost not only with respect to the transactions with the social world, but also from the first-person perspectival point of view.

Schizophrenia as 'lack of resonance', as an empathic disorder, has been a constant theme in the reflections of phenomenologically inspired psychiatry. Blankenburg (1971) characterizes the autistic dimension of schizophrenia as a global crisis of 'common sense', an incapacity to pre-reflexively grasp the meaning of the world, a world that looks terribly unfamiliar and strange to the schizophrenic's eyes. Parnas and Bovet (1991) have argued that schizophrenic autism derives from a transformation of the structure of subjectivity in its tripartite dimensions: self-awareness, intentionality and intersubjectivity. A lack of attunement would be at the origin of the incapacity of schizophrenics to draw a coherent and meaningful picture of their social world. In a more recent paper Parnas *et al.* (2002, p. 133) argue that in schizophrenics '. . . experience is more observed than lived', most likely because of the incapacity to attain a '. . . non-reflective, tacit sensibility, procuring a background texture or organization to the field of experience'. This is exactly the same level of pre-reflexive, non-propositional experiential understanding of the world of interpersonal relations that I have been characterizing throughout the paper, under the heading of 'shared manifold of intersubjectivity'.

More recently, along a similar phenomenologically inspired vein, Stanghellini (2000, 2002) pointed out that the interpersonal disorders observed in schizophrenic patients constitute a fundamental aspect of their psychosis. 'Defective attunement', the incapacity to engage oneself in meaningful relations with others and the impossibility of establishing non-inferential, 'intuitive' interpersonal bonds, would represent a major feature of schizophrenia.

The 'defective attunement' hypothesis of phenomenological psychiatry is highly consonant with the picture I presented here. A disruption of the multilevel simulation processes characterizing the shared manifold might be a possible cause of 'defective intentional attunement' in schizophrenic patients. The ineffable nature of schizophrenics' estrangement is just a negative sign of their core problem. There are no words or propositions available to describe what healthy individuals directly and pre-verbally experience. If the mechanisms enabling us to constitute the implicit certainties we normally entertain about the world do not function properly, we are left in need of purposively attributing a sense to a world that looks totally strange.

24.9 Psychopathological implications of intentional attunement: autism

A similar proposal can be made for the autistic syndrome of children. The autistic syndrome is a severe and chronic developmental disorder, characterized by social and communicative deficits and by a reduced interest in the environment, towards which restricted and often stereotyped initiatives are taken (Dawson *et al.*, 2002). To be an autistic child means, with variable degrees of severity, to be incapable of establishing meaningful social communications and bonds, of establishing visual contact with the world of others, of sharing attention with the others, to be incapable of imitating others' behaviour or of understanding others' intentions, emotions and sensations.

I would like to briefly focus on some of the early-onset symptoms. Towards the end of the first year of life, autistic children experience difficulties with orientation, or even find it impossible, on the basis of cues provided by others. They are incapable of sharing attention with others; incapable of reacting in a congruent fashion to others' emotions. They are also highly impaired in recognizing human faces or in displaying imitative behaviours. All of these early manifestations of autism share a common root: the cognitive skills required to establish meaningful bonds with others are missing or seriously impaired.

My hypothesis is that these deficits are to be ascribed to a deficit or malfunction of 'intentional attunement'. If it is true – as held throughout the paper – that at the basis of our social competence is *in primis* the capacity to constitute an implicit and directly shared interpersonally meaningful space, enabling us to establish a link with the multiple intentional relations instantiated by others, then it follows that a disruption of this shared manifold should be the core problem of the autistic mind. The incapacity to develop a full and comprehensive intentional attunement with others implies as a consequence the development of an incomplete or malfunctioning shared manifold.

The lack of a full-blown intentional attunement will produce various and diversified cognitive and executive deficits, all sharing the same functional origin: a lack or malfunctioning of embodied simulation routines, likely underpinned by impairments in connectivity and/or functioning of the mirror neurone system. If my hypothesis is correct, the posited intentional attunement deficit should become manifest at the various levels of social cognition it normally underpins. A series of experimental data seem to suggest this to be the case.

A recent study investigating postural adjustments in autistic children has shown that at difference with healthy individuals, they use motor strategies basically relying on feedback information, rather than on feed-forward modes of control. Such disturbance of executive control strategies prevent autistic children from adopting anticipatory postural adjustments (Schmitz et al., 2003). Given the functional characterization of forward models as simulation-based, it is difficult not to interpret these data as evidence of a simulation deficit. Such postural deficits are not intrinsically social; however, they stem from a disruption within the executive control domain of a functional mechanism – simulation – that I propose to be at the root of the constitution of the shared experiential interpersonal space.

A further exemplification of simulation deficits in the autistic syndrome is exemplified by imitation deficits. Autistic children have problems in both symbolic and non-symbolic imitative behaviours, in imitating the use of objects, in imitating facial gestures and in vocal imitation (see Rogers, 1999). These deficits characterize both high- and low-functioning forms of autism. Furthermore, imitation deficits are apparent not only in comparison with the performances of healthy subjects, but also with those of mentally retarded non-autistic subjects. According to my hypothesis, imitation deficits in autism are determined by the incapacity to establish a motor equivalence between demonstrator and imitator, most likely due to a malfunctioning of the mirror neurone system, or because of disrupted emotional/affective regulation of the same system. Imitation deficits thus can be characterized as further examples of a disrupted shared manifold.

Let me now briefly turn to emotional-affective deficits. Several studies reported the severe problems autistic children experience in the facial expression of emotions and its understanding in others (Hobson et al., 1988, 1989; Snow et al., 1988; Yirmiya et al., 1989). Furthermore, Hobson and Lee (1999) reported that autistic children score much worse than healthy controls in reproducing the affective qualities of observed actions. All these deficits can be framed as affective attunement deficits, hence as further instantiations of a lacunose shared manifold.

My hypothesis, to interpret the autistic syndrome as an intentional attunement deficit, is quite divergent from many of the mainstream ideas concerning the origin of this developmental disorder. One of the most credited theories on autism, in spite of its different – not always congruent – articulations, posits that autism is caused by a deficit of a specific mind module, the Theory of Mind module, selected in the course of evolution to build theories about the mind of others (Baron-Cohen, 1988, 1995; Baron-Cohen *et al.*, 1985). One of the problems of this theory is that it can be barely reconciled with what we learn from the reports of some high-functioning autistic individuals. What they claim is that in order to understand how they supposedly should feel in given social contexts, and what others supposedly feel and think in those same contexts, they must rely on theorizing. What these reports seem to suggest is that theorizing about the other's mind is not quite the basic deficit, but the only compensating strategy available in the absence of more elementary and basic cognitive skills enabling a direct experiential take on the world of others.

The shared manifold of intersubjectivity constitutes a general hypothesis on social cognition (see also Gallese, 2005; Gallese *et al.*, 2004) that can be empirically tested at multiple levels, both in healthy and psychotic individuals. Furthermore, this proposal and the approaches it generates have the merit of disclosing the possibility of establishing more insightful therapeutic bonds with psychotic patients.

24.10 Conclusions

The main point of the present paper is that we have discovered some of the neural mechanisms mediating between the multilevel personal knowledge we hold of our lived body, and the *implicit certainties* we simultaneously hold about others. Such personal body-related knowledge enables us to directly understand the actions performed by others, and to decode the emotions and sensations they experience. Our seemingly effortless capacity to conceive of the acting bodies inhabiting our social world as *goal-oriented persons* like us depends on the constitution of a shared meaningful interpersonal space. I propose that this shared manifold space can be characterized at the functional level as embodied simulation, a specific mechanism likely constituting a basic functional feature by means of which our brain/body system models its interactions with the world. Embodied simulation constitutes the crucial functional mechanism in social cognition, and it can be neurobiologically characterized. The mirror neurone matching systems represent the sub-personal instantiation of simulation. With this mechanism we do not just 'see' an action, an emotion, or a sensation. Side by side with the sensory description of the observed social stimuli, internal representations of the body states associated with these actions, emotions and sensations are evoked in the observer, 'as if' he/she would be doing a similar action or experiencing a similar emotion or sensation.

The neuroscientific evidence reviewed here suggests that social cognition is tractable at the neural level of description. This level is implicit, though, when the organism is confronting the intentional behaviour of others, it produces a specific phenomenal state of 'intentional attunement'. This phenomenal state generates a peculiar quality of familiarity with other individuals, produced by the collapse of the others' intentions into the observer's ones. This seems to be what being empathic is about.

The sharp distinction, classically drawn between the first- and third-person perspective of acting and experiencing emotions and sensations, appears to be much more blurred at the level of the subpersonal mechanisms mapping it. The gap between the two perspectives is bridged by the way the intentional relation is functionally mapped at the neural-body level. Any intentional relation can be mapped as a relation holding between a subject and an object. The mirror neural circuits described in this paper map the different intentional relations in a compressed and indeterminate fashion, which is neutral about the specific quality or identity of the agentive/subjective parameter. By means of a shared functional state realized in two different bodies that nevertheless obey to the same morpho-functional rules, the 'objectual other' becomes 'another self'.

The shareability of the phenomenal content of intentional relations as mediated by sensory-motor multimodally integrated neural circuits has interesting consequences – from both theoretical and empirical points of view – for the debate on how semantics is mapped in the brain. The picture conveyed by the neuro-scientific data I reviewed here suggests the necessity of cutting across the widely endorsed dichotomy between distinct semantic and pragmatic cognitive domains. Social meaning is primarily the object of practical concern, and not of theoretical judgement (see Millikan, 2004). It relies on non-inferential mechanisms, which do not require the explicit use of rationality. As proposed by Gordon (2005), the implicit recognition of conspecifics as intentional agents is a case of procedural rather than declarative knowledge.

Furthermore, if embodied simulation and its neural counterpart – the mirror neurone circuits – do indeed constitute an automatic, non-propositional mechanism for social meaning attribution, the sharp dichotomy between a semantic/pragmatic division of labour among brain areas recipient of the ventral and dorsal visual streams (see Goodale & Milner, 1992; Jacob & Jeannerod, 2003) should also be questioned.

Social cognition is not only thinking about the contents of someone else's mind. Our brains, and those of other primates, appear to have developed a basic functional mechanism, embodied simulation, which gives us an experiential insight of other minds. This mechanism may provide the first unifying perspective of the neural basis of social cognition.

Acknowledgments

This work was supported by MIUR and, as part of the European Science Foundation EUROCORES Programme OMLL, was supported by funds to V. G. from the Italian C. N. R. and the EC Sixth Framework Programme under Contract no. ERAS-CT-2003-980409.

REFERENCES

Adolphs, R. (2002). Neural systems for recognizing emotion. *Current Opinion in Neurobiology*, **12(2)**, 169–177.

Adolphs, R. (2003). Cognitive neuroscience of human social behaviour. *Nature Review Neuroscience*, **4(3)**, 165–178.

Adolphs, R., Damasio, H., Tranel, D., Cooper, G., & Damasio, A. R. (2000). A role for somatosensory cortices in the visual recognition of emotion as revealed by three-dimensional lesion mapping. *Journal of Neuroscience*, **20**, 2683–2690.

Adolphs, R., Tranel, D., & Damasio, A. R. (2003). Dissociable neural systems for recognizing emotions. *Brain and Cognition*, **52(1)**, 61–69.

Baron-Cohen, S. (1988). Social and pragmatic deficits in autism: cognitive or affective? *Journal of Autism and Developmental Disorders*, **18**, 379–402.

Baron-Cohen, S. (1995). *Mindblindness. An Essay on Autism and Theory of Mind*. Cambridge, Mass.: MIT Press.

Baron-Cohen, S., Leslie, A. M., & Frith, U. (1985). Does the autistic child have a 'theory of mind'? *Cognition*, **21**, 37–46.

Blankenburg, W. (1971). Der Verlust der natürlichen Selbstverständlichkeit. *Ein Beitrag zur Psychopathologie symptomarmer Schizophrenien*. Stuttgart: Enke.

Bleuler, E. (1911). Dementia Praecox oder Gruppe der Schizophrenien. In: G. Aschaffenburg, (ed.), *Handbuch der Psychiatrie*. Leipzig: Deuticke.

Bruce, C., Desimone, R., & Gross, C. G. (1981). Visual properties of neurons in a polysensory area in superior temporal sulcus of the macaque. *Journal of Neurophysiology*, **46**, 369–384.

Buccino, G., Binkofski, F., Fink, G. R., *et al.* (2001). Action observation activates premotor and parietal areas in a somatotopic manner: an fMRI study. *European Journal of Neuroscience*, **13**, 400–404.

Buccino, G., Lui, F., Canessa, N., *et al.* (2004). Neural circuits involved in the recognition of actions performed by nonconspecifics: an fMRI study. *Journal of Cognitive Neuroscience*, **16**, 114–126.

Calder, A. J., Keane, J., Manes, F., Antoun, N., & Young, A. W. (2000). Impaired recognition and experience of disgust following brain injury. *Nature Neuroscience*, **3**, 1077–1078.

Carr, L., Iacoboni, M., Dubeau, M. C., Mazziotta, J. C., & Lenzi, G. L. (2003). Neural mechanisms of empathy in humans: a relay from neural systems for imitation to limbic areas. *Proceedings of the National Academy of Science of the USA*, **100(9)**, 5497–5502.

Cochin, S., Barthelemy, C., Lejeune, B., Roux, S., & Martineau, J. (1998). Perception of motion and qEEG activity in human adults. *Electroencephalography and Clinical Neurophysiology*, **107**, 287–295.

Damsaio, A. R. (1994). *Decartes's Error: Emotion, Reason and the Human Brain*. New York: Putnam.

Damasio, A. R. (1999). *The Feeling of What Happens: Body and Emotion in the Making of Consciousness*. New York: Harcourt Brace & Company.

Dawson, G., Webb, S., Schellenberg, G. D., *et al.* (2002). Defining the broader phenotype of autism: genetic, brain, and behavioral perspectives. *Development and Psychopathology*, **14**, 581–611.

Decety, J., & Grèzes, J. (1999). Neural mechanisms subserving the perception of human actions. *Trends in Cognitive Sciences*, **3**, 172–178.

Decety, J., Grèzes, J., Costes, N., *et al.* (1997). Brain activity during observation of actions. Influence of action content and subject's strategy. *Brain*, **120**, 1763–1777.

Ehrsson, H. H., Geyer, S., & Naito, E. (2003). Imagery of voluntary movement of fingers, toes, and tongue activates corresponding body-part-specific motor representations. *Journal of Neurophysiology*, **90(5)**, 3304–3316.

Fadiga, L., Fogassi, L., Pavesi, G., & Rizzolatti, G. (1995). Motor facilitation during action observation: a magnetic stimulation study. *Journal of Neurophysiology*, **73**, 2608–2611.

Ferrari, P. F., Gallese, V., Rizzolatti, G., & Fogassi, L. (2003). Mirror neurons responding to the observation of ingestive and communicative mouth actions in the monkey ventral premotor cortex. *European Journal of Neuroscience*, **17**, 1703–1714.

Gallese, V. (2000). The acting subject: towards the neural basis of social cognition. In T. Metzinger, (ed.), *Neural Correlates of Consciousness. Empirical and Conceptual Questions* (pp. 325–333). Cambridge, Mass.: MIT Press.

Gallese, V. (2001). The 'Shared Manifold' Hypothesis: from mirror neurons to empathy. *Journal of Consciousness Studies*, **8**, No. 5–7; 33–50.

Gallese, V. (2003a). The manifold nature of interpersonal relations: the quest for a common mechanism. *Philosophical Transactions of the Royal Society of London, Series B*, **358**, 517–528.

Gallese, V. (2003b). The roots of empathy: the shared manifold hypothesis and the neural basis of intersubjectivity. *Psychopathology*, **36**, No. 4, 171–180.

Gallese, V. (2003c). A neuroscientific grasp of concepts: from control to representation. *Philosophical Transactions of the Royal Society of London, Series B*, **358**, 1231–1240.

Gallese, V. (2005). 'Being like me': self-other identity, mirror neurons and empathy. In S. Hurley, & N. Chater (eds.), *Perspectives on Imitation: From Cognitive Neuroscience to Social Science* (Vol. 1). Cambridge, Mass.: MIT Press.

Gallese, V., Fadiga, L., Fogassi, L., & Rizzolatti, G. (1996). Action recognition in the premotor cortex. *Brain*, **119**, 593–609.

Gallese, V., Fogassi, L., Fadiga, L., & Rizzolatti, G. (2002). Action representation and the inferior parietal lobule. In W. Prinz, & B. Hommel, (eds.), *Attention and Performance XIX* (pp. 247–266). Oxford: Oxford University Press.

Gallese, V., & Goldman, A. (1998). Mirror neurons and the simulation theory of mind-reading. *Trends in Cognitive Sciences*, **12**, 493–501.

Gallese, V., Keysers, C., & Rizzolatti, G. (2004). A unifying view of the basis of social cognition. *Trends in Cognitive Sciences*, **8**, 396–403.

Gallese, V., & Lakoff, G. (2005). The brain's concepts: the role of the sensory-motor system in reason and language. *Cognitive Neuropsychology*, **22**, 455–479.

Gallese, V., & Metzinger, T. (2003). Motor ontology: the representational reality of goals, actions, and selves. *Philosophical Psychology*, **13**, No. 3, 365–388.

Goldman, A. (1989). Interpretation psychologized. *Mind and Language*, **4**, 161–185.

Goldman, A. (1992a). In defense of the simulation theory. *Mind and Language*, **7**, 104–119.

Goldman, A. (1992b). Empathy, mind, and morals: presidential address. *Proceedings and Addresses of the American Philosophical Association*, **66**, 17–41.

Goldman, A. (1993a). The psychology of folk psychology. *Behavioral Brain Sciences*, **16**, 15–28.

Goldman, A. (1993b). *Philosophical Applications of Cognitive Science*. Boulder, Colo.: Westview Press.

Goldman, A. (2000). The mentalizing folk. In D. Sperber (ed.), *Metarepresentation*. Oxford: Oxford University Press.

Goldman, A., & Gallese, V. (2000). Reply to Schulkin. *Trends in Cognitive Sciences*, **4**, 255–256.

Goldman, A., & Sripada, C. S. (2005). Simulationist models of face-based emotion recognition. *Cognition*, **94**, 193–213.

Goodale, M. A., & Milner, A. D. (1992). Separate visual pathways for perception and action. *Trends in Neuroscience*, **15**, 20–25.

Gordon, R. (1986). Folk psychology as simulation. *Mind and Language*, **1**, 158–171.

Gordon, R. (1995). Simulation without introspection or inference from me to you. In M. Davies, & T. Stone (eds.), *Mental Simulation* (pp. 53–67). Oxford: Blackwell.

Gordon, R. (1996). 'Radical' simulationism. In P. Carruthers, & P. Smith (eds.), *Theories of Theories of Mind* (pp. 11–21). Cambridge: Cambridge University Press.

Gordon, R. (2005). Intentional agents like myself. In S. Hurley, & N. Chater (eds.), *Perspectives on Imitation: From Cognitive Neuroscience to Social Science* (Vol. 2). Cambridge, Mass.: MIT Press.

Grafton, S. T., Arbib, M. A., Fadiga, L., & Rizzolatti, G. (1996). Localization of grasp representations in humans by PET: 2. Observation compared with imagination. *Experimental Brain Research*, **112**, 103–111.

Hari, R., Forss, N., Avikainen, S., *et al.* (1998). Activation of human primary motor cortex during action observation: a neuromagnetic study. *Proceedings of the National Academy of Science of the USA*, **95**, 15061–15065.

Hobson, R. P., & Lee, A. (1999). Imitation and identification in autism. *Journal of Child Psychology and Psychiatry*, **40**, 649–659.

Hobson, R. P., Ouston, J., & Lee, A. (1988). Emotion recognition in autism: coordinating faces and voices. *Psychological Medicine*, **18**, 911–923.

Hobson, R. P., Ouston, J., & Lee, A. (1989). Naming emotion in faces and voices: abilities and disabilities in autism and mental retardation. *British Journal of Developmental Psychology*, **7**, 237–250.

Husserl, E. (1989). *Ideas pertaining to a pure phenomenology and to a phenomenological philosophy, Second Book: Studies in the Phenomenology of Constitution.* Dordrecht: Kluwer Academic Publishers.

Iacoboni, M., Woods, R. P., Brass, M., *et al.* (1999). Cortical mechanisms of human imitation. *Science*, **286**, 2526–2528.

Jacob, P., & Jeannerod, M. (2003). *Ways of Seeing – The Scope and Limits of Visual Cognition.* Oxford: Oxford University Press.

Keysers, C., Wickers, B., Gazzola, V., *et al.* (2004). A touching sight: SII/PV activation during the observation and experience of touch. *Neuron*, **42**, April 22, 1–20.

Kohler, E., Keysers, C., Umiltà, M. A., *et al.* (2002). Hearing sounds, understanding actions: action representation in mirror neurons. *Science*, **297**, 846–848.

Krolak-Salmon, P., Henaff, M. A., Isnard, J., *et al.* (2003). An attention modulated response to disgust in human ventral anterior insula. *Annals of Neurology*, **53**, 446–453.

Lambie, J. A., & Marcel, A. J. (2002). Consciousness and the varieties of emotion experience: a theoretical framework. *Psychological Reviews*, **109**, 219–259.

Leslie, A. M. (1987). Pretence and representation. The origins of 'theory of mind'. *Psychological Reviews*, **94**, 412–426.

Metzinger, T., & Gallese, V. (2003). The emergence of a shared action ontology: building blocks for a theory. *Consciousness and Cognition*, **12**, 549–571.

Millikan, R. G. (2004). *Varieties of Meaning.* Boston, Mass.: MIT Press.

Minkowski, E. (1927). *La Schizophrénie. Psychopathologie des Schizoides et des Schizophrènes.* Paris: Payot.

Parnas, J., & Bovet, P. (1991). Autism in schizophrenia revisited. *Comprehensive Psychiatry*, **32**, 7–21.

Parnas, J., Bovet, P., & Zahavi, D. (2002). Schizophrenic autism: clinical phenomenology and pathogenetic implications. *World Psychiatry*, **1/3**, 131–136.

Penfield, W., & Faulk, M. E. (1955). The insula: further observations on its function. *Brain*, **78**, 445–470.

Perrett, D. I., Rolls, E. T., & Caan, W. (1982). Visual neurones responsive to faces in the monkey temporal cortex. *Experimental Brain Research*, **47**, 329–342.

Rizzolatti, G., Fadiga, L., Gallese, V., & Fogassi, L. (1996a). Premotor cortex and the recognition of motor actions. *Cognitive Brain Research*, **3**, 131–141.

Rizzolatti, G., Fadiga, L., Matelli, M., *et al.* (1996b). Localization of grasp representations in humans by PET: 1. Observation versus execution. *Experimental Brain Research*, **111**, 246–252.

Rogers, S. (1999). An examination of the imitation deficit in autism. In J. Nadel, & G. Butterworth (eds.), *Imitation in Infancy* (pp. 254–279). Cambridge: Cambridge University Press.

Schmitz, C., Martineau, J., Barthélemy, C., & Assaiante, C. (2003). Motor control and children with autism: deficit of anticipatory function? *Neuroscience Letters*, **348**, 17–20.

Schneider, K. (1955). *Klinische Psychopathologie.* Stuttgart: Thieme Verlag.

Snow, M. E., Hertzig, M. E., & Shapiro, T. (1988). Expression of emotion in young autistic children. In S. Chess, A. Thomas, M. E. Hertzig (eds.), *Annual Progress in Child Psychiatry & Child Development* (pp. 514–522). New York: Brunner/Mazel Inc.

Stanghellini, G. (2000). Vulnerability to schizophrenia and lack of common sense. *Schizophrenia Bulletin*, **26**, 775–787.

Stanghellini, G. (2002). Psycopathology of common sense. Unpublished manuscript.

Terenius, L. (2000). Schizophrenia: pathophysiological mechanisms – a synthesis. *Brain Research Reviews*, **31**, 401–404.

Umiltà, M. A., Kohler, E., Gallese, V., *et al.* (2001). 'I know what you are doing': a neurophysiological study. *Neuron*, **32**, 91–101.

Watkins, K. E., Strafella, A. P., & Paus, T. (2003). Seeing and hearing speech excites the motor system involved in speech production. *Neuropsychologia*, **41**(8), 989–994.

Wicker, B., Keysers, C., Plailly, J., *et al.* (2003). Both of us disgusted in my insula: the common neural basis of seeing and feeling disgust. *Neuron*, **40**, 655–664.

Yirmiya, N., Kasari, C., Sigman, M., & Mundy, P. (1989). Facial expressions of affect in autistic, mentally retarded and normal children. *Journal of Child Psychology & Psychiatry & Allied Disciplines*, **30**, 725–735.

Using literature and the arts to develop empathy in medical students

Johanna Shapiro

Department of Family Medicine, University of California Irvine, School of Medicine

25.1 The problematic role of empathy in medicine

Medicine has had a mixed history where empathy is concerned. Although there is a tradition stretching from Hippocrates through to the current epoch of sympathy and compassion as defining qualities of medical professionalism, modern medicine has been dominated by a reductive, rationalist approach to clinical practice (Halpern, 2003). The modernist framing of professionalism engendered by this perspective presumes that impersonality, neutrality and detachment are needed to achieve objective medical care that does not favour one patient over another. In this view, the metaphor of medicine as science predominates, and the rationalist attributes of the successful scientist are transferred wholesale to the physician. Less often stated but also influential to this line of thinking is the assumption that allowing oneself feeling for patients can be emotionally overwhelming and leads to exhaustion and burn-out.

In terms of empathy, these conceptualizations have led either to its downgrading, culminating in the call for a 'de-empathization' of medicine in order to enable physicians to make sound, scientifically based medical decisions (Landau, 1993), or for a restricted definition of empathy as essentially a cognitive process based on the achievement of a purely logical understanding of the other. As an outgrowth of this position, medical school curricula now routinely attempt to teach empathy to students as a set of cognitive and behavioural skills (Winefield & Chur-Hansen, 2000). Although this interpretation and resultant method of instruction have produced certain positive pedagogic outcomes, concerns have also been expressed about whether this approach is sufficient to bring into being truly empathic physicians (Henry-Tillman *et al.*, 2002).

Such uneasiness calls into question the proper definition of empathy. Our English term empathy is derived from the German *Einfuhlung*, a word coined by

Empathy in Mental Illness, eds. Tom F. D. Farrow and Peter W. R. Woodruff. Published by Cambridge University Press. © Cambridge University Press 2007.

Theodor Lipps in his discussion of aesthetic experience, which means something like 'feeling one's way into the subjective experience of another'. Martin Buber, the great twentieth century philosopher, provided the striking image of empathy as 'a bold swinging ... into the life of the other'. However, these descriptions of 'sympathetic merging' grow out of aesthetic and philosophical, rather than clinical, traditions.

From a clinical perspective, the argument has been made that while empathy should be more than rational analysis, cold intelligence and aloof observation, it should not imply losing oneself in the other. Halpern introduces the term 'clinical empathy' (Halpern, 1993) to describe the special sort of empathy needed by physicians that derives from a detailed *experiential* as well as cognitive understanding of what the patient is feeling. Clinical empathy is neither detachment nor immersion, but rather requires an ongoing double movement of emotional resonance and compassionate curiosity about the meaning of the clinical situation to the patient. It may best be defined as the capacity to participate deeply in the patient's experience, while not losing sight of the fact that this imaginative projection is not, in fact, one's own experience but that of another. Accordingly, physicians should have the capacity to be affected by, but also to be able to contain, the patient's distress. In other words, the clinician must possess the 'negative capability' not to be overwhelmed by the patient's plight while simultaneously being moved by his or her suffering (Coulehan, 1995).

This expansive revisioning of empathy suggests more broadly conceived potential outcomes than those used in studies determining the empirical efficacy of training in behavioural empathic techniques. The expression of clinical empathy by physicians is assumed to engender trust in patients, thereby making it easier for them to tell their stories fully and honestly. Similarly, clinical empathy is conceived to be key to successful medical intervention and treatment, because it is only when patients feel deeply understood that they are willing to engage with the doctor's recommendations. Empathic connection is even viewed as potentially healing for patients, emotionally if not physically, because it helps them imagine possibilities for themselves that are more bearable than their current predicament. Finally, empathic connection gives the patients the sense that they are not alone, that someone understands them, recognizes them (Berger, 1967), and is not afraid to accompany them on the difficult journey of illness that lies ahead (Broyard, 1992).

Regardless of the debate regarding the definition, nature and parameters of empathy, most professional bodies in medicine, such as the Accreditation Council for Graduate Medical Education and the Association of American Medical Colleges, have identified empathy as a component of professionalism and specify that medical education must include curriculum whose goal is the development of empathy in learners (Larson & Yao, 2005). A survey of 533 medical residents ranked empathy as among the top three attributes associated with professionalism (Brownell & Cote, 2001). However, although empirical research has linked learner empathy not only to patient satisfaction (Smith *et al.*, 1995) but to clinical competence (Hojat *et al.*, 2002), other evidence suggests that various humanistic traits, including empathy, either stagnate (Branch, 2000) or actually decline over the course of undergraduate medical education (Newton *et al.*, 2000). As has been poignantly observed, 'medical students start out with empathy and love ... they learn detachment and equanimity ...' (Spiro, 1993).

25.2 Theorizing a humanities-based approach to train empathy

If empathy is as much art as science (Misch, 2002), then perhaps it may be developed through the study of humanities and arts (Charon, 2000), as well as through more skill-based, analytic procedures. The humanities and arts engage the emotions as well as the intellect, thereby creating the potential to achieve deep experiential understanding of and insight into the human condition (Charon, 2001). From a theoretical perspective, the potential value of the humanities as a curricular option in medical education arises out of a post-modernist conceptualization of medicine itself.

This post-modernist view contrasts with the still-dominant modernist medical paradigm, whose most widely endorsed metaphor depicts the body as a machine, disease as a malfunction, the doctor as an emotionally detached expert and the patient as a passive object; and the goal of intervention as a return of the patient to normalcy (Morris, 1998). The only desirable, indeed acceptable, modernist medical narrative is the restitution story (Frank, 1995), in which an individual suffers temporary breakdown due to disease, is diagnosed and treated by an authoritative but distant physician, and ultimately is restored to perfect, pre-disease status. What the restitution story omits are all the 'left-over aspects' of the ill person's experience, i.e. those elements that cannot be transformed or fixed by medical intervention. 'Re/covering' in this sense often 'erases' significant portions of the experience of the survivor (Wagner, 2000). The modernist position does not leave room for understanding the complex relations patients have with their illnesses; it does not allow for the reality that, once ill, people are inevitably changed by their experience, in ways both good and bad.

The post-modern interpretation of medicine, found more often in the writings of social scientists, humanists and 'boundary-crossing' physicians (Aull & Lewis, 2004) than in the actual practice of clinicians or the actual education of medical students, stresses the unity of mind and body: the limits and fallibility of the physician, as well as physician expertise; patient self-knowledge and testimony; and the need to replace detachment in the doctor-patient relationship with a certain emotional closeness (Morris, 1998). The pedagogical usefulness of literature and art that address themes and content broadly related to patients' experiences of illness and/or the doctor–patient relationship lies in their capacity to develop in learners the attitude of empathy implied in the post-modern perspective. Literature and the arts can help students see that there may be other dimensions to illness that are 'not allowed in' to the official modernist discourse. They provide additional ways in which individuals suffering from illness, as well as their families and friends, can contribute to the production of knowledge about their own conditions by raising their subjective, particularistic voices and authoring their own accounts that tell other, more ambiguous, stories than those of restitution.

25.3 A theoretical model

We have little empirical evidence, or indeed evidence of any kind (see below), to guide our understanding of the process by which literature and art might stimulate empathy in medical students. However, based on long-term observation of and interaction with learners, it is possible to theorize the following five-step model (see Figure 25.1). When medical students are exposed to literature and the arts (**step 1**), for example in a literature and medicine seminar, they achieve a psychological **zone of safety (step 2)** (Stein, 1996). One dimension of this zone of safety is that, while they are studying literature, learners have ***no direct clinical responsibilities***. The intense pressure of patient-care duties, especially for neophyte learners, not surprisingly produces stress and anxiety, emotions antithetical to the cultivation of empathy. Students are so consumed by managing their own problematic feelings that they have few emotional resources left over from which to evoke empathy for patients. Further, since in a sense patients are the cause of these negative emotions, it becomes easy for students to blame them, even unconsciously, for the confusion and misery they often experience on the wards, rather than empathize with their condition.

Reading, or viewing art, removes the direct-action component of clinical care, giving students the opportunity to reflect on, *and empathize with*, the situations or emotions portrayed in a given story, poem, or painting. In this respect, literature and art produce catharsis because they allow learners to confront horror and suffering without being contaminated by it. Learners can pay closer attention to the complexities and nuances of a fictional character's experience than they can to those of a real patient, without worry that doing so might distract them from medical issues critical to that patient's recovery. Learners also experience a sense of **emotional safety** because a protective barrier, the text or picture, has been interposed between them and the patient. Learners no longer have to be concerned

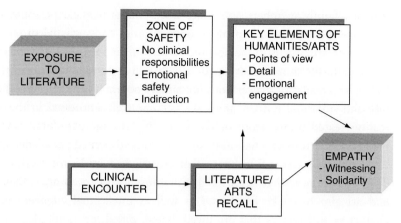

Figure 25.1. A theoretical model illustrating how literature works to create empathy in learners

that either their physical or emotional well-being is threatened by the suffering of the patient. They are free to feel and to reflect, to risk 'entering into' the world of the patient (Shapiro & Rucker, 2004).

A second component of the zone of safety is its favouring ***indirection*** as a means of bringing learners to a response of empathy rather than self-protection. Given the potential intensity of affect surrounding patient care, it becomes difficult to adequately deal with learner issues in this domain in a meaningful way. Direct probing and confrontation of prejudices, negative stereotypes, frustration, and even outright hostility in the learner generally result in denial and politically correct assertions. Literature and the arts offer the advantage of allowing learners to probe deeply into a problematic situation without, at least initially, having to reflect on themselves, and on personal attitudes and behaviours that may feel embarrassing or shameful. By focusing the discussion on an imagined creation, students feel safe in offering commentary about what 'the physician' or 'the patient' may be feeling without risk of negative personal consequences involving the intersubjective region between doctors and patients (Apprey & Stein, 1993). Interestingly, while such discussions start in the third person, they regularly move to the first person, as learners begin to feel secure enough to feel their way into their own patients' experiences, including their patients' perceptions of illness and of the medical system.

Once a zone of safety has been created through the removal of clinical respon-sibility and the use of indirection, three **key elements** characteristic of both literature and the arts emerge which tend to trigger empathy in learners (**step 3**). First is their unique ability to bring to life ***differing points of view*** (Charon, 2001), especially those that are either silenced or ignored by a medical hierarchy that privileges physician voices of authority and expertise, often at the expense of patients, family members and other lower status medical personnel. Personal narrative, poetry and art provide opportunities for such disenfranchised and unwilling participants in the health care discourse to express their perspectives.

Secondly, literature and art are unusually rich in ***particularistic detail*** (Downie, 2002). The reader or viewer does not simply obtain a general sense of character, plot and situation. Rather, he or she is completely immersed in the alternative reality created by the story or painting. This attention to detail helps learners recognize and respect what otherwise are easily dismissed particulars of patients' lives, singular facets of existence that are deemed irrelevant to the differential diagnosis but nevertheless are filled with idiosyncratic meaning. Finally, literature and art aim to evoke ***emotional*** as well as intellectual ***engagement***, creating characters and images that are loved, hated, pitied, or admired, and situations and symbols that evoke pathos, tragedy, or humour. Students studying literature and the arts have an opening to concentrate on deepening their understanding, emotionally and cognitively, of the experiences of others. They can become more versatile in recognizing, understanding and working with difficult emotions of anger, resentment, frustration, fear, hopelessness, despair and disgust in others (and themselves) in more skillful, conscious and compassionate ways.

Even if empathy can be successfully elicited in the context of a literature/arts-based teaching session, we must further ask how or whether it generalizes to an actual clinical encounter (**step 4**). Anecdotal evidence suggests that it does (Charon *et al.*, 1996). We hypothesize that affective and cognitive **recall** of these teaching sessions (**step 5**) is a partial explanatory mechanism for how this transference might occur. Students who have participated in literature and medicine or visual-arts seminars describe a process in which contact with particular patients associationally triggers recollections of poems or art representing a similar dilemma or difficulty. The students are then able to conjure up both the insights and the empathy that were evoked by the particular poem or painting, and bring them fruitfully into the clinical present.

Two specific dimensions of empathy promoted by this pedagogical use of literature are ***witnessing*** and ***solidarity***. *Witnessing* is a term that grew out of the Holocaust literature, when questions arose as to whether it was possible to record or listen to accounts of the unimaginable suffering that occurred in Nazi concentration camps with any sort of moral integrity. In the context of this article, 'witnessing' refers to the necessity of receiving with the utmost respect, compassion, lack of negative judgement and empathy the 'testimony' of patients, accepting their stories not as means to an end (in the case of medicine, the end of making an appropriate differential diagnosis), but as ends in themselves. *Solidarity* with the patient implies the ability, through an act of empathic imagination, to see a person initially perceived to be wholly 'other' as simultaneously sharing similarities and commonalities with the self and also possessing certain critical irreducible differences. Attitudes of witnessing and solidarity encourage a repositioning of the student in the direction of respect and empathy for the patient's subjective experience and lived reality.

25.4 Translational applications

The observational, hermeneutic and interpretive skills that can be achieved through study of the humanities and arts have important implications for patient care. The translational applications most obviously related to empathy are: the close observational skills from which inferences about the patient's mood and state of mind are derived; the capacity to identify and appreciate multiple coexisting, and often conflicting, perspectives and points of view; the ability to imagine the patient's encounter with illness within the context of his or her lived life; and a familiarity with the emotional, psychological and symbolic worlds uniquely accessed by illness and modified by both individual experience and culture. In an appeal for practising a more narrative-based medicine, Charon observes that 'physicians sometimes lack the capacities to recognize the plights of their patients, to extend empathy toward those who suffer, and to join honestly and courageously with patients in their illness' (2001; p. 1897). She asserts that it is only through narrative competence that physicians will be able to understand the meaning and significance of their patients' stories.

In literature-based sessions, learners are often asked to respond to a story from the points of view of the various characters. This strategy helps break down the tendency to intellectualize or assume an omniscient expert perspective regarding a particular clinical dilemma, the perspective they are trained to adopt as part of their medical education. To illustrate this point, in the story 'Fathering' by Indian-American writer Bharati Mukherjee (1990), learners are likely to quickly jump to diagnostic labelling (the child in the story, an Amerasian little girl named Eng, appears to be suffering from post-traumatic stress disorder). The diagnosis per se is probably not wrong, but it does highlight the medical expert's emphasis on identifying pathology and then treating it, conveniently by-passing any need for empathy in the process. This view sees patients 'from the outside in', at a safe professional distance. When learners employ not the third-person voice ('Eng needs psychiatric help') but the first person ('I saw my grandma get shot by Yankee soldiers'), they discover more understanding, insight and empathy for the character's troubles. As they become immersed in the details of her horrific past, as they begin to imagine experientially what it might be like to live through such events, Eng becomes not just a diagnosis, but a whole person, a survivor worthy of respect and caring as well as assistance (Shapiro, 2003).

A similar account of using visual arts to increase empathy in medical learners is reported by Stein (2003). He describes presenting the painting 'The Gleaners' by Jean Francois Millet (1857) to a group of family practice residents who initially express disdain and resentment toward their population of indigent patients, living as they do on the margins of society. In Millet's painting, humble figures gather up the remains of a wheat field, following the biblical injunction (Leviticus 19:9–10) that allows the poor the residual portion of a harvested crop. For these physicians-in-training, mostly products themselves of the Great Plains, the painting evokes many personal memories of ripe fields of plenty. As the residents begin to describe emerging associations of the scene depicted with their faith and families, their emotions soften and empathy replaces scorn.

25.5 State of the research on the humanities and empathy

Although the humanities have been held up as an exemplar for improving empathy in medical learners, few data as yet exist to support this claim. In part, this is because the humanities espouse different methodologies for demonstrating veracity than those found in the social and medical sciences. Therefore, research into this question has been lacking. Pragmatic issues, including the adequacy of measures to assess empathy, the difficulty of appropriate designs and lack of funding, have played a part as well in inhibiting such investigations. A modest research programme at my home institution studying the relationship between medical student exposure to the humanities and arts and increased empathy has produced suggestive results, although the sample sizes are small and the designs limited.

For example, in one study examining the effects of a literature and medicine course on 22 first-year medical students (Shapiro *et al.*, 2004), we found significant improvement in self-reported empathy, with a scaled treatment effect in the moderate range and statistically significant pre-to-post changes. Qualitative data from this same study indicated that student understanding of the patient's perspective became more detailed and complex after the literature-based intervention.

Another study analysed second-year students' writing samples in response to a prose-poem prompt describing the death of a patient from a heart attack (Shapiro & Lie, 2004). The analysis found that two kinds of written language used by students, i.e. expressing high positive emotion and expressing distancing emotion in ways that lacked empathy for the clinical situation, were related to 'detached' coping methods. Standardized patients rated students who used highly positive emotional language lacking in empathy as having poorer professionalism and communication skills. Students who endorsed 'accepting' (more empathic) coping were perceived as more professional.

A descriptive study at the same institution examining third-year medical students' use of writing and other creative media to reflect on problematic, challenging, or memorable patient encounters during an internal medicine clerkship showed that the large majority of these imaginative works by students expressed empathy for the patient, and frequently adopted the patient's point of view in their writing (Rucker & Shapiro, 2003). A final study exposed third-year medical students to three presentations on classical art and dance, and afterwards found that students reported increased empathy for others' predicaments (Shapiro *et al.*, 2006).

Other research shows similar small-scale, but promising results. A project presenting the drama *Wit* as a way of training empathy and compassion in medical students also concludes that such exposure can be used to promote positive attitude change (Deloney & Graham, 2003). A qualitative study of reflective writing concluded that, although emotionally challenging for participants, it was an effective way to increase learner empathy (DasGupta & Charon, 2004). By and large, however, much work remains to be done before we can definitively establish that exposure to the humanities and arts is an effective method for enhancing empathy in medical student learners.

25.6 Mental illness as an exemplar of 'otherness'

The remainder of this chapter examines how literature can be used specifically to help undergraduate students, medical students and family practice residents develop greater empathy for persons with mental illness. (I have not personally employed art in this manner, although intuitively art would seem to lend itself well to such an endeavour, e.g. Munch's *The Scream*.) Although the topic of mental illness meshes neatly with the theme of this book, it is selected as a focus for a more important reason. Mental illness is a condition that epitomizes the sense of 'otherness' that can take form in student-physicians (as well as more experienced physicians) toward patients, especially patients who are marginalized and devalued because of factors of race (non-white), gender (female or gay, bisexual, or transgender), socioeconomic status (poor), educational attainment (low), or medical condition (AIDS, alcoholism). Disturbances of the mind can come to represent all that is fearful, alien and threatening in medical practice. Instead of feeling empathy toward mental patients, students may begin to experience distancing, fearfulness and rejection.

'Otherness' is a construct studied by philosophers, psychologists and other social scientists (Lacan, 1977). It refers to the identification of someone or a group of persons as 'not-self'; in other words, falling outside the boundaries of one's identity. In terms of individual psychological needs, defining certain persons or groups of persons as 'other' creates a sense of distance between them and the individual doing the boundary-setting, thus establishing a means of self-protection from feared 'contamination' or 'pollution' of the self's 'clean and proper body' (Kristeva, 1982). Distance becomes the mechanism to avoid contamination by the feared object. In this way, the ill other helps us define our own boundaries of normality and health (Crawford, 1994). Since otherness is a construct of exclusivity, it is also potentially a tool of social control. By maintaining attitudes of otherness toward persons who are ill (as well as toward other stigmatized, minority and disadvantaged groups), society promotes homogeneity and certain standards of belongingness. Therefore, on both the individual and the societal level, otherness can be seen as fulfilling certain reassuring and cohesive functions. But otherness designations also create in-groups and out-groups, shunning, shaming, avoidance and attack. To deny our own vulnerability, to quiet our own anxiety, we engage in distancing from, silencing and isolating the diseased or different other.

Mental illness adds an additional layer of potential alienation between student-physician and patient because of the stigma still attached to mental health problems. Historically, mental illness was associated with moral deficiency or punishment from God. Its sufferers were therefore automatically placed in a despised and loathsome category, to be avoided at all costs. Even today, mental illness can create disgust and fear, because many people, including well-educated medical students, still see it as somehow shameful, a personal failing, despite scientific explanations involving neurotransmitters, synapses and brain chemicals. [As has been pointed out, such biological explanations both console and humiliate, because they place responsibility for very personal behaviours and experiences outside of the control of the individual (Lewis, 2003).] Although mental illness is not viewed as 'contagious', it does appear as somewhat contaminating (Shildrick, 2000). The construct of otherness insulates the non-mentally ill from the fragility and vulnerability that the possibility of 'incurring' mental illness might otherwise engender.

Contemporary biopsychiatry defines mental health and illness based on assumptions of Cartesian logic. Certain modes of thinking and feeling are designated as normal, while the various categories of mental aberration compiled in DSM-IV are considered deviant and abnormal. It has been observed that binarism is never value-free, but implies superior-inferior relationships (Grosz, 1989), so that this original bifurcated analysis of mental wellness and illness leads to other even more disturbing dualisms: good/bad; desirable/undesirable; pure/contaminated; doctor/patient; self/other, all of which become inextricably associated with mental illness. Biopsychiatry also minimizes the contributions of factors such as social injustice, lack of resources and systematic denigration to the development and exacerbation of mental illness, thereby locating the cause of mental illness exclusively in the individual rather than the society, while privileging the domination of the interests of powerful pharmaceutical companies in defining treatment (Lewis, 2003). In the biopsychiatric discourse, suffering itself has become deviant (Epstein, 1995), so that it no longer holds a legitimate place in the human experience. Instead, suffering is translated as 'depression', thereby becoming a medicalized, dysfunctional, *and treatable* (therefore curable) phenomenon that serves to separate 'normal' people from 'abnormal' people. All of these factors work together to confirm perceptions of otherness about individuals with mental illness, and reduce attitudes of empathy.

25.7 Mental illness as a curricular challenge

Encouraging medical learners to develop empathy, and its components of witnessing and solidarity, toward psychiatric patients does not imply a romanticized view of mental illness. It does not suggest that there are no differences between people with mental illness and people without these diagnoses, or that mentally ill people do not experience real misery and anguish, although it does insinuate that the inherent suffering brought about by mental illness is often compounded by societal attitudes and behaviour. Nor do attitudes of empathy imply that persons with mental illness should not be treated with the whole range of treatment options produced by biotechnology. However, such attitudes do recognize that the only non-threatening story about mental illness from society's point of view is one which either relegates mentally ill persons to the category of irreducible 'otherness' or places them within the context of a restitution plot, so that they are returned to normalcy as fully functioning members of society. Empathy, especially in the form of witnessing and solidarity, enables students to enter into the grey area between these two extremes that so many psychiatric patients inhabit.

The medical humanities courses I teach (usually in collaboration with a physician partner) are either university or medical school electives, designed for undergraduate freshmen, or first- and second-year medical students. At this point in their education, students have little or no exposure to patients with mental illness. Their beliefs, attitudes and expectations are generally formed through a combination of popular media, previous academic study, and occasionally personal experience. The topic of mental illness is also addressed in a family medicine residency monthly seminar. In this case, all participants have already graduated from medical school, and by the end of their first (of three) years of training are licensed physicians. Consequently, they have considerably more experience than medical students with patients suffering from psychiatric disorders, and require a somewhat more clinically oriented approach.

These literature and medicine electives are broad-ranging in terms of subject matter, and cover a spectrum of issues of concern to student- and resident-physicians such as difficult patients, breaking bad news, death and dying, and the doctor–patient relationship. Of 12–15 sessions, generally only 1 or 2 focus on mental health issues. Within a given module examining psychiatric disorders, I include readings on various diagnoses, e.g. schizophrenia, major depressive disorder, bipolar disorder, anxiety disorders and personality disorders. These are all conditions that are frequently seen in low-income primary care clinics, so are relevant to learners' present or future clinical encounters. Sessions are held as small groups (between 10 and 15 learners), generally occur monthly, and last anywhere from 45 min to 1½ hours. Readings are sometimes assigned outside class, but more commonly are read on-site. Discussion ensues, and follows these guidelines:

1. Basic orientation questions, such as who is telling the story?; what is the setting?; what is happening; when is the action taking place?; what is the tone of the selection?
2. Summary and justification of the points of view expressed in the selection's 'message', themes, or main points.
3. Eliciting differing opinions and points of view about the selection.
4. Expression of personal feelings about the characters, events, and situations portrayed.
5. Take-home messages for clinical practice.

25.8 Literature relevant to specific psychiatric diagnoses

I now offer some examples of how specific literary selections about mental illness make certain points or raise certain issues that may enhance empathy in learners. The power of literature is that it provides equal validity to the voice of the physician, the voice of the patient, the voice of the family member, and anyone else who chooses to express their viewpoint. The accounts of mental illness examined below are usually attempts by an author to create a more experientially authentic image of persons with mental illness, rather than keeping hidden those aspects that do not fit a restitution plot or are viewed as socially unacceptable.

In a way that a psychiatric textbook cannot, literature raises the question of what is sanity and what is insanity. *Aberrants* (Biggs, 1992) explores the notion of the social construction of insanity. In this poem, the narrator has a chance encounter with the husband of a friend, who explains why he recently had his wife committed to a mental institution. She was doing 'crazy' things, the husband complains, such as walking at night, talking to the stars, listening to Bach, running naked and generally recognizing the craziness of the world. The husband seems glad to be rid of this troublesome spouse. The narrator's final thought, by contrast, is that, according to these criteria, she too is not far from insanity. This is an interesting poem because, in the minds of students, there is usually a clear dividing line between people who are 'crazy' and people who are not. Because the sympathies and point of view of the reader are filtered through the eyes of the friend of the committed woman, the poem invites us to reconsider how madness is defined, by whom, and for what ends.

In another poem, *The Invisible Woman* (Morgan, 1994), we see madness from an insider's perspective. An insane woman, locked up in an asylum, is convinced she is invisible. Because her doctor tries to tell her she *isn't* invisible, the patient concludes *he* himself must be quite mad. To comfort the doctor, she momentarily assumes visibility, body and voice, out of pity that the doctor is not strong enough to confront his own derangement. This poem, too, probes the relationship between psychological normalcy and abnormality. In addition, it challenges the view of mental patient as passive object acted upon by the patronizingly benevolent physician. Here, we hear only the patient's voice, judgements and assessments. What is most remarkable about the poem is the way the narrator responds with compassion and caring to her psychiatrist's perceived insanity. Her act of generosity provokes perceptive exchanges among students about mutuality in the doctor–patient relationship.

The Walking Woman (Grant, 1990) also hints at the aspect of social control present in defining mental illness. Elaine lives her own life, singing, cursing, communing with UFOs, lost in a glamorous fantasy existence, parading up and down the street. She is that homeless person so well-recognized, yet so little known, by most of the students. The merchants of the area circulate a petition to lock her away, but at the writing of the poem she remains crazy and free. This poem serves as a trigger for students to share stories of personal experiences with persons who are homeless, both negative and positive. The poem is also a useful stimulus for considering how the plight of the homeless can be glamorized as a carefree existence freed from the constraints and norms of society, ignoring the real suffering, psychological and physical, that most homeless persons endure.

In *Differences* (Shepherd, 1990), the narrator is a schizophrenic man who is hospitalized, treated and 'normalized', but feels he has lost some part of himself in the process. The man insists he is happy following 'his way', but family, doctor and psychiatrists force him into treatment which leaves him 'less crazy' but 'so much alone'. This perspective adds to a more nuanced interpretation of the nature of madness. Painful and distressing as mental illness is, it is also intimately wrapped up with personal identity, and shedding its signs and symptoms is often no easy matter. The poem is also useful in provoking discussion of 'forced treatment' for mentally ill individuals, and whether this violates their rights, or serves as a critical protection for society.

In Amy Bloom's moving *Silver Water* (Bloom, 2000), the story opens with the narrator describing her sister's amazing voice, a voice so beautiful it is like water poured from a silver pitcher. It is a beautiful, extraordinary image, and as a first introduction binds the reader emotionally to sister Rose who, we discover as we read on, is also psychotically violent, unpredictable and generally out of control. Although some first-person accounts of mental illness fault family for their difficulties, in this story the parents are concerned, loving and caring, good people who try to do the best for their daughter. *Silver Water* is also useful in its portrayal of both bad and good family therapists. The examples in the story motivate engaged discussions about how health professional behaviour can ameliorate or exacerbate the torments of patient and family. Eventually, Rose commits suicide and her sister, although aware of what is happening, does not try to save her. Remarkably, the mother is able to find within herself an understanding for the anguished choices of both of her daughters, to whom she refers as 'warrior queens'. The grim conclusion is not the happily-ever-after ending that medical students often expect medicine can provide through stories of restitution. Instead, it leads them to reflect on the limitations of medical care, and to confront the possibility that medical intervention cannot always stave off suffering and tragedy. Students also struggle to understand the feelings and consequent decisions of sisters and mother. There is strong disagreement about whether these are moral acts, but the eloquence of the perspectives represented enables students to approach the family with respect and empathy.

William Styrone's *Darkness Visible* (1990) is a compelling evocation of the experience of depression. Although it is possible to extract from this account the requisite symptoms necessary to make a DSM-IV diagnosis, more importantly it provides a window into the lived nature of the author's suffering. Especially in the era of selective serotonin re-uptake inhibitors (SSRIs), physician learners tend to regard depression as a rather prosaic disease, easily managed by psychopharmacologic intervention. They often overlook the intense and constant psychic pain it causes, as well as the variable individual response to medication. Styrone's ability to describe his sense of dread, of no exit, of being among the walking wounded, and of experiencing without surcease the 'despair beyond despair' helps learners gain experiential knowledge of the devastating effects of major depressive disorder.

Sylvia Plath's account of her own descent into madness – *Under the Bell Jar* (1971), although somewhat dated, is also useful in depicting the lived experience of depression. Her small book offers yet another portrayal of patient and psychiatrist, the latter presented in a highly unfavourable light precisely because he seems such a perfect individual, with the requisite good looks, education, wife and children. Plath plumbs the inevitable gap that exists between doctor and patient and suggests that, when it is too large, and not bridged by empathy, a healing relationship cannot be constructed. Plath's vivid description of the psychiatrist often leads to a discussion of vulnerability and mutuality versus authority and unilaterality in the doctor–patient relationship.

An Unquiet Mind by Kay Jamison (1995), a leading researcher on bipolar disorder as well as someone who herself suffers from this disease, courageously describes her cycling of manic and depressive episodes, which for many years she keeps hidden in fear and shame. Her brutally honest recounting of spending sprees, hallucinations, and her own physical violence, as well as her descriptions of the beauty and excitement of the early phases of a manic episode make the experience of bipolar disorder accessible to learners on a human level. Particularly valuable is Jamison's history of her own non-compliance with medication as both a denial of her illness and a fear that she was consigning herself to a bland, robotic existence. In a profound insight, Jamison acknowledges that despite her suffering, her disease has taught her to feel more deeply, experience events more intensely, appreciate life more and find the courage to explore 'new corners of her mind and heart'. Students are struck by the complexity of the relationship between the disease and the person *with* the disease. Instead of seeing mental illness only as bad, or something to 'be gotten rid of', they begin to appreciate how integral it is in shaping a person's life, and how controlling such illness produces many consequences, some desirable and some surprisingly problematic.

The poem *Therapy* by physician-poet John Wright (1998) strikes a wise, balanced and hopeful note regarding the complex process of treating depression. Written in the voice of a physician, the poem directly addresses his patient as 'you'. Doctor and patient seem to be discussing the patient's symptomatic improvement from a major depression. While the physician credits only pharmacology for the patient's recovery, the patient perceives healing to be a more complex process. In contrast with the logico-scientific, reductive model of his doctor, the patient gives 'half the credit' to the hope of rebirth and renewal symbolized by the pear tree blossoming outside the physician's window; and to the human warmth of the physician himself. Reading this poem reminds students that, although medication is often necessary, healing powers exist within the therapeutic relationship itself.

Anxiety Wins a Round by Marge Piercy (2000) describes generalized anxiety disorder. The narrator tells of a fear that is so grinding, oppressive like a stone, throbbing like a toothache, that it produces the sense of being completely overwhelmed and swept away, as in a flood. She also talks openly about the dissolution of self, and how the old familiar anchors cannot reassure her. In vivid imagery, it is as though she is 'impaled' by this experience of anxiety – lost, overwhelmed, reduced to a rat in a maze. The range and depth of metaphors, the uncompromising detail offered by the poem make it impossible for learners to avoid or intellectualize the pain of pervasive anxiety. Despite the patient's well-documented misery, the poem is essentially optimistic. The title suggests that dealing with anxiety is an ongoing process, and the narrator is hopeful she can overcome her demons and regroup in the morning. These words enable students to see treatment of mental illness as an ongoing process, one which requires commitment and perseverance from both patient and physician.

Another poem, *Agoraphobia* by Susan Hahn (1994), describes the psychiatric condition of fear of open spaces and crowds. In this first-person rendering, the narrator reveals an encroaching isolation, so that her encounters with the outside world become increasingly reduced to the realm of memory. Her world steadily shrinks until the only safe place is the bed and TV, a classic agoraphobic outcome. The narrator anchors herself in this small realm by listening to news of disasters, which confirms her sense that venturing out is unacceptably dangerous. Although pleasurable events are tempting, she can now experience them only in her mind. The chronology of the narrator's illness enables learners to 'walk with' her as her agoraphobia progresses and begins to dominate her life. Yet it also becomes apparent to the learners that, from the patient's perspective, her responses are logical and sensible. Again, seeing the world through the eyes of the patient evokes compassion and additional insight into what reassurances this patient might need in order to accept treatment.

Arthur Kleinman's classic work, *The Illness Narratives* (1988), contains perceptive sketches of hypochondriasis and panic disorder, as well as other psychosomatic ailments. Arnie Springer is convinced, despite all evidence to the contrary, that he has cancer. Although medicine can reassure him, it cannot unequivocally guarantee that he will never develop cancer, so Arnie remains perpetually terrified. A systems analyst, he has lost his ability to deal with the uncertainty and inherent disorder of the world. Kleinman also describes Wolf Segal, who regularly presents in emergency rooms, convinced he is having a heart attack, with accompanying symptoms of chest pain, numbness in his hands, shortness of breath, rapid breathing and palpitations, as well as the sensation that he is going to die. In fact, there is nothing wrong with his heart; Wolf is experiencing a typical panic attack. Hypochondriasis and panic disorder can easily be dismissed by medical students as 'non-illnesses'. Kleinman's brilliance lies in the way he reveals these patients not as cases, but as *stories*, involving readers in their narratives, and forcing them to see through the eyes of these patients.

25.9 Limitations, possibilities and conclusions

Literature is not a panacea for helping learners to become more empathetic toward patients with mental disorders, or other illnesses. One problem with its use is that it may idealize or glamorize the illness experience in a simplistic fashion, creating an exaggerated identification or advocacy in learners rather than clear-sighted empathy. For example, the efforts of persons with mental illness, or their supporters, to present an alternative perspective to the dominant discourse may sometimes convey the impression that mental disorder is an invention of the medical establishment. This radical conceptualization is not helpful to either students or patients. However, the awareness that there are *multiple* perspectives about how to interpret mental illness, or the illness experience overall, is revelatory for medical students. To guard against over-simplification, it is useful to expose learners to a wide range of texts.

Other potential problems are more subtle in nature. How the humanities are taught in medical schools is of critical importance in influencing their efficacy. If they are perceived as simply additional bodies of knowledge to be mastered, they will be unlikely to help learners become more empathetic. Although it is, of course, legitimate to approach the study of literature or art as a purely intellectual inquiry, this will do little if anything to help students be moved by their patients' suffering. It is not the specialized erudition of literary or aesthetic analysis that stimulates empathy in medical learners, but rather the fundamental insights and knowledge about the human condition that can be acquired through becoming fully engaged on multiple cognitive, emotional and spiritual levels with a text or painting. Humanities succeed best in promoting empathy when they offer opportunities for thoughtful reflection, rather than concentrating solely on transmitting academic information (Koppelman, 1999).

In a somewhat different way, curricular error also occurs when the humanities are 'quarantined' (Stempsey, 1999) from the core of medical education, much as psychiatric disease is quarantined from less stigmatized medical conditions. When literature and the arts are not part of the standard curriculum, they will be regarded by learners as tangential and low status. Whatever they attempt to convey to learners about the importance and value of empathy will similarly be devalued, or perceived as irrelevant to 'real' patient care. This method cannot produce humane physicians because learners will see the experience as too limited and ivory-tower (Greaves, 2001).

In an ideal world, the humanities and arts would become integrated into the overall medical school curriculum (Gorovitz, 1998), where they would be viewed as an equally legitimate, although different, method of accessing important knowledge about doctors and patients. In this utopian medical school, students learning anatomy would be just as likely to read a poem about a cadaver as to examine a bone. The patient chart would include not only the history of present illness, physical findings, a SOAP (subjective, objective, assessment and plan) note and treatment plan, but also would be enriched by a personal narrative written by the patient, and perhaps a poem by an orderly, nurse, or physician who was moved to reflect creatively about the patient. Attending physicians would model encouraging patients to write a letter to their diabetes, sharing their frustrations and fears, while medical students would keep journals documenting their own socialization experiences into the medical profession. The corridors and walls of the hospital wards would be filled with the photography, paintings, sculptures and poems of students, physicians, patients and staff. In the hospital courtyard a volunteer medical student orchestra might serenade off-duty nurses, residents, patients and family members, while in a lecture hall across the way cancer patients, students and physicians might attend a performance of the play *Wit*, about an English professor dying of ovarian cancer (Edson, 1993). The efficacy of all of these activities to reduce stress, promote mutual compassion and increase healing would be evaluated by innovative combined quantitative and qualitative methodologies that gave credence to experiential as well as abstract knowledge (Saunders, 2001) and to particular, individual perceptions as well as statistically significant group differences. It is as an equal partner of this as yet non-existent educational system that the humanities and arts might best help medical students develop the necessary empathy to compassionately and wisely address the needs of patients with mental illness, and indeed the needs of all patients.

In summary, the role of empathy in medicine has been a longstanding but ambivalent one. The concept of clinical empathy makes a significant contribution toward defining the proper relationship between doctor and patient, including as it does a balance between emotional steadiness and tenderness. Because of the limitations of teaching empathy to medical learners strictly as a behavioural skill set, the possibilities of integrating literature and the arts as pedagogical supplements to the standard curriculum are intriguing in terms of promoting empathy.

A theoretical model of the relationship between exposure to literature and the arts and empathy posits creating a zone of practical and emotional safety through removal of clinical responsibilities. The use of indirection allows learners to attend to issues of multiple perspectives, individual particularity, and emotional engagement that literature and arts uniquely address. In subsequent clinical encounters, these experiences are vividly recalled, and incline the learner toward actual expression of greater empathy toward patients, particularly in the form of witnessing and solidarity. At this point in time, little research exists to substantiate this model, although preliminary investigations do find a relationship between study of fictional and first-person narrative literature related to illness and increases in self-reported student empathy.

Although empathy is a necessary component of all patient–physician interactions, it is acutely relevant in the case of psychological disorders, where issues of otherness and stigma are especially in evidence. Using literary examples to teach medical students about schizophrenia, depression and anxiety heightens learner understanding on dimensions of point of view, particularistic details and emotional connection. Such an approach challenges the omnipresent restitution story as the only acceptable story about mental illness, and offers learners the opportunity to listen closely to the voice of the patient. The result is often increased empathy and understanding.

While literature and the arts have great potential in medical education, their value is by no means guaranteed. Problems that compromise the pedagogic goal of promoting empathy in learners arise when the arts present too one-sided a view of illness; when they are taught as a purely academic subject; and when they are marginalized within the curriculum. Nevertheless, literature and the arts offer great potential for helping medical learners understand how to be more empathic toward their patients.

REFERENCES

Apprey, M., & Stein, H. F. (1993). *Intersubjectivity, Projective Identification and Otherness*. Pittsburgh: Dusquesne University Press.

Aull, F., & Lewis, B. (2004). Medical intellectuals: resisting medical orientalism. *Journal of Medical Humanities*, **25**, 87–108.

Berger, J. (1967). *A Fortunate Man: The Story of a Country Doctor*. New York: Vintage Books.

Biggs, M. K. (1992). Aberrants. In S. B. Walker, & R. D. Roffman (eds.) *Life on the Line: Selections on Words & Healing* (p. 582). Mobile, Ala.: Negative Capability Press.

Bloom, A. (2000). Silver water. In R. V. Cassill, & Richard Bausch (eds.), *Norton Anthology of Short Fiction,* 6th edn. New York: W.W. Norton & Co.

Branch, W. T. Jr. (2000). Supporting the moral development of medical students. *Journal of General Internal Medicine*, **15**, 503–508.

Brownell, A. K., & Cote, L. (2001). Senior residents' views on the meaning of professionalism and how they learn about it. *Academic Medicine*, **76**, 734–737.

Broyard, A. (1992). *Intoxicated by my Illness: and other Writings about Life and Death*. New York: Fawcett Columbine.

Charon, R. (2000). Literature and medicine: origins and destinies. *Academic Medicine*, **75**, 23–27.

Charon, R. (2001). Narrative medicine: a model for empathy, reflection, profession, and trust. *Journal of the American Medical Association*, **286**, 1897–1902.

Charon, R., Brody, H., Clark, M. W., *et al.* (1996). Literature and ethical medicine: five cases from common practice. *Journal of Medical Philosophy*, **21**, 243–265.

Coulehan, J. L. (1995). Tenderness and steadiness: emotions in medical practice. *Literature and Medicine*, **14**, 222–236.

Crawford, R. (1994). The boundaries of the self and the unhealthy other: reflections on health, culture, and AIDS. *Social Science & Medicine*, **38**, 1347–1375.

DasGupta, S., & Charon, R. (2004). Personal illness narratives: using reflective writing to teach empathy. *Academic Medicine*, **79**, 351–356.

Deloney, L. A., Graham, C. J. (2003). Wit: using drama to teach first-year medical students about empathy and compassion. *Teaching and Learning in Medicine*, **25**, 247–251.

Downie, G. (2002). Telling: detail and diagnosis in medical poetry. *Medical Humanities Review*, **16**, 9–17.

Edson, M. (1993). *Wit*. New York: Faber and Faber.

Epstein, J. (1995). *Altered Conditions: Disease, Medicine, and Storytelling*. New York: Routledge.

Frank, A. W. (1995). *The Wounded Storyteller: Body, Illness, and Ethics*. Chicago, Ill.: University of Chicago Press.

Gorovitz, S. (1998). Healthcare under siege. *Health Decisions*, **5**, 1–2.

Grant, P. (1990). The walking woman. In R. Charach (ed.), *The Naked Physician: Poems About the Lives of Patients and Doctors* (p. 74). Ontario: Quarry Press.

Greaves, D. (2001). The nature and role of the medical humanities. In M. Evans & I. G. Finlay (eds.), *Medical Humanities* (pp. 13–22). London: BMJ Books.

Grosz, E. (1989). *Sexual Subversions: Three French Feminists*. Sydney: Allen & Unwin.

Hahn, S. (1994). Agoraphobia. In J. Mukand (ed.), *Articulations: The Body and Illness in Poetry* (p. 277). Iowa City: University of Iowa Press.

Halpern, J. (1993). Empathy: using resonance emotions in the service of curiosity. In R. Selzer, H. Spiro, M. G. McCrea-Curnen, E. Peschel & D. St. James (eds.), *Empathy and the Practice of Medicine* (pp. 160–173). Yale: Yale University Press.

Halpern, J. (2003). *From Detached Concern to Empathy: Humanizing Medical Practice*. Oxford: Oxford University Press.

Henry-Tillman, R., Deloney, L. A., Savidge, M., Graham, C. J., & Klimberg, V. S. (2002). The medical student as patient navigator as an approach to teaching empathy. *American Journal of Surgery*, **183**, 659–662.

Hojat, M., Gonnella, J. S., Mangione, S., *et al.* (2002). Empathy in medical students as related to academic performance, clinical competence and gender. *Medical Education*, **36**, 522–527.

Jamison, K. R. (1995). *An Unquiet Mind: A Memoir of Moods and Madness*. New York: Vintage Books.

Kleinman, A. (1988). *The Illness Narratives: Suffering, Healing, and the Human Condition*. New York: Basic Books.

Koppelman, L. M. (1999). Values and virtues: how should they be taught? *Academic Medicine*, **74**, 1307–1310.

Kristeva, J. (1982). *Powers of Horror: An Essay on Abjection*. New York: Columbia University Press.

Lacan, J. (1977). *Ecrits: A Selection* (A. Sheridan, trans). London: W. W. Norton.

Landau, R. L. (1993). And the least of these is empathy. In R. Selzer, H. Spiro, M. G. McCrea-Curnen, E. Peschel, & D. St. James (eds.), *Empathy and the Practice of Medicine* (pp. 103–109). Yale: Yale University Press.

Larson, E. B., & Yao, X. (2005). Clinical empathy as emotional labor in the patient-physician relationship. *Journal of the American Medical Association*, **295**, 1100–1106.

Lewis, B. E. (2003). Prozac and the post-human politics of cyborgs. *Journal of Medical Humanities*, **24**, 49–63.

Misch, D. A. (2002). Evaluating physicians' professionalism and humanism: the case for human-ism 'connoisseurs'. *Academic Medicine*, **77**, 489–495.

Morgan, R. (1994). The invisible woman. In J. Mukand (ed.), *Articulations: The Body and Illness in Poetry* (p. 301). Iowa City: University of Iowa Press.

Morris, D. B. (1998). *Illness and Culture in the Postmodern Age*. Berkeley, Calif.: University of California Press.

Mukherjee, B. (1990). Fathering. In J. Mukand (ed.), *Vital Lines: Contemporary Fiction About Medicine* (pp. 135–142). New York: St. Martin's Press.

Newton, B. W., Savidge, M. A., Barber, L., *et al.* (2000). Differences in medical students' empathy. *Academic Medicine*, **75**, 1215.

Piercy, M. (2000). Anxiety wins a round. In D. Walders (ed.), *Using Poetry in Therapeutic Settings: A Resource Manual & Poetry Collection* (p. 35). Bethesda, Md.: The Children's Inn at NIH.

Plath, S. (1971). *The Bell Jar*. New York: Bantam Books.

Rucker, L., & Shapiro, J. (2003). Becoming a physician: students' creative projects in a third-year IM clerkship. *Academic Medicine*, **78**, 391–398.

Saunders, J. (2001). Validating the facts of experience in medicine. In M. Evans, & I. G. Finlay (eds), *Medical Humanities* (pp. 223–235). London: BMJ Books.

Shapiro, J. (2003). New points of view: fiction in residency teaching [Literature and Medicine feature column]. *American Society for Bioethics and Humanities Exchange*, **1** (Spring), 3.

Shapiro, J., & Lie, D. (2004). A comparison of medical students' written expressions of emotion and coping and standardized patients' ratings of student professionalism and communication skills. *Medical Teacher*, **26**, 733–735.

Shapiro, J., Morrison, E. H., & Boker, J. (2004). Teaching empathy to first year medical students: evaluation of an elective literature and medicine course. *Education for Health*, **17**, 73–84.

Shapiro, J., & Rucker, L. (2004). The Don Quixote effect: why going to the movies can help develop professionalism in medical students and residents. *Families, Systems, & Health*, **22**, 445–452.

Shapiro, J., Rucker, L., & Beck, J. (2006). Training the clinical eye and mind: using the arts to develop medical students' observational and pattern recognition skills. *Medical Education*, **40**, 263–268.

Shepherd, R. W. (1990). Differences. In R. Charach (ed.), *The Naked Physician: Poems About the Lives of Patients and Doctors* (p. 68). Ontario: Quarry Press.

Shildrick, M. (2000). Becoming vulnerable: contagious encounters and the ethics of risk. *Journal of Medical Humanities*, **21**, 215–227.

Smith, R. C., Lyles, J. S., Mettler, J. A., *et al.* (1995). A strategy for improving patient satisfaction by the intensive training of residents in psychosocial medicine: a controlled, randomized study. *Academic Medicine*, **70**, 729–732.

Spiro, H. M. (1993). What is empathy and can it be taught? In R. Selzer, H. Spiro, M. G. McCrea-Curnen, E. Peschel, D. St. James (eds.), *Empathy and the Practice of Medicine* (pp. 7–14). Yale: Yale University Press.

Stein, H. F. (1996). *Prairie Voices: Process Anthropology in Family Medicine*. Westport, Conn.: Bergin & Garvey.

Stein, H. F. (2003). Ways of knowing in medicine: seeing and beyond. *Families, Systems, & Health*, **21**, 29–35.

Stempsey, W. E. (1999). The quarantine of philosophy in medical education: why teaching the humanities may not produce humane physicians. *Medicine, Health Care, and Philosophy*, **2**, 3–9.

Styrone, W. (1990). *Darkness Visible: A Memoir of Madness*. New York: Random House.

Wagner, A. T. (2000). Re/covered bodies: the sites and stories of illness in popular media. *Journal of Medical Humanities*, **21**, 15–27.

Winefield, H. R., & Chur-Hansen, A. (2000). Evaluating the outcomes of communication skill teaching for entry-level medical students: does knowledge of empathy increase? *Medical Education*, **34**, 90–94.

Wright, J. (1998). Therapy. In A. Belli & J. L. Coulehan (eds.), *Blood & Bone: Poems by Physicians* (p. 54). Iowa City: University of Iowa Press.

Index